D1758928

IMAGING IN
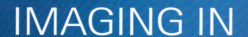

ABDOMINAL SURGERY

FEDERLE | LAU

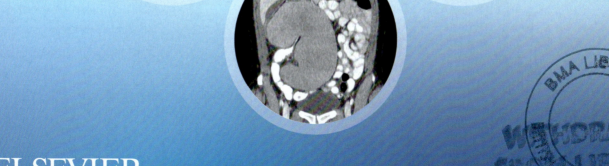

ELSEVIER

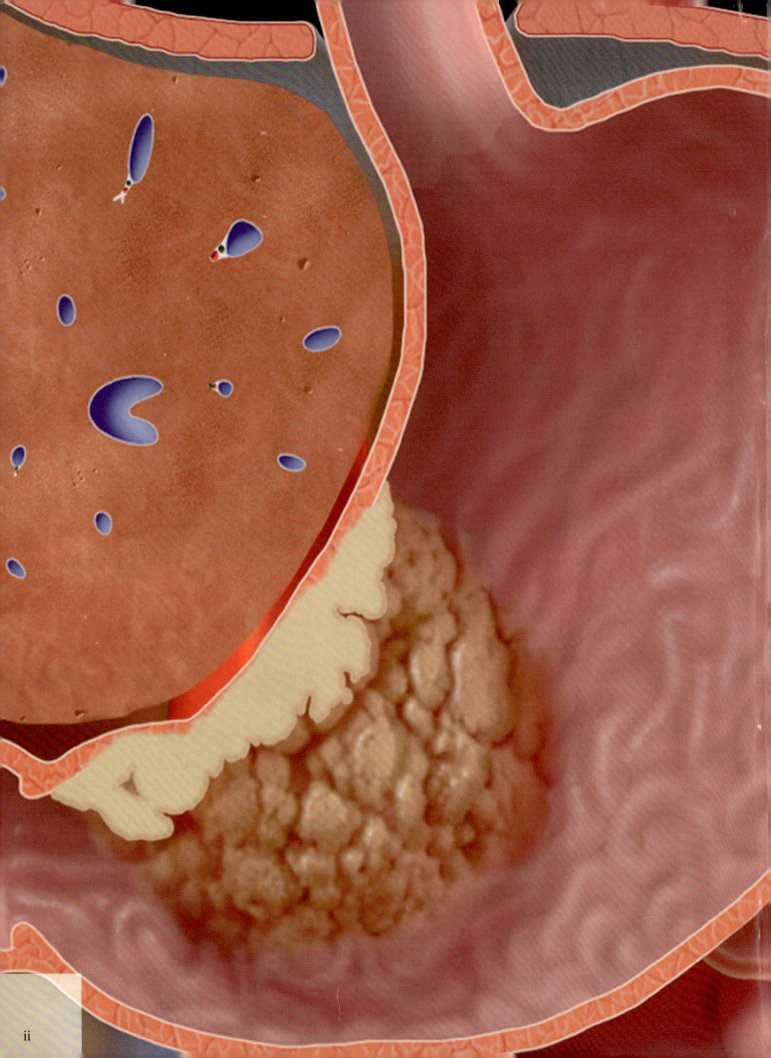

IMAGING IN

ABDOMINAL SURGERY

Michael P. Federle, MD, FACR

Professor of Radiology
Department of Radiology
Stanford University School of Medicine
Stanford, California

James N. Lau, MD, MHPE, FACS

Clinical Professor of Surgery
Stanford University School of Medicine
Stanford, California

ELSEVIER

1600 John F. Kennedy Blvd.
Ste 1800
Philadelphia, PA 19103-2899

IMAGING IN ABDOMINAL SURGERY

ISBN: 978-0-323-61135-0

Notices

Knowledge and best practice in this field are constantly changing. As new research and experience broaden our understanding, changes in research methods, professional practices, or medical treatment may become necessary.

Practitioners and researchers must always rely on their own experience and knowledge in evaluating and using any information, methods, compounds, or experiments described herein. In using such information or methods they should be mindful of their own safety and the safety of others, including parties for whom they have a professional responsibility.

With respect to any drug or pharmaceutical products identified, readers are advised to check the most current information provided (i) on procedures featured or (ii) by the manufacturer of each product to be administered, to verify the recommended dose or formula, the method and duration of administration, and contraindications. It is the responsibility of practitioners, relying on their own experience and knowledge of their patients, to make diagnoses, to determine dosages and the best treatment for each individual patient, and to take all appropriate safety precautions.

To the fullest extent of the law, neither the Publisher nor the authors, contributors, or editors, assume any liability for any injury and/or damage to persons or property as a matter of products liability, negligence or otherwise, or from any use or operation of any methods, products, instructions, or ideas contained in the material herein.

Publisher Cataloging-in-Publication Data

Names: Federle, Michael P. | Lau, James N.
Title: Imaging in abdominal surgery / [edited by] Michael P. Federle and James N. Lau.
Description: Salt Lake City, UT : Elsevier, Inc., [2018] | Includes bibliographical
  references and index.
Identifiers: ISBN 978-0-323-61135-0
Subjects: LCSH: Abdomen--Radiography--Handbooks, manuals, etc. | Abdomen--Surgery--Handbooks,
  manuals, etc. | MESH: Abdomen--diagnostic imaging--Atlases. | Abdomen--surgery--
  Atlases. | Radiography--Atlases.
Classification: LCC RC944.I43 2018 | NLM WI 900 | DDC 617.5507572--dc23

International Standard Book Number: 978-0-323-61135-0

Cover Designer: Tom M. Olson, BA

Printed in Canada by Friesens, Altona, Manitoba, Canada

Last digit is the print number: 9 8 7 6 5 4 3 2 1

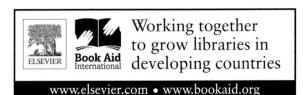

Dedications

To Lynne, Andrew, and Tim,
who continue to inspire me to do my best.

MPF

My affability and sense of a greater contribution to others
comes from seeing these characteristics in my wife, Patricia, and in
my amazing children, Raphael and Jamie. I yearn to be more like them every day.

JNL

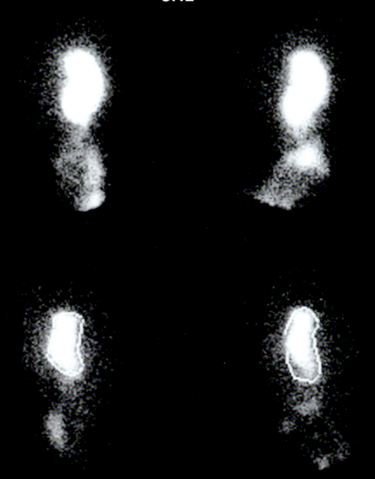

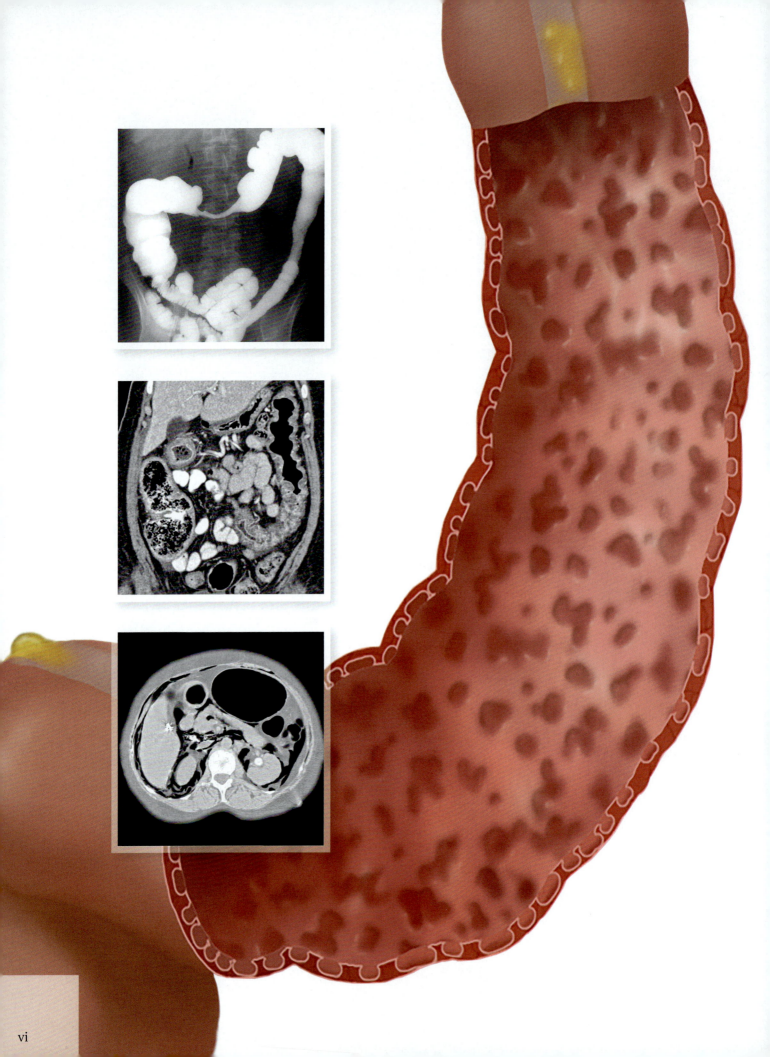

Contributing Authors

Amir A. Borhani, MD

Assistant Professor of Radiology
Abdominal Imaging Section
University of Pittsburgh School of Medicine
Pittsburgh, Pennsylvania

R. Brooke Jeffrey, MD

Professor and Vice Chairman
Department of Radiology
Stanford University School of Medicine
Stanford, California

Peter D. Poullos, MD

Clinical Associate Professor, Radiology
Clinical Associate Professor, Medicine—Gastroenterology & Hepatology
Stanford University School of Medicine
Stanford, California

Siva P. Raman, MD

Bay Imaging Consultants
Walnut Creek, California

Mitchell Tublin, MD

Professor and Vice Chair of Radiology
Chief, Abdominal Imaging Section
University of Pittsburgh School of Medicine
Pittsburgh, Pennsylvania

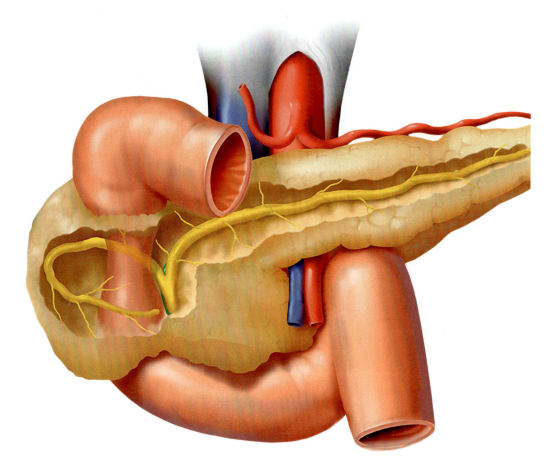

Foreword

I had the privilege of working closely with Mike Federle for nearly a decade when he was Chief of Radiology at San Francisco General Hospital; I was a busy trauma and general surgeon, and later Chief of Surgery at the same institution. He and his radiology colleagues organized a weekly conference for surgery residents and faculty at which they would collect the unusual and interesting cases for the week and then review and discuss them in an open interactive session with a view to educating both specialties in the most effective and efficient way to diagnose and manage a wide variety of problems, while at the same time significantly enhancing the surgeons' abilities to interpret radiologic images. It was one of the few conferences surgery residents did not have to be nudged to attend, as the extraordinary level of professional interaction and unique learning value was apparent to all.

Mike and his coauthor, Jim Lau, Clinical Professor of Surgery at Stanford, have brought the same level of cross-disciplinary discussion of abdominal surgical problems to this text. It is not just a compendium of radiologic images, but a merger of radiologic information correlated with surgical anatomy, surgical procedures, and surgical complications. The text is further enhanced because of the encyclopedic amount of information that is included and the remarkable quality of the anatomic drawings and radiologic images. There is virtually no problem in abdominal diagnosis that a surgeon will encounter that is not covered in this text, usually with multiple images relative to the problem.

The book begins with two overview sections: The first deals with common symptoms, signs, and conditions, and the second with disorders affecting multiple organs. Most of the first section includes common issues, such as pain, nausea and vomiting, GI bleeding, jaundice, etc., but it also includes imaging of bariatric surgery, imaging during pregancy and lacatation, and postoperative and postprocedure bowel imaging. The second section deals with multisystem disorders, including HIV/AIDS, IgG4-related disease, vasculitis, and scleroderma, but this section also includes treatment-related surgical problems, including postoperative free air and fluid, abdominal incision and injection sites, and foreign bodies, which again illustrates the specific relevance for surgeons.

Following these two initial sections, the book adopts a traditional structure, with anatomy being the primary level of organization, types of conditions the secondary level (infectious, inflammatory, and degenerative; trauma; vascular disorders; benign neoplasms; malignant neoplasms), and specific diagnoses the tertiary level. When appropriate, sections on embryology, normal variants and artifacts, and treatment-related conditions are added at the secondary level. This structure makes it extremely easy to reference any particular problem or diagnosis that the clinician wishes to investigate and find the needed material. As noted earlier, the conditions referenced here are comprehensive and will cover virtually anything the surgeon is likely to encounter.

This book is not one that can be skimmed nor quickly read from cover to cover, but rather one that will be picked up whenever a clinician has a particular problem and wishes to investigate it in depth, or when a resident is rotating on a particular service and wishes to acquire extensive knowledge of the various problems and imaging that he or she is likely to encounter in that specialty area. It will be of special value to the surgeon who insists on always seeing his own patient's diagnostic studies, takes pride in his or her radiologic skills and seeks to continually improve them, and who is occasionally able to challenge the radiologist's interpretations in a difficult case.

This is a lovely and valuable contribution to the surgical radiologic literature, and it represents a further contribution to the very high-quality radiologic library that Dr. Federle and his colleagues have assembled over the last decade and a half through the organization and operation of Amirsys, a physician-run radiologic publishing house, and the later integration of this into Elsevier. The special hallmarks of the book are: (1) Its combination of surgical and radiologic information into an integrated presentation, (2) the exquisite quality and detail of the anatomic and radiologic images, (3) the comprehensive coverage of surgical subjects, and (4) the density and detail of the information presented. I highly recommend it to both budding and established surgeons, from medical student to experienced practitioner, and feel it will enhance the diagnostic skills of anyone who spends some dedicated time studying it.

Frank R. Lewis, Jr., MD, FACS
Executive Director Emeritus
American Board of Surgery

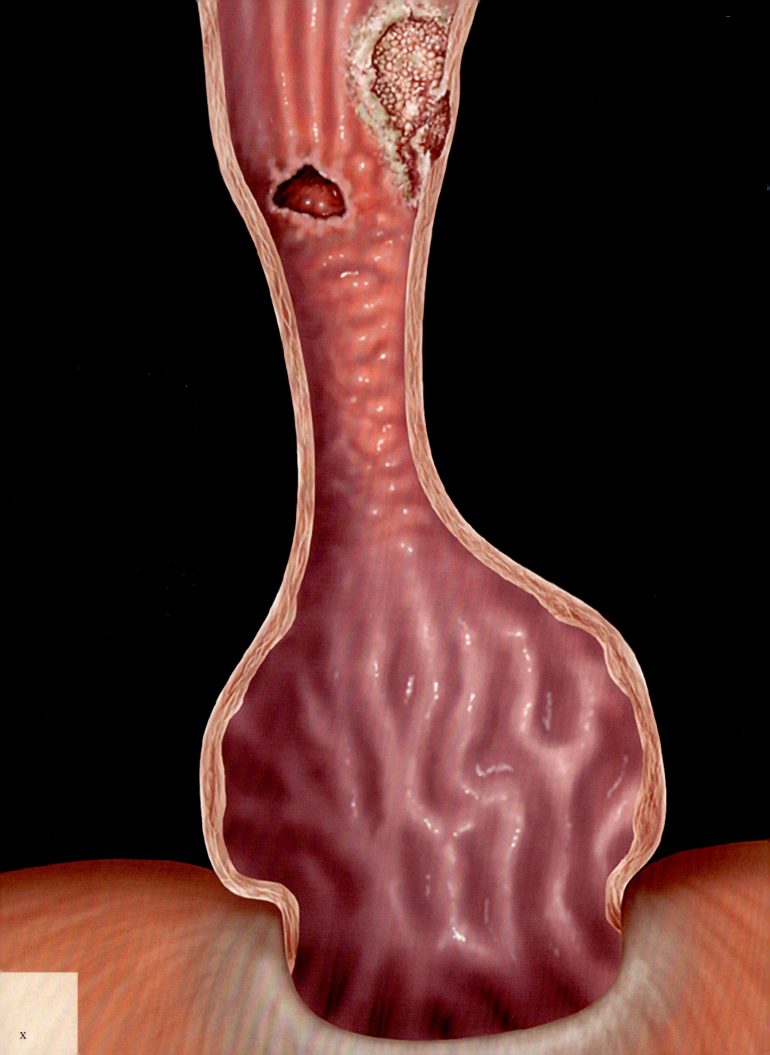

Preface

The field of abdominal imaging has changed dramatically over the past 15 years. Traditional mainstays, such as plain film radiography and fluoroscopy, have lost much of their relevance with the proliferation of endoscopy and cross-sectional imaging, including ultrasonography, computed tomography, and magnetic resonance imaging. Rapid and ongoing technical advances in imaging equipment, contrast media, and protocols make it extremely difficult for even recently trained physicians to keep abreast of developments that may have important implications for the evaluation and treatment of abdominal disorders. Our premise and goal in writing this book is that surgeons and other physicians caring for patients with disorders of the bowel, pancreas, or hepatobiliary system would benefit from a review of pertinent cross-sectional imaging anatomy, as well as the principles underlying the optimal selection of imaging modalities and protocols.

We provide individual chapters on essentially all of the important disorders that affect the GI tract, whether congenital, infectious, inflammatory, or neoplastic. These are presented in the classic Amirsys/Elsevier format of bulleted text, allowing us to present more than twice as much text as the equivalent traditional prose format textbook in an easily readable style. We also utilize high-quality medical illustrations and representative imaging studies to an extent rarely found in medical texts. We have, however, used a more informal prose format for the Overview and Introductory portions to help readers grasp the essential anatomical issues, imaging protocols, and general approaches to the most common and important disorders affecting each organ system.

Our book is intended to be complementary, not competitive, to other texts, such as the *Sabiston Textbook of Surgery*, which cover in great detail the pathophysiology, clinical evaluation, and treatment of disease. We cover most of the same symptom complexes and disorders but focus on the role of imaging. Every chapter in this book had the input of experienced abdominal radiologists as well as surgeons to assure accuracy and relevance. Additional features include numerous lists of differential diagnoses based on symptom complex (such as "right lower quadrant pain") or imaging finding (such as "cystic pancreatic mass"). Reference to specific chapters on the most likely candidates will then quickly lead to a more accurate and specific diagnosis.

Fluoroscopy in the modern era (endoscopy and CT) has evolved to focus primarily on the pre- and postoperative evaluation of patients for surgical alterations of the GI tract. Therefore, we have deemphasized the more esoteric aspects of fluoroscopic diagnosis of abdominal disorders in favor of more expansive coverage of topics such as bariatric surgery, antireflux procedures, esophageal and bowel resections, and so forth. Additional detailed diagnostic material, images, and references are included in Elsevier's eBook, Expert Consult, which accompanies the print version of *Imaging in Abdominal Surgery*.

We hope that this will be a welcome and unique addition to your library.

Michael P. Federle, MD, FACR
Professor of Radiology
Department of Radiology
Stanford University School of Medicine
Stanford, California

James N. Lau, MD, MHPE, FACS
Clinical Professor of Surgery
Stanford University School of Medicine
Stanford, California

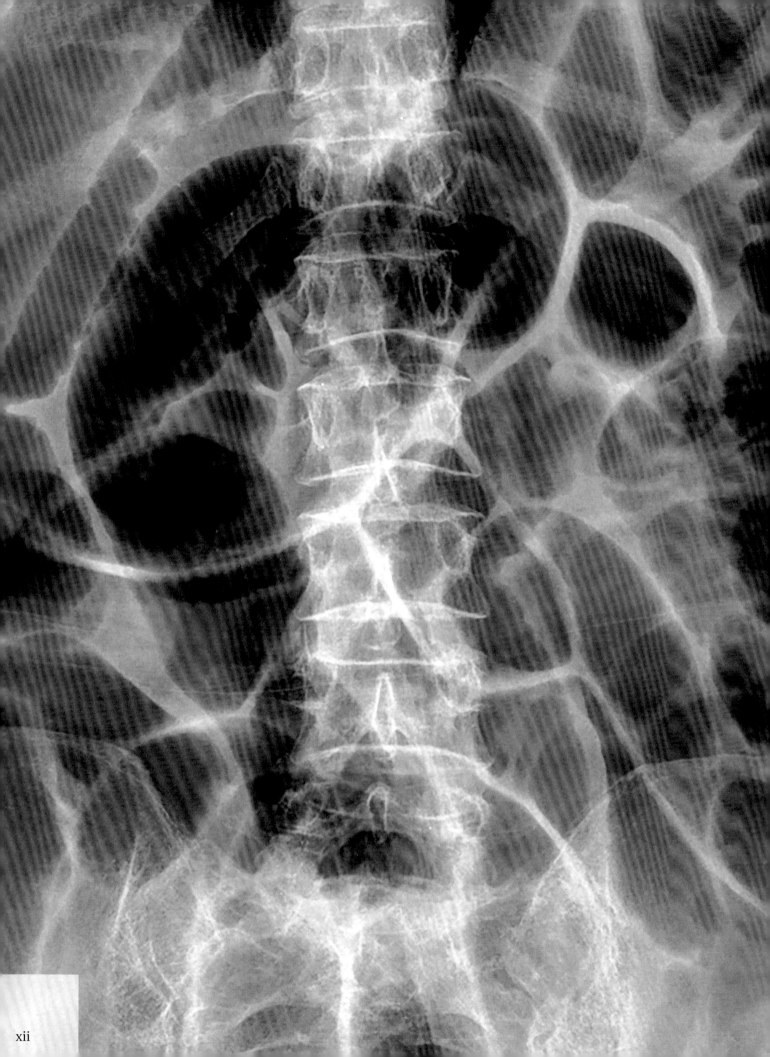

Acknowledgments

Lead Editor

Lisa A. Gervais, BS

Text Editors

Arthur G. Gelsinger, MA
Rebecca L. Bluth, BA
Nina I. Bennett, BA
Terry W. Ferrell, MS
Matt W. Hoecherl, BS
Megg Morin, BA

Image Editors

Jeffrey J. Marmorstone, BS
Lisa A. M. Steadman, BS

Illustrations

Richard Coombs, MS
Lane R. Bennion, MS
Laura C. Wissler, MA

Art Direction and Design

Tom M. Olson, BA

Production Coordinators

Angela M. G. Terry, BA
Emily C. Fassett, BA

ELSEVIER

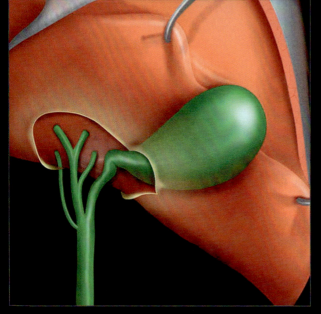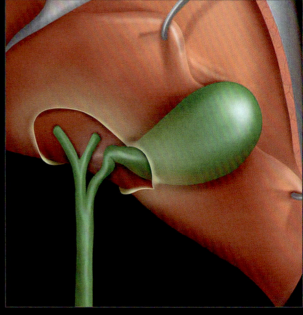
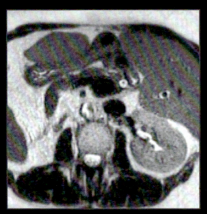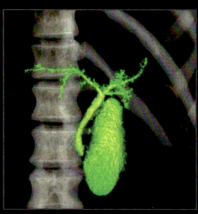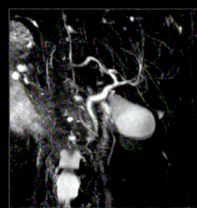
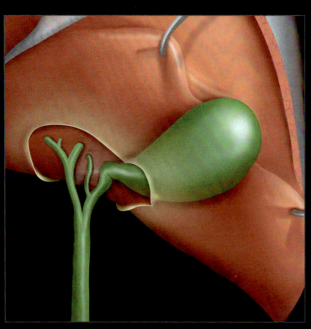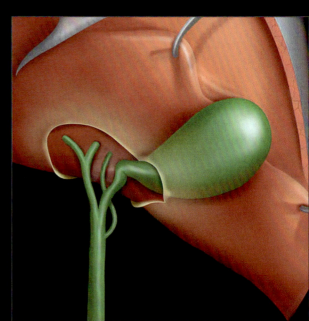

Sections

TABLE OF CONTENTS

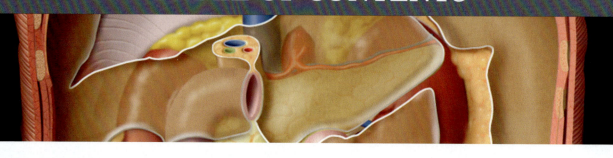

TABLE OF CONTENTS

TABLE OF CONTENTS

TABLE OF CONTENTS

TABLE OF CONTENTS

TABLE OF CONTENTS

18F FDG: F-18 fluorodeoxyglucose

A

ADC: apparent diffusion coefficient

AP: anteroposterior

C

CBD: common bile duct

CECT: contrast-enhanced computed tomography

CT: computed tomography

CTA: computed tomography angiography

D

DWI: diffusion-weighted imaging

DWI MR: diffusion-weighted imaging using MR

E

ERCP: endoscopic retrograde
   cholangiopancreatography

EUS: endoscopic ultrasound

F

FSE T2: T2 fast spin-echo imaging

G

GB: gallbladder

GRE: gradient-echo

H

HU: Hounsfield unit

I

IHBD: intrahepatic bile duct(s)

IPMN: intraductal papillary mucinous neoplasm

M

MCN: mucinous cystic neoplasm (pancreas)

MIP: maximum intensity projection

MPD: main pancreatic duct

MR: magnetic resonance

MR T1: magnetic resonance T1

MRA: magnetic resonance angiography

N

NECT: nonenhanced computed tomography

P

PA: posteroanterior

PET: positron emission tomography

PSC: primary sclerosing cholangitis

PTLD: post-Tx lymphoproliferative disorder

S

SMA: superior mesenteric artery

SMV: superior mesenteric vein

SPECT: single-photon emission computed tomography

STIR: short tau inversion recovery

STIR MR: short tau inversion recovery MR

SWI: susceptibility weighted imaging

T

T1: spin lattice or longitudinal relaxation time
   (MR scan)

T1 C+: T1 contrast-enhanced

T1 C+ FS: T1 contrast-enhanced with fat suppression

T1WI: T1-weighted imaging

T2: spin-spin or transverse relaxation time

T2*: T2 star, observed or effective T2

T2* GRE: gradient-echo T2 star

T2* SWI: T2 star susceptibility weighted imaging

T2WI: T2-weighted imaging

T2WI FS MR: T2-weighted magnetic resonance
   imaging with fat suppression

Tc-99m: technetium-99m

TPN: total parenteral nutrition

IMAGING IN

ABDOMINAL SURGERY

FEDERLE | LAU

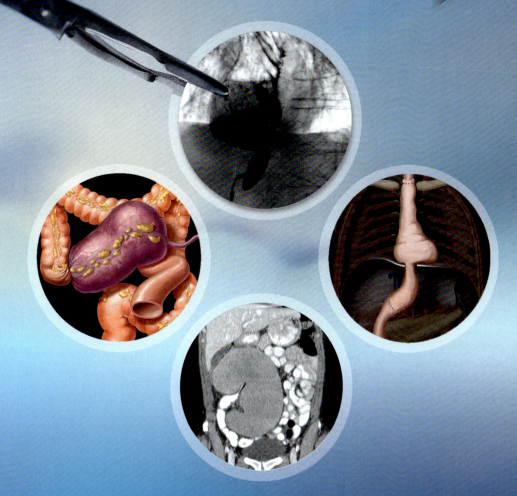

SECTION 1
Common Symptoms, Signs, and Conditions

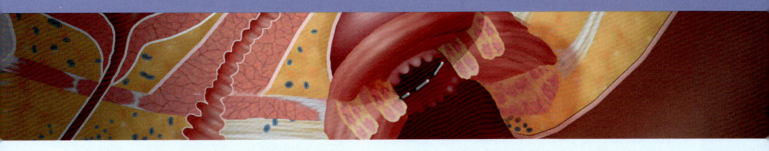

Overview

Within the past 20 years, the various imaging tools used to evaluate patients with abdominal symptoms have changed dramatically. In this era with relatively easy access to cross-sectional imaging and endoscopy, plain radiography and fluoroscopic ("barium") exams have lost much of their utility, though not all. Ultrasonography (US), computed tomography (CT), and magnetic resonance (MR) are now the dominant modalities in common use.

Many surgeons and other physicians caring for patients with hepatobiliary, pancreatic, or gastrointestinal (GI) disorders are likely to have received relatively little formal instruction in cross-sectional imaging anatomy or its appearance on imaging studies during medical school or residency. Moreover, the continuing rapid evolution of imaging equipment and scan protocols may make it difficult for radiologists, and nearly impossible for other physicians, to keep abreast of newer and important developments. With this introductory chapter and the rest of this book, we hope to make our readers more knowledgeable and comfortable in understanding the proper role and interpretation of various imaging tools for evaluation of abdominal disorders.

We will start with a brief overview of individual imaging modalities and an assessment of their strengths and limitations, acknowledging that there are legitimate reasons for considerable variability in practice patterns based on the training of physicians and the availability of specific equipment.

Imaging Modalities and Equipment

Radiography

Plain radiography has undergone the least technical advancement and the most drastic decline in use over the past 2 decades. Like other imaging techniques, "plain films" are now acquired and displayed digitally, which offers advantages in image quality, lower radiation does, and ease of distribution throughout the medical environment. No longer do physicians need to physically visit the radiology department to view or check out an abdominal film of their patient. Film reporting is now done by voice recognition, allowing almost immediate availability of the formal interpretation, obviating the need to hear the interpretation directly from a radiologist or waiting (hours or even days) for the paper report to make it to the patient's chart. On balance, these changes are good, but all of us "senior" radiologists miss the opportunity to discuss individual patients with referring physicians. Without question, the most ideal setting is one in which the referring physician selects the ideal imaging modality based on the patient's clinical presentation, and the radiologist interprets the study with a full understanding of the concerns and questions to be addressed in his or her report. Regrettably, this is rarely the case today.

The most common indication for an abdominal plain film today is to check the position of a feeding tube or other device. For this, a supine portable film is sufficient and accurate. A term sometimes used as a synonym for a plain film is a KUB (meaning kidneys, ureters, bladder), and this reflects the prior belief that such films were quite accurate in detecting calculi within the renal collecting system. A similar belief that plain films reliably depicted free intraperitoneal air (bowel perforation) and bowel obstruction persisted until CT came into widespread use, causing us to conclude that we had been missing a lot of disease on plain films.

If plain films are to be used to detect any abdominal disorder other than tube malposition, the study **must include supine and either upright (not sitting) or decubitus views**. The latter are essential in order to detect free intraperitoneal air or air-fluid levels.

Fluoroscopy

The other major "victim" of the modern era has been the fluoroscopic study of the GI tract. During the senior author's training and earlier practice, air-contrast barium studies of the entire GI tract were commonly employed to diagnose almost the whole spectrum of inflammatory, infectious, ischemic, and neoplastic disorders. Today, in most industrialized countries, most fluoroscopic studies are performed to evaluate patients before and after surgical procedures. Among the more common of these are antireflux (GERD), such as fundoplication, and bariatric surgical procedures, such as sleeve gastrectomy and Roux-en-Y gastric bypass. For patients who have had all or part of the colon resected, some form of contrast enema is generally performed to ensure there is no anastomotic stricture or leak.

Fluoroscopy has retained a primary role in evaluation of patients with dysphagia or symptoms of GERD and is complementary to various endoscopic and manometric procedures. These protocols and disorders are discussed at length in the Esophagus section of this book.

Ultrasonography

US has become the most widely utilized imaging study in the world, owing to its portability, affordability, and lack of ionizing radiation. Some physicians consider US an extension of the physical exam and encourage its use by practitioners of all sorts. This trend has been accelerated by the availability of small, inexpensive US units that can be used in the office, clinic, or emergency department. At the same time, some caution is warranted. Although some conditions and disorders may be readily apparent to even the infrequent US practitioner, such as large amounts of fluid in the peritoneal cavity, other conditions require considerable experience and expertise in US for accurate assessment.

US has at least 2 inherent limitations: A rather small field of view and its inability to image structures "hidden" by overlying bone or air. Although these can, to some extent, be overcome by repositioning the patient, US imaging of the GI tract will always be technically challenging. US has a primary role in evaluation of hepatobiliary disorders, as discussed at length in subsequent chapters.

Endoscopic US has attained an important role in evaluation of hepatobiliary and pancreatic disorders. A high-frequency US transducer placed near the tip of an endoscope provides direct visualization and high-resolution images of the bile ducts and pancreas, along with the ability to biopsy or otherwise retrieve tissue or fluid samples for laboratory analysis.

US equipment and protocols have evolved along 2 somewhat diverging paths: The simple but cheap and the complex but more expensive. The latter includes developments such as power Doppler, harmonic imaging, and even US contrast agents. Recently approved for use in the USA as well as in Europe and Asia are US "bubble" contrast agents. Real-time US imaging of the abdomen following IV bolus injection of one of these agents has shown great promise in evaluation of the vascularity and etiology of many neoplastic and other disorders. For more comprehensive and sophisticated applications of US, considerable expertise and experience are demanded for both its performance and interpretation.

Computed Tomography

CT has assumed a dominant role in evaluation of abdominal disorders of almost any etiology. With current CT scanners, high-resolution images can be obtained through the abdomen and pelvis in much less time than a minute with almost instantaneous "reconstruction" of the images available in any desired plane, such as coronal or sagittal (**multiplanar CT**). We routinely review all CT studies of the abdomen and pelvis in at least the axial and coronal planes. Curved planar reformations can be extremely instructive in evaluation of structures, such as the biliary and pancreatic ducts and blood vessels, as will be illustrated in multiple chapters. The ability of modern scanners to quickly acquire thousands of submillimeter-thick axial sections, coupled with powerful computers, has also led to the development of specific applications, such as **CT enterography, colonography**, and **angiography**, each of which has important uses in abdominal imaging.

The newer generation of CT scanners also provides CT hardware and software that has **markedly decreased the dose of ionizing radiation** to patients with many CT protocols now resulting in an effective dose that is less than yearly background radiation. Many educational and decision-support tools are available on the internet that can help guide referring physicians in ordering the most appropriate imaging studies, including those offered by the American College of Radiology and the American Board of Internal Medicine (through its Choosing Wisely campaign). Referring physicians should always weigh the risk:reward ratio in evaluation of any diagnostic or therapeutic procedure, and consultation with radiologists in a particular case is very useful in choosing the most appropriate imaging test and protocol.

Unlike other imaging studies, CT need not be limited to evaluation of a single organ or region, such as the right upper quadrant, and it is equally effective in depicting the spectrum of inflammatory, infectious, vascular, and neoplastic disorders that may affect any of the thoracic, abdominal, pelvic, or retroperitoneal organs. For almost all CT protocols, with the exception of suspected renal calculi, abdominal CT scans are most informative when performed during the rapid bolus **infusion of iodinated contrast medium**. Newer contrast agents can be administered safely, even to patients with renal insufficiency, utilizing smaller volumes of contrast media, newer CT scan protocols (e.g., lower kilovoltage tube current), and adequate hydration of the patient before and after the study. The **prevalence of contrast-induced nephropathy (CIN) from IV administration of contrast for CT is extremely low**, especially in adequately hydrated patients. There have been numerous, well-designed studies of CIN and its relationship to CT scanning, and there is broad agreement that the risk of CIN from CT has been greatly exaggerated. We agree with the recommendations of the Mayo Clinic and the American College of Radiology that **IV contrast media should not be withheld when it is deemed necessary for accurate CT diagnosis**.

Another technical advance in CT has been the faster acquisition and display of images, allowing selective imaging through large structures or regions (e.g., the entire liver or abdomen) in the arterial, venous, &/or delayed phase of contrast passage and uptake. Such **multiphasic contrast-enhanced CT protocols** have greatly improved our ability to detect disorders, such as GI bleeding, as well as hypervascular tumors and their metastases. We will discuss and illustrate specific uses of multiphasic CT in subsequent chapters.

Magnetic Resonance

No imaging modality has undergone more rapid and varied development over the last decade than MR. MR is inherently more sensitive to slight differences in tissue contrast than CT or US and can directly depict the body in any plane of section. Individual MR sequences and protocols can be utilized to display and quantitate, for example, the fat or iron content of the liver, the presence of hemorrhage, or many other characteristic features that allow more accurate diagnoses of abdominal disorders. Owing to the length of most abdominal MR protocols (> 30 minutes), MR is less optimal for imaging clinically unstable patients or larger anatomic regions (e.g., chest, abdomen, and pelvis). Because of its expense and more limited distribution, MR may be reserved for more detailed analysis of a disorder 1st suggested by CT or US, but it is assuming a more prominent role as the 1st-line imaging study in many cases, as discussed throughout this book.

As with CT and US, MR protocols have evolved to include the use of novel contrast agents. For abdominal MR protocols, the most important of these is **gadoxetate** disodium, commercially known in North America as **Eovist** and elsewhere as **Primovist**. Gadoxetate differs from most other gadolinium-based contrast agents in having substantial (~ 50%) hepatobiliary excretion. Gadoxetate-enhanced MR protocols are of proven value in allowing improved quality MR cholangiography and in helping to characterize certain hepatic disorders and masses, as addressed in subsequent chapters.

Nuclear Medicine

Radionuclide scintigraphy is inherently limited in its spatial resolution but offers unique physiologic properties that allow it to retain an important role in abdominal imaging. Foremost among these is the pairing of the physiologic display of glucose metabolism (radiolabeled FDG) and the anatomic display of CT into combined ("fused") PET/CT studies. PET/CT has achieved a critical role in oncologic imaging and is uniquely valuable in the initial staging, evaluation of response to treatment, and ongoing surveillance of GI malignancies. Unique PET tracers have been designed for specific targets, such as somatostatin analogues. Gallium 68-DOTATATE PET/CT is of proven superiority in detection and staging of neuroendocrine tumors, as discussed in other chapters. PET/MR is already entering clinical practice and will find its place in abdominal imaging as well.

Selected References

1. McDonald RJ et al: Intravenous contrast material-induced nephropathy: causal or coincident phenomenon? Radiology. 278(1):306, 2016
2. Parakh A et al: CT radiation dose management: a comprehensive optimization process for improving patient safety. Radiology. 280(3):663-73, 2016
3. McDonald RJ et al: Controversies in contrast material-induced acute kidney injury: closing in on the truth? Radiology. 277(3):627-32, 2015
4. Edinger B: Statistical sins of CIN (contrast material-induced nephropathy). Radiology. 270(3):938, 2014
5. Mayo-Smith WW et al: How I do it: managing radiation dose in CT. Radiology. 273(3):657-72, 2014
6. Newhouse JH et al: Quantitating contrast medium-induced nephropathy: controlling the controls. Radiology. 267(1):4-8, 2013
7. Balemans CE et al: Epidemiology of contrast material-induced nephropathy in the era of hydration. Radiology. 263(3):706-13, 2012
8. Nakaura T et al: Abdominal dynamic CT in patients with renal dysfunction: contrast agent dose reduction with low tube voltage and high tube current-time product settings at 256-detector row CT. Radiology. 261(2):467-76, 2011

(Left) US demonstrates the normal appearance of the gallbladder (GB). Note the thin GB wall ➡ (which should measure < 3 mm) and the clear, anechoic bile ➡ distending its lumen. (Right) The GB fundus ➡ is its distal tip, whereas the neck ➡ represents the proximal portion of the GB, which tapers toward the junction of the GB with the cystic duct. The cystic duct ➡ is not routinely visualized well on US but is seen here as a tubular, tortuous structure.

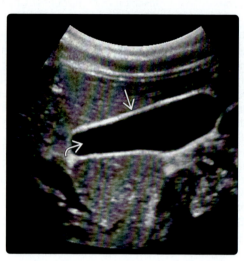
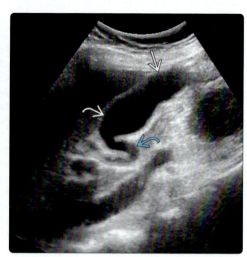

(Left) Sagittal US section shows the normal look and relationships of collecting bile duct (CBD) ➡ and portal vein (PV) ➡. The hepatic artery ➡ lies between the CBD and PV. The CBD is normally ~ 40% the diameter of the accompanying branch of the PV. (Right) Sagittal US through the liver shows its homogeneous echogenicity with interspersed vessels ➡ and small intrahepatic bile ducts. The right kidney ➡ and liver have similar echogenicity, which helps determine whether the liver is abnormally echogenic, suggesting steatosis.

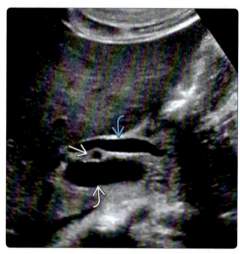
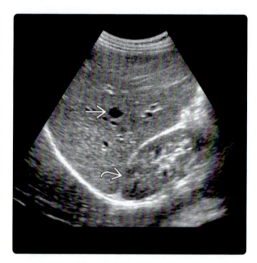

(Left) US shows the confluence of the hepatic veins ➡ with the inferior vena cava (IVC) ➡. Note the uniform, low-level echogenicity of the normal hepatic parenchyma. The diaphragm is marked ➡. (Right) Transverse US demonstrates the normal right ➡ and left ➡ PVs, both of which have the thick echogenic wall that is characteristic of the portal venous system (and allows PVs to be easily differentiated from hepatic veins).

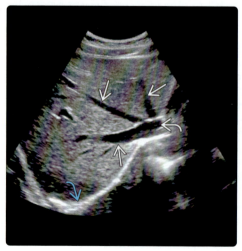
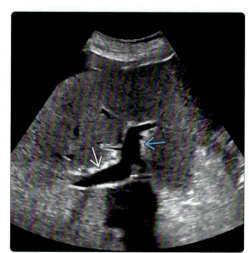

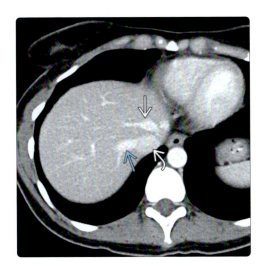
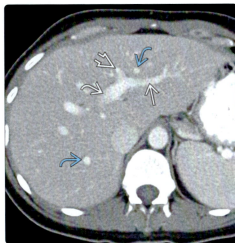

(Left) *First of 6 axial CECT images through a normal liver shows the middle ➡ and right ➡ hepatic veins joining the IVC ➡.* (Right) *More caudal CT section shows the lateral ➡ and medial ➡ segments of the left PV ➡. The hepatic veins ➡ travel in a more cephalocaudal direction and are seen in short axis on this axial image.*

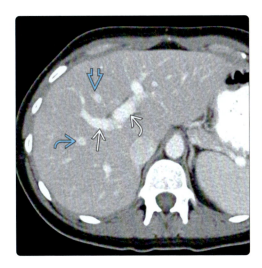
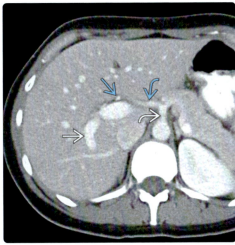

(Left) *More caudal section shows the anterior branch ➡ of the right PV and the undivided left PV ➡. The middle ➡ and right ➡ hepatic veins are seen in cross section. The hepatic veins tend to have a more vertical course, unlike the more horizontal course of the PVs.* (Right) *More caudal section shows the posterior branch ➡ of the right PV as well as the right hepatic artery ➡. The common hepatic artery ➡ branches from the celiac trunk ➡ along with the splenic and left gastric arteries.*

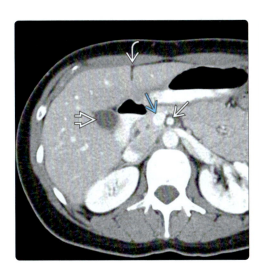
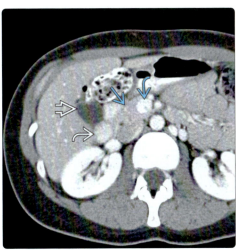

(Left) *More caudal section shows the falciform ligament cleft ➡, separating the medial and lateral segments of the left lobe. Also noted are the GB ➡ and superior mesenteric artery ➡ and vein ➡.* (Right) *More caudal section shows the inferior segments of the right hepatic lobe and GB ➡. The pancreatic head ➡ lies between the superior mesenteric vein ➡ and the 2nd portion of the duodenum ➡.*

(Left) *First of 3 arterial-phase contrast-enhanced T1 MR sections shows the homogeneously enhancing hepatic parenchyma and the enhanced left PV ➡. The middle and right hepatic veins ➡ are not yet enhanced on this early phase of imaging and appear dark.* **(Right)** *More caudal section shows the anterior branch ➡ of the right PV as well as the nonenhanced hepatic veins ➡. The falciform ligament cleft ➡ is also seen.*

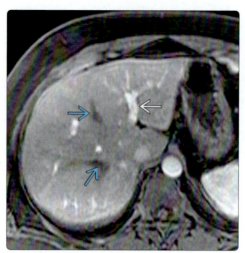 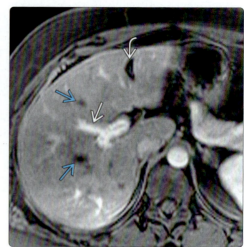

(Left) *More caudal section shows the posterior branch of the right PV ➡. Also note the celiac trunk ➡ and brisk enhancement of the pancreatic body ➡.* **(Right)** *First of 3 axial fat-suppressed nonenhanced T2 MR sections shows normal, low-intensity liver parenchyma and very low signal (flow void) within vessels, such as the right hepatic vein ➡, IVC ➡, and aorta ➡. Note bright signal from static fluid within the intrahepatic bile ducts ➡ and cerebrospinal fluid ➡ within the spinal canal.*

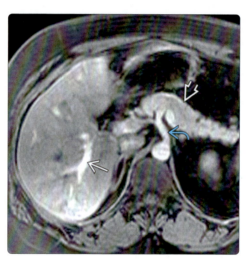 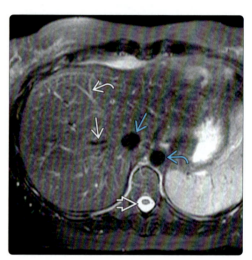

(Left) *More caudal MR section shows bright signal within the right hepatic duct ➡, which lies immediately anterior to the right PV ➡. The intrahepatic bile ducts are the branching, high-intensity (bright) foci within the liver.* **(Right)** *More caudal MR section shows bright signal from bile within the neck of the GB ➡ and the right hepatic duct ➡. Low-signal flow voids mark the hepatic artery ➡, PV ➡, and celiac trunk ➡.*

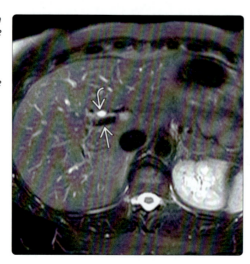 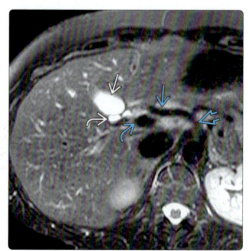

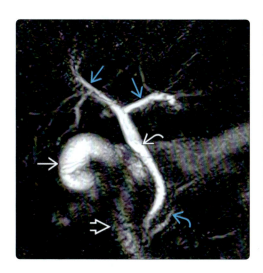

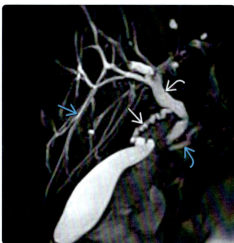

(Left) *Coronal MRCP, obtained without the use of contrast media, shows bright signal from fluid within the GB ➡, common duct ➡, and intrahepatic bile ducts ➡. A portion of the pancreatic duct ➡ and fluid-filled duodenum ➡ are also seen on this plane of section.* (Right) *Section from an MRCP study shows the GB, cystic duct ➡, and common hepatic ➡ and intrahepatic ducts ➡ as well as a portion of the pancreatic duct ➡, which was better seen on other planes of section.*

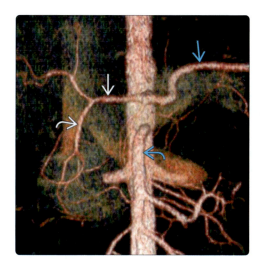

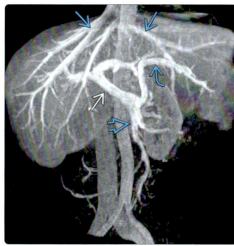

(Left) *CT angiogram shows enhancing arteries, including the common hepatic ➡, gastroduodenal ➡, splenic ➡, and superior mesenteric arteries ➡. CT and MR angiography usually make catheter angiography unnecessary for diagnosis, reserving this for interventions.* (Right) *Venous-phase, contrast-enhanced MR angiogram shows bright enhancement of venous structures, including the PVs ➡ and hepatic veins ➡. Portions of the splenic ➡ and superior mesenteric vein ➡ are included in this plane.*

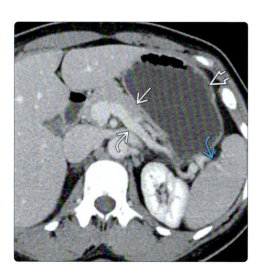

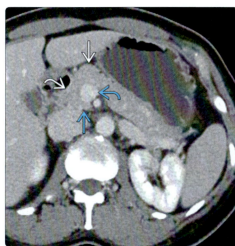

(Left) *In this 1st axial CECT, the normal pancreas is seen as a homogeneous, soft tissue density viscus lying just ventral to the splenic vein ➡, which lies in a groove along the dorsal surface of the pancreatic body ➡. The pancreatic tail lies on a more cephalic plane and inserts into the hilum of the spleen ➡. The stomach ➡ lies just ventral to the pancreas.* (Right) *More caudal section shows most of the pancreas, including the body, neck ➡, head ➡, and uncinate process ➡, which lies dorsal to the superior mesenteric vein ➡.*

Overview

The evaluation of the adult patient with abdominal pain is often challenging for the primary care, emergency physician, or surgeon. While occasional abdominal pain is experienced by almost all adults and is usually self-limited, it can herald serious disorders, demanding immediate diagnosis and treatment.

Much has been written about the clinical evaluation of acute abdominal pain and will be covered here only briefly, allowing us to focus on the appropriate role of imaging. Evaluation begins with a thorough history, determining, for instance, whether the pain is new or recurrent, its location and nature, what aggravates or alleviates the pain, associated GI (or GU) symptoms, etc. The physical exam includes the vital signs as well as auscultation for bowel sounds, percussion and palpation for tenderness, and signs of peritonitis or trauma. Women of reproductive age require specific screening for pregnancy, sexually transmitted diseases, and a pelvic exam, if lower abdominal or pelvic pain is part of the presentation. Laboratory studies can be tailored to specific symptom complexes, such as evaluation of liver function tests in patients with right upper quadrant (RUQ) pain, but should always include a complete blood count with differential, serum electrolytes, BUN, creatinine and glucose, and lipase &/or amylase. Women of reproductive age and almost any acute type of abdominal or pelvic pain should have a serum pregnancy test (β HCG) and urinalysis.

Whether a patient with acute abdominal pain can be evaluated safely and effectively in the outpatient or office setting is an essential decision to be made quickly. Patients with unstable vital signs or evidence of peritonitis on physical exam, or in whom there are concerns for a life-threatening disorder (e.g., ruptured aortic aneurysm, ectopic pregnancy, mesenteric ischemia), should be referred immediately to an emergency department with consideration for urgent surgery.

Abdominal pain may be relatively diffuse and poorly localized with many possible etiologies. In addition, localized pain and tenderness may be present in sites other than those usually associated with a particular disorder. Examples include right colonic diverticulitis, causing right lower quadrant, rather than the more common left lower quadrant (LLQ), pain and tenderness. Similarly, acute appendicitis may present as RUQ or even LLQ pain in patients who have a long, mobile appendix or malposition of the cecum. For this, among other reasons, any list of differential diagnostic possibilities, including those provided below, will not include every possible etiology. For the same reasons, strong consideration should be given to clinical and imaging evaluation beyond a narrow focus limited to a portion of the abdomen or pelvis.

Acute vs. Chronic Pain

There is no strict temporal criterion that will reliably classify pain or its etiology with some exceptions. Pain that has remained essentially unchanged for months or years may be safely classified as chronic, while pain that has worsened progressively over hours to days up to the point of presentation is clearly acute. Most obstetric and gynecologic disorders, urolithiasis (renal stones), or ruptured abdominal aortic aneurysm are much more likely to have an acute onset. Other patients have a pattern best considered as "acute on chronic" or recurring pain, with periodic exacerbations, with inflammatory bowel disease being a typical example. Many of the disorders listed in the following tables of differential

diagnoses for abdominal pain may have an acute, subacute, recurring, or even chronic mode of presentation. For these reasons, we will not present a separate set of differential diagnoses for chronic pain.

Evaluation of patients with **chronic abdominal pain** is particularly challenging. Those who have a specifically treatable structural or organic etiology can often be diagnosed with a combination of clinical and imaging evaluation. Diagnosis of a "functional GI disorder," almost by definition, cannot be made by imaging and is made only after excluding organic or structural etiologies. Among the common causes are irritable bowel syndrome, diabetic neuropathy, neurogenic abdominal pain (abdominal migraine or epilepsy), functional dyspepsia, and functional abdominal pain syndrome. Imaging, especially nuclear medicine scintigraphic studies, can play an important role in evaluation of a few nonstructural disorders, such as gastroparesis and sphincter of Oddi or gallbladder dysfunction.

Another category of disease generally regarded as a clinical rather than imaging diagnosis is metabolic disorder, such as porphyria or lead poisoning, though these cases may not be referred for evaluation by a surgeon.

Role of Imaging

Plain film radiography has a limited but important role in evaluating patients with acute abdominal pain, mainly for detection of small bowel or colonic obstruction or perforation (free air). **Plain film evaluation must include both supine and upright (or left lateral decubitus) films**; the latter are essential to detect free intraperitoneal air and air-fluid levels. If the referring physician has determined that abdominal CT is needed to evaluate a particular patient, plain films can be considered redundant, as CT detects nearly all abdominal disorders with greater sensitivity and specificity.

Imaging evaluation of young women or patients with acute RUQ pain or pelvic pain should begin with **ultrasonography (US)**. Many of the potential causes for RUQ or pelvic pain can be made or excluded with a combination of US and clinical evaluation. Moreover, US can effectively exclude the presence of an intrauterine pregnancy in a woman who may need additional evaluation by computed tomography (CT), thus alleviating concerns for radiation exposure of a fetus. US is highly operator dependent. While some diagnoses, such as acute cholecystitis, are relatively straightforward, many other conditions, including acute appendicitis and most obstetric and gynecologic disorders, require considerable expertise for both performance and interpretation. The increasing diffusion of sonography among various physicians in different clinical settings with limited US training is a matter of some concern, and quality control monitoring is important.

Once a patient has been found to have significant abdominal pain of uncertain etiology, **abdominal-pelvic CT** (to include the chest in some cases) is the mainstay of imaging evaluation. While we wish that all patients have a thorough clinical evaluation prior to ordering CT evaluation, this is not the most common practice. At the very least, one should determine the pregnancy status of female patients and the renal function of all patients. It is essential to have at least some reasonable differential diagnosis in mind (and communicated along with the CT requisition) in order to get the most useful CT protocol and correct interpretation. With the exception of the evaluation of renal colic, **nearly all GI and GU disorders are evaluated much more easily and accurately by CT following**

Abdominal Pain

the administration of intravenous contrast media. Some diagnoses, such as ischemic injury of the bowel, spleen, or kidneys, cannot be made on the basis of a nonenhanced CT scan. For some disorders, such as GI bleeding, aneurysms, and arterial occlusion, **CT angiography** is the technique of choice, and this is different than the standard contrast-enhanced CT in that scans are obtained during the arterial (rather than venous) phase of enhancement. A properly performed and interpreted abdominal-pelvic CT scan is extremely accurate in the diagnosis or exclusion of structural/organic causes of abdominal pain, especially those requiring urgent medical or surgical intervention. Far fewer patients are discharged from the emergency department with "nonspecific abdominal pain" as the diagnosis and the "exploratory laparotomy" has essentially been eliminated.

A somewhat counterintuitive principle is that the **administration of "positive" (radiopaque) oral or enteric contrast medium is rarely necessary for evaluation of the acutely ill patient and may be contraindicated**. The presence of high-density material in the gut makes it difficult or impossible to determine the presence and extent of GI mucosal enhancement, which is a critical criterion for enteric ischemia, infection, or inflammation. Even for suspected bowel obstruction, we do not recommend administration of oral contrast material for several reasons: Patients are usually nauseated and reluctant to drink; the lumen of obstructed bowel is sufficiently distended with normal enteric fluid; and we want to see vessel and mucosal enhancement to aid recognition of complications of bowel obstruction, such as volvulus and ischemia.

The following tables list most of the common and less common causes for abdominal or pelvic pain based on the primary focus of pain &/or tenderness. It is apparent that many etiologies appear on more than 1 list or location.

Differential Diagnosis

Right Upper Quadrant Pain
Common
- Acute or chronic cholecystitis
- Choledocholithiasis or cholangitis
- Gallbladder or sphincter of Oddi dysfunction
- Acute hepatitis or passive congestion
- Hepatic abscess
- Hepatic steatosis (fatty liver)
- Fitz-Hugh-Curtis syndrome
- Acute pancreatitis

Less Common
- Acute colitis
- Appendicitis
- Omental infarct
- Pyelonephritis
- Thoracic infection or infarction
- Cardiac ischemia or pericarditis
- Hepatic tumor

Epigastric Pain
Common
- Functional dyspepsia
- Acute esophageal inflammation or obstruction
- Gastritis or ulcer (gastric or duodenal)
- Gastroparesis
- Gastric tumor
- Acute or chronic cholecystitis
- Choledocholithiasis or cholangitis

- Acute or chronic pancreatitis
- Pancreatic tumor
- Gastroenteritis or colitis
- Acute appendicitis
- Small bowel obstruction
- Crohn's disease
- Eosinophilic gastroenteritis
- (Sclerosing) mesenteritis
- Angioedema (hereditary or drug induced)
- Hepatic inflammation, infection, or tumor
- Abdominal hernia (external and internal)
- Hiatal hernia ± gastroesophageal reflux disease
- Coronary artery disease
- Psychosomatic disorders

Right Lower Quadrant Pain
Common
- Appendicitis
- Crohn's disease
- Gynecologic and obstetric causes
- Pyelonephritis
- Obstructing ureteral stone
- Mesenteric enteritis/adenitis
- Infectious or ischemic colitis

Less Common
- Neutropenic colitis (typhlitis)
- Diverticulitis
- Omental infarction or epiploic appendagitis
- Cecal volvulus
- Colon carcinoma
- Renal infection or infarction
- Abdominal wall hematoma
- Intussusception
- Meckel diverticulitis
- Mucocele of appendix

Left Lower Quadrant Pain
Common
- Diverticulitis
- Colon carcinoma
- Epiploic appendagitis
- Infectious or ischemic colitis
- Ulcerative or Crohn's colitis
- Fecal impaction/stercoral colitis
- Gynecologic and obstetric causes
- Obstructing ureteral stone
- Sigmoid volvulus

Less Common
- Abdominal abscess or peritonitis
- Renal infection, infarction, or tumor
- Renal tumor
- Coagulopathic ("retroperitoneal") hemorrhage
- External or internal hernias
- Appendicitis

Pelvic Pain in Nonpregnant Women
Common
- Ovarian follicular cyst
- Ovarian corpus luteum
- Ovarian hemorrhagic cyst
- Pelvic inflammatory disease
- Ovarian torsion
- Complicated paraovarian cyst

Less Common
- Endometriosis or endometritis

- Ovarian tumor
- Complications of uterine leiomyomas
- Complications of mature cystic teratoma
- Ovarian hyperstimulation syndrome
- Hematosalpinx

Selected References

1. Pandharipande PV et al: CT in the emergency department: a real-time study of changes in physician decision making. Radiology. 278(3):812-21, 2016
2. Revzin MV et al: Pelvic inflammatory disease: multimodality imaging approach with clinical-pathologic correlation. Radiographics. 36(5):1579-96, 2016
3. Patel NB et al: Multidetector CT of emergent biliary pathologic conditions. Radiographics. 33(7):1867-88, 2013
4. Parker RA 3rd et al: MR imaging findings of ectopic pregnancy: a pictorial review. Radiographics. 32(5):1445-60; discussion 1460-2, 2012
5. Pooler BD et al: Alternative diagnoses to suspected appendicitis at CT. Radiology. 265(3):733-42, 2012
6. Spalluto LB et al: MR imaging evaluation of abdominal pain during pregnancy: appendicitis and other nonobstetric causes. Radiographics. 32(2):317-34, 2012
7. Heverhagen JT et al: MR imaging for acute lower abdominal and pelvic pain. Radiographics. 29(6):1781-96, 2009
8. Stoker J et al: Imaging patients with acute abdominal pain. Radiology. 253(1):31-46, 2009
9. Jaffe TA et al: Abdominal pain: coronal reformations from isotropic voxels with 16-section CT–reader lesion detection and interpretation time. Radiology. 242(1):175-81, 2007
10. Lazarus E et al: CT in the evaluation of nontraumatic abdominal pain in pregnant women. Radiology. 244(3):784-90, 2007
11. Pedrosa I et al: MR imaging of acute right lower quadrant pain in pregnant and nonpregnant patients. Radiographics. 27(3):721-43; discussion 743-53, 2007
12. Singh AK et al: Acute epiploic appendagitis and its mimics. Radiographics. 25(6):1521-34, 2005
13. O'Malley ME et al: US of gastrointestinal tract abnormalities with CT correlation. Radiographics. 23(1):59-72, 2003
14. Ahn SH et al: Acute nontraumatic abdominal pain in adult patients: abdominal radiography compared with CT evaluation. Radiology. 225(1):159-64, 2002
15. Bennett GL et al: Gynecologic causes of acute pelvic pain: spectrum of CT findings. Radiographics. 22:785-801, 2002
16. Cognet F et al: Chronic mesenteric ischemia: imaging and percutaneous treatment. Radiographics. 22(4):863-79; discussion 879-80, 2002
17. Boudiaf M et al: Ct evaluation of small bowel obstruction. Radiographics. 21(3):613-24, 2001

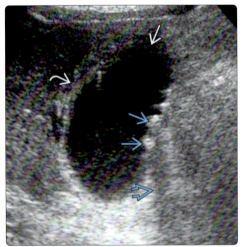
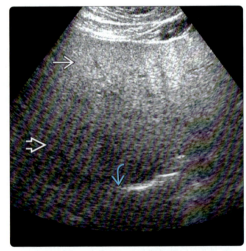

(Left) In this woman with acute RUQ pain and fever, US shows a distended gallbladder ➡ with diffuse wall thickening ⇗ and multiple gallstones ⇨ with posterior acoustic shadows ⇨. The sonographic Murphy sign was positive, all classic features of acute cholecystitis. (Right) In this woman with acute RUQ pain due to steatohepatitis, US shows severe, diffusely increased hepatic echogenicity ➡ with loss of signal from deeper tissue ⇗. The intrahepatic vessels and most of the diaphragm ⇗ cannot be seen.

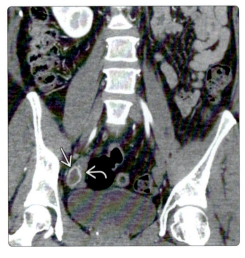
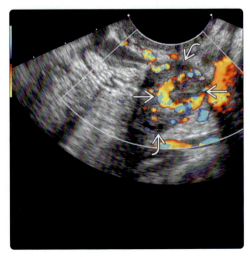

(Left) In this 47-year-old woman with RLQ pain, a coronal CT section shows a ring-enhancing, cystic structure ➡ with surrounding blood ⇗, diagnostic of a ruptured corpus luteum, a common cause of acute pain in women of reproductive age. (Right) In this young woman with acute lower abdominal and pelvic pain, color Doppler sonography shows a ring of hypervascularity ➡ within a normal-sized ovary ⇗, diagnostic of a corpus luteum cyst. US should be the 1st-line imaging test for abdominal or pelvic pain in young women.

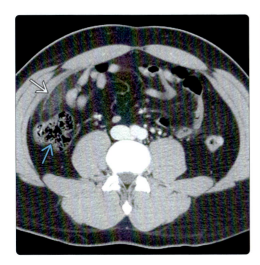

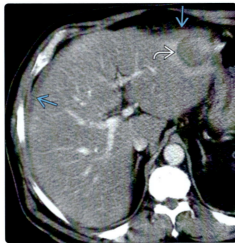

(Left) *In this young man with acute right abdominal pain, CT shows an encapsulated, oval, fatty "mass"* ➡ *adjacent to a normal-appearing ascending colon* ➡*; findings are diagnostic of acute omental infarction.* (Right) *In this man with acute epigastric pain, CT shows an encapsulated, heterogeneous mass* ➡ *that had ruptured through the hepatic capsule, causing hemoperitoneum* ➡*. Hepatocellular carcinoma was found and resected at surgery.*

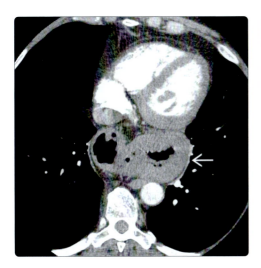

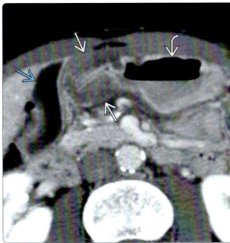

(Left) *In this 50-year-old man with epigastric pain, axial CECT shows a retrocardiac herniation of much of the stomach* ➡*, a large (paraesophageal) hiatal hernia.* (Right) *In this man with acute epigastric pain, CT shows marked thickening and submucosal edema of the gastric antral wall* ➡ *resulting in compression of the gastric lumen. The more proximal stomach* ➡ *and gallbladder* ➡ *are normal. Antral gastritis was confirmed on EGD.*

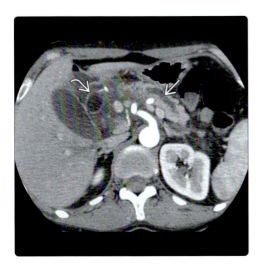

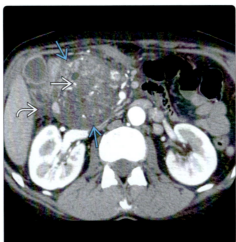

(Left) *In this woman with acute and recurring abdominal pain, CT shows dilation of the pancreatic* ➡ *and common bile duct* ➡*.* (Right) *In the same patient, another CT section shows marked enlargement of the pancreatic head* ➡*, peripancreatic edema or fluid* ➡*, and multifocal calcifications* ➡*. These findings are diagnostic of acute exacerbation of chronic pancreatitis. The mass is the fibroinflammatory process often seen in chronic pancreatitis.*

(Left) *In this patient with abdominal pain, nausea, and vomiting, a supine film of the abdomen shows no obvious dilation of bowel loops.* (Right) *In the same patient, an upright film shows multiple air-fluid levels ➡ and several "strings of pearls" ➡ that indicate small collections of gas floating on top of fluid within distended segments of small bowel (SB).*

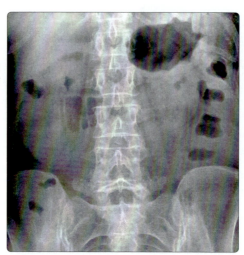 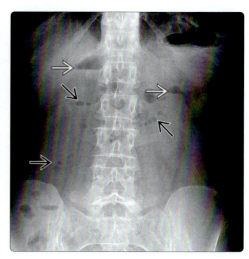

(Left) *In the same patient, a coronal reformatted CECT shows massively dilated, fluid-filled proximal SB ➡ and collapsed distal SB segments ➡. (Right) In the same patient, axial CT shows massively dilated and fluid-distended segments of proximal and mid SB ➡, while the colon ➡ is collapsed.*

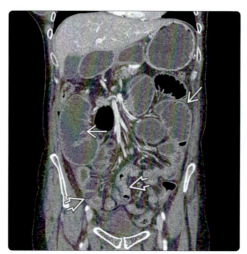 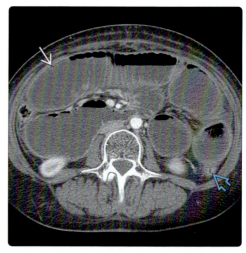

(Left) *In the same patient, another CT section shows both dilated, fluid-distended, proximal SB ➡ as well as collapsed distal SB segments ➡. (Right) Another CT section in the same patient shows the point of transition ➡ between the dilated ➡ and collapsed ➡ SB segments. The findings are characteristic of adhesive SB obstruction. Note that "oral" (enteric) contrast material was not given nor needed, as the fluid content of the SB makes it easy to identify normal SB mucosal enhancement.*

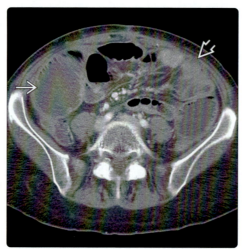 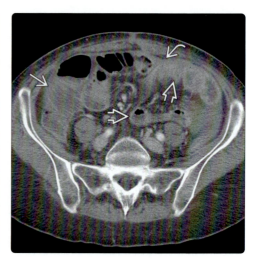

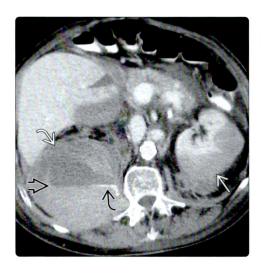

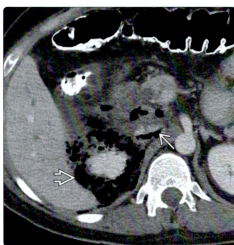

(Left) In this patient, CT shows high-density hemorrhage involving multiple anatomic spaces and planes, including the left perirenal ➡ and right retroperitoneal ➡. Note the fluid-fluid, or "hematocrit," level ⬚ in the iliopsoas hematoma, which also shows a focus of active extravasation of blood ➡. These findings are diagnostic of a coagulopathic hemorrhage. (Right) CT shows gas bubbles surrounding the retroperitoneal portions of the duodenum ➡, extending into the perirenal space ➡ via the renal hilum, due to a perforated duodenal ulcer.

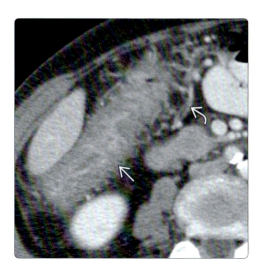

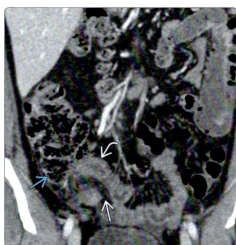

(Left) In this elderly woman with abdominal pain and diarrhea, CT shows marked, edematous thickening of the wall of the hepatic flexure ➡ and engorged blood vessels ➡. Similar findings were present throughout the colon and rectum, diagnostic of acute infectious colitis. (Right) In this young woman with acute abdominal pain, coronal CT shows a thick-walled, dilated appendix ➡ arising from the tip of the cecum ➡. The periappendiceal fat is inflamed ➡; findings are diagnostic of acute appendicitis.

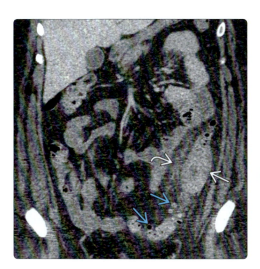

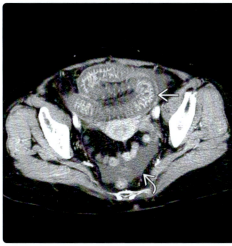

(Left) In this 33-year-old woman with acute LLQ pain, coronal CT shows mural thickening of the descending colon ➡, multiple diverticula ➡, and infiltration of the adjacent pericolonic fat ➡, diagnostic of acute diverticulitis. (Right) In this elderly woman with repeated episodes of severe abdominal pain, CT shows ascites ➡ and marked mural thickening and submucosal edema in a long segment of SB ➡. The history and CT findings are typical of ACE-inhibitor-induced intestinal angioedema.

Overview

Nausea and vomiting are experienced by almost everyone, and most episodes and causes are self-limited, rarely coming to medical attention. Patients are often aware of the common causes, such as acute viral infections, "traveler's" nausea and diarrhea, or the after effects of excessive alcohol consumption, and self-medicate or wait for the symptoms to pass. Other episodes are sufficiently severe or atypical that patients seek medical care.

Certain clinical features may be characteristic enough for the clinician to make a confident diagnosis as to the cause of the patient's nausea and vomiting without reliance on sophisticated laboratory or imaging tests. A complete history and physical examination are necessary in order to choose among the myriad potential causes of the patient's symptoms, including whether these are an initial, acute, recurring, or chronic event, and whether they are accompanied by extraabdominal signs and symptoms. A list of prescribed or otherwise consumed drugs is also mandatory, as adverse drug effects are a common cause of nausea and vomiting.

Tables listing some principal causes of nausea and vomiting, along with examples, are listed here.

Principal Causes of Nausea and Vomiting

Abdominal Causes
- (See 2nd table for details)

Drugs
- Aspirin and other NSAIDs
- Antimicrobial medications
- Cancer chemotherapy
- Others

Infectious Causes
- Acute gastroenteritis
- Systemic infections

Metabolic and Endocrine Disorders
- Diabetes
- Thyroid disorders
- Pregnancy
- Others

Neurological Causes
- Migraine headaches
- Inner ear disturbance
- Brain disorders
- Others

Other Causes
- Cardiac disease
- Collagen vascular disease
- Postoperative conditions
- Psychological disorders
- Others

Common Abdominal Causes of Nausea and Vomiting

Mechanical Obstruction
- Gastric outlet obstruction (e.g., peptic ulcer; gastric or duodenal carcinoma)
- Small bowel obstruction
- Incarcerated hernias
- Superior mesenteric artery syndrome

Motility Disorders
- Gastroparesis
- Functional dyspepsia
- Chronic intestinal pseudoobstruction

Others
- Acute gastroenteritis
- Gastroesophageal reflux
- Acute appendicitis
- Acute cholecystitis or cholelithiasis
- Renal calculi
- Acute hepatitis
- Mesenteric (bowel) ischemia
- Crohn's disease
- Peptic ulcer disease
- Bezoar (gastric or intestinal)
- Pancreatitis and pancreatic tumors
- Peritonitis and carcinomatosis
- Mesenteric and retroperitoneal disorders
- Obstetric and gynecologic conditions

Role of Imaging

Following the initial assessment of the patient, some form of imaging is usually warranted if the clinician considers any of the common abdominal etiologies for nausea or vomiting to be a likely source.

Plain Abdominal Radiography

Plain films can be helpful in diagnosing or ruling out conditions, such as bowel perforation, obstruction, or renal calculi. These should include both **supine and upright films**. However, we have learned that the plain film diagnosis of even free air, renal calculi, and bowel obstruction is limited. Moreover, even when plain films correctly suggest the presence of these and other disorders, clinicians typically require more specific and detailed imaging information on which to base management. For instance, most cases of mechanical small bowel obstruction no longer result in immediate surgery. Important criteria, such as the degree and cause of the obstruction and presence of complications, such as bowel ischemia, are not answered with sufficient accuracy by plain films alone. If a clinician has decided that abdominal-pelvic CT is to be obtained, there is usually little to be gained by preceding this with plain radiography.

Ultrasonography

If the clinical differential diagnosis includes acute biliary disorders, **US** is the 1st-line imaging study, being highly accurate in depicting gallstones, acute cholecystitis, and biliary obstruction, while also offering evaluation of many other abdominal and retroperitoneal disorders, such as renal calculi, hydronephrosis, and pancreatic disorders.

Computed Tomography

CT is the most versatile imaging modality in the initial evaluation of almost all abdominal, "mechanical" causes of nausea and vomiting, including inflammatory, infectious, ischemic, and neoplastic disorders of any of the abdominal viscera. Sensitivity and specificity vary to a degree for specific etiologies, but CT is highly accurate (> 90%) in detecting or excluding conditions that warrant urgent medical or surgical attention. Multiple studies have demonstrated that the use of CT in the emergency department setting is highly cost-effective in avoiding unnecessary hospital admission and surgery; conversely, disorders in need of urgent intervention are recognized with confidence and efficiency.

For almost all CT evaluations of acute abdominal disorders, **IV contrast-enhanced CT with multiplanar viewing** of images is mandatory. **The administration of radiopaque oral/enteric contrast material is not generally helpful** and actually impedes the ability to assess for GI mucosal enhancement, an important criterion in diagnosing or excluding inflammatory and infectious GI disorders. Even for suspected gastric outlet or bowel obstruction, oral contrast medium should not be given for a number of reasons; the normal gastric and small bowel secretions are sufficient to allow distention and identification of these organs.

Individual chapters address the detailed findings for all the disorders listed in the table of differential diagnoses (above) along with other disorders that may have nausea and vomiting as part of their clinical presentation.

Magnetic Resonance Imaging

While **MR** is highly accurate and useful in diagnosing specific abdominal disorders, such as choledocholithiasis and pancreatic neoplasms, it is most often employed as a problem-solving modality for a disorder 1st identified by US or CT, which are less expensive and more widely available.

Information provided by US or CT can direct attention to a specific organ or finding (e.g., dilated common bile duct), allowing a more focused MR protocol to be employed.

Radionuclide Scintigraphy

"Nuclear medicine" imaging tests are limited by spatial (anatomic) resolution but play an important role in some patients with nausea and vomiting. The biphasic (solid and liquid food, labeled with a radiotracer) gastric emptying study provides valuable objective measures of delayed emptying of the stomach. The technetium "HIDA" scan is an important 2nd-line test (behind US) in evaluation of patients with suspected gallbladder disease.

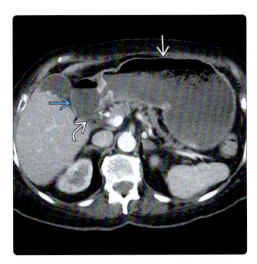
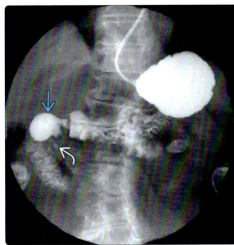

(Left) Axial CT in an elderly woman with persistent nausea and vomiting shows distention of the stomach ➡ and duodenal bulb ➡ with abrupt narrowing of the postbulbar duodenum ➡; no mass was seen. (Right) Spot film from an upper GI series in the same patient shows a dilated and deformed duodenal bulb ➡ and an ulcer ➡ in the postbulbar duodenum that caused the gastric outlet obstruction, confirmed by endoscopy.

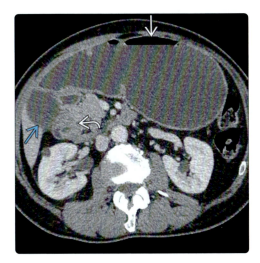
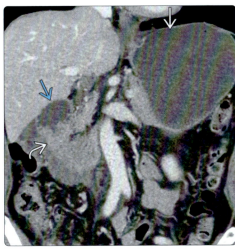

(Left) Axial CT in a 60-year-old man with persistent nausea and vomiting shows distention of the stomach ➡ and duodenal bulb ➡ with a mass ➡ encircling the 2nd portion of the duodenum and compressing its lumen. (Right) Coronal reformation of the CECT in the same patient shows the distended stomach ➡ and duodenal bulb ➡ and an "apple core" constricting mass ➡ of the 2nd portion of the duodenum, a primary duodenal carcinoma.

(Left) In this 50-year-old woman with progressive nausea and vomiting, a coronal CECT shows markedly distended proximal small bowel segments ➡ and a collapsed distal small bowel ⇨ and colon. (Right) In the same patient, an axial CT section shows the point of transition ➡ between the dilated and collapsed small bowel. On this and other sections, the bowel seemed to come to an abrupt, pointed narrowing, typical of adhesive small bowel obstruction, confirmed on subsequent surgery.

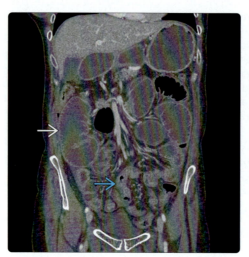
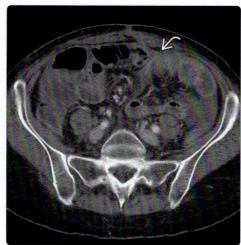

(Left) In this young woman with persistent nausea and vomiting, axial CT shows marked distention of the stomach ⇨ and proximal duodenum ➡ with abrupt compression of the 3rd duodenum ➡ between the aorta and SMVs. (Right) Coronal CT (same patient) shows the dilated stomach ⇨ and 2nd duodenum ➡. The distal duodenum and proximal small bowel ➡ were normal. The pinching of the duodenum between the aorta and SMA is the classic imaging appearance of "SMA syndrome."

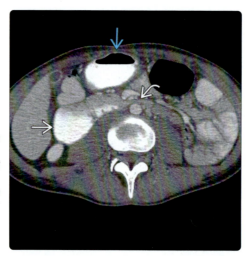
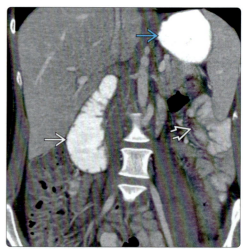

(Left) Four coronal images from a gastric-emptying scintiscan, taken 1, 2, 3, and 4 hours after ingestion of radiolabelled food, show significantly delayed emptying of the stomach ⇨ at each interval, consistent with gastroparesis. (Right) In this patient with diabetes, a film from a UGI series shows stasis of the barium in the stomach (20-minute delay), indicating delayed gastric emptying (gastroparesis). The large filling defect ➡ within the stomach that conforms to the shape of the stomach is a bezoar.

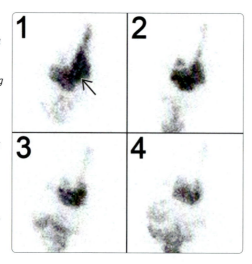
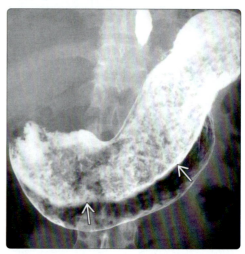

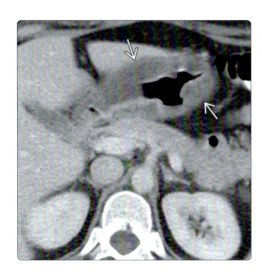

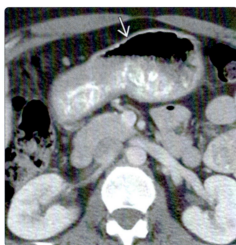

(Left) *In this young man with nausea and abdominal pain, axial CECT shows massive thickening and edema of the gastric wall ➡. He was using large doses of NSAIDs to relieve pain from athletic injuries.* (Right) *Repeat CECT study in the same patient following cessation of NSAID use 4 weeks later shows a completely normal stomach ➡, supporting the diagnosis of NSAID-induced gastritis.*

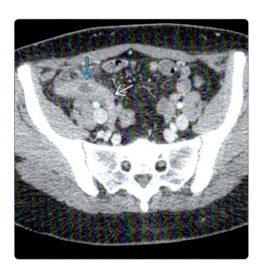

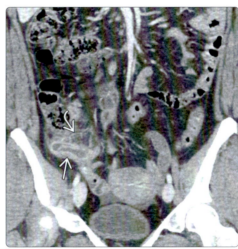

(Left) *In this 32-year-old woman, axial CECT shows a thick-walled appendix ➡ with infiltration of the surrounding fat and probable perforation of its wall ➡.* (Right) *Coronal CECT in the same patient shows the thick-walled appendix ➡ with hyperenhancement of its mucosal lining and infiltration of the mesenteric fat ➡. Acute perforated appendicitis was confirmed at surgery.*

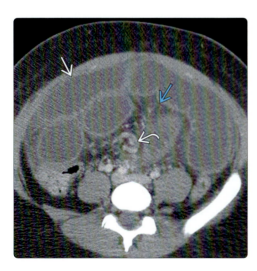

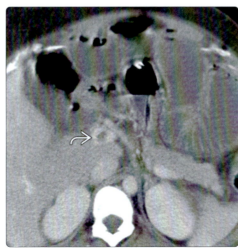

(Left) *In this young woman with severe nausea and abdominal pain, CT shows a dilated, fluid-filled small bowel ➡, mesenteric infiltration ➡, and clot within the SMV ➡.* (Right) *Contrast-enhanced CT in the same patient shows the SMV clot extending up into the portal vein ➡. The bowel ischemia and clot resolved with thrombolytic therapy; the patient was later diagnosed with a prothrombotic condition.*

Overview

Diarrhea is a symptom experienced by nearly everyone, generally considered an increase in the volume, fluidity, &/or frequency of stools. Most episodes are transient and self-limited or self-treated with nonprescription medications. However, diarrhea may be persistent or complicated by pain, fever, rectal bleeding, or other factors that bring patients to medical attention. Chronic diarrhea may affect ~ 5% of people in industrialized countries, and acute or chronic infectious diarrhea remains an important cause of morbidity and mortality in developing countries.

Diarrhea often represents a protective response to a variety of intestinal infections and toxins and is of value, at least acutely. Diarrhea may result from abnormalities of intestinal motility or length (e.g., short gut syndrome; effects of vagotomy) but more commonly is due to an excess of stool water resulting from abnormal epithelial function (water and electrolyte transport); this is referred to as "secretory diarrhea." Causes include various drugs, exogenous secretagogues, such as cholera enterotoxins, or endogenous secretagogues, such as intestinal neuroendocrine tumor (carcinoid). Diffuse intestinal mucosal disease, such as celiac or Crohn's disease, or infectious enteritis or colitis may cause diarrhea, as can intestinal ischemia.

The most common cause of acute secretory diarrhea is infection. Enterotoxins are produced primarily by bacteria but also by parasites, protozoa, and viruses. Clinicians can classify or categorize diarrheal states using a variety of terms, including watery, inflammatory, or fatty diarrhea. Chronic inflammatory diarrhea may result from a diverse group of infectious, idiopathic inflammatory, or neoplastic processes, as listed below. It may also be useful to consider diarrhea that occurs in specific clinical settings, such as travelers, epidemics, patients with HIV/AIDS, or institutionalized patients, as listed below.

Role of Imaging

Following the initial thorough history and physical exam, imaging can play an important role in establishing the cause of diarrhea. Structural disorders, such as short gut, postoperative alterations, or extensive small bowel diverticulosis, are readily evident on routine contrast-enhanced CT scans with multiplanar reformations being especially revealing. Most causes of infectious or inflammatory small intestinal or colonic disease result in mucosal hyperenhancement and submucosal edema, often associated with infiltration and hyperemia of surrounding tissues. Common and less common etiologies for bowel wall thickening are listed in tables of differential diagnosis below. These findings are especially evident on CT and MR enterography with multiphasic (arterial and venous) and multiplanar imaging. Many of these, such as Crohn's disease and *Clostridium difficile* (pseudomembranous) colitis, have imaging findings so distinctive as to suggest a specific diagnosis, as detailed in individual chapters on each entity.

Imaging can be of greater value if the radiologist is informed of the main clinical concerns to be addressed. For CT or MR evaluation of almost any acute intestinal or colonic disorder, the administration of IV contrast is almost mandatory, while **giving "positive" oral contrast agents is not only unnecessary but contraindicated**, as these make evaluation of mucosal enhancement and other findings difficult or impossible. If Crohn's disease is a major consideration, **CT or MR enterography** is the preferred imaging modality.

Conversely, for suspected mesenteric ischemia, CT angiography is the ideal noninvasive test.

Chronic Diarrhea: Common Causes

Fatty Diarrhea (Malabsorption or Maldigestion)
- Mesenteric (bowel) ischemia
- Mucosal diseases (e.g., celiac disease, Whipple disease)
- Short bowel syndrome
- Small intestinal bacterial overgrowth
- Pancreatic exocrine insufficiency

Inflammatory Diarrhea
- Infectious enteritis (e.g., yersiniosis, cytomegalovirus, amebiasis)
- Infectious colitis
- Inflammatory bowel disease (Crohn's, ulcerative colitis)
- Ischemic colitis
- Colon cancer or lymphoma
- Radiation enteritis or colitis
- Diverticulitis

Others (Examples)
- Postoperative states (e.g., bowel resection; bariatric surgery; cholecystectomy)
- Endocrinopathies
- Laxative abuse
- Vasculitis

Diarrhea: Common Causes in Specific Settings

Travelers
- Bacterial, protozoal or parasitic infection

Epidemics or Outbreaks
- Bacterial infection (e.g., *Escherichia coli* colitis)
- Protozoal infection (e.g., *Giardia*)
- Viral infection (e.g., rotavirus)

Patients With Diabetes
- Altered bowel motility
- Celiac disease (associated)
- Pancreatic insufficiency
- Small intestinal bacterial overgrowth
- Drug side effects

Patients With HIV/AIDS
- Drug side effects
- Opportunistic infections
- Lymphoma

Hospitalized or Institutionalized Patients
- Infectious (including *C. difficile*) colitis
- Drug side effects
- Fecal impaction with "overflow" diarrhea
- Ischemic colitis
- Enteric tube feeding

Differential Diagnosis

Colonic Submucosal Wall Thickening
Common
- Diverticulitis
- Infectious colitis
- Ischemic colitis
- Portal hypertension
- Ulcerative colitis
- Crohn's disease
- Obesity (mimic)

Less Common
- Colon carcinoma

Diarrhea

- Typhlitis (neutropenic colitis)
- Chemical proctocolitis
- Colonic metastases and lymphoma
- Intramural hemorrhage
- Pneumatosis of intestine
- Hemolytic uremic syndrome
- Intestinal angioedema

Segmental or Diffuse Small Bowel Wall Thickening

Common
- Crohn's disease
- Infectious enteritis
- Ischemic enteritis
- Intramural hemorrhage
- Shock bowel (hypotensive complex)
- Portal hypertension
- Hypoalbuminemia

Less Common
- Radiation enteritis
- Opportunistic intestinal infections
- Vasculitis
- Metastases and lymphoma, intestinal
- Carcinoid tumor
- Angioedema, intestinal
- Lymphangiectasia, intestinal
- Endometriosis
- Graft-vs.-host disease

Irregular Diffuse Small Bowel Fold Thickening

Common
- Celiac disease
- Malabsorption conditions
- Opportunistic intestinal infections
- Portal hypertension, varices

Less Common
- Ischemic enteritis
- Metastases and lymphoma, intestinal

Rare but Important
- Lymphangiectasia, intestinal
- Whipple disease
- Eosinophilic gastroenteritis
- Amyloidosis
- Mastocytosis
- Tropical sprue
- Abetalipoproteinemia
- Waldenstrom macroglobulinemia

Selected References

1. Masselli G et al: Diagnosis of small-bowel diseases: prospective comparison of multi-detector row CT enterography with MR enterography. Radiology. 279(2):420-31, 2016
2. Wallihan DB et al: Diagnostic performance and dose comparison of filtered back projection and adaptive iterative dose reduction three-dimensional CT enterography in children and young adults. Radiology. 276(1):233-42, 2015
3. Del Gaizo AJ et al: Reducing radiation dose in CT enterography. Radiographics. 33(4):1109-24, 2013
4. Scholz FJ et al: CT findings in adult celiac disease. Radiographics. 31(4):977-92, 2011
5. Elsayes KM et al: CT enterography: principles, trends, and interpretation of findings. Radiographics. 30(7):1955-70, 2010
6. Lee SS et al: Crohn disease of the small bowel: comparison of CT enterography, MR enterography, and small-bowel follow-through as diagnostic techniques. Radiology. 251(3):751-61, 2009
7. Bodily KD et al: Crohn Disease: mural attenuation and thickness at contrast-enhanced CT Enterography--correlation with endoscopic and histologic findings of inflammation. Radiology. 238(2):505-16, 2006
8. Booya F et al: Active Crohn disease: CT findings and interobserver agreement for enteric phase CT enterography. Radiology. 241(3):787-95, 2006
9. Hara AK et al: Crohn disease of the small bowel: preliminary comparison among CT enterography, capsule endoscopy, small-bowel follow-through, and ileoscopy. Radiology. 238(1):128-34, 2006
10. Maglinte DD: Science to practice: do mural attenuation and thickness at contrast-enhanced CT enterography correlate with endoscopic and histologic findings of inflammation in Crohn disease? Radiology. 238(2):381-2, 2006
11. Paulsen SR et al: CT enterography as a diagnostic tool in evaluating small bowel disorders: review of clinical experience with over 700 cases. Radiographics. 26(3):641-57; discussion 657-62, 2006
12. Thoeni RF et al: CT imaging of colitis. Radiology. 240(3):623-38, 2006
13. Boudiaf M et al: Small-bowel diseases: prospective evaluation of multi-detector row helical CT enteroclysis in 107 consecutive patients. Radiology. 233(2):338-44, 2004
14. Wold PB et al: Assessment of small bowel Crohn disease: noninvasive peroral CT enterography compared with other imaging methods and endoscopy–feasibility study. Radiology. 229(1):275-81, 2003
15. Horton KM et al: CT evaluation of the colon: inflammatory disease. RadioGraphics 20: 399-418, 2000
16. Balthazar EJ et al: Ischemic colitis: CT evaluation of 54 cases. Radiology. 211(2):381-8, 1999
17. Philpotts LE et al: Colitis: use of CT findings in differential diagnosis. Radiology. 190(2):445-9, 1994

(Left) *In this 18-year-old woman with bloody diarrhea, coronal CECT shows pancolitis with marked submucosal edema, mostly marked in the right side of the colon ➡, while the entire colon is fluid distended ➡, indicating a diarrheal state. Escherichia coli (type O157: H7) was the etiology of this infectious colitis.* **(Right)** *Axial CT in the same patient shows excess fluid throughout the colon ➡ and massive submucosal edema ➡ in the colonic wall, diagnostic of infectious colitis.*

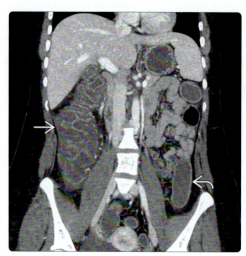
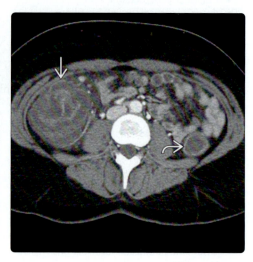

(Left) *This 65-year-old woman had chronic diarrhea due to small intestinal bacterial overgrowth. A film from a small bowel (SB) follow-through shows multiple large duodenal and SB diverticula ➡ that were also seen on CT.* **(Right)** *CT in the same patient shows multiple large, gas-filled SB diverticula ➡ without signs of active inflammation. Bacterial overgrowth within the diverticula accounted for the small intestinal bacterial overgrowth syndrome.*

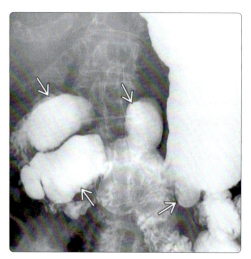
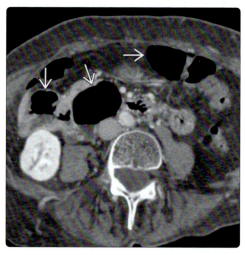

(Left) *In this elderly man with chronic diarrhea, CT shows fluid distention of the SB ➡ and a short-segment, nonobstructing intussusception ➡ with a target appearance and intraluminal mesenteric fat.* **(Right)** *In the same patient, CT shows more of the intussusception ➡ and an abnormal fold pattern of the ileum ➡ that was much more prominent than that of the jejunum, a reverse of the normal situation. These are characteristic features of celiac disease.*

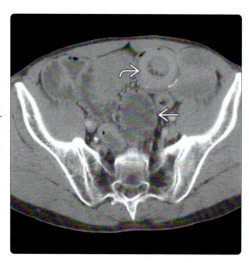
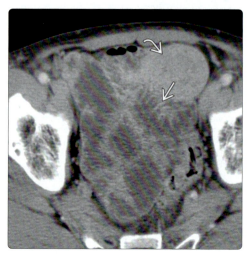

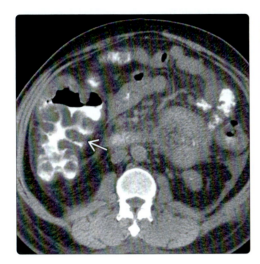

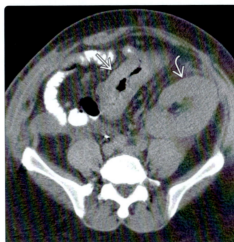

(Left) *Following renal transplantation, this man developed severe diarrhea. CT shows massive thickening of the wall of the entire colon (pancolitis) with some segments having a thumbprinted appearance* ➡ *due to Clostridium difficile colitis.* (Right) *Axial CT in the same patient shows the renal allograft* ➡ *and mural edema of the sigmoid colon* ➡. *C. difficile colitis typically causes more submucosal edema than does ulcerative colitis.*

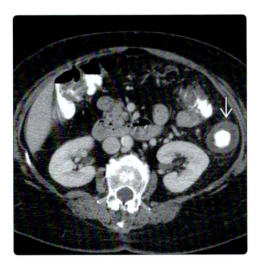

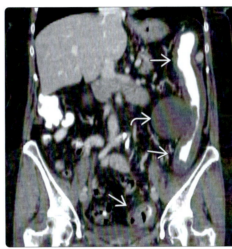

(Left) *In this elderly woman with cardiac disease, axial CECT shows diffuse, circumferential, low-attenuation mural thickening of the descending colon* ➡. (Right) *In the same patient, a coronal CT shows mural thickening of the entire descending and sigmoid colon* ➡, *but the rectum was spared. These are typical clinical and CT features of ischemic colitis due to hypoperfusion. A renal cyst is noted, incidentally* ➡.

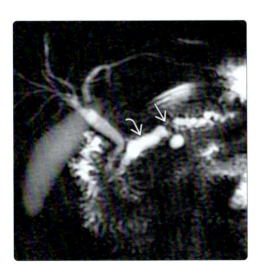

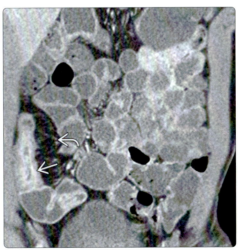

(Left) *This woman has chronic alcohol abuse and fatty diarrhea. MRCP shows a signal void representing a main duct calculus* ➡ *within an irregularly dilated pancreatic duct* ➡, *consistent with chronic pancreatitis.* (Right) *This 42-year-old man has acute and chronic abdominal pain and diarrhea. Coronal CT enterography shows luminal stenosis, mucosal hyperenhancement, and mural thickening of the terminal ileum* ➡ *as well as mesenteric fibrofatty proliferation* ➡, *classic features of Crohn's disease.*

Clinical Classification of Functional Constipation

Category	Features	Physiologic and Imaging Test Results
Normal-transit constipation	Incomplete evacuation; abdominal pain may be present but not predominant feature	Normal; may show excessive stool in colon
Slow-transit constipation	Infrequent stools (e.g., ≤ 1/week), lack of urge to defecate, poor response to fiber and laxatives, generalized symptoms (e.g., malaise, fatigue); more prevalent in young women	Delay in colonic transit [e.g., retention throughout colon of > 20% of radiopaque markers (Sitzmarks) 5 days after ingestion]
Defecatory disorder	Frequent straining, incomplete evacuation, need for manual maneuvers to facilitate defecation	Abnormal balloon expulsion test &/or anorectal manometry; abnormal fluoroscopic or MR defecography

Overview

Constipation is a common complaint that may be intermittent or chronic, mild, or disabling. The American College of Gastroenterology defines constipation as unsatisfactory defecation characterized by infrequent stools, difficult stool passage, or both. Chronic constipation is defined as the presence of symptoms for at least 3 months. Risk factors include female gender, advanced age, nonwhite ethnicity, low levels of income and education, and a low level of physical activity. Other risk factors include diet and lifestyle, use of certain medications, and certain underlying medical conditions. Commonly implicated medications include those in widespread use as prescription and "over-the-counter" drugs, such as calcium supplements, antacids, diuretics, and opioid agonists. Metabolic and endocrinologic disorders, including diabetes, hypothyroidism, and pregnancy and numerous diseases, such as multiple sclerosis, parkinsonism, and stroke, are recognized etiologies. Constipation may also be the result of mechanical narrowing or obstruction of the colon or functional constipation. In the postoperative setting, constipation and ileus may coexist or mimic each other, but usually resolve quickly, often hastened by administration of stool softeners.

Imaging Protocols

Imaging can play an important role in detecting or excluding a **mechanical obstruction** (e.g., colorectal cancer; sigmoid volvulus) or functional abnormality of the colon or rectum. Plain film radiography may show colonic distention with gas &/or formed stool. In general, there should be no continuous column of gas or stool throughout the colon. The transverse colon is generally no more than 6 cm in diameter and the cecum ≤ 9 cm. The presence of excessive gas or stool suggests one of the etiologies listed in the differential diagnosis table for colonic ileus or dilation.

An especially severe and dangerous complication of constipation is **stercoral colitis**, though many physicians underestimate its prevalence and importance. Impacted stool within the rectosigmoid colon can adhere to the bowel wall and produce ulceration with possible colonic perforation. While the diagnosis may be suggested by plain films, CT is definitive, documenting the extent and consistency of fecal impaction along with infiltration or frank perforation into surrounding tissues.

The presence or absence of a mechanical obstructing lesion as the etiology for constipation has traditionally been a major indication for a **fluoroscopic contrast enema**. Colon carcinoma, sigmoid or cecal volvulus, and diverticulosis or diverticulitis can be diagnosed with confidence. If distal colonic obstruction or fecal impaction is suspected, a water-contrast fluoroscopic exam can outline the colonic length and width (increases of which can contribute to constipation) and may demonstrate an obstructing mass. Moreover, the hypertonic nature of the contrast media tends to draw water into the colon and often results in easier and more complete evacuation of feces. More recently, CT and colonoscopy have largely replaced the barium enema as 1st-line diagnostic studies, and **multiplanar, contrast-enhanced CT** is very accurate and noninvasive in this setting.

More often, constipation is due to disordered function of the colon or rectum. **Functional constipation** can be divided into 3 broad categories: Normal-transit constipation, slow-transit constipation, and defecatory or rectal evacuation disorders. In one large study of 1,000 patients with functional constipation, 59% were found to have normal-transit constipation, 25% had defecatory disorders, 13% had slow-transit constipation, and 3% had a combination of a defecatory disorder and slow-transit constipation.

The mean **colonic transit time** in healthy volunteers is 35 hours with 72 hours as an an upper limit. An objective measure of colonic transit time involves the oral administration of **radiopaque markers** (Sitzmarks) with a plain film of the abdomen obtained at 5 &/or 7 days after ingestion. The presence of > 20% of the opaque rings is an abnormal finding; if the rings are distributed throughout the colon, the patient most likely has hypomotility or colonic inertia. If most of the rings are gathered in the rectosigmoid, the patient most likely has functional outlet obstruction, and some means of evaluation for a defecatory disorder is warranted.

Disorders of defecation are commonly attributed to weakness or disordered contraction of muscles comprising the pelvic floor and can be objectively assessed by anorectal manometry, the "balloon expulsion test," and imaging studies, including the fluoroscopic barium defecography exam or MR pelvic floor imaging. **Defecography (evacuation proctography)** is a fluoroscopic study that involves imaging of rectal evacuation of a barium paste. While it is simple to perform and interpret, it is not in widespread use. Following insertion of barium paste into the rectum, the patient is seated upright on a commode attached to a fluoroscopic table in the Radiology Department. Videofluoroscopy and spot filming take place with the patient in a lateral position, making note of the anorectal configuration and pelvic floor position at rest with Valsalva and Kegel maneuvers and during evacuation. Modifications of the technique may include administration of contrast medium into the bladder &/or

vagina, though these are not in common use. The barium defecography exam is quite useful for documenting disorders, such as rectoceles, varying degrees of rectal mucosal intussusception or prolapse, abnormally prominent or deficient pelvic floor descent, and obstructed defecation due to spasm of the puborectalis sling.

Within the past decade, there has been increasing interest and utilization of **MR** to evaluate not only constipation but other disorders of the female pelvic floor. Rectal paste or gel can be administered to perform MR defecography, which may be as useful as fluoroscopic barium defecography, though patients are usually lying supine within the MR magnet, and the rectal gel is not meant to mimic the consistency of stool. MR offers the distinct advantage of simultaneous evaluation of all 3 pelvic "compartments." Women with pelvic floor weakness often have a combination of complaints, such as urinary incontinence, fecal incontinence, and vaginal or uterine prolapse that can be displayed very effectively by dynamic MR imaging.

Differential Diagnosis

Colonic Ileus or Dilation

Common
- Ileus
- Colon carcinoma
- Rectal carcinoma
- Sigmoid volvulus
- Cecal volvulus
- Diverticulitis
- Ogilvie syndrome
- Fecal impaction

Less Common
- Ischemic colitis
- Toxic megacolon
- Endocrine disorders
- Distended urinary bladder
- Neuromuscular disorders

Selected References

1. García Del Salto L et al: MR imaging-based assessment of the female pelvic floor. Radiographics. 34(5):1417-39, 2014
2. Colaiacomo MC et al: Dynamic MR imaging of the pelvic floor: a pictorial review. Radiographics. 29(3):e35, 2009

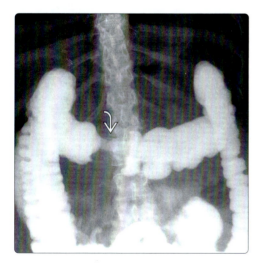

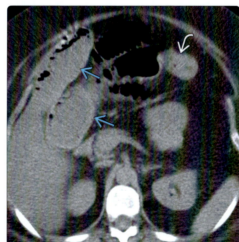

(Left) *In this patient with constipation and abdominal pain, a contrast enema shows an "apple core"-type constricting mass* ⮫ *of the transverse colon, consistent with colon carcinoma.* (Right) *In the same patient, nonenhanced CT confirms the obstructing mass* ⮫ *along with dilation of the proximal colon and small bowel* ⮕.

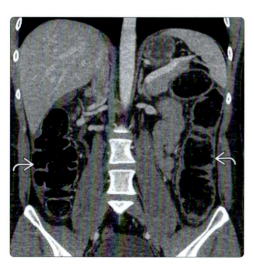

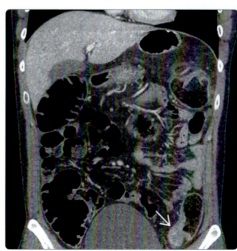

(Left) *In this 31-year-old man with chronic constipation, a coronal CECT shows the colon* ⮫ *is grossly dilated with stool and gas.* (Right) *Another coronal CECT in the same patient shows the dilated colon narrowing abruptly at an "apple core" lesion* ⮫ *at the junction of the descending and sigmoid colon, a proven primary colon cancer.*

(Left) *In this elderly constipated man with acute abdominal pain, axial CT shows the colon* ➡ *markedly distended with stool and gas plus free intraperitoneal air* ➡. **(Right)** *Coronal CECT in the same patient shows the dilated colon* ➡ *that is pinched and obstructed as it enters a large inguinal hernia* ➡. *This perforation proved fatal.*

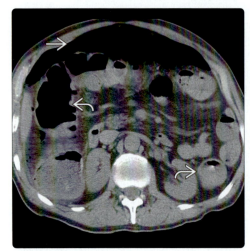
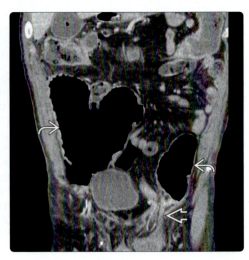

(Left) *Abdominal film shows marked dilation of the sigmoid colon* ➡. *The apposed walls of the redundant sigmoid colon* ➡ *form the "seam" of the coffee-bean shape. The sigmoid extends into the upper abdomen above the transverse colon* ➡. **(Right)** *Coronal CECT in the same patient shows twisting and displacement of the base of the sigmoid colon and its mesentery* ➡, *confirming sigmoid volvulus.*

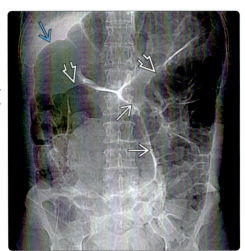
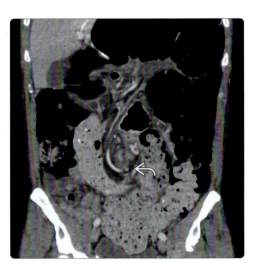

(Left) *This 85-year-old woman had chronic constipation and presented with acute abdominal pain. Axial CECT shows massive distention of the rectum by solid feces* ➡ *and infiltration of perirectal fat planes* ➡. **(Right)** *Sagittal CECT in the same patient shows fecal distention of the rectum and sigmoid colon* ➡, *with perforation of the latter, causing free intraperitoneal air* ➡ *indicating stercoral colitis, which was fatal.*

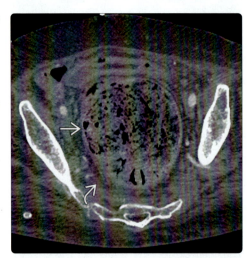
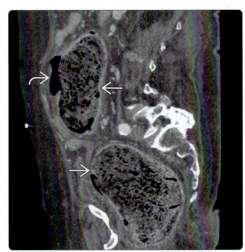

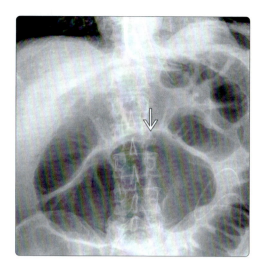

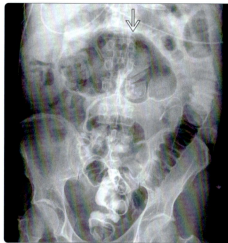

(Left) *In this elderly constipated woman, a plain supine abdominal film taken 1 day after hip surgery shows a medially displaced, dilated cecum* ➡ *and generalized gaseous distention of the colon. The cecum measures 15 cm in diameter and appears to be folded upon itself, a cecal bascule or simply colonic ileus (Ogilvie syndrome).* **(Right)** *Following placement of an NG tube and administration of IV neostigmine in the same patient, a repeat abdominal film demonstrates substantially less cecal distention* ➡.

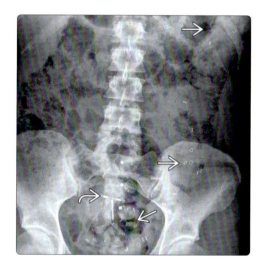

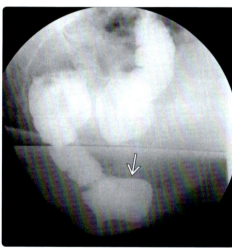

(Left) *In a 36-year-old woman with chronic constipation, an abdominal film shows the presence of ~ 20 radiopaque markers* ➡ *(Sitzmarks) throughout a gas- and stool-filled colon. A packet of 24 Sitzmarks was ingested by patient 7 days prior; this degree and pattern of retention is diagnostic of colonic inertia. An IUD is also noted* ➡. **(Right)** *Lateral film from a defecography study (same patient) shows anterior rectocele* ➡ *and other abnormalities on the dynamic study (not shown) indicating functional outlet obstruction.*

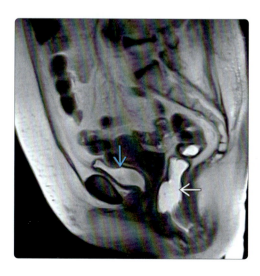

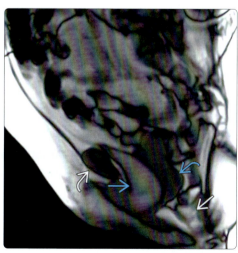

(Left) *In this young woman with chronic constipation and incontinence, a sagittal T2 MR from the pelvic floor evaluation shows the gel-filled rectum* ➡ *and the urinary bladder* ➡ *with the patient at rest.* **(Right)** *In the same patient during evacuation, the T2 MR shows marked descent of the pelvic floor with the bladder* ➡, *vagina* ➡, *and rectum* ➡ *prolapsing well below the symphisis* ➡. *MR evaluates all 3 pelvic compartments, unlike standard barium defecography.*

Introduction

Gastrointestinal bleeding (GIB) is a common clinical problem, the presentation of which may be acute or chronic. GIB is classified as arising from the upper (proximal to ligament of Treitz) or lower (distal to the ligament of Treitz) GI tract.

Classically, **acute upper GIB** (UGIB) presents with overt hematemesis or melena, while **acute lower GIB** (LGIB) presents with hematochezia, although there is substantial overlap in clinical presentation, particularly with a very brisk UGIB causing hematochezia. Chronic GIB may manifest as anemia and heme-positive stools, ± perceptible changes in appearance of the stool, and thus can be further subclassified into "overt" or "occult" presentations.

Overt GIB designates visible blood in the stool, whereas **occult GIB** implies that the stool has a normal appearance despite the presence of detectable blood products. Another important definition is that of **"obscure" GIB**, which means that after a thorough evaluation by **esophagogastroduodenoscopy (EGD)** and **colonoscopy**, the cause of bleeding remains unidentified. This usually indicates a source beyond the reach of the standard endoscopes, i.e., the small bowel, and it has been proposed recently that the term "suspected small bowel bleeding" replace "obscure GIB," and the "obscure" designation be reserved for causes of bleeding, which remain unknown after a thorough investigation of the **entire** GI tract. This reflects the fact that in recent years we have developed more effective tools (video capsule endoscopy, deep enteroscopy, and radiologic imaging) to diagnose small bowel bleeding.

In the past, acute UGIB was more common than LGIB; however, there has been a striking decrease in upper GI events and increase in lower GI events, which are now nearly equal in incidence. The most common causes of UGIB are **peptic ulcers**, gastroduodenal erosions, esophagitis, **esophageal and gastric varices**, **Mallory Weiss tears**, and vascular malformations. The diagnosis and management of variceal hemorrhage are outside the scope of this chapter. Therefore, UGIB subsequently will refer to nonvariceal UGIB. The most common causes of LGIB depend on the age group. In younger people, inflammatory bowel disease (IBD) and Meckel diverticulum are most prevalent. In older individuals, diverticular hemorrhage, angiodysplasia, and colon cancer are most common.

In the evaluation of patients with acute GIB, most commonly encountered in the emergency department, the 1st step is to do a thorough history, physical, and laboratory evaluation. This should include a digital rectal examination, as well as placement of a nasogastric tube, in an attempt to determine if the hemorrhage has an upper GI source. Hemodynamic stabilization and resuscitation, correction of coagulopathy if present, administration of available pharmacologic treatments (e.g., somatostatin, acid suppression, etc.), and gastroenterology consultation are prioritized in preparation for an efficient and focused diagnostic evaluation. In appropriately risk-stratified patients with suspected UGIB, the 1st step is usually EGD, while in LGIB, the 1st step is more variable and may include EGD, colonoscopy, or radiologic testing depending on the clinical situation and local practice patterns.

Acute Gastrointestinal Bleeding

EGD has sensitivity and specificity over 90% for the diagnosis of causes of UGIB and allows treatment of identified lesions. However, there are situations where EGD may be unsuccessful in diagnosing or treating lesions or where, because of hemodynamic instability or medical comorbidities (especially recent myocardial infarction), the procedure is contraindicated. In this case, other diagnostic and therapeutic options must be considered.

Radiologic procedures used in the diagnosis of GIB include **nuclear scintigraphy**, **transarterial angiography with embolization (TAE)**, and **CT angiography (CTA)**. The choice of radiologic test depends on the clinical situation.

When there is acute UGIB in a patient too unstable to undergo EGD, urgent catheter angiography (TAE) is the procedure of choice for diagnosis and treatment. When the site of bleeding is identified on EGD but cannot be controlled, TAE should again be the next step in management. A major advantage of TAE over endoscopy is that it is not adversely affected by the presence of endoluminal hemorrhage, which can severely limit visualization at EGD. CTA is a diagnostic alternative to TAE in this situation and can be used to guide further therapy.

When EGD visualizes blood but not the source, TAE or CTA are both acceptable next steps. CTA is highly sensitive and specific in the diagnosis of UGIB and can make some diagnoses that EGD cannot: Mesenteric pseudoaneurysms, aortoenteric fistulas, submucosal masses, or causes of hemobilia, such as intrahepatic tumors or arterial-biliary fistulas. The last scenario to consider is that of a patient with postsurgical GIB where CTA is the procedure of choice to detect anastomotic bleeding, pseudoaneurysms, or other iatrogenic complications.

For acute LGIB, the best 1st diagnostic step is less well established. Because patients with suspected LGIB and hemodynamic instability may actually have an upper source, EGD is the appropriate 1st-line test before any further testing. In stable patients, colonoscopy is recommended as the 1st-line test.

However, although colonoscopy has potential for diagnosis and treatment, poor visibility from hemorrhage and the lack of bowel preparation is problematic. The yield of colonoscopy for acute LGIB is highly variable in the literature, and the evidence that colonoscopy should be the initial diagnostic exam in all patients with acute LGIB is weak.

The role of radiology as a 1st-line test is more firmly established in the setting of LGIB than in UGIB. A thorough understanding of the choices of radiologic diagnostic and therapeutic examinations, along with advantages and disadvantages, is essential to optimal patient management.

Imaging Acute Gastrointestinal Bleeding

Nuclear scintigraphy utilizing the patient's own red blood cells (RBC) tagged with technetium-99m is potentially the most sensitive diagnostic test in the setting of acute LGIB. It can detect low bleeding flow between 0.05 and 0.20 mL per minute, and because images can be obtained over minutes to hours, intermittent bleeding can also be detected. The traditional role of scintigraphy has been as a screening or triage exam to demonstrate the presence and location of bleeding to guide further angiographic, endoscopic, or surgical treatments. For example, if a sigmoid colonic

Advantages and Disadvantages of Radiologic Exams in GI Bleeding

Radiologic Test	Advantages	Disadvantages
Tagged red blood cell nuclear scintigraphy	Most sensitive test for very slow bleeding rates; can image or reimage over several hours; may increase the yield of angiography	Inaccurate for determining site and etiology of bleeding
Transarterial angiography with embolization	Potential for treatment	Invasive exam with potential for complications; can only detect brisk active bleeding
CT angiogram	Fast and readily available; noninvasive; accurate in identifying location and etiology of bleeding	Low sensitivity for slow bleeding and intermittent bleeding

hemorrhage is identified, the angiographer could proceed immediately to inferior mesenteric artery injection without injecting the superior mesenteric artery 1st.

Although some studies have demonstrated that a preceding tagged RBC scan increases the yield of angiography and facilitates targeted contrast injection, others have shown that it has little effect. Moreover, it is lacking in the ability to accurately pinpoint the site and, especially, the etiology.

Accuracy rates vary widely across studies, which have shown a significant portion of the exams incorrectly localize sites of bleeding. Bleeding can sometimes only be localized to a generalized area within the abdomen, which may be misleading in cases where structures overlap. For example, in a patient with hemorrhage within a low-lying cecum, this might simulate rectal bleeding, which would have serious diagnostic and therapeutic implications. An additional disadvantage of scintigraphy is that availability is limited, especially after hours.

At conclusion of a scintigraphic exam, if no bleeding is identified, further diagnostic testing with angiography is unlikely to be helpful, as the lower limit of flow rate detection for an arteriogram is 0.5 mL per minute, less sensitive than scintigraphy. However, if active bleeding is identified at scintigraphy, angiography is an appropriate next step for potential intraarterial embolic therapy to accomplish hemostasis. The patient should be transferred immediately from the nuclear medicine department to the angiography suite to optimize the chance that the bleeding will still be ongoing, visible, and therefore treatable. Angiography can localize the source of the lower GI bleed in 25-70% of patients.

In a study of patients with diverticular hemorrhage undergoing therapeutic angiography, hemostasis was accomplished in 40-100% of patients with a rate of rebleeding from 0-50%. The primary complication was bowel ischemia. Given the potential complications and the fact that angiography can only detect active bleeding, it should only be utilized in patients with high-volume, ongoing hemorrhage.

CTA has evolved in recent years to be a 1st-line test for the diagnosis of acute GIB with a sensitivity of 91% and specificity of 99%. The blood flow sensitivity for CTA is somewhere between that of scintigraphy and angiography, likely 0.3 mL per minute or slower.

But CTA has other advantages over scintigraphy; it is more available, especially after hours; image acquisition is much faster (seconds instead of minutes or hours); and it is very accurate in identifying the location and cause of bleeding. The 1 disadvantage is lower sensitivity for very slow bleeding and intermittent bleeding.

Adherence to proper technique in the performance of CTA in the setting of GIB is essential. In contrast to conventional single-phase CTA obtained for other indications, such as aortic dissection, CTA for GI bleeding requires 3 phases. After obtaining a noncontrast set of images, IV contrast medium is injected at high flow rates (4-5 mL per second), and the patient is reimaged in arterial and venous phases (at 30- and 60-second delay, respectively). The diagnosis of GI bleeding will be based on the detection of a "blush" or spurt of IV contrast leaving the splanchnic blood vessels and entering the lumen of the GI tract on the angiographic-phase images, so-called "active extravasation."

High-density material already present in the lumen before contrast administration, such as pill fragments, retained oral contrast from prior studies, milk of magnesia, or blood clot, can simulate or mask active extravasation, but this pitfall can be avoided by acquiring noncontrast images 1st, allowing the radiologist to compare images side by side and determine what is hemorrhage and what is not. Of course, the **administration of positive oral contrast is strictly contraindicated** as it would make detection of hemorrhage impossible.

The venous images are essential to obtain after the arterial phase as they allow for better evaluation of the bowel wall as well as the rest of the abdominal organs. They are most important, however, for confirmation of active extravasation because the shape of the blush or spurting will characteristically change between phases, enlarging or defusing within the bowel. Slower bleeds are also more visible in the venous phase because more time has passed after contrast injection, permitting a larger volume to pool within the bowel.

Multiplanar reformations, as well as maximum-intensity projection and volume-rendered images, are very helpful for the radiologist. If the location and cause of bleeding is identified, the patient can then be triaged to the appropriate therapy. The accuracy of CT for the diagnosis of cause of acute GIB is 80-100%. Diverticular hemorrhage, benign or malignant tumors, infection, inflammation, and vascular abnormalities, such as angioectasia, are some of the etiologies effectively diagnosed with CTA.

Once the source of the bleed has been identified, the patient can undergo appropriate endoscopic, angiographic, or surgical evaluation and treatment.

Imaging Chronic Gastrointestinal Bleeding

The evaluation of patients with chronic obscure GIB, who often have abnormalities in the small bowel, can also be accomplished using readily available radiologic examinations, most typically **CT and MR enterography (CTE and MRE)**.

These tests are complementary to the examinations performed by gastroenterologists, specifically **video capsule endoscopy** and **double balloon enteroscopy**.

Capsule endoscopy compares favorably in the detection of vascular abnormalities and mucosal lesions. CTE and MRE perform better in the detection of mass lesions, especially submucosal masses. Another advantage is that there is no risk of obstruction in contradistinction to the capsule, which can be trapped by a stricture.

CTE is a mainstay of small bowel imaging. In addition to detecting causes of chronic bleeding, it is frequently employed for the initial evaluation and follow-up of individuals with IBD. MRE is especially appealing for longitudinal follow-up given that there is no radiation exposure to these typically young patients who may have a multitude of studies throughout their life. The most important factor in obtaining a good quality CTE or MRE is accomplishing adequate distention of the small bowel using so-called "neutral" or "negative" oral contrast, such as very dilute 0.1% weight/volume barium sulfate (VoLumen, Bracco Diagnostics). Patients typically ingest 1.5 L over the 1.5 hours before the examination. Adequate distention of the small bowel is important because collapsed loops can simulate bowel wall thickening, and these "pseudolesions" are a common cause of false-positive examinations. Also, collapsed loops can mask small lesions, causing false-negative examinations. Importantly, negative oral contrast is not indicated in the setting of acute GIB, as it would cause unnecessary delay, and it is not necessary for the detection of active bleeding.

The rapid bolus IV injection of an iodinated contrast agent is essential (4-5 mL per second), with image acquisition at 40-50 seconds post injection, intended to capture maximum SB mucosal enhancement. This is considered the late arterial phase, in contrast to the early arterial or angiographic phase obtained with an actual CTA. The decision whether to obtain a 2nd phase depends on the suspected etiology of the chronic bleeding. In patients with suspected Crohn's disease (CD), a 2nd phase is not typically performed. For obscure GIB, a 2nd scan through the abdomen should be acquired in the portal venous phase in case active bleeding is detected.

Abnormalities causing chronic GIB of small bowel origin detectable by CTE include IBD, such as **CD**, which is accurately diagnosed by CT. **Angiodysplasia** of the small bowel is the most common cause of occult GIB in patients older than 40 years. The appearance is that of a strongly enhancing mural nodule or plaque ± an early draining vein. Other detectable etiologies include vascular malformations, **tumors**, and **Meckel diverticulum**. The appearance of tumors on CTE depends on histology, but CT is quite accurate in diagnosis and distinction among these tumors.

Differential Diagnosis

Occult Gastrointestinal Bleeding
Common
- Angiodysplasia
- CD

Less Common
- Primary and metastatic tumors
- Vasculitis
- Ischemic enteritis or colitis
- Meckel diverticulum
- Mesenteric varices

- Radiation enteritis

Acute Upper Gastrointestinal Bleeding
- Peptic ulcer disease
- Esophageal and gastric varices
- Esophagitis, gastritis, or duodenitis
- Tumors
- Mallory Weiss tear
- Angiodysplasia

Acute Lower Gastrointestinal Bleeding
- Diverticular hemorrhage
- Tumors
- Anorectal disorders
- Ischemic colitis
- Infectious colitis
- IBD
- Angiodysplasia
- Meckel diverticulum

Selected References

1. Appropriateness Criteria. ACR appropriateness criteria for non-variceal upper gastrointestinal bleeding. https://acsearch.acr.org/docs/69413/Narrative. Reviewed June 19, 2017. Accessed June 19, 2017.
2. Strate LL et al: ACG clinical guideline: management of patients with acute lower gastrointestinal bleeding. Am J Gastroenterol. 111(5):755, 2016
3. Gerson LB et al: ACG clinical guideline: diagnosis and management of small bowel bleeding. Am J Gastroenterol. 110(9):1265-87; quiz 1288, 2015
4. Soto JA et al: Gastrointestinal hemorrhage: evaluation with MDCT. Abdom Imaging. 40(5):993-1009, 2015
5. Artigas JM et al: Multidetector CT angiography for acute gastrointestinal bleeding: technique and findings. Radiographics. 33(5):1453-70, 2013
6. Geffroy Y et al: Multidetector CT angiography in acute gastrointestinal bleeding: why, when, and how. Radiographics. 31(3):E35-46, 2011
7. Lee SS et al: Obscure gastrointestinal bleeding: diagnostic performance of multidetector CT enterography. Radiology. 259(3):739-48, 2011
8. Graça BM et al: Gastroenterologic and radiologic approach to obscure gastrointestinal bleeding: how, why, and when? Radiographics. 30(1):235-52, 2010
9. Lanas A et al: Time trends and impact of upper and lower gastrointestinal bleeding and perforation in clinical practice. Am J Gastroenterol. 104(7):1633-41, 2009
10. Zink SI et al: Noninvasive evaluation of active lower gastrointestinal bleeding: comparison between contrast-enhanced MDCT and 99mTc-labeled RBC scintigraphy. AJR Am J Roentgenol. 191(4):1107-14, 2008
11. Scheffel H et al: Acute gastrointestinal bleeding: detection of source and etiology with multi-detector-row CT. Eur Radiol. 17(6):1555-65, 2007
12. Howarth DM: The role of nuclear medicine in the detection of acute gastrointestinal bleeding. Semin Nucl Med. 36(2):133-46, 2006
13. Yoon W et al: Acute massive gastrointestinal bleeding: detection and localization with arterial phase multi-detector row helical CT. Radiology. 239(1):160-7, 2006
14. Kuhle WG et al: Detection of active colonic hemorrhage with use of helical CT: findings in a swine model. Radiology. 228(3):743-52, 2003

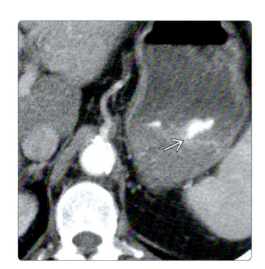

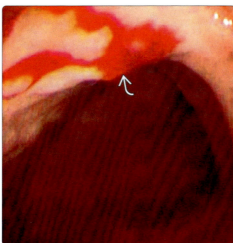

(Left) *In this elderly man with hematemesis, arterial-phase CT shows active extravasation ➡, indicating bleeding into the stomach. No oral contrast agent had been given. Note that the extravasated blood is isodense with the aorta. No ulcers, masses, or varices were seen.* (Right) *In the same patient, esophagogastroduodenoscopy shows a flat lesion with active bleeding, representing an arteriovenous malformation ➡.*

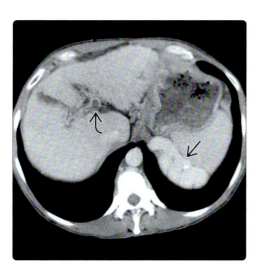

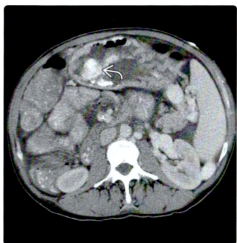

(Left) *In this man with cirrhosis and hematemesis, CT shows thrombosis of the portal vein ➡, a cirrhotic liver, and huge upper abdominal varices ➡.* (Right) *In the same patient, CT shows a hyperdense collection within the gastric lumen ➡ represents active bleeding from gastric varices. Note that only water was given as an "oral contrast" agent.*

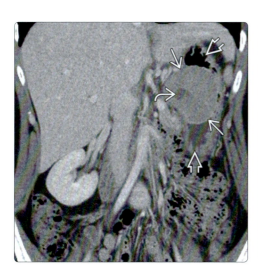

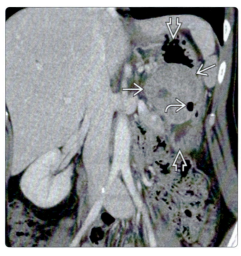

(Left) *In this young woman with vague abdominal discomfort and 1 episode of hematemesis, coronal CT shows a large, exophytic mass ➡ arising from the stomach ➡. The mass is encapsulated with central necrosis ➡.* (Right) *In the same patient, coronal CT shows the large mass ➡, which deforms the lumen of the stomach ➡. Gas ➡ within the mass indicates communication with the gastric lumen, all typical features for a gastric stromal tumor (GIST).*

(Left) *In this patient with obscure GI bleeding, CT reformatted into the coronal plane shows extravasation of contrast-opacified blood ➡ within the jejunum.* (Right) *In the same patient, volume-rendered CT proved optimal for demonstrating the jejunal vessels ➡ and the active bleeding ➡ into the jejunal lumen. Angiodysplasia was confirmed at surgery as the source of hemorrhage.*

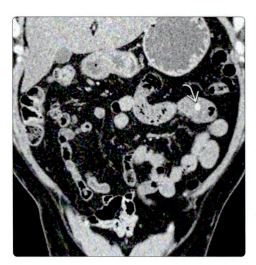
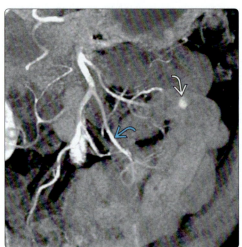

(Left) *In this patient with an obscure cause for hematochezia, CT enterography shows a brightly enhancing mass ➡ arising from the ileum. Within the affected segment of bowel, there are high-density foci of extravasated contrast material ➡, indicating active bleeding from the mass.* (Right) *In the same patient, coronal CT better demonstrates the distal small bowel ➡ origin of the bleeding submucosal mass ➡. At surgery, a small bowel GIST was resected, as suggested preoperatively by CT.*

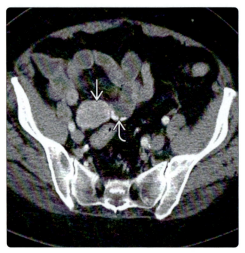
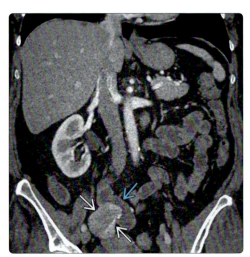

(Left) *In this elderly man who had hematemesis months after surgical repair of an aortic aneurysm, CECT shows the native, calcified aortic wall ➡ wrapped around the synthetic graft. Ectopic gas ➡ is present around the aortic graft and between the graft and the duodenum ➡.* (Right) *In the same patient, sagittal reformation of the CT shows the perigraft gas ➡ and a rind of soft tissue ➡ between the graft and the duodenum ➡, indicating an aortoenteric fistula, confirmed at surgery.*

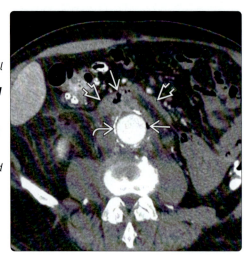
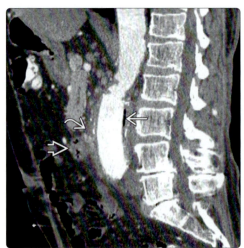

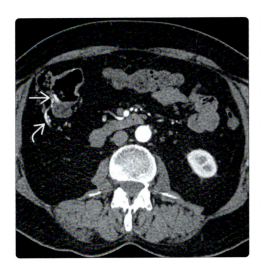

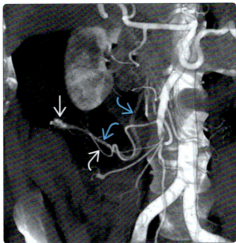

(Left) In this elderly man with melena and a low hematocrit, axial CECT shows a prominent ileocolic artery ⮡ leading to a small, hyperenhancing focus ➡ within the wall of the ascending colon. (Right) In the same patient, 3D reformation of the CECT demonstrates the ileocolic artery ⮡ and early filling of the ileocolic vein ➡ as well as the colonic lesion ➡ that has the appearance of a small tangle of blood vessels.

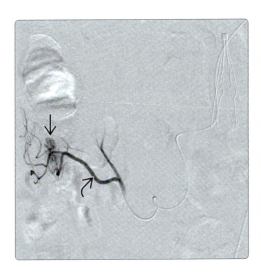

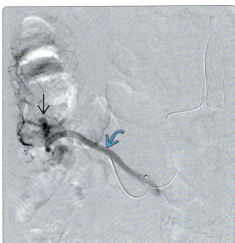

(Left) In the same patient, a catheter angiogram of the ileocolic artery ➡ shows this vessel feeding a vascular lesion ➡ within the ascending colon, having the typical appearance of angiodysplasia. (Right) Another film from the catheter angiogram shows the colonic lesion ➡ and early filling of an enlarged ileocolic vein ➡. Findings are diagnostic of arteriovenous malformation or angiodysplastic lesion of the colonic wall, a relatively common cause of GI bleeding in older adults.

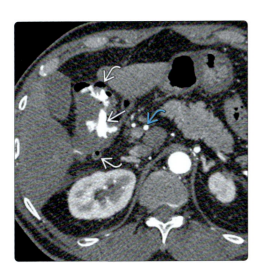

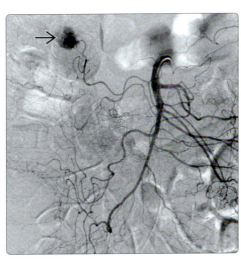

(Left) In this 75-year-old man with hematochezia, arterial-phase axial CECT shows right colonic diverticula ⮡. Within the lumen of the colon is a collection of fluid ➡ that has the same density as blood in the aorta and mesenteric arteries ➡, indicating active bleeding from diverticulosis. (Right) In the same patient, a film from a catheter superior mesenteric angiogram confirms active bleeding ➡ from the ileocolic artery. During the same procedure, the bleeding was successfully treated with embolization.

Overview

Jaundice (icterus) is a condition characterized by yellow discoloration of the skin and mucus membranes resulting from deposition of bilirubin, a pigmented metabolite of heme. Jaundice is most commonly due to disorders of the liver or bile ducts, but precise diagnosis and management may be challenging. Patients may have isolated disorders of bilirubin metabolism (e.g., hemolysis, congenital or acquired errors of hepatocellular uptake or conjugation); acute, subacute, or chronic hepatocellular disease; or biliary obstruction or inflammation.

Diagnosis begins with a thorough history and physical exam, including any history of drug use known to be associated with hepatic injury (hepatotoxins). Laboratory testing plays a key role, including "toxic screens," measures of hepatocellular injury and those associated with biliary obstruction. Specific clinical conditions are known to be associated with jaundice, including pregnancy and critical illnesses of various sorts, including hepatic ischemia, blood transfusions, hepatotoxic drugs, and sepsis.

Role of Imaging

Cross-sectional imaging plays an important role in helping to distinguish among the many causes of jaundice, especially hepatocellular injury, infiltrative disease, and bile duct disorders. Acute injury to the liver may not be evident on imaging, although some abnormalities are commonly seen. Acute alcoholic and nonalcoholic **steatosis** results in widespread decreased attenuation on CT and increased echogenicity on US. The most specific imaging finding for steatosis is found on gradient-echo (GRE) MR, where opposed-phase imaging shows selective loss of signal from foci of steatosis. Similar CT and US findings less commonly result from other inflammatory or ischemic injury, infectious, and neoplastic (e.g., lymphoma) processes, as listed in tables below. Acute **viral hepatitis** has no specific findings on imaging, although periportal edema, gallbladder wall thickening, and porta hepatis lymphadenopathy are frequently noted. Patients who have received a stem cell transplantation or chemotherapy (particularly oxaliplatin) are at risk for **sinusoidal obstruction syndrome** (venoocclusive disease), which may cause pain and jaundice. A characteristic pattern has been described on gadoxetate (Eovist)-enhanced MR that may suggest this diagnosis. **Cirrhosis** can be diagnosed reliably on imaging; findings include surface and parenchymal nodularity, volume loss of the right lobe with hypertrophy of the caudate and lateral segments, widened fissures, and signs of portal hypertension. **Hepatic tumors**, primary or metastatic, can be detected and characterized very well by multiphasic contrast-enhanced CT and MR with greater reliability and less operator dependence than US. Hepatic tumors may cause jaundice by diffuse replacement of liver parenchyma &/or by obstructing intrahepatic bile ducts (IHBDs).

US plays a primary role in evaluation of the jaundiced patient with suspected hepatobiliary disease. US has positive and negative predictive values of over 90% in distinguishing obstructive from nonobstructive jaundice. Dilation of the common bile duct is a sensitive sign of extrahepatic biliary obstruction, though this is commonly seen in older patients who have had a prior cholecystectomy. In this setting, correlation with clinical and laboratory signs of biliary obstruction is mandatory in order to obviate unnecessary

additional imaging or intervention. **Painless jaundice** is a classic presentation of pancreatic carcinoma (or, less commonly, other malignancies), while acute onset of pain and biliary obstruction is most commonly due to choledocholithiasis. US demonstrates nearly all stones within the gallbladder but only ~ 70% of those within the common duct. **CT** has a similar accuracy for diagnosis of choledocholithiasis but shows fewer gallbladder stones, especially cholesterol stones that may be isodense to bile. MR/MRCP shows nearly all biliary stones.

While US and CT can demonstrate dilation of IHBDs, MR and direct cholangiography (ERCP or transhepatic cholangiography) provide more detailed depiction of the presence, extent, level, and cause of dilated IHBDs, as listed in tables below. **MR with MRCP** is the **best single modality for depicting both hepatic and biliary causes of jaundice**. The accuracy of MRCP is such that ERCP is often reserved for treatment of obstructing lesions (e.g., removal of common duct stones or stenting of ductal obstruction due to tumor). **ERCP and endoscopic US** also provide direct visualization of the ampulla and permit needle or brush sampling of suspected neoplasms. **Percutaneous transhepatic cholangiography** provides most of the same diagnostic and therapeutic advantages as ERCP and is particularly valuable in cases of proximal bile duct obstruction and when ERCP is technically challenging.

Nuclear scintigraphy plays a secondary role in the diagnosis of acute cholecystitis, but its value in the setting of jaundice is quite limited. Diminished hepatobiliary excretion of the radiotracer and inherently limited spatial resolution are major drawbacks.

Differential Diagnosis

Widespread Low Attenuation Within Liver (on CT)
Common
- Steatosis (fatty liver)

Less Common
- Hepatitis
- Toxic hepatic injury
- Hepatic metastases and lymphoma
- Sinusoidal obstruction syndrome
- Budd-Chiari syndrome
- Hepatic sarcoidosis
- Opportunistic infections, hepatic
- Hepatocellular carcinoma
- Hepatic infarction
- Wilson disease
- Radiation hepatitis
- Glycogen storage disease

Hyperechoic Liver, Diffuse (on US)
Common
- Steatosis (fatty liver)
- Cirrhosis
- Hepatitis
- Metastases and lymphoma, hepatic
- Technical artifact (mimic)

Less Common
- Hepatocellular carcinoma
- AIDS, hepatic involvement
- Hepatic sarcoidosis
- Miliary tuberculosis
- Schistosomiasis, hepatic
- Biliary hamartomas

- Mononucleosis
- Glycogen storage disease
- Wilson disease

Dilated Common Bile Duct
Common
- Postcholecystectomy
- Senescent change, common bile duct
- Choledocholithiasis
- Pancreatic ductal carcinoma
- Chronic pancreatitis

Less Common
- Other pancreatic neoplasms
- Gallbladder carcinoma
- Pancreatic pseudocyst
- Ascending cholangitis
- Recurrent pyogenic cholangitis
- Porta hepatis adenopathy
- Porta hepatis varices
- Biliary trauma (including iatrogenic)
- Small bowel obstruction
- Choledochal cyst

Asymmetric Dilation of Intrahepatic Bile Ducts
Common
- Primary sclerosing cholangitis
- Cholangiocarcinoma
- Ascending cholangitis
- Hepatocellular carcinoma
- Hepatic metastases and lymphoma
- AIDS cholangiopathy

Less Common
- Recurrent pyogenic cholangitis
- Pancreatobiliary parasites
- Hepatic hydatid cyst
- Intraductal papillary mucinous neoplasm, biliary

Biliary Strictures, Multiple
Common
- Primary sclerosing cholangitis
- Ascending cholangitis
- Autoimmune (IgG4-related) cholangitis
- Posttransplant liver
- Cirrhosis (mimic)

Less Common
- AIDS cholangiopathy
- Cholangiocarcinoma
- Recurrent pyogenic cholangitis
- Congenital hepatic fibrosis
- Caroli disease
- Chemotherapy-induced cholangitis
- Hepatic metastases (mimic)
- Pancreatobiliary parasites

Widened Hepatic Fissures
Common
- Cirrhosis
- Focal confluent fibrosis
- Senescent change
- Postsurgical (mimic)

Less Common
- Congenital absence of hepatic segments
- Liver metastases
- Primary sclerosing cholangitis
- Congenital hepatic fibrosis

- Schistosomiasis

Dysmorphic Liver With Abnormal Bile Ducts
Common
- Primary sclerosing cholangitis
- Cirrhosis (mimic)
- Hepatitis
- Peribiliary cysts
- Portal vein thrombophlebitis (mimic)
- Diverticulitis
- Hepatic pyogenic abscess
- Cholangiocarcinoma, intrahepatic or hilar

Less Common
- Budd-Chiari syndrome (mimic)
- Chemotherapy cholangitis
- Ascending cholangitis
- AIDS cholangiopathy
- Fibropolycystic liver diseases
- Congenital hepatic fibrosis
- Caroli disease
- Choledochal cyst
- Biliary hamartomas
- Autosomal dominant polycystic disease, liver
- Recurrent pyogenic cholangitis
- Hepatic hydatid disease

Selected References

1. Choi SH et al: Intrahepatic cholangiocarcinoma in patients with cirrhosis: differentiation from hepatocellular carcinoma by using gadoxetic acid-enhanced MR imaging and dynamic CT. Radiology. 282(3):771-781, 2017
2. Tanabe M et al: Imaging outcomes of liver imaging reporting and data system version 2014 category 2, 3, and 4 observations detected at CT and MR imaging. Radiology. 281(1):129-39, 2016
3. Darnell A et al: Liver imaging reporting and data system with MR imaging: evaluation in nodules 20 mm or smaller detected in cirrhosis at screening US. Radiology. 275(3):698-707, 2015
4. Choi JY et al: CT and MR imaging diagnosis and staging of hepatocellular carcinoma: part I. Development, growth, and spread: key pathologic and imaging aspects. Radiology. 272(3):635-54, 2014
5. Davenport MS et al: Repeatability of diagnostic features and scoring systems for hepatocellular carcinoma by using MR imaging. Radiology. 272(1):132-42, 2014
6. Kim YK et al: Hypovascular hypointense nodules on hepatobiliary phase gadoxetic acid-enhanced MR images in patients with cirrhosis: potential of DW imaging in predicting progression to hypervascular HCC. Radiology. 265(1):104-14, 2012
7. Purysko AS et al: LI-RADS: a case-based review of the new categorization of liver findings in patients with end-stage liver disease. Radiographics. 32(7):1977-95, 2012
8. Chung YE et al: Varying appearances of cholangiocarcinoma: radiologic-pathologic correlation. Radiographics. 29(3):683-700, 2009
9. Hussain SM et al: Cirrhosis and lesion characterization at MR imaging. Radiographics. 29(6):1637-52, 2009
10. Marin D et al: Hepatocellular carcinoma in patients with cirrhosis: qualitative comparison of gadobenate dimeglumine-enhanced MR imaging and multiphasic 64-section CT. Radiology. 251(1):85-95, 2009
11. Iannaccone R et al: Hepatocellular carcinoma in patients with nonalcoholic fatty liver disease: helical CT and MR imaging findings with clinical-pathologic comparison. Radiology. 243(2):422-30, 2007
12. Watanabe Y et al: MR imaging of acute biliary disorders. Radiographics. 27(2):477-95, 2007
13. Teefey SA et al: Detection of primary hepatic malignancy in liver transplant candidates: prospective comparison of CT, MR imaging, US, and PET. Radiology. 226(2):533-42, 2003
14. Han JK et al: Cholangiocarcinoma: pictorial essay of CT and cholangiographic findings. Radiographics. 22(1):173-87, 2002
15. Han JK et al: Hilar cholangiocarcinoma: thin-section spiral CT findings with cholangiographic correlation. Radiographics. 17(6):1475-85, 1997
16. Kim TK et al: Peripheral cholangiocarcinoma of the liver: two-phase spiral CT findings. Radiology. 204(2):539-43, 1997
17. Lacomis JM et al: Cholangiocarcinoma: delayed CT contrast enhancement patterns. Radiology. 203(1):98-104, 1997

(Left) In this patient with jaundice, a T2WI MR section shows innumerable subcentimeter hypointense nodules ➡ throughout the liver, diagnostic of cirrhotic regenerative nodules. Also noted is an enlarged spleen ⇨. **(Right)** In this patient with jaundice, a contrast-enhanced T1WI MR section shows multiple signs of cirrhosis and portal hypertension, including a shrunken liver with widened fissures, large varices ➡, and splenomegaly with hypointense Gamna-Gandy bodies ➡.

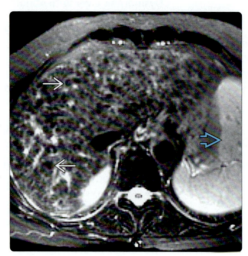
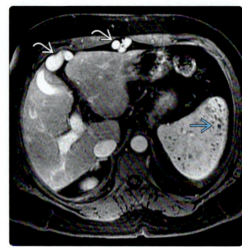

(Left) In this patient with primary sclerosing cholangitis (PSC) and jaundice, CT shows an atrophic peripheral liver ➡ with hypertrophy of the deep right and caudate segments ➡. The intrahepatic bile ducts (IHBDs) are irregularly dilated ➡ especially within the lateral segment. Large varices are seen ➡. The findings are typical of biliary cirrhosis due to PSC. **(Right)** In the same patient, ERCP shows both focal and long strictures ➡ of the IHBDs, characteristic of PSC. A dominant stricture causes marked dilation of the left lateral hepatic duct ➡.

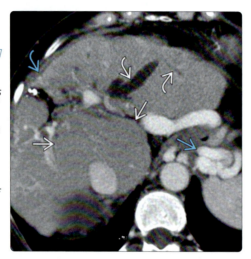
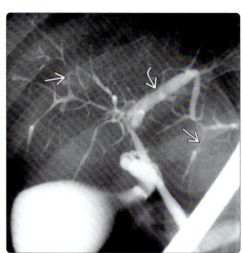

(Left) This 59-year-old man with liver metastases developed painful jaundice while receiving oxaliplatin chemotherapy. Delayed-phase gadoxetate-enhanced (Eovist) MR shows 1 of 2 small liver metastases ➡ as well as a peculiar enhancement pattern of the liver. **(Right)** Another axial image from the delayed-phase gadoxetate-enhanced MR shows diffuse, reticular hypodensity throughout the periphery of the liver, suggesting sinusoidal obstruction syndrome, which was confirmed on biopsy.

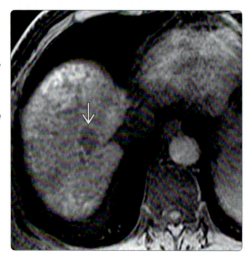
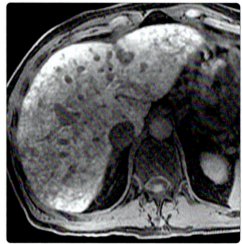

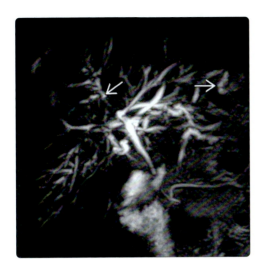

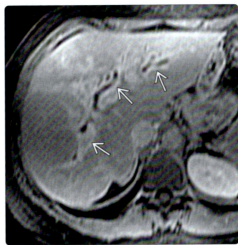

(Left) Coronal MRCP demonstrates irregular beading and dilation of the IHBDs ➡ in a patient with PSC. Many more IHBDs are visualized than on a normal MRCP, indicating intrahepatic dilation and strictures. (Right) Axial contrast-enhanced MR in the same patient demonstrates mural thickening and hyperenhancement of the dilated IHBDs ➡ diffusely throughout the liver, indicating active inflammation, characteristic features of PSC.

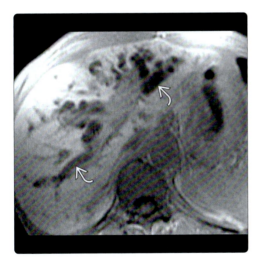

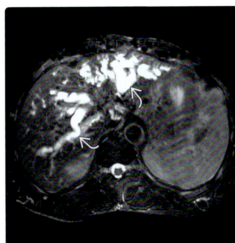

(Left) In this man with jaundice and pruritis, nonenhanced T1WI MR shows massive dilation of IHBDs ➡ but no apparent mass or stone. (Right) In the same patient, axial T2WI MR again shows dilated IHBDs ➡ but no mass. This degree of dilation of IHBDs usually indicates a malignant biliary obstruction, in this case, at the confluence of the main right and left bile ducts.

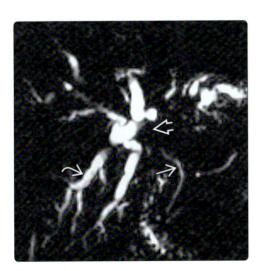

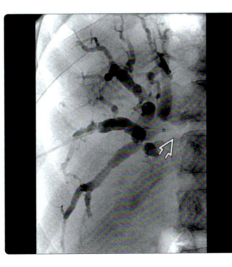

(Left) In the same case, MRCP shows gross dilation of the IHBDs ➡ but a normal-sized common duct ➡. There is no large mass evident at the site of obstruction ➡, a finding characteristic of a hilar, Klatskin-type, cholangiocarcinoma. (Right) Transhepatic cholangiography shows complete obstruction at the confluence of the main right and left hepatic ducts ➡, characteristic of a Klatskin-type cholangiocarcinoma.

(Left) *In this 65-year-old man with painless jaundice, arterial-phase CT shows a well-defined, encapsulated, and hypervascular mass ➡. The IHBDs ➡ are grossly dilated.* **(Right)** *In the same patient, venous-phase CT shows contrast washout from the mass ➡, as well as an enhancing mass ➡ within the common duct, representing direct intraductal invasion by an hepatocellular carcinoma.*

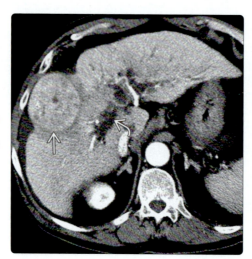
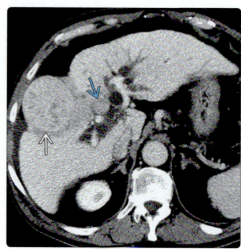

(Left) *In this 49-year-old woman with jaundice and a history of thyroid cancer, contrast-enhanced T1WI MR shows multiple ring-enhancing hepatic metastases ➡ and marked dilation of IHBDs ➡.* **(Right)** *In the same case and study, MRCP shows massive dilation of the IHBDs ➡ with abrupt cutoff ➡ where a metastasis had invaded the bile duct.*

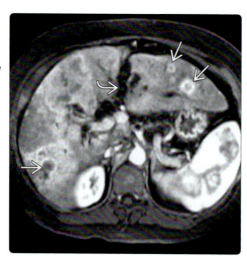
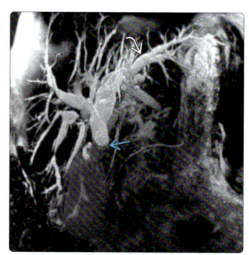

(Left) *In this man with painless jaundice, coronal CT shows dilation of the bile ducts ➡ and pancreatic duct ➡ by a mass ➡ in the pancreatic head, a classic presentation for pancreatic head carcinoma.* **(Right)** *MRCP in the same patient shows abrupt obstruction of the distal pancreatic ➡ and bile ➡ ducts by the pancreatic cancer, the double duct sign.*

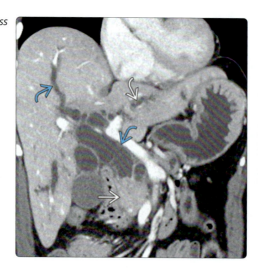
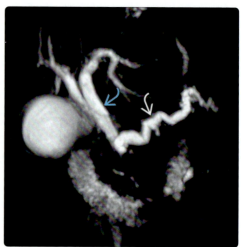

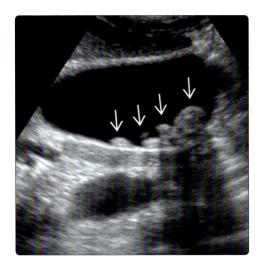
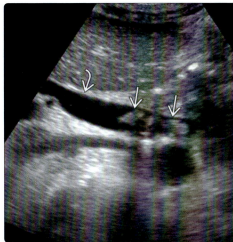

(Left) *In this man with RUQ pain and elevated serum bilirubin, US shows multiple echogenic, shadowing stones* ➡ *within an otherwise normal-appearing gallbladder.* (Right) *In the same patient, US shows a dilated common duct* ➡ *with numerous intraductal calculi* ➡. *US visualization of common duct stones is often limited by bowel gas, which blocks the US beam.*

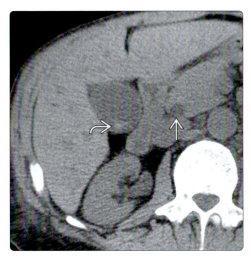
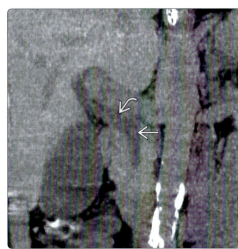

(Left) *In the same patient, nonenhanced CT shows subtle hyperdensity within the gallbladder* ➡ *and common duct* ➡ *stones.* (Right) *In the same patient, a coronal CT of the dilated common duct* ➡ *shows subtle evidence of rim-calcified stones* ➡ *within the common duct. CT diagnosis of gallstones is limited by the low density (attenuation) of cholesterol stones. Multiple stones were confirmed and extracted at ERCP.*

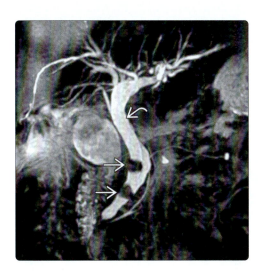
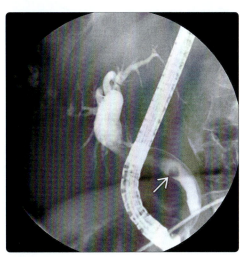

(Left) *MRCP shows 2 stones as signal voids* ➡ *within the mildly dilated common bile duct* ➡. (Right) *In the same patient, ERCP was performed to remove the calculi* ➡ *and to place a temporary biliary stent. ERCP can generally be reserved for treatment of calculi or other causes of jaundice confidently diagnosed by noninvasive imaging, such as MR.*

Common Symptoms, Signs, and Conditions

IMAGING

- CT of chest, abdomen, and pelvis can be performed in < 1 minute of scan time
  - Multiplanar, multiphasic CECT shows extent of bowel and solid visceral injuries and bleeding
  - Evaluation of brain and spine injuries can be done quickly in the same setting
- "Sentinel clot": High density (> 60 HU); near the source of bleeding
- "Active extravasation": Isodense to enhanced arteries
  - Active bleeding from spleen, liver, or kidney is usually treated effectively with transcatheter coil embolization by interventional radiologists (IR)
- Splenic trauma
  - Parenchymal laceration ± devitalized tissue (wedge- or oval-shaped focus of nonenhanced tissue)
  - Active bleeding from spleen → coil embolization as optimal therapy in most cases
- Hepatic and biliary trauma

- Deep laceration may injure large vessels or bile ducts
- Active bleeding is usually best treated with coil embolization in IR
- Biliary injuries are confirmed and treated via ERCP with stent placement
- Pancreatic trauma
  - CT can often distinguish contusion from transection
  - MRCP or ERCP are more definitive
- Bowel and mesenteric
  - Missed more often than injuries to solid organs
  - Free intra- or retroperitoneal gas may be absent even with transection of small bowel
- Focused assessment with sonography in trauma (FAST)
  - Main value: Quick assessment of hemodynamically unstable patients for hemoperitoneum
  - Does not depict source nor severity of hemorrhage
  - Misses bowel, pelvic, retroperitoneal injuries

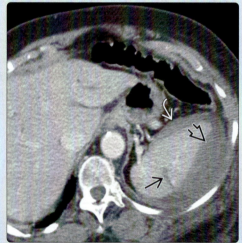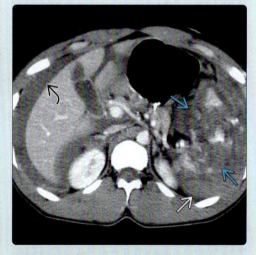

(Left) Axial CECT in an 87-year-old woman who fell at a nursing home demonstrates a splenic parenchymal laceration ⬎ and intraperitoneal blood ⬈ as well as a lentiform heterogeneous subcapsular hematoma ⬊. No intervention was required. (Right) Axial CECT in a 23-year-old man injured in a motor vehicle accident shows a shattered spleen ➡ surrounded by a sentinel clot ➡ in the perisplenic region and a large hemoperitoneum ⬊. Splenectomy was required.

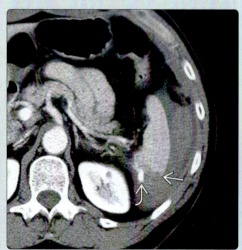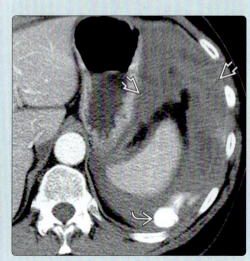

(Left) Axial CECT shows a splenic laceration with active extravasation. Note the fracture of the lower pole ➡ featuring a site of high-attenuation arterial extravasation ➡. (Right) Axial CECT in the same patient demonstrates a large perisplenic hematoma ➡ and extensive arterial extravasation ➡. Transcatheter coil embolization of the bleeding vessel was successful in avoiding splenectomy.

TERMINOLOGY

Definitions

- Abdominal or pelvic visceral injury resulting from blunt trauma

IMAGING

CT Findings

- **CT of chest, abdomen, and pelvis can be performed in < 1 minute of scan time**
  - Evaluation of brain and spine injuries can be done in same setting very quickly
  - Multiplanar, multiphasic CECT shows extent of bowel and solid visceral injuries and bleeding
- CT protocol
  - If brain scan is needed, do this before administration of IV contrast medium
  - Spine images can be reconstructed in any plane from standard axial images through neck, thorax, abdomen, and pelvis
  - No oral contrast medium is needed in most cases
  - IV contrast medium injected at 3-4 mL/second
  - If chest is to be evaluated, start scanning at thoracic inlet 30 seconds after initiation of IV contrast bolus
  - Start scanning top of abdomen through pelvis at 70 seconds from initiation of IV bolus
  - **Do not request CT angiogram of abdomen**
    - Scan delay for a CTA is ~ 18 seconds, too early to allow optimal identification of abdominal visceral injuries and active bleeding
    - Blood vessels, visceral injuries, and active bleeding are all demonstrated well with 70-second delay through abdomen and pelvis
- General principles
  - Hemoperitoneum: Lower density, more homogeneous fluid (30-45 HU)
    - Amount and location are readily apparent on CT
  - "Sentinel clot": High density (> 60 HU)
    - Heterogeneous clot accumulates near source of bleeding
  - "Active extravasation": Active arterial bleeding is isodense to enhanced arteries
    - Active bleeding from spleen, liver, or kidney is usually treated effectively with transcatheter coil embolization by interventional radiologists (IR)
  - Splenic trauma
    - Parenchymal laceration ± devitalized tissue
      - Appears as wedge-shaped or oval segment of nonenhancing tissue
    - Sentinel clot surrounds spleen
    - Subcapsular hematoma: Lentiform clot flattens splenic contour
    - Active bleeding from spleen → coil embolization as optimal therapy in most cases
      - Effective at stopping bleeding and avoiding surgery in > 90% of cases
    - Shattered spleen usually requires urgent surgery
  - Hepatic and biliary trauma
    - Usually right lobe laceration
    - Deep laceration may injure large vessels

- Active bleeding: Best treated with coil embolization
  - May also injure bile ducts: Confirm and treat via ERCP ± stent
  - Left lobe laceration is often accompanied by injury to other midline organs (e.g., pancreas and duodenum)
  - Pancreatic trauma
    - Contusion: Peripancreatic infiltration or hematoma
    - Laceration: Discrete, linear, hypodense cleft through pancreas, from ventral surface to splenic vein
    - Fracture: Larger laceration with clear separation of 2 sections of gland
    - Key determination is whether pancreatic duct is transected
      - May not be evident on CT; may require MRCP or ERCP for confirmation
  - Bowel and mesenteric trauma
    - Found in 2-5% of patients having surgery for blunt abdominal trauma
    - Occur more frequently in association with direct contusion of anterior abdominal wall
    - **Bowel and mesenteric injuries are missed by clinicians and radiologists much more often than injuries to solid viscera**
      - Most common: Duodenum and proximal jejunum
    - Common combination of findings suggesting bowel injury
      - Sentinel clot in bowel wall &/or mesentery
      - Bowel wall thickening (> 3 mm)
      - ↑ or ↓ enhancement of bowel wall
      - Ascites or sentinel clot: Between bowel loops; higher than water density
    - Active bleeding (extravasation) from bowel or mesentery
      - Requires surgical intervention to evaluate bowel integrity
      - Coil embolization of mesenteric vessels may cause bowel ischemia
    - Free intra- or retroperitoneal gas
      - May be absent even with transection of small bowel
      - Pneumothorax may mimic or extend to free intraperitoneal air

Ultrasonographic Findings

- **Focused assessment with sonography in trauma (FAST)**
  - Main value: Quick assessment of hemodynamically unstable patients for hemoperitoneum
  - Drawbacks; does not reliably detect:
    - Source of hemorrhage nor active bleeding
    - Bowel, retroperitoneal, or pelvic injuries

SELECTED REFERENCES

1. Patlas MN et al: Abdominal and Pelvic Trauma: Misses and Misinterpretations at Multidetector CT: Trauma/Emergency Radiology. Radiographics. 37(2):703-704, 2017
2. Dreizin D et al: Multidetector CT for Penetrating Torso Trauma: State of the Art. Radiology. 277(2):338-55, 2015
3. Sadro CT et al: Geriatric Trauma: A Radiologist's Guide to Imaging Trauma Patients Aged 65 Years and Older. Radiographics. 35(4):1263-85, 2015
4. Soto JA et al: Multidetector CT of blunt abdominal trauma. Radiology. 265(3):678-93, 2012

(Left) *CT in a 37-year-old man who sustained blunt abdominal trauma in a motor vehicle accident shows a large right lobe hepatic injury (laceration ➡ and infarct or parenchymal hematoma) with high-attenuation active arterial extravasation ➡.* (Right) *Selective right hepatic artery angiogram in the same patient confirms active bleeding ➡, which was successfully treated with coil embolization. The patient made an uneventful recovery without the need for surgery or blood transfusion.*

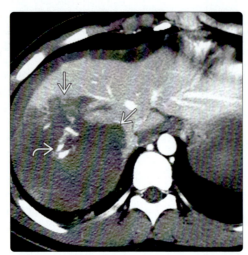
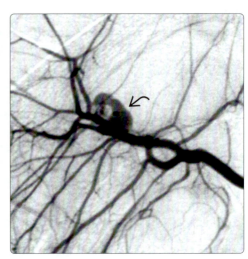

(Left) *Axial CECT obtained in a 19-year-old man who sustained multiple injuries after a motorcycle accident demonstrates a right lobe hepatic laceration ➡ with active bleeding ➡.* (Right) *Axial CECT in the same patient shows extension of active bleeding ➡ into the peritoneal cavity along the hepatic capsule. Due to the acute intraperitoneal bleeding, urgent surgery was performed, which revealed an actively bleeding capsular artery.*

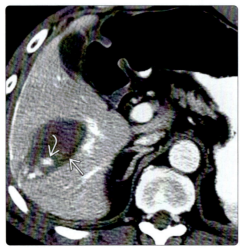
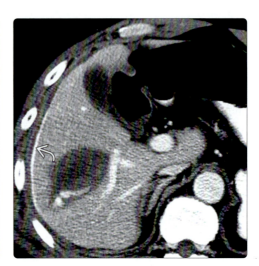

(Left) *Axial CECT shows a laceration through the left lobe of the liver ➡.* (Right) *Axial CECT in the same patient demonstrates a fracture plane through the pancreatic neck ➡ extending completely through the gland to the splenic vein ➡, where active bleeding is evident ➡. Injuries to the left lobe of the liver are often associated with injuries to other midline organs.*

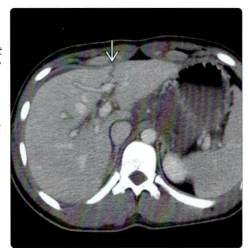
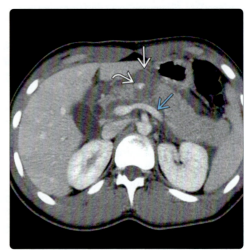

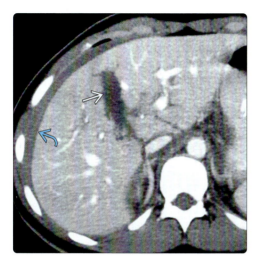

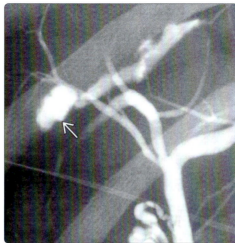

(Left) Axial CECT in a patient after blunt trauma demonstrates a deep liver laceration ➡ and small hemoperitoneum ➔. The depth of the laceration raised concern for biliary transection. The patient developed signs of bile peritonitis. (Right) ERCP in the same patient shows extravasation of contrast from a transected bile duct ➡. The patient was successfully treated with biliary stenting without surgery. The biliary and hepatic injuries resolved.

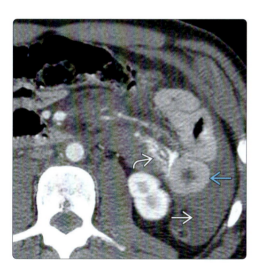

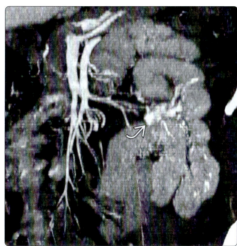

(Left) Axial CECT in a 24-year-old man injured in a motor vehicle crash shows a sentinel clot ➡, adjacent to thick-walled jejunum ➔, and active bleeding as evidenced by the contrast extravasation ➔, all characteristic findings in intestinal trauma. (Right) Coronal CECT in the same patient shows an injured branch of the superior mesenteric artery with a large focus of contrast extravasation ➡. The mesenteric injury was surgically repaired and a segment of small intestine was resected.

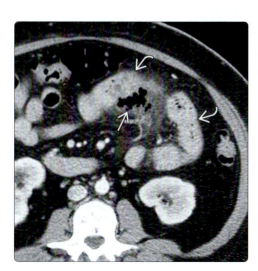

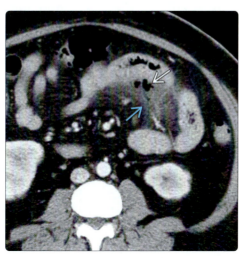

(Left) Axial CECT in a 28-year-old man who was injured in an motor vehicle crash demonstrates ectopic gas ➡ adjacent to a thick-walled jejunal segment ➔, indicative of transmural laceration or perforation. (Right) Axial CECT in the same patient demonstrates mesenteric gas ➡ and stranding ➔, characteristic findings in the setting of intestinal trauma. The transected jejunal segment was resected.

TERMINOLOGY

- Localized abdominal collection of pus or infected fluid

IMAGING

- **CT is imaging test of choice**: Low density, loculated, encapsulated fluid collection with peripheral rim enhancement
  - Simple fluid density (0-10 HU) or slightly hyperdense
  - Internal gas in absence of intervention/drainage highly suspicious for infected collection
  - "Abscess" suggests discrete, drainable fluid collection: Differentiate from ill-defined inflammation and fluid that is not drainable (i.e., phlegmon)
  - Adjacent fat stranding, edema, and fascial thickening due to inflammation
  - Intraparenchymal abscess (liver, kidney, etc.) often surrounded by low-density parenchymal edema
- **US**: Complex fluid collection with internal low-level echoes, membranes, or septations
  - Increasing complexity within abscess fluid suggests thicker, more viscous contents
  - Greater complexity on US often implies greater difficulty in drainage (especially with small-caliber catheters)
  - Center of abscess avascular on color Doppler imaging with peripheral hyperemia

PATHOLOGY

- Many different causes, including postoperative setting, enteric perforation, generalized bacteremia, and trauma

CLINICAL ISSUES

- Increased incidence in diabetics, immunocompromised patients, and postoperative patients

DIAGNOSTIC CHECKLIST

- Differentiating abscess from noninfected collections after surgery may be difficult and requires correlation with clinical symptoms of infection or fluid aspiration

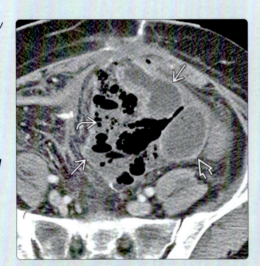
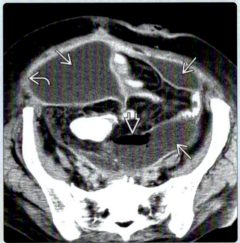

(Left) *Axial CECT in an elderly postoperative patient demonstrates a rounded complex fluid collection ➡ with gas bubbles ➡ and an enhancing capsule ➡, findings diagnostic for an abdominal abscess.* (Right) *Axial CECT in an elderly postoperative patient demonstrates multiple loculated fluid collections ➡ with prominently enhancing capsules ➡ and mass effect on adjacent structures, representing abdominal abscesses. Note the air-fluid level ➡ within one of the abscesses.*

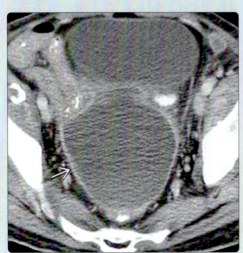
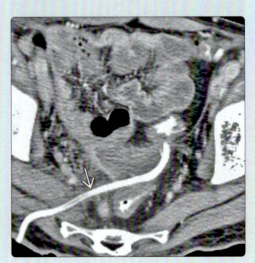

(Left) *Axial CECT shows a large pelvic abscess ➡ following hysterectomy. Note the presence of a discrete enhancing rim and mass effect on adjacent loops of bowel and the bladder.* (Right) *Axial CECT shows placement of a percutaneous drainage catheter ➡ using a transgluteal approach. The abscess has almost completely resolved following drainage.*

Abdominal Abscess

TERMINOLOGY

Definitions

- Localized abdominal collection of pus or infected fluid

IMAGING

General Features

- Best diagnostic clue
  - Loculated, encapsulated fluid collection with peripheral rim enhancement ± gas bubbles or air-fluid level on CECT
- Location
  - Can occur anywhere within abdominal cavity, including intraperitoneal space, extraperitoneal spaces, or intraparenchymal
- Size
  - Highly variable
    - 2-15 cm in diameter, microabscesses < 2 cm

CT Findings

- Low density, loculated, encapsulated fluid collection with peripheral rim enhancement
  - May be simple fluid density (0-10 HU) or slightly hyperdense
  - Often adjacent fat stranding, edema, and fascial thickening due to inflammation
  - Intraparenchymal abscess (liver, kidney, spleen, etc.) often shows surrounding low-density parenchymal edema
- Presence of internal gas (~ 50% of cases) in absence of intervention highly suspicious for infected collection
- Term "abscess" suggests discrete, **drainable** fluid collection: Differentiate from ill-defined inflammation and fluid that is not drainable (i.e., phlegmon)
- Can be difficult to distinguish infected from noninfected (e.g., seroma, lymphocele, hematoma) collections

MR Findings

- Typically central core of abscess demonstrates fluid signal (low-signal T1WI, high-signal T2WI)
  - Internal complexity may slightly alter signal characteristics (e.g., hemorrhage, proteinaceous content)
- Enhancing peripheral rim on T1WI C+ images
- Abscesses anywhere in abdomen tend to show restricted diffusion (high signal on DWI with low ADC values)
  - Lower ADC values than noninfected fluid collections
    - However, lack of restricted diffusion cannot exclude possibility of abscess (overlap in ADC values with necrotic tumors and noninfected collections)
- Usually evidence of adjacent soft tissue edema around abscess (high T2 signal)

Ultrasonographic Findings

- Complex fluid collection with internal low-level echoes, membranes, or septations on US
  - Dependent echoes represent debris within abscess
    - Increasing complexity within abscess fluid suggests thicker, more viscous contents
    - Greater complexity on US often implies more difficult drainage (especially with small-caliber catheter)
  - Posterior acoustic through transmission may vary depending on composition of fluid in abscess
    - Abscesses with thick, viscous, proteinaceous fluid may have relatively little through transmission
  - Center of abscess is typically avascular on color Doppler imaging with peripheral hyperemia
  - Fat surrounding abscess may appear markedly echogenic due to inflammation
    - Inflamed fat hyperemic on color Doppler
  - Internal echogenic foci with ring-down artifact and posterior "dirty" acoustic shadowing suggest presence of gas

Radiographic Findings

- Radiography
  - Soft tissue "mass" or density ± internal ectopic gas (~ 50% of cases) or air-fluid levels
    - May be associated with loss of soft tissue-fat interface
  - Dilated bowel loops due to focal ileus
  - Subphrenic abscess often results in adjacent pleural effusion and lower lobe atelectasis

Fluoroscopic Findings

- Abscess sinogram
  - Useful after percutaneous drainage to assess presence of residual abscess cavity
  - Defines catheter position and communication with abscess
  - Identifies fistulization of abscess with adjacent bowel, pancreas, or biliary tree

Nuclear Medicine Findings

- Ga-67 scan
  - Most often utilized for chronic infections and fever of unknown origin
  - Nonspecific, as Ga-97 may demonstrate uptake with tumors, such as lymphoma, as well as chronic granulomatous processes (i.e., sarcoidosis)
- In-111 or Tc-99m-labelled white blood cell (WBC) scan
  - Most often utilized for acute infections or inflammatory bowel disease

Imaging Recommendations

- Best imaging tool
  - Contrast-enhanced, multiplanar CT

DIFFERENTIAL DIAGNOSIS

Postoperative Lymphocele

- History of lymph node dissection with collection adjacent to surgical clips along lymphatic drainage pathways
- Loculated collection of simple fluid attenuation without peripheral enhancement or internal gas

Biloma

- Fluid collection adjacent to biliary tree in patient with history of biliary or hepatic surgery
- Usually simple fluid attenuation without peripheral enhancement or internal gas (unless superinfected)

Postoperative Seroma

- Simple fluid attenuation without peripheral enhancement

- May be loculated or contain internal gas due to recent surgery

Loculated Ascites

- Often in patients with cirrhosis, chronic liver disease, chronic renal failure, or other underlying cause for ascites
- Simple fluid attenuation with minimal mass effect, no peripheral enhancement, and no internal gas
- May demonstrate complexity (e.g., septations) on US or MR but appear simple on CT

Pancreatic Pseudocyst

- Clinical history or imaging stigmata of prior pancreatitis
- Location highly variable, but most often within pancreatic parenchyma, lesser sac, anterior pararenal space, or transverse mesocolon
- Pseudocyst usually requires several weeks to develop peripheral pseudocapsule

Abdominal Hematoma

- Attenuation variable depending on age of blood products, but clot is typically high attenuation (> 45 HU) in acute setting and gradually decreases in attenuation over time
- May demonstrate weak peripheral enhancement as it evolves (without necessarily being infected)

Retained Oxidized Cellulose (Surgicel)

- Placed at surgery to induce hemostasis and appears as collection of gas bubbles without much fluid
- May mimic abscess, but no discrete fluid collection

PATHOLOGY

General Features

- Etiology
  - Many different causes, including enteric perforation (e.g., perforated appendicitis, diverticulitis), postoperative setting, generalized bacteremia, and trauma
    - Postoperative abscess may be variably located depending on site of surgery, but most often occurs in intraperitoneal spaces, such as cul-de-sac, Morison pouch, subphrenic spaces
- Genetics
  - Risk increased if genetically altered immune response
  - Diabetics have ↑ incidence of gas-forming abscesses

CLINICAL ISSUES

Presentation

- Most common signs/symptoms
  - Fever, chills, abdominal pain
  - Tachycardia and hypotension in setting of sepsis
- Clinical profile
  - Leukocytosis, positive blood cultures, elevated ESR
  - Elderly and immunocompromised patients may not have fever or ↑ WBC

Demographics

- Epidemiology
  - Most commonly in postoperative setting
  - Increased incidence in diabetic and immunocompromised patients

- Microabscesses due to fungal infections in immunocompromised patients

Natural History & Prognosis

- Variable depending on extent of abscess, patient's immune system status, and other comorbidities
- Overall excellent prognosis if treated appropriately

Treatment

- Options, risks, complications
  - Percutaneous abscess drainage (PAD)
    - 80% success rate, with patient selection critical for success
    - Best candidates have well-defined, encapsulated, fluid-filled abscesses > 3 cm with safe catheter access route
    - Drainage can be performed under CT or US guidance with multiple approaches possible (transcutaneous, transgluteal, transrectal, transvaginal)
    - Complex abscess (i.e., multiseptated) or abscess with enteric fistula may take weeks or months to drain, but most abscesses can be drained in 10-14 days
    - Catheter removed when drainage < 10 cc per shift or when abscess cavity resolves on imaging
  - Contraindications for PAD related to patient coagulopathy (elevated INR or low platelet count)
  - Contraindications for PAD related to abscess
    - Poorly defined collection (i.e., phlegmon) rather than discrete drainable abscess
    - No safe access route for catheter insertion due to intervening bowel, adjacent vital organs, or pleura
      - Crossing colon is greater risk than traversing small bowel or stomach
      - Crossing sterile collections (such as hematoma) or sterile pleural effusion should be avoided due to risk of superinfection
    - Echinococcal cyst (due to risk of leakage and resultant anaphylaxis)
  - Surgery indications
    - Extensive intraperitoneal abscesses
    - Debridement of necrotic infected tissue
    - Failed percutaneous drainage
  - Small abscesses (usually < 3 cm) may be treated conservatively with antibiotic therapy

DIAGNOSTIC CHECKLIST

Consider

- Differentiating abscess from noninfected collections in postoperative setting (e.g., seroma, lymphocele, hematoma) may be difficult and requires correlation with clinical symptoms of infection or fluid aspiration

SELECTED REFERENCES

1. Chang ST et al: Molecular and Clinical Approach to Intra-abdominal Adverse Effects of Targeted Cancer Therapies. Radiographics. 37(5):1461-1482, 2017
2. Hartung MP et al: Mimics of Malignancy in Abdominal Imaging: Multisystem Radiology. Radiographics. 37(7):2202-2203, 2017
3. Sheedy SP et al: MR Imaging of Perianal Crohn Disease. Radiology. 282(3):628-645, 2017
4. Elagili F et al: Predictors of postoperative outcomes for patients with diverticular abscess initially treated with percutaneous drainage. Am J Surg. ePub, 2014

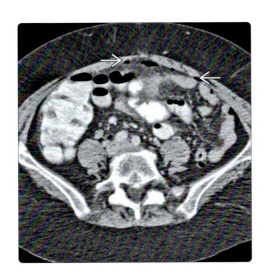
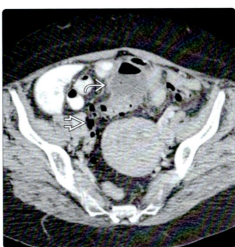

(Left) Axial CECT in a woman who presented with lower abdominal pain, fever, and tenderness shows extensive free intraperitoneal gas ➡. (Right) Axial CECT in the same patient shows a loculated abscess ➡ immediately adjacent to a segment of sigmoid colon with extensive diverticulosis ➡, which proved to be the source of the free air and abscesses.

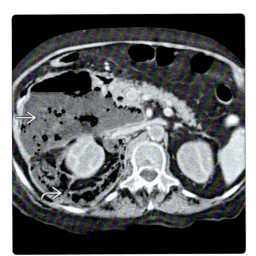
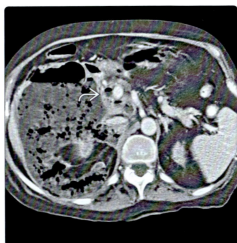

(Left) Axial CECT in an elderly woman after ERCP and papillotomy shows a large collection of gas and fluid ➡ dissecting through the retroperitoneal spaces, especially the anterior pararenal space and the interfascial plane ➡. (Right) Axial CECT in the same patient demonstrates the retroperitoneal abscess. The perforation site was the 2nd portion of the duodenum ➡ at the papillotomy site.

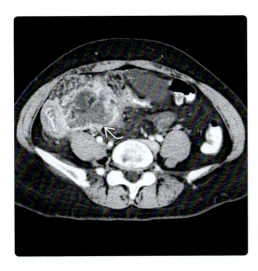
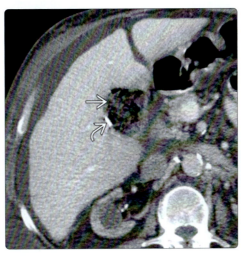

(Left) Axial CECT in a young woman with progressive fever and abdominal pain over several days reveals a large periappendiceal abscess ➡ with mass effect displacing the small bowel, bladder, and uterus. (Right) Axial CECT in a patient who underwent a cholecystectomy shows a collection of gas ➡, but very little fluid, in the cholecystectomy bed. Surgical clips ➡ are also seen. This represents oxidized cellulose (Surgicel), which was placed for hemostasis at surgery, and not an abscess.

KEY FACTS

TERMINOLOGY

- Patient injury caused by improper feeding tube placement
- Feeding tubes
  - Small, soft enteric tubes
  - Some with flexible metallic tips
  - Tip of feeding tube should be located beyond stomach (distal duodenum or jejunum)
- Nasogastric tubes
  - Large bore, moderately stiff
  - Used for temporary gastric and bowel decompression
  - Tip placed in pylorus can cause outlet obstruction
- Gastrostomy and jejunostomy tubes
  - Balloon-tipped catheters should not be placed into small bowel (may obstruct lumen)
  - Small amount of free air after placement is common and usually does not require intervention

IMAGING

- Malposition is most frequent complication of feeding tubes
  - Can be visualized on chest or abdominal radiograph
  - **Auscultation over abdomen is not reliable method for confirming proper tube placement**

CLINICAL ISSUES

- 1-3% of feeding tubes enter tracheobronchial tree
  - Anywhere from trachea to pleural space
  - Can perforate lung with significant morbidity and mortality
- Tube may penetrate esophagus or duodenum with fatal results
  - Often through diverticula (e.g., Zenker), due to thin wall
- High-risk patients
  - Altered mental status
  - Absent gag reflex
  - Multiple or repetitive insertion attempts
- Treatment
  - Reposition feeding tube if in incorrect location
  - Perforation of lung or bowel may require surgery

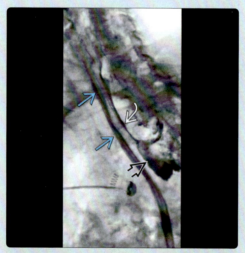
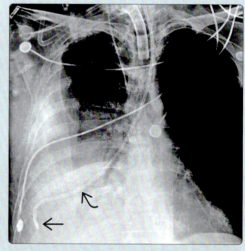

(Left) Esophagram shows a retroesophageal collection of gas and contrast medium ⊟ resulting from perforation of a Zenker diverticulum by attempted placement of a feeding tube whose track ⊟ runs parallel to the proximal esophagus ⊟. (Right) Chest radiograph shows a feeding tube ⊟ that has entered the right bronchus and perforated the lung though a lower lobe bronchus. The tip ⊟ lies in the pleural space, a procedural complication that may be fatal, especially if food is given through the tube.

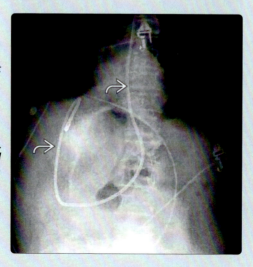
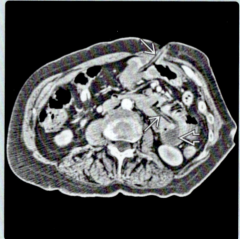

(Left) Frontal radiograph shows the peculiar course of the feeding tube ⊟ with abrupt upper deviation of its distal portion. CT showed that the tube had perforated the duodenum and had been advanced with its wire in place. (Right) Axial CECT shows a feeding gastrostomy tube ⊟ entering the stomach. The balloon tip of the tube ⊟ has migrated into the jejunum where it is partially occluding its lumen.

TERMINOLOGY

Definitions

- Patient injury caused by improper feeding tube placement
- Feeding tubes
  - Small, soft enteric tubes
  - Some with flexible metallic tips
  - Used for feeding chronically ill patients
  - Can be used for long periods of time
- Nasogastric tubes
  - Large-bore, moderately stiff
  - Used for temporary bowel decompression or fluid sampling
  - Tip placed in pylorus can cause gastric outlet obstruction
- Gastrostomy and jejunostomy tubes
  - Placed surgically, endoscopically, or percutaneously
  - Used for long-term, possibly permanent, feeding
  - Use imaging to visualize tube balloon, surgical clips, and cuff
    - Cuff initiates soft tissue reaction to anchor tube to abdominal wall
  - PEG button can replace tube several weeks post placement
    - Placed in anterior abdominal wall
  - Balloon-tipped catheters should not be placed into small bowel
    - Likely to obstruct bowel lumen

IMAGING

General Features

- Best diagnostic clue
  - Malposition is most frequent complication of feeding tubes
    - Check on chest or abdominal radiograph
  - Usual course: Nares/mouth → esophagus → stomach → small bowel
- Location
  - Tip of feeding tube should be located beyond stomach
    - In distal duodenum or proximal jejunum

Imaging Recommendations

- Best imaging tool
  - Chest or abdominal radiograph
  - Radiography is most accurate way to detect malposition/complications
    - Obtain chest film after initial placement, followed by abdominal film
  - Electromagnetically guided placement systems are also in use
  - **Auscultation over abdomen is not reliable method for detecting proper tube placement**

Radiographic Findings

- Inadvertent placement in airways
  - Metal tip or stiffening wire can perforate lung
  - Administration of formula → empyema
- Malposition in esophagus
  - Can enter stomach and then coil back into esophagus
- Aspiration of gastrointestinal contents

- Secondary to malposition in esophagus, pharynx, or stomach
- Clue: Bilateral pulmonary infiltrates
- Perforation of gastrointestinal tract
  - Can perforate esophagus (e.g., Zenker diverticulum) or duodenum
- Gastrointestinal hemorrhage
  - May irritate and ulcerate mucosa
- Knotted tubing
  - Due to coiling, often within stomach
  - Can result in tube malfunction due to obstruction
- Complications of PEG tubes
  - Free intraperitoneal air
    - Usually does not require intervention
  - Injury to abdominal structures (liver, colon)
  - Gastrointestinal obstruction
    - Secondary to migration of balloon tip into pylorus or duodenum
    - Do not put Foley catheter through PEG tube track

CLINICAL ISSUES

Presentation

- Other signs/symptoms
  - Respiratory distress
    - Cough, dyspnea, cyanosis
    - Not always present
  - Aberrant pH of aspirate
    - Limited by use of proton-pump inhibitors

Demographics

- Epidemiology
  - 1-3% of feeding tubes lodge in airways
- High-risk patients
  - Altered mental status
  - Absent gag reflex
  - Multiple or repetitive insertion attempts

Treatment

- Reposition feeding tube if in incorrect location

DIAGNOSTIC CHECKLIST

Consider

- Radiographic confirmation is best way to ascertain proper tube position
- Feeding tubes can move spontaneously
  - Position should be confirmed on each radiograph

SELECTED REFERENCES

1. Ojo O: Problems with use of a Foley catheter in enteral tube feeding. Br J Nurs. 23(7):360-2, 364, 2014
2. Gor P: Placement of nasogastric tubes must be checked thoroughly. Nurs Stand. 27(43):32, 2013
3. Khasawneh FA et al: Nasopharyngeal perforation by a new electromagnetically visualised enteral feeding tube. BMJ Case Rep. 2013, 2013
4. Marco J et al: Bronchopulmonary complications associated to enteral nutrition devices in patients admitted to internal medicine departments. Rev Clin Esp (Barc). 213(5):223-8, 2013
5. Simons SR et al: Bedside assessment of enteral tube placement: aligning practice with evidence. Am J Nurs. 112(2):40-6; quiz 48, 47, 2012

KEY FACTS

IMAGING

- CT and upper GI radiography have complementary roles
- **Laparoscopic adjustable gastric banding** (LAGB) procedure (a.k.a. "lap band")
  - Less effective for sustained weight loss
  - Complications: Less common and less varied
  - May be too tight or too loose
  - Band may erode into stomach or esophagus
- **Sleeve gastrectomy (gastric sleeve)**
  - 75% of stomach is removed by dividing stomach along its long axis
    - Complications: Less or comparable to LAGB, less than Roux-en-Y gastric bypass
    - Leak: Early complication seen in < 1%
    - Stricture in mid stomach (transient or persistent)
- **Roux-en-Y Gastric Bypass (RYGB)**
  - Gastrointestinal complications occur in ~ 10%
  - Anastomotic stricture

- Dilation of gastric pouch, spherical shape, air-fluid-contrast material levels, delayed emptying
- Anastomotic leaks
  - Most commonly at gastrojejunal anastomosis
  - CT may demonstrate major and minor leaks; fluid collections not evident on upper GI series
- Marginal ulcers; rate of 0.5-1.4% after RYGB
  - Usually result of ischemia
- Small bowel obstruction
  - Most common etiology: Internal hernias (IH) and adhesions
  - IH: CT appearance depends on location
  - Clustering of small bowel loops; congestion, crowding, twisting of mesenteric vessels
  - Displacement of jejunal anastomotic staple line
- Obstruction of excluded stomach and biliopancreatic limb
  - Cannot be diagnosed with upper GI series; CT is key
  - May progress to perforation (often fatal)

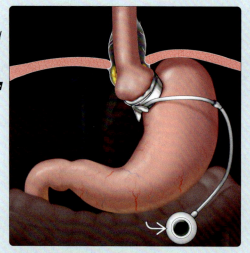 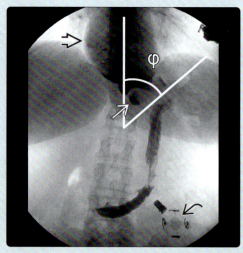

(Left) *Graphic depicts the gastric banding procedure in which a silicone band is looped around the proximal stomach. A tube connects the inflatable liner of the band to a subcutaneously placed port ➡ that can be accessed and inflated or deflated with injections of fluid.* **(Right)** *Spot film from an esophagram shows the gastric band ➡ in its expected position with a "Phi" angle of ~ 45° (normal). The dilated, slowly emptying esophagus ➡ indicates that the band is too tight and fluid will be removed from the access port ➡.*

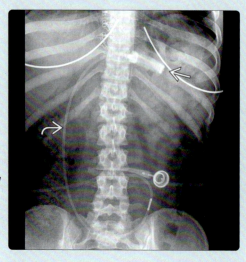 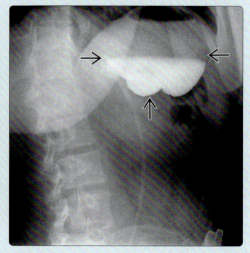

(Left) *Radiograph shows an abnormal position of the gastric band ➡, which has slipped inferiorly and rotated clockwise. The connecting tubing ➡ has also migrated into a more rightward position than expected.* **(Right)** *Upright film from an esophagram in the same patient shows dilation of a larger than expected portion of the proximal stomach ➡ with air-fluid-contrast levels, indicating stasis. Slip and rotation of the band often result in obstruction and require revision.*

TERMINOLOGY

Definitions

- Imaging techniques and findings used to evaluate possible complications of surgical procedures meant to induce weight loss

IMAGING

General Features

- Morphology
  - **Laparoscopic adjustable gastric banding (LAGB) procedure**
    - Silicone band with inflatable cuff is looped around fundus, 2-3 cm below gastroesophageal (GE) junction
    - Opening (stoma) is adjustable by accessing subcutaneous port connected to inflatable cuff
      - Fluid is injected into or removed from port to inflate or deflate cuff
    - Complications: Less common and less varied than in laparoscopic **R**oux-en-**Y g**astric **b**ypass (RYGB) procedure
    - May be too tight (→ nausea, dehydration, excessive weight loss) or too loose (→ insufficient restriction of food intake)
    - Twisting or displacement of band (4-13% of patients)
      - Should lie at "phi" angle (between vertical line and horizontal axis of band) between 30-60°
      - May slip down and twist, partially obstructing gastric lumen through band
      - Signs of slip: Phi angle > 60°
        - Distended stomach above band with slow emptying (air-fluid levels)
        - O sign: On frontal image, gastric band is en face seen as O rather than seen in profile
    - May erode into stomach (1-14% of patients)
      - Partial erosion: May have nonspecific symptoms
        - Oral contrast coats intragastric band; may not extravasate beyond stomach
      - Complete erosion: May see intraperitoneal spill of contrast medium (CT or upper GI)
    - Leak from stomach may occur even without erosion of band into stomach (early complication)
    - May be less effective for sustained weight loss than other procedures
  - **Sleeve gastrectomy (gastric sleeve)**
    - 75% of stomach is removed by dividing stomach along its long axis
      - Removes greater curvature portion of fundus, body, and proximal antrum
      - Remaining stomach only holds volume of ~ 100 mL
    - Complications: Less or comparable to LAGB, less than RYGB
      - Leak: Early complication seen in < 1%
        - Usually along proximal end of staple line
        - Extends laterally from greater curvature
      - Stricture: Early or late complication
        - Focal narrowing in mid gastric pouch, at end of staple line
        - May be transient or require stent or revision
      - GE reflux (in 20% of patients)
  - **Laparoscopic RYGB**
    - Surgeon divides stomach into small (~ 30-mL) gastric pouch (parts of cardia and fundus) and much larger excluded stomach (gastric remnant)
    - Excluded stomach (gastric remnant) empties into duodenum as usual, now referred to as biliopancreatic limb
    - Pouch is anastomosed to Roux limb of jejunum (alimentary limb) that is 75-150 cm long
      - Roux limb is usually placed in antegastric and antecolic location
    - Roux (alimentary) and biliopancreatic limbs are joined side to side [jejunojejunal (J-J) anastomosis]
    - Normal postoperative upper GI study
      - Usually performed within 48 hours of surgery to exclude leak or obstruction
      - Esophagus and pouch should empty rapidly into Roux limb
      - Blind end of Roux limb should not be mistaken for leak or ulcer
      - Enteric contrast usually opacifies intestine to and beyond J-J anastomosis
        - Helps to exclude stricture at or near J-J anastomosis
    - Complications: More varied and common than with other bariatric procedures
      - Spasm or stricture at pouch-enteric anastomosis
        - Early (spasm) or late (stricture) complication
        - Recognized by dilated pouch with air-fluid level and slow emptying
        - Fairly common but may resolve or respond to balloon dilation
    - Leak: Usually at pouch-enteric anastomosis (up to 5% of cases)
      - Early (within 10 days) complication
      - Detected with upper GI or CT (complementary) by extravasation of water-soluble contrast medium
      - May be contained; look for opacification of surgical drain lumen
      - May extend into larger spaces, usually left subphrenic and around spleen
    - Marginal ulcer
      - Reported in 3-10% (more common after revision of prior gastric surgery)
      - May result from reflux of acid up Roux limb or ischemic injury
      - Usually appears as fixed collection of barium with adjacent fold thickening
      - Near pouch-enteric anastomosis
    - Gastrogastric fistula
      - Opening of staple line meant to divide gastric pouch from excluded stomach
      - Evident by orally administered contrast material entering excluded stomach
      - May account for failure to lose expected weight, but this is relatively rare complication
    - Small bowel obstruction (affects 5-10% of RYGB patients)
      - Any site of obstruction may be due to adhesions or internal hernia (IH)
      - Think "ABC"

□ A = alimentary (Roux) limb is dilated
  □ Often down to near J-J anastomosis
□ B = biliopancreatic limb (excluded stomach, duodenum, and proximal jejunum)
  □ **This is closed loop obstruction and will not be detected by upper GI series (CT is essential)**
  □ Risk of perforation of stomach or duodenum; usually constitutes surgical emergency
□ C = common channel of bowel beyond J-J anastomosis
– IHs are as common as adhesive obstructions in some reports
  □ CT is more sensitive and specific than fluoroscopic barium studies for diagnosis of IH
  □ CT signs of IH
    □ Cluster of small bowel loops in abnormal location
      □ Through defect in small bowel or transverse colon mesentery
      □ Or between mesentery of Roux limb and transverse colon (Peterson hernia)
    □ **Twisted, displaced, ± dilated mesenteric vessels**
    □ **Displacement of J-J anastomotic staple line** (from expected left mid abdomen to right side of abdomen usually)

Imaging Recommendations

- Best imaging tool
  ○ CT and upper GI radiography; complementary roles
    – Some cases of leaks and obstructions will be more evident on one study than another
    – Fluoroscopy is better at detecting marginal ulcers and pouch-enteric anastomotic strictures
    – CT is better for diagnosis of IH, obstruction of biliopancreatic limb, and complications such as abscess following anastomotic leak
- Protocol advice
  ○ Upper GI series with water-soluble contrast material; performed routinely within 24 hours after surgery
    – If leak is suspected but not shown on study with water-soluble contrast medium, barium may be administered to detect subtle leak
  ○ CT used if small bowel obstruction or intraabdominal abscess suspected
    – In all patients with unexplained fever, pain, abdominal distension following bariatric surgery

CLINICAL ISSUES

Presentation

- Leaks: Incidence of 1-6% after laparoscopic RYGB or LAGB
  ○ Most dreaded complication of bariatric surgery
    – May result in sepsis or death
  ○ Leaks usually occur within first 10 days of surgery
  ○ May present with only tachycardia, abdominal discomfort, with no signs of peritonitis or fever
  ○ High index of suspicion; especially if respiratory distress and tachycardia > 120 beats per minute
- Small bowel obstruction
  ○ Reported in 4-5% of patients after RYGB

○ Laparoscopic approach associated with less trauma; fewer adhesions
  – ↑ prevalence of IH (3%), however
○ Early obstructions within 3 days to 3 months of surgery; more commonly due to adhesions
  – IH develops later (in 90% > 1 month after surgery)
○ Clinical symptoms of IH: Nonspecific nausea, pain
  – IH: Prone to volvulus and strangulation of small bowel
○ May result in closed loop obstruction; can be lethal
- Stenosis at gastrojejunostomy; due to relative ischemia
  ○ Incidence: Up to 27% after RYGB
  ○ Dysphagia, vomiting, dehydration, excessive weight loss; diagnosis usually made with endoscopy
  ○ Late complication; months after surgery
  ○ Usually treatable with endoscopic balloon dilation

Demographics

- Epidemiology
  ○ During last 3 decades, incidence of overweight American adults nearly tripled to 35% (> 12 million)
  ○ Gastric sleeve has become most common bariatric procedure
    – RYGB is next most common
  ○ Gastric banding has decreased markedly within past few years

Natural History & Prognosis

- Advantages of bariatric surgery: Significant, sustained weight loss
  ○ Control or reversal of some obesity-related health problems
    – e.g., diabetes, arthritis, sleep apnea
- Advantages of RYGB: Greater weight loss than other procedures
  ○ Good long-term weight loss and patient tolerance
  ○ Acceptable short- and long-term complication rates
- Advantages of laparoscopic approach to RYGB: ↓ postoperative pain and complications; shorter hospital stay; faster recovery
  ○ Less invasive; especially benefits high-risk morbidly obese patients with multiple comorbidities
- Mortality: < 1% after laparoscopic RYGB, gastric sleeve, or LAGB

DIAGNOSTIC CHECKLIST

Consider

- Nonspecific clinical presentation of some gastrointestinal complications of bariatric surgery
  ○ CT and UGI series are important and complimentary
  ○ Radiologist is often 1st to recognize complications

SELECTED REFERENCES

1. Gaetke-Udager K et al: A guide to imaging in bariatric surgery. Emerg Radiol. 21(3):309-19, 2014
2. Levine MS et al: Imaging of bariatric surgery: normal anatomy and postoperative complications. Radiology. 270(2):327-41, 2014
3. Ni Mhuircheartaigh J et al: Imaging features of bariatric surgery and its complications. Semin Ultrasound CT MR. 34(4):311-24, 2013
4. Sonavane SK et al: Laparoscopic adjustable gastric banding: what radiologists need to know. Radiographics. 32(4):1161-78, 2012
5. Kawamoto S et al: Adjustable laparoscopic gastric banding: demonstrated on multidetector computed tomography with multiplanar reformation and 3-dimensional imaging. J Comput Assist Tomogr. 33(2):288-90, 2009

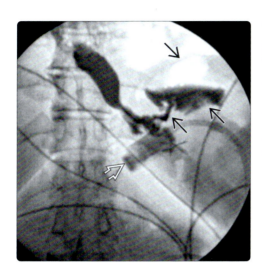

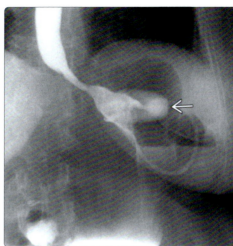

(Left) *Spot film from an esophagram shows a leak* ➡ *of gas and contrast medium following placement of a gastric band* ➡ *around the gastric fundus.* (Right) *Upright film from esophagram shows an abnormally inferior and clockwise-rotated position of the gastric band* ➡. *The oral contrast medium flows over (rather than through) the band, which is sharply outlined by gas within the stomach, indicating intragastric erosion. Perigastric scarring prevented free intraperitoneal spill of contrast medium.*

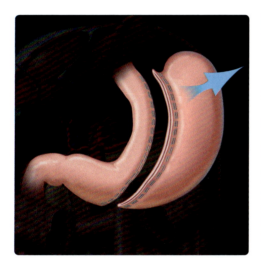

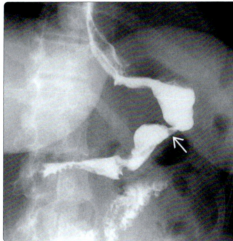

(Left) *Graphic demonstrates the gastric sleeve (sleeve gastrectomy) procedure in which 75% of the stomach is removed by dividing it along its long axis. The remaining stomach is banana-shaped and only ~100 mL in volume.* (Right) *Upright film from an upper GI series in a patient who recently had a gastric sleeve procedure shows the stomach as small and banana-shaped with a focal stricture* ➡ *at the end of the gastric staple line. These strictures are often transient and mild, although this instance required stent dilation.*

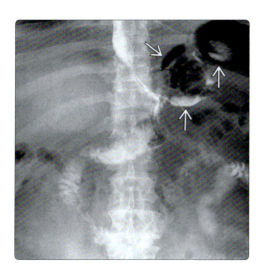

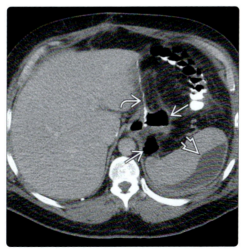

(Left) *This patient had a gastric sleeve procedure 24 hours prior to this upper GI series, which shows extraluminal collections of contrast medium and gas* ➡, *apparently leaking from the gastric staple line.* (Right) *CT scan the same day shows collections of gas and contrast medium* ➡ *adjacent to the gastric staple line* ➡. *Also noted is a subcapsular hematoma* ➡, *likely caused by a retractor injury during surgery.*

(Left) *Graphic shows the typical procedure for a Roux-en-Y gastric bypass (RYGB) procedure with a small gastric pouch* ➡ *anastomosed to a Roux limb that is 75-150 cm long and that is anastomosed side to side with the "biliopancreatic" limb* ➡ *~ 35-45 cm beyond the ligament of Treitz. (Right) Upper GI series in an RYGB patient shows a minor anastomotic leak, evident only as opacification of the surgical drain* ➡ *that was placed near the gastric pouch* ➡ *. The pouch-enteric anastomosis* ➡ *is noted.*

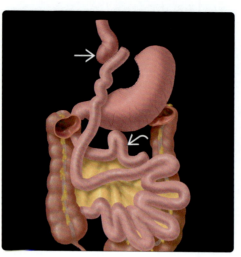
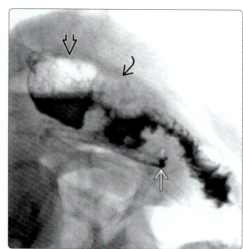

(Left) *Upper GI series in a patient with a major leak days after RYGB shows a large collection of extraluminal contrast material* ➡ *and gas* ➡ *in the left subphrenic space. There is almost no opacification of the small bowel. This is an unusually large leak from the pouch-enteric anastomosis, but the location and timing are typical. Surgical drainage and revision were required. (Right) Film from an upper GI series shows an extraluminal collection of contrast medium* ➡ *in a patient following RYGB.*

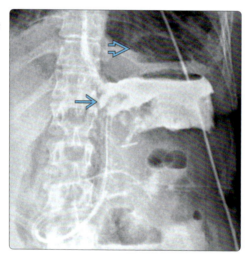
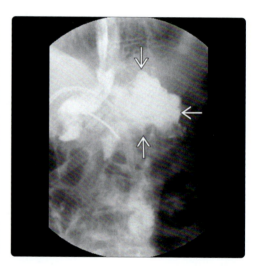

(Left) *CT in the same patient shows the pouch-enteric anastomosis* ➡ *and extraluminal collections* ➡ *of oral contrast medium, gas, and fluid. (Right) Another CT section shows more of the extravasated fluid and gas* ➡ *. These often collect around the spleen, as in this case.*

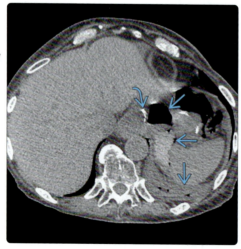
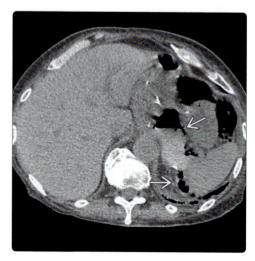

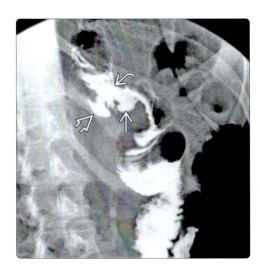

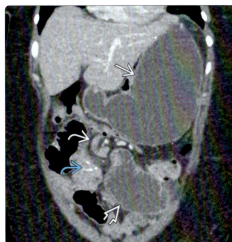

(Left) *Film from an upper GI series shows a marginal ulcer* ➡ *within the Roux limb just beyond the anastomosis* ➡ *with the gastric pouch. The ulcer was a fixed, featureless collection of barium, unlike the blind end* ➡ *of the Roux limb.* (Right) *Coronal reformatted CT following RYGB shows massive dilation of the excluded stomach* ➡ *and biliopancreatic limb* ➡. *The jejunojejunal (J-J) anastomosis* ➡ *is displaced to the right of midline, and the mesenteric vessels* ➡ *are twisted.*

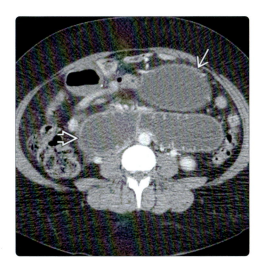

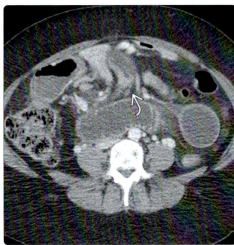

(Left) *Axial CT in the same patient shows the dilated excluded stomach* ➡ *and biliopancreatic limb* ➡. (Right) *Another CT section shows the twisted, engorged mesenteric vessels* ➡ *to the dilated loop. These passed through a defect behind the Roux limb (Peterson internal hernia).*

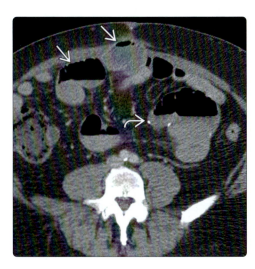

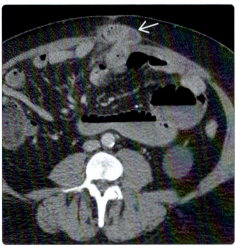

(Left) *CT shows dilation of small bowel, including both the Roux loop and the biliopancreatic limb. The bowel is dilated* ➡ *past the J-J anastomosis* ➡. (Right) *Another CT section shows that the point of obstruction at the midline laparoscopic port site* ➡, *through which the bowel has herniated. Bowel obstruction can result from several circumstances particular to the RYGB technique, including anastomotic strictures and internal and external hernias, some at laparoscopic port sites, as in this case.*

Terminology

Within the past 10 years, the use of CT and MR has more than doubled for pregnant and lactating women with an acute abdominal or pelvic disorder. Conversely, some women have declined or been denied access to needed imaging due to misinformation or an overabundance of caution, resulting in missed diagnoses and other tragic outcomes, including advice to terminate their pregnancy. Our goal in this chapter is to review the accepted and evolving guidelines for the use of imaging and contrast media during pregnancy and lactation.

Risks to Fetus From Radiation Exposure

The leading concern when a pregnant woman is considering an imaging study is the risk related to radiation exposure. This risk can be considered in terms of deterministic and stochastic effects of radiation.

Deterministic effects are those which result from radiation damage to many cells with a threshold before damage occurs. These include teratogenic malformations, growth or intellectual disability, and death. The most vulnerable stage of embryo development in terms of teratogenesis is between the 2nd and 20th week of gestation. In its 2007 recommendations, the International Committee on Radiological Procedures concluded that no deterministic effects of significance would be expected to occur below a dose of 100 mGy. [The average accumulated background radiation dose to an individual in the USA is 1 milligray (1 mGy)]. The unit for equivalent dose is millisievert (mSv). For the purpose of comparing the radiation effects of CT scanning, the 2 terms are interchangeable. **There is essentially no diagnostic imaging study in current use that would result in a risk of fetal death, malformation, or intellectual disability (see table 1).**

Stochastic effects originate from damage to a single cell and can lead to carcinogenesis. While there is considerable controversy about the existence or extent of damage with low doses of radiation, the risk of damage increases with radiation dose. The risk of childhood cancer in the general population is estimated to be 1 in 500. Fetal radiation doses of up to 1 mGy are considered to be acceptable, being associated with an estimated incremental risk of carcinogenesis of < 1 in 10,000. Most radiologic examinations of anatomic structures above the diaphragm or below the knees fall into this category and should not be withheld from pregnant women who would benefit from the information provided. (Many institutions, including our own, do not require informed consent for these very low-dose procedures.) Most radiologic procedures increase the theoretical risk of childhood cancer by < 1 in 1,000. With larger doses (e.g., a fetal dose of 10-25 mGy received during abdominopelvic CT), the risk of carcinogenesis may increase by ~ a factor of 2 (i.e., 2 in 1,000), although it remains very low in absolute terms (see table 2). Placed in another context, the chance that any child would not develop childhood cancer is 99.9%; the **probability of no childhood cancer is still over 99% for those who have received in utero radiation exposure**, as addressed in table 2. Most institutions require informed consent to perform an imaging procedure with moderate to higher dose examinations, and this consent should be obtained by a physician who is well-informed about these issues. As endorsed by the American College of Obstetricians and Gynecologists, along with leading authorities within Radiology and Radiation Physics, **women should be counseled that x-ray exposure to a single diagnostic procedure (resulting in < 50 mGy) does not result in harmful fetal effects.**

Imaging Protocols

Plain Film Radiography

For imaging evaluation of the chest and for extremity trauma, plain radiography exposes the fetus to minimal (< 0.1 mGy) radiation dose. Lead apron shielding of the abdomen decreases this even more but is not considered necessary. Abdominal radiography is associated with a radiation dose from ~ 0.1-3.0 mGy. Because plain films are uncommonly diagnostic or sufficient to evaluate most clinically significant abdominal and pelvic disorders, these are rarely performed in pregnant patients in most institutions.

Ultrasonography

Ultrasonography (US) is the 1st choice for evaluation of pregnant patients with almost any acute abdominal or pelvic disorder, given its lack of ionizing radiation. In the setting of blunt abdominal trauma, US may help identify free intraperitoneal blood and some solid visceral injuries. For gallstones and acute cholecystitis, US is often both sufficient and diagnostic. For other acute, nontraumatic abdominal disorders, such as appendicitis, diverticulitis or bowel obstruction, US usually is not diagnostic, in part due to distortion of abdominal and pelvic anatomy during pregnancy. For most obstetric and gynecologic disorders occurring in pregnant women, US is the 1st-line imaging modality, though MR is assuming an increasing role, as addressed below.

Nuclear Medicine

Unlike radiography and CT, for which the fetus is exposed to ionizing radiation essentially only when the abdomen or pelvis is being imaged, radionuclides are distributed throughout the body and result in fetal radiation, albeit in relatively low doses, regardless of the intended "target" (e.g., a lung, bone, or brain scan). Because of their limited value during pregnancy and because better alternatives exist, radionuclide scintigraphy is rarely requested or performed during pregnancy nor in lactating mothers.

Computed Tomography

For computed tomography (CT), the dose to the fetus varies according to many factors, including patient size, anatomic region being scanned, and CT technical factors. Neither head nor extremity CT is a significant source of fetal radiation (dose near 0 mGy). Some estimated and typical doses from a single CT acquisition are provided in table 1. CT protocols should be tailored to address the clinical concern while limiting radiation dose. Newer CT scanners feature many dose-reducing technical features (e.g., automated exposure control) that substantially reduce radiation dose below levels reported using earlier CT models. In general, multiphasic CT protocols (scanning the same body part during arterial, venous, &/or delayed phases) should not be utilized in pregnant patients, as these result in a substantial increase in dose. Conversely, multiplanar reformations (coronal, sagittal, etc.) are extremely useful and result in no additional radiation dose.

Pulmonary Embolism

Venous thromboembolism is 10x more common in pregnant and recently postpartum women than in the general population and is a leading cause of mortality in this group. Plain chest radiography can help exclude pneumothorax and pneumonia as diagnostic considerations. For pregnant women

Fetal Radiation Doses Associated With Common Radiologic Examinations

Type of Examination	Fetal Dose (in mGY)*
Very Low-Dose Examinations (< 0.1 mGy)	
Cervical spine radiography (anteroposterior and lateral views)	< 0.001
Radiography of extremity	< 0.001
Mammography (2 views)	0.001-0.010
Chest radiography (2 views)	0.0005-0.0100
Low- to Moderate-Dose Examinations (0.1-10.0 mGy)	
Abdominal radiography	0.1-3.0
Lumbar spine radiography	1.0-10
Intravenous pyelography	5-10
Head or neck CT	0.0-0.1
Chest CT or CT-pulmonary embolism study	0.01-0.20
Lung ventilation-perfusion scintigraphy	0.1-0.5
Limited CT pelvimetry (single axial section through femoral heads)	< 1
Technetium-99m bone scintigraphy	4-5
Higher Dose Examinations (10-50 mGy)	
Abdominal CT	1.3-25.0
Pelvic CT	10-25
F-18 PET/CT whole-body scintigraphy	10-50

Note: Annual average background radiation = 1.1-2.5 mGy, F-18 = 2-[fluorine-18] fluoro-2-deoxy-D-glucose, PET = positron emission tomography.
*Fetal exposure varies with gestational age, maternal body habitus, and exact acquisition parameters.

Table adapted and modified from Tremblay E et al: Quality initiatives: guidelines for use of medical imaging during pregnancy and lactation. Radiographics. 32(3):897-911, 2012.

Probability of Birth With No Malformation and No Childhood Cancer

Dose to Fetus (mGy)	No Malformation (%)	No Childhood Cancer (%)	No Malformation and No Childhood Cancer (%)
0.0	96.000	99.930	95.930
0.5	95.999	99.926	95.928
1.0	95.998	99.921	95.922
2.5	95.995	99.908	95.910
5.0	95.990	99.890	95.880
10.0	95.980	99.840	95.830
50.0	95.900	99.510	95.430
100.0	95.800	99.070	94.910

Table directly adapted from McCollough CH et al: Radiation exposure and pregnancy: when should we be concerned? Radiographics. 27(4):909-17; discussion 917-8, 2007.

suspected to have an acute pulmonary embolism, a contrast-enhanced "CT-PE protocol" is the imaging test of choice. CT in this setting has very high sensitivity and specificity (> 90%) and has a similar or lower fetal radiation dose (~ 0.2 mGy) than a radionuclide ventilation-perfusion scan in all 3 trimesters.

Abdominal Trauma

Trauma affects 5-7% of all pregnancies, is often due to assault, and remains the leading cause of nonobstetric maternal and fetal death. Prompt, accurate diagnosis and management are essential. Sonography, including the "FAST" protocol, may be of value in initial screening of the pregnant patient who has suffered significant abdominal trauma, although the accuracy of sonography is decreased in the setting of late pregnancy.

Sonographic evaluation of the fetus and uterus is essential to determine fetal age, injury, and viability as well as placental abruption. Almost regardless of the sonographic findings, contrast-enhanced CT remains the best means of evaluation for significant maternal injury, as well as for uterine injuries, including uterine rupture and placental abruption. CT is of proven safety and accuracy in evaluation of pregnant women who have suffered significant abdominal trauma. CT evaluation of the abdomen and pelvis (plus chest, if indicated) can be achieved without exceeding the threshold of 50 mGy. The use of IV contrast media improves detection of maternal and fetal injuries, including visceral, vascular, and placental. IV iodinated contrast media are not considered (by the USA Food and Drug Administration and other authorities) to have any known adverse effects on the fetus. Based on published experience with hundreds of cases, CT seems to have similar high sensitivity and specificity for detecting traumatic injuries in pregnant patients as in the general population. While no adverse effects of oral or rectal contrast have been reported, we reserve the use of these for evaluation of patient with penetrating torso injuries.

MR is not considered appropriate for evaluation of pregnant patients with blunt or penetrating trauma for many reasons, including the length of the examination, difficulty in monitoring and resuscitating patients within the MR scan room, and lack of a proven, safe IV contrast medium for use in this setting.

Acute Abdominal Pain

A wide variety of disorders, including gastrointestinal, genitourinary, and gynecologic, can present as acute abdominal or pelvic pain in pregnancy with appendicitis being the most common. Clinical and laboratory findings are less definitive in pregnant patients than in the general population. If sonographic evaluation of a pregnant woman with acute abdominal pain is not definitive, CT or MR evaluation should be considered and have been reported to have high sensitivity and specificity in this setting.

For pregnant patients suspected of having an obstructing **renal/ureteral calculus**, imaging evaluation begins with US. While hydronephrosis may be found, this is of less diagnostic value in pregnant women who often have caliectasis and a dilated ureter related to pregnancy, not a real stone. US may demonstrate an echogenic renal stone, but these are rarely the source of symptoms, and ureteral calculi are not well detected by sonography. Lack of a sonographic "ureteral jet" ipsilateral to the side of abdominal or flank pain is supportive of the diagnosis of ureteral calculus. Many patients are best evaluated by a noncontrast-enhanced "renal stone protocol CT." It is especially useful for clinicians to convey renal stone as a leading diagnostic consideration, as this CT protocol is very different than the "acute abdomen CT" protocol. Because renal calculi are very dense, they are easily detected on low-dose, nonenhanced CT scans, which may not be sufficient to diagnose other conditions.

To rule out **appendicitis** and other **infectious/inflammatory conditions**, an IV contrast-enhanced CT of the abdomen and pelvis is performed with multiplanar reformations offering valuable additional information without increased radiation dose. CT signs of appendicitis are the same as reported in the nonpregnant population, namely a distended, thick-walled appendix usually with periappendiceal inflammation and often with a visible appendicolith.

More recently, MR has been found to be an accurate means of diagnosing appendicitis and other conditions during pregnancy. MR is considered to be safe in pregnancy regardless of the trimester. Limiting factors include reduced availability, less experience in performance and interpretation, and the understandable reluctance to administer gadolinium-based contrast media intravenously to a pregnant woman, given concerns about potential gadolinium toxicity to the fetus. The MR signs of acute appendicitis are essentially the same as those on CT. While contrast enhancement of the appendiceal wall cannot be evaluated, other MR features can act as surrogate findings of acute inflammation (e.g., bright signal on diffusion-weighted and T2W MR). MR does not detect appendicoliths as well as CT, though this may not be a major limitation.

The list of **other disorders** accounting for acute abdominal pain in pregnancy diagnosed by CT and MR grows steadily, including small bowel and colonic obstruction, diaphragmatic and abdominal wall hernias, and diverticulitis. Patients with inflammatory bowel disease (Crohn's disease or ulcerative colitis) are generally evaluated better by MR than by CT, although this has been established in the nonpregnant population for the most part. Similarly, there is extensive validation of the accuracy and utility of MR for acute gynecologic causes of abdominal/pelvic pain, such as endometriosis, torsed and degenerated fibroids, and adnexal masses, though experience within the subset of pregnant patients is much more limited.

Known or Suspected Abdominal or Pelvic Malignancy

It is uncommon, but not rare, to encounter a pregnant woman with a palpable abdominal or pelvic mass, or clinical/laboratory signs of malignancy, raising concern for a primary or metastatic focus within the abdomen. As with other conditions, the decision concerning the choice and timing of an imaging study must weigh multiple factors, including fetal age and radiation dose. As noted above, imaging of the abdomen and pelvis can be accomplished with individual or even combined studies that result in fetal radiation dose considered to have small to negligible danger to the fetus. The health and well-being of the mother should also be weighed carefully, including the danger of a delayed or missed diagnosis of abdominal malignancy.

Use of Contrast Media in Lactating Mothers

The benefits of breastfeeding are well established, and physicians should do their part in its encouragement. Even a temporary cessation of breastfeeding may lead to complete cessation. Many drugs are excreted into breast milk, though predominantly those of low molecular weight. Because iodinated and gadolinium-based contrast media are of high molecular weight, nonionized, and water soluble, there is minimal excretion into breast milk. As a general rule, a drug can be considered safe for breast-fed babies if the dose that reaches the infant is < 10% of its therapeutic dose. For iodinated (CT) and gadolinium-based (MR) contrast media, < 1% of the contrast medium reaches the breast milk, and even this amount falls rapidly within a few hours of administration to the lactating mother. Therefore, **there is no valid medical reason to discourage a lactating mother who has had a recent enhanced CT or MR scan from breastfeeding** her infant. Some physicians, acting with extreme caution, encourage the mother to consider discarding breast milk for one feeding ("pump and dump").

Selected References

1. Tirada N et al: Imaging pregnant and lactating patients. Radiographics. 35(6):1751-65, 2015
2. Tremblay E et al: Quality initiatives: guidelines for use of medical imaging during pregnancy and lactation. Radiographics. 32(3):897-911, 2012
3. McCollough CH et al: Radiation exposure and pregnancy: when should we be concerned? Radiographics. 27(4):909-17; discussion 917-8, 2007

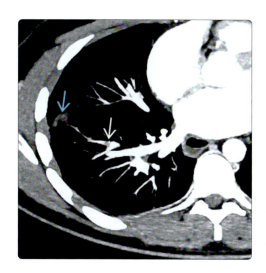

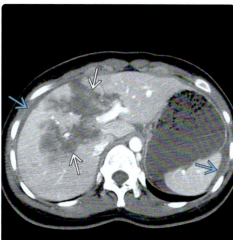

(Left) *In this young woman with chest pain & hypoxemia, PE protocol CT scan shows 1 of several pulmonary emboli* ➡ *& infarcted lung tissue* ➡. *Pulmonary emboli are diagnosed confidently & safely during pregnancy by CT.* (Right) *In this woman injured by a motor vehicle crash during her 2nd trimester, the FAST exam showed hemoperitoneum. CT shows hemoperitoneum* ➡ *and a deep, complex hepatic laceration* ➡. *The absence of active bleeding on CT helped direct successful nonoperative management.*

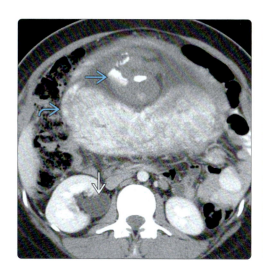

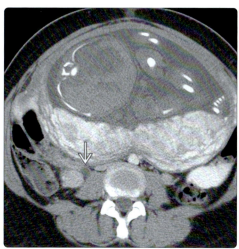

(Left) *In this young woman with flank pain and sonographic evidence of hydronephrosis during her 2nd trimester, axial CECT section shows the gravid uterus, placenta* ➡, *and fetus* ➡. *The right renal pelvis is dilated* ➡, *but the kidneys enhance normally and symmetrically.* (Right) *In the same patient, this and other CT sections show the dilated ureter* ➡ *but no obstructing stone or mass. Symptoms resolved soon after completion of the CT scan.*

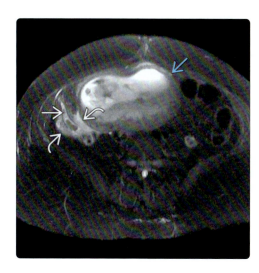

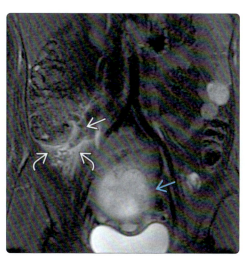

(Left) *In this young woman with acute abdominal pain and fever during her 2nd trimester, MR shows the gravid uterus* ➡, *and a dilated appendix* ➡ *surrounded by inflamed fat* ➡ *and marked by bright signal on this T2-weighted image, diagnostic of acute appendicitis.* (Right) *In the same woman, coronal MR section also shows the dilated appendix* ➡ *and adjacent inflammation* ➡ *as well as the gravid uterus* ➡.

(Left) *In this woman with acute right abdominal pain and fever during her 3rd trimester, a coronal CECT section shows 2 of many right-sided diverticula* ➡ *with inflammation of the pericolonic fat* ➡, *indicating acute diverticulitis.* (Right) *In this young woman with abdominal pain in her 3rd trimester, sonography had demonstrated stones in the gallbladder but no signs of acute inflammation. MRCP shows the gallstones* ➡ *as well as stones* ➡ *within a dilated common bile duct.*

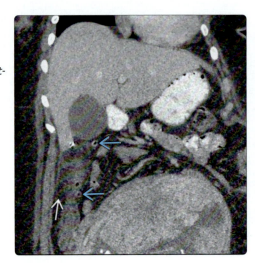
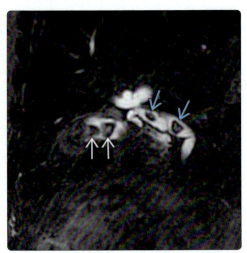

(Left) *In this young woman with acute abdominal pain and diarrhea during her 2nd trimester, MR enterography shows fluid distention of the bowel* ➡ *and colon* ➡. *The wall of the entire colon is thickened with engorged colonic vessels* ➡. (Right) *In the same patient, the engorged mesenteric vessels* ➡, *fluid-distended colon, and its thickened wall* ➡ *are again noted, along with the gravid uterus* ➡. *Ulcerative colitis was confirmed.*

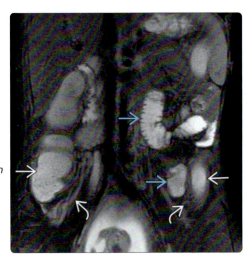
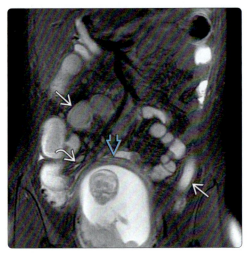

(Left) *In this young woman with right abdominal pain and hypotension during her 3rd trimester, coronal MR shows the fetal brain* ➡ *within the gravid uterus and a normal gallbladder* ➡. *A large hemorrhagic mass* ➡ *is surrounded by fluid* ➡ *and indents the liver.* (Right) *Another coronal T2W MR shows the large mass* ➡ *displacing the kidney* ➡ *inferiorly. A hemorrhagic adrenal cyst was surgically removed.*

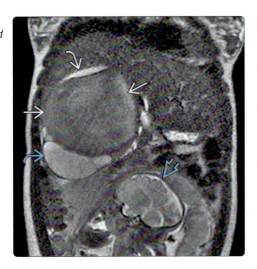
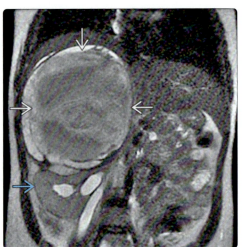

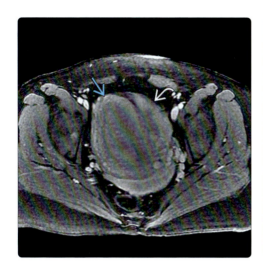
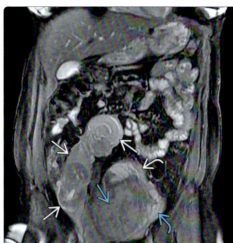

(Left) *In this woman with abdominal pain in her 3rd trimester, axial T1W MR shows an enlarged but empty uterus →. The placenta → is implanted on the outer surface of the uterus.* (Right) *In the same case, coronal MR shows the fetus → lying within the peritoneal cavity, an intraabdominal ectopic pregnancy in an unusually advanced state. The placenta → and its engorged vessels → lie on the surface of the enlarged but empty uterus →.*

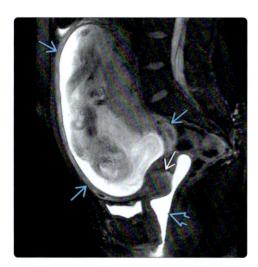
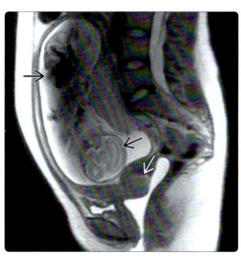

(Left) *In this woman with a visible and palpable cervical mass found during her 3rd trimester, sagittal, fat-suppressed T2WI MR shows the gravid uterus → with the vagina marked and distended with sonographic gel →. A solid cervical mass → is identified.* (Right) *In the same patient, another T2WI MR, without fat suppression, shows the fetus → within the gravid uterus and the cervical mass →, which proved to be an invasive carcinoma.*

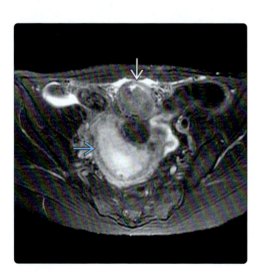
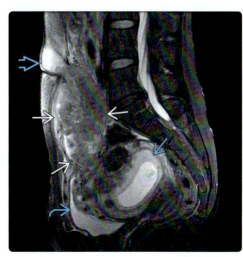

(Left) *In this 36-year-old woman with a palpable abdominal mass and a 1st trimester pregnancy, axial T2WI MR section shows part of the gravid uterus → and part of the midline abdominal-pelvic mass →.* (Right) *In the same patient, sagittal T2WI MR shows the gravid uterus → and a large midline mass → that extends from the bladder → to the umbilicus → representing a urachal carcinoma.*

Common Symptoms, Signs, and Conditions

IMAGING

- Afferent loop (AL) syndrome
  - AL becomes obstructed by adhesions, recurrent tumor, internal hernia, etc.
  - CT is better than fluoroscopic studies for this diagnosis
- Colonoscopy and other endoscopic procedures
  - Prevalence of complications is 1-2%
  - CT shows perforation best and more safely
- Enterectomy and anastomosis
  - Low rectal anastomoses are especially prone to ischemia, stricture, leak, and fistulas
- Small bowel anastomoses
  - Side-to-side anastomosis may simulate obstruction or "aneurysmal dilation"
  - Identify metallic staple lines on CT
- Ileoanal pouch
  - Create reservoir (pouch) of ileum that is anastomosed to distal rectum or anal sphincter

- Fluoroscopic and CT studies are complementary and essential to diagnose complications
  - Usually perform "pouchogram" (fluoroscopic-controlled contrast injection of ileoanal pouch through anus)
  - Performed whenever leak or stricture is suspected
  - Performed prior to takedown of diverting ileostomy
- For fluoroscopic retrograde contrast injection
  - Use soft catheter with balloon inflated within healthy portion of bowel
- Enteroclysis: May show subtle adhesive obstruction or leak missed by other modalities
- CT enterography (ingested contrast medium) or enteroclysis (pump-injected contrast medium)
- CT has advantage of better delineation of disease beyond bowel wall (e.g., abscess)
  - **IV contrast is essential for CT evaluation; uncommonly need oral/enteric contrast**

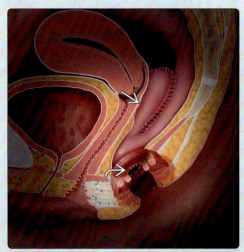 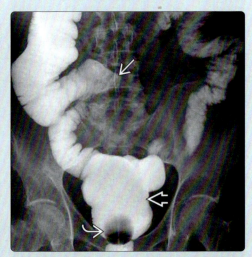

(Left) Lateral view of the pelvis shows the results of a prior proctocolectomy with creation of a J-shaped ileal pouch ➡ that has been anastomosed to the anal sphincter ➡. (Right) "Pouchogram" shows evidence of the prior colectomy with an ileoanal pouch ➡. The balloon tip of the catheter ➡ used to inject the contrast medium is just above the ileoanal anastomosis. The sharp angulation and tethered appearance of a segment of small bowel (SB) ➡ are typical of an adhesive SB obstruction (SBO).

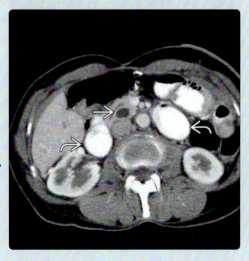 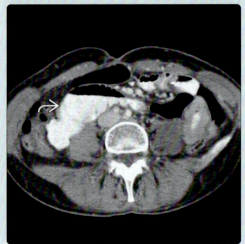

(Left) Axial CECT in a patient with afferent loop syndrome following Billroth II procedure shows dilated bile ducts ➡ down to the ampulla. The afferent limb (duodenum) ➡ is dilated due to a stricture that caused partial bowel obstruction. (Right) Dilated duodenum ➡ (same patient) is filled with oral contrast medium, which is somewhat unusual since a stricture at the gastroenteric anastomosis often precludes filling of this segment. The elevated intraluminal pressure within the duodenum contributed to the biliary obstruction.

TERMINOLOGY

Definitions

- Enterotomy: Surgical entry of bowel to remove polyp, foreign body, etc., or to insert enteric tube
- Enteroplasty: Surgical alteration of bowel, usually to open strictured segment
- Plication: Alteration of bowel to relieve obstruction
- Enterectomy: Resection of damaged or neoplastic segment of bowel
- Colectomy: Resection of damaged or neoplastic segment of colon
- Ostomy: Temporary or permanent opening of bowel onto surface of abdomen for feeding or drainage purposes

IMAGING

General Features

- **Upper gastrointestinal surgery**
  - Involves resection of some portion of stomach and proximal bowel with creation of gastroenteric anastomosis
    - e.g., Billroth II partial gastrectomy, Whipple procedure (pancreaticoduodenectomy)
  - Dumping syndrome
    - Loss of pyloric sphincter allows rapid emptying of hyperosmotic gastric contents into jejunum
    - Symptoms: Nausea, urgent diarrhea, lightheadedness immediately after eating
    - Imaging: Nonspecific; may show dilation and hyperperistalsis of jejunum
  - Afferent loop (AL) syndrome
    - AL becomes obstructed by adhesions, recurrent tumor, internal hernia, etc.
    - AL varies by type of surgical procedure
      - Billroth II: AL = duodenum
      - Whipple: AL = Roux jejunal loop
      - Roux-en-Y gastric bypass: AL = duodenum and proximal jejunum ("pancreaticobiliary limb")
    - Symptoms: Nonspecific; no bilious vomiting; dilation of AL may result in progressive dilation of AL and perforation; may lead to malnutrition, jaundice
    - Imaging: Plain films and barium fluoroscopic exams often miss this complication as AL is fluid-distended and oral contrast medium does not enter AL
    - CT shows dilation of AL and any complications (e.g., dilated bile ducts, recurrent tumor, perforation)
- **Colonoscopy and other endoscopic procedures**
  - Complication rate is low but varies by clinical setting, type of procedure, and experience of endoscopist
  - Perforation
    - Can occur with or without biopsy
    - Prevalence is < 1% for "routine" colonoscopy
    - Prevalence after polypectomy ~ 1-2%
    - CT detects extraluminal gas and fluid more accurately than plain radiography
  - Bleeding
    - Occurs in 30-50% who have polypectomy
      - Usually resolves without specific treatment
  - Postpolypectomy syndrome
    - Due to burn of colonic wall during polyp removal by "hot wire" snare
    - Symptoms: Pain, fever, leukocytosis
    - Usually resolves with medical and supportive therapy
- **Enterectomy and anastomosis**
  - Any resection and anastomosis done in setting of peritoneal contamination or borderline viability of bowel is prone to dehiscence or stricture
    - **Low rectal anastomoses are especially prone to ischemia, stricture, leak, and fistulas**
      - Vascular supply is tenuous and surgical exposure of operative field is limited
  - Small bowel (SB) anastomoses
    - May be end-to-end, end-to-side, side-to-side
    - End-to-end is most physiologic but most prone to anastomotic stricture
    - End- or side-to-side anastomoses have lower prevalence of stricture or obstruction but higher rate of stasis within "blind segments"
      - May cause bacterial overgrowth problems
    - Side-to-side: Bowel appears at least twice diameter of normal bowel
      - May simulate "aneurysmal dilation" but no thickening of wall (unlike SB lymphoma, metastases, or gastrointestinal stromal tumor, other causes of aneurysmal dilation)
    - Imaging
      - CT usually shows metallic staples at anastomotic suture line
      - Water-soluble contrast medium can be administered orally, rectally, or through ostomy to visualize anastomosis and other bowel segments
  - Short bowel syndrome
    - Follows resection of critical length of SB
      - Jejunal length < 200 cm usually necessitates nutritional support
      - Loss of ileum leads to deficiency of vitamin and bile salt absorption
      - Usual reasons for loss of SB: Recurrent surgery for Crohn's disease, intestinal ischemia, strangulated internal hernia, Gardner syndrome with mesenteric desmoids
      - Can be treated with long-term parenteral nutrition or small bowel transplantation
      - Fluoroscopic small bowel study and CT are used to estimate length and health of remaining bowel
- **Enterostomy**
  - Often for placement of jejunal feeding tube for long-term enteral nutrition
  - Pneumatosis in this setting does not necessarily indicate bowel infarction or ischemia
  - Complications: Leak of enteric contents; obstruction
  - Caution: Use of balloon-tipped catheter within SB is associated with risk of intussusception and obstruction
  - Concern for leak can be assessed with contrast injection through jejunostomy tube plus plain film, fluoroscopy, or CT to follow
- **Ileostomy**
  - Conventional (end) ileostomy
    - Distal ileum brought (permanently) to skin surface
    - Leads to fecal incontinence, requires ileostomy bag

- o "Loop" (double-barrel, diverting) ileostomy
  - – Usually intended as temporary diversion of most or all of fecal stream
  - – Usually performed in setting of recent distal bowel anastomosis
  - – Diverting ostomy decompresses bowel to protect distal anastomosis until healing is complete
  - o Complications
    - – Adhesions, recurrent disease, parastomal herniation (of fat ± bowel)
- **Small bowel reservoirs**
  - o Continence-preserving surgical procedures
  - o Preferred technique to restore function and body image following colectomy
  - o Koch-type continent ileostomy (uncommonly performed)
    - – Complex surgical procedure that results in internal ileal reservoir and continence (no bag) but requires periodic emptying of reservoir by intubation of stoma
  - o Ileoanal pouch
    - – Preferred procedure following colectomy
    - – 2 important components
      - □ Remove mucosa of rectum/anus (to prevent recurrence of original disease)
      - □ Create reservoir (pouch) of ileum that is anastomosed to distal rectum or anal sphincter
    - – Simplest to illustrate and perform is "J" pouch
      - □ Pouch created by taking distal 25 cm of ileum and forming into "J" shape with side-to-side anastomosis of adjacent segments
      - □ Dependent part of pouch is anastomosed to rectum or anus
    - – Diverting ileostomy is usually performed to protect anastomotic staple lines for several months
      - □ Contrast enema (through rectum or ileostomy) or CECT is performed to establish patency and integrity of anastomosis
      - □ Following confirmation of intact pouch and anastomosis, diverting ostomy is closed (about 8-12 weeks after surgery)
    - – Complications
      - □ Anastomotic strictures or dehiscence, abscess, adhesions, fistulas, "pouchitis"
      - □ Ileoanal pouch "failure" (need for permanent end ileostomy) in ~10%
    - – Caution
      - □ Surgeon may leave blind-ending pouch that communicates with main pouch
      - □ Enteric contrast ± gas may fill this and mimic leak of extraluminal contents
    - – Imaging evaluation
      - □ Usually perform "pouchogram" (fluoroscopic-controlled contrast injection of ileoanal pouch through anus)
      - □ Performed whenever leak or stricture is suspected
      - □ Performed prior to takedown of diverting ileostomy

Imaging Recommendations

- Protocol advice

- o For fluoroscopic inspection of bowel using retrograde contrast injection
  - – Use soft balloon-tipped catheter with balloon inflated within healthy portion of bowel
  - – Water soluble (iodinated) contrast material is used
- o Fluoroscopic enteroclysis
  - – Best technique for detailed depiction of bowel anatomy
    - □ May show subtle adhesive obstruction or leak missed by other modalities
- o CT enterography (ingested contrast medium) or enteroclysis (pump-injected contrast medium)
  - – Probably equivalent to fluoroscopic enteroclysis for evaluation of bowel
  - – CT has advantage of better delineation of disease beyond bowel wall
    - □ Abscess, fistula, etc.
- o **Multiplanar reformations of CT and IV contrast administration are essential**
  - – Coronal and other planes frequently help delineate pertinent anatomy and pathology

DIAGNOSTIC CHECKLIST

Image Interpretation Pearls

- Radiologist must know specific surgical procedure performed in order to conduct and interpret imaging study correctly
  - o Postoperative anatomy may be complicated and confusing, especially in patients with multiple prior bowel resections

SELECTED REFERENCES

1. Farinella E et al: Modified H-pouch as an alternative to the J-pouch for anorectal reconstruction. Colorectal Dis. 16(9):O332-4, 2014
2. Sanada Y et al: Recurrent cholangitis by biliary stasis due to non-obstructive afferent loop syndrome after pylorus-preserving pancreatoduodenectomy: report of a case. Int Surg. 99(4):426-31, 2014
3. Lee WY et al: Endoscopic treatment of efferent loop syndrome with insertion of double pigtail stent. World J Gastroenterol. 19(41):7209-12, 2013
4. Hoda KM et al: Predictors of pouchitis after ileal pouch-anal anastomosis: a retrospective review. Dis Colon Rectum. 51(5):554-60, 2008
5. Kiran RP et al: Complications and functional results after ileoanal pouch formation in obese patients. J Gastrointest Surg. 12(4):668-74, 2008
6. Pfefferkorn U et al: Recurrent pancreatitis as only presenting symptom of intermittent small bowel obstruction after biliopancreatic diversion with duodenal switch. Surg Obes Relat Dis. 4(2):202-4, 2008
7. Power N et al: CT assessment of anastomotic bowel leak. Clin Radiol. 62(1):37-42, 2007
8. Crema MD et al: Pouchography, CT, and MRI features of ileal J pouch-anal anastomosis. AJR Am J Roentgenol. 187(6):W594-603, 2006
9. Sandrasegaran K et al: CT findings for postsurgical blind pouch of small bowel. AJR Am J Roentgenol. 186(1):110-3, 2006
10. Sandrasegaran K et al: CT of acute biliopancreatic limb obstruction. AJR Am J Roentgenol. 186(1):104-9, 2006
11. Sandrasegaran K et al: Small-bowel complications of major gastrointestinal tract surgery. AJR Am J Roentgenol. 185(3):671-81, 2005
12. Hui GC et al: Small-bowel intussusception around a gastrojejunostomy tube resulting in ischemic necrosis of the intestine. Pediatr Radiol. 34(11):916-8, 2004
13. Blake MF et al: Intestinal obstruction following biliopancreatic diversion. Dig Dis Sci. 48(4):737-40, 2003
14. Kim HC et al: Afferent loop obstruction after gastric cancer surgery: helical CT findings. Abdom Imaging. 28(5):624-30, 2003
15. Carucci LR et al: Evaluation of patients with jejunostomy tubes: imaging findings. Radiology. 223(1):241-7, 2002

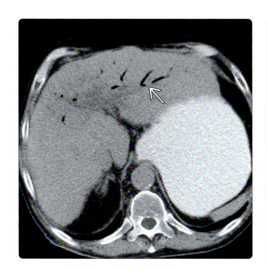

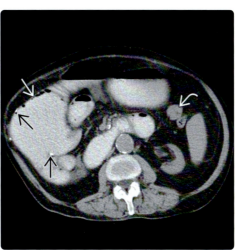

(Left) *Axial NECT shows portal venous gas* ➡️ *in this patient with recurrent bowel obstruction following prior enterectomy.* (Right) *Axial CECT in the same patient shows marked dilation of a segment of SB* ➡️*, but the presence of surgical staples* ➡️ *and absence of a bowel wall mass indicate that this is the result of a prior side-to-side anastomosis. The proximal SB is dilated, while the distal bowel is collapsed* ➡️*. The obstruction and portal venous gas resolved without surgery and were presumed to have resulted from adhesive SBO.*

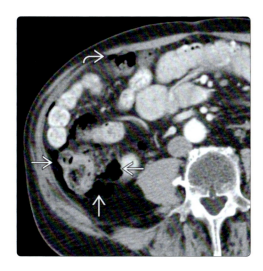

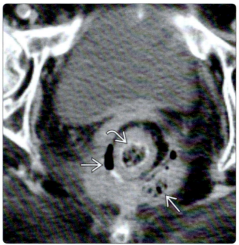

(Left) *Axial CECT in a patient with abdominal pain following colonoscopy and biopsy of a cecal mass shows extraluminal gas* ➡️ *near the cecum that is both retroperitoneal and intraperitoneal* ➡️*. The biopsy had shown adenocarcinoma of the cecum, and this and the perforation were confirmed at surgery.* (Right) *Axial CECT in a patient with pain and fever following proctocolectomy for diverticulitis shows metallic staples at the site of the sigmoid anastomosis* ➡️ *and extraluminal gas, fluid, and enteric contrast media* ➡️*, indicating anastomotic leak.*

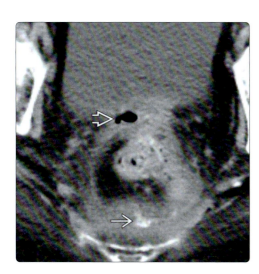

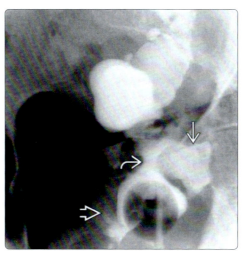

(Left) *Axial CECT in the same patient shows more of the extraluminal gas and contrast medium* ➡️*, including some that has entered the vagina* ➡️*, indicating colovaginal fistula from an anastomotic breakdown.* (Right) *Spot film from a contrast enema in the same patient shows narrowing at the level of the anastomosis* ➡️*, retrorectal extravasation* ➡️*, and filling of the vagina* ➡️*. Anastomotic leaks often result in infection and further breakdown of the anastomosis; abscesses and fistulas commonly result.*

Disorders Affecting Multiple Organs

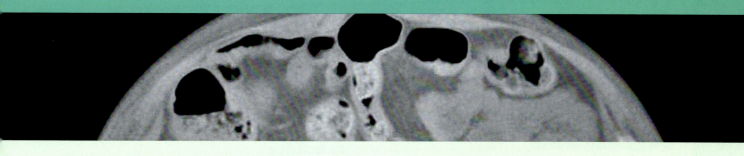

KEY FACTS

TERMINOLOGY

- Abdominal opportunistic infections and neoplasms resulting from HIV/AIDS-related immunodeficiency

IMAGING

- **Liver and spleen**
  - Small hypodense nodules may be microabscesses
  - Larger hypodense lesions might be infectious, but AIDS-related lymphoma should be considered
  - *Pneumocystis* may result in tiny calcifications
- **Biliary tree**
  - Cholangitis or acalculous cholecystitis caused by opportunistic infections
- **Stomach, small bowel, and large bowel**
  - Wall thickening raises concern for opportunistic infection, which can involve any segment of GI tract
  - Mural thickening of esophagus suggests esophagitis, often due to candidiasis, CMV, or HSV
  - Proctitis in homosexual men related to sexual activity may be due to *Neisseria gonorrhoeae*, *Chlamydia*, or HSV
  - Focal mass-like wall thickening in GI tract should raise concern for malignancy (lymphoma, Kaposi sarcoma)
- **Lymph nodes**
  - Mild generalized lymphadenopathy (usually < 1.5 cm) is typically reactive and may be 1st clue to HIV infection
  - More significant adenopathy (> 1.5 cm) suggests opportunistic infection or AIDS-related lymphoma
- **Kidneys**
  - Bilateral large kidneys (↑ echogenicity on US) with urothelial thickening due to HIV nephropathy

PATHOLOGY

- Infections more common in HIV patients even with CD4 > 200, although risk ↑ substantially with lower CD4 counts
- Incidence of AIDS-defining malignancies (AIDS-related non-Hodgkin lymphoma, Kaposi sarcoma) has dramatically decreased with effective antiretroviral therapy

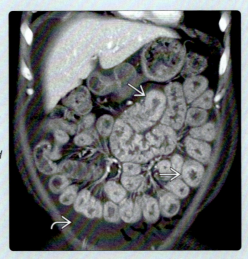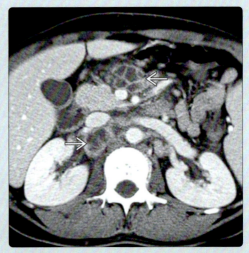

(Left) Coronal volume-rendered CECT in an AIDS patient with low CD4 count demonstrates diffuse wall thickening of the small bowel ➡ with ascites ➡. The bowel appeared similar on several subsequent studies, and this was found to be infection with MAI. (Right) Axial CECT in an HIV(+) patient presenting with 3 weeks of fever, diarrhea, and weight loss shows multiple sites of low-attenuation lymphadenopathy ➡ involving retroperitoneal and mesenteric nodes. Biopsy confirmed MAI.

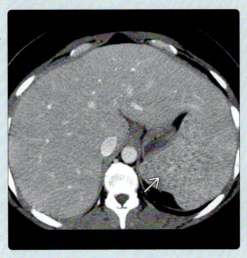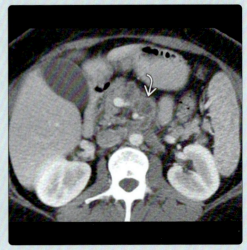

(Left) Axial CECT shows innumerable small hypodense foci in the spleen ➡ and, more subtly, in the liver. Both the liver and spleen are enlarged. All findings were due to disseminated mycobacterial infection. (Right) Axial CECT in the same patient demonstrates multiple low-density enlarged lymph nodes ➡. This constellation of findings was found to represent disseminated mycobacterial infection.

TERMINOLOGY

Abbreviations

- Acquired immune deficiency syndrome (AIDS)
- Human immunodeficiency virus (HIV)

Definitions

- Abdominal opportunistic infections and neoplasms resulting from HIV/AIDS-related immunodeficiency

IMAGING

General Features

- Location
  - Can affect visceral organs, GI tract, genitourinary tract, and lymph nodes
- Size
  - Variable: Ranges from microabscesses (< 1 cm) to large masses due to lymphoma or Kaposi sarcoma

Imaging Recommendations

- Best imaging tool
  - CECT

CT Findings

- **Liver**
  - Liver may appear nodular and cirrhotic due to strong demographic overlap of HIV and chronic viral hepatitis
  - Small hypodense nodules scattered throughout liver suggests microabscesses [often due to *Mycobacterium avium-intracellulare* (MAI), tuberculosis, histoplasmosis, *Candida*, *Pneumocystis*, etc.]
  - Liver may appear globally enlarged without focal lesions due to infiltrative infections (e.g., MAI)
  - *Pneumocystis* (and rarely CMV or MAI) can result in multiple tiny calcifications throughout liver
    - Calcifications do not signify inactive disease
  - Liver is involved in up to 1/4 of patients with AIDS-related lymphoma with hypodense nodules of variable size
- **Biliary tree**
  - Cholangitis may be caused by opportunistic infections
    - Intrahepatic and extrahepatic biliary strictures with papillary stenosis: Bile ducts may appear thickened and enhancing
    - Bile ducts may have beaded appearance very similar to primary sclerosing cholangitis
  - Acalculous cholecystitis may due to opportunistic infections (e.g., CMV, *Cryptosporidium*)
    - Thickened gallbladder with pericholecystic fluid and stranding
- **Spleen**
  - Splenomegaly in up to 3/4 of AIDS patients even without infection or tumor
  - Small tiny hypodense foci (microabscesses) usually due to disseminated infection (e.g., *Candida*, MAI, tuberculosis, *Pneumocystis*, etc.)
  - Larger hypodense lesions might still be infectious, but AIDS-related lymphoma should also be considered
  - Small calcifications (similar to liver) from *Pneumocystis*
- **Stomach, small bowel, and large bowel**
  - Bowel wall thickening, mucosal hyperemia, and fat stranding surrounding bowel should always raise concern for infection (including opportunistic infections)
    - CMV-related ulcerations of bowel may lead to GI tract perforation (one of most common reasons for emergent abdominal surgery in AIDS patients)
  - Most opportunistic infections can involve any segment of GI tract (*Cryptosporidium*, CMV, MAI, tuberculosis, microsporidium, *Clostridium difficile*, amebiasis, etc.)
    - Difficult to predict pathogen based on distribution, but some organisms have predisposition for certain locations
      - CMV and TB tend to involve ileum
      - *Giardia*, microsporidium tend to involve proximal small bowel
      - Colon infections often due to CMV, *C. difficile*, *Campylobacter*, amebiasis, *Salmonella*, and *Shigella*
  - Mural thickening of esophagus suggests esophagitis, often due to candidiasis, CMV, or herpes simplex
  - Proctitis in homosexual men due to sexual activity may be due to *Neisseria gonorrhoeae*, chlamydia, or HSV
  - Focal mass-like wall thickening anywhere in GI tract should raise concern for malignancy (AIDS-related lymphoma, Kaposi sarcoma)
    - Lymphoma associated with intussusceptions
- **Lymph nodes**
  - Mild generalized lymphadenopathy (< 1.5 cm) is usually reactive and may be 1st clue to HIV infection
    - May persist for years in absence of symptoms (i.e., persistent generalized lymphadenopathy)
  - More significant adenopathy (> 1.5 cm) suggests opportunistic infection (MAI, tuberculosis) or AIDS-related lymphoma/Kaposi sarcoma
    - Necrotic mesenteric nodes from MAI or tuberculosis
    - Hyperenhancing lymph nodes in Kaposi sarcoma
  - AIDS-related lymphoma may be associated with discrete lesions in liver/spleen or focal mass in GI tract
    - GI tract most common extranodal site of involvement (75%), most often involving colon, ileum, and stomach
- **Kidneys**
  - Bilateral large kidneys with urothelial thickening due to HIV nephropathy
  - Focal hypodense lesions could reflect infection (tuberculosis, MAI, fungus) or AIDS-related lymphoma
  - Calcifications may be present in setting of *Pneumocystis* (similar to liver and spleen) or rarely MAI/CMV
- **Pancreas**
  - Opportunistic infections can cause acute pancreatitis and pancreatic duct strictures (e.g., CMV, *Cryptococcus*, etc.)

Ultrasonographic Findings

- **Kidneys**
  - HIV nephropathy: Normal sized or enlarged kidneys with increased echogenicity (kidney > liver)
    - May be associated with urothelial thickening in pelvis/intrarenal collecting system
    - Parenchymal heterogeneity and loss of corticomedullary differentiation
  - Hyperechoic foci or calcifications without posterior acoustic shadowing due to *Pneumocystis*, MAI, or CMV
- **Gallbladder**

- o GB wall thickening may be reactive due to hepatitis or secondary to opportunistic acute acalculous cholecystitis
- o Wall thickening and dilation of extrahepatic &/or intrahepatic bile ducts due to AIDS cholangiopathy
- **Liver**
  - o Opportunistic infections present as small hypoechoic nodules (microabscesses) scattered throughout liver
  - o *Pneumocystis* may result in small hypoechoic nodules or tiny echogenic foci
- **Lymph nodes**
  - o Necrotic nodes most often due to MAI or tuberculosis

DIFFERENTIAL DIAGNOSIS

Lymphoma Unrelated to HIV/AIDS

- Nodal involvement more common, unlike AIDS, where extranodal involvement is disproportionately common
- AIDS-related lymphoma often aggressive with widespread dissemination, whereas non-AIDS related lymphoma may present with early stage disease confined to nodes

Biliary Hamartomas

- Multiple small cystic lesions scattered throughout liver
- May mimic hepatic microabscesses, but patients are asymptomatic without signs of infection

Sarcoidosis

- May present with multiple small hypodense lesions in liver and spleen (mimicking microabscesses)
- Upper abdominal adenopathy frequently present, and may be mistaken for HIV-related adenopathy
- Mediastinal and hilar lymphadenopathy as well as characteristic lung disease may allow distinction

PATHOLOGY

General Features

- Etiology
  - o HIV results in immunodeficiency through infection and lysis of CD4(+) T cells
  - o HIV-infected patients have increased risk of developing malignancies, particularly when coinfected by Epstein-Barr virus, herpesvirus, or papillomavirus
    - Incidence of AIDS-defining malignancies (AIDS-related non-Hodgkin lymphoma, Kaposi sarcoma) has dramatically ↓ with effective antiretroviral therapy
    - HIV-infected patients are at risk of other malignancies, which are often atypically aggressive and occur at younger ages than usual
    - **Non-Hodgkin lymphoma**
      - □ AIDS-defining malignancy (usually CD4 count < 100) that includes several types of lymphoma, including diffuse large B-cell and Burkitt lymphoma
      - □ Strong tendency to arise in extranodal sites (especially GI tract), involve unusual locations, and present with advanced disease
    - **Kaposi sarcoma**
      - □ Low-grade soft tissue sarcoma of vascular origin associated with HHV-8 infection
  - o Infections more common in HIV patients even with CD4 counts > 200, although risk increases substantially with lower CD4 counts

- Many different AIDS-defining infections, including disseminated MAI, tuberculosis, *Pneumocystis* infection, recurrent bacterial pneumonias, persistent *Cryptosporidium* infection, chronic HSV, etc.
  - □ Most occur when CD4 count < 200 but can rarely occur at higher CD4 counts

CLINICAL ISSUES

Presentation

- Most common signs/symptoms
  - o Acute HIV infection may resemble mononucleosis with fever, headaches, and body aches
  - o Many patients with chronic HIV infection asymptomatic when effectively treated with antiretrovirals
    - Skin abnormalities and mild constitutional symptoms possible even without immunosuppression
  - o Patients with advanced HIV/AIDS and immunosuppression may experience symptoms related to opportunistic infections (diarrhea, cough/shortness of breath, abdominal pain, etc.)
    - Some patients experience wasting syndrome with profound weight loss and chronic diarrhea
- Other signs/symptoms
  - o Patients with low CD4 counts frequently pancytopenic (anemia, thrombocytopenia, and lymphopenia)
  - o Generalized lymphadenopathy and splenomegaly common even in absence of active infection
- Clinical profile
  - o Clinical profile varies from country to country
    - HIV in developing world spreads primarily by vaginal sex (small proportions due to IV drug abuse and perinatal transmission)
    - HIV in USA disproportionately associated with IV drug abuse and homosexual sexual contact

Demographics

- Age
  - o Primarily adults, but perinatal transmission possible
- Gender
  - o Worldwide most cases in heterosexuals, with F > M
- Epidemiology
  - o > 35 million affected worldwide

Natural History & Prognosis

- Multiple opportunistic infections and AIDS-related tumors are likely unless antiretroviral drugs used to suppress HIV
- AIDS defined as CD4 < 200 or development of AIDS-defining illness (either infection or malignancy)

Treatment

- Antiretroviral drugs to preserve immune status
- Antibiotics for bacterial infections and antiviral drugs for CMV infection

SELECTED REFERENCES

1. Tonolini M et al: Mesenterial, omental, and peritoneal disorders in antiretroviral-treated HIV/AIDS patients: spectrum of cross-sectional imaging findings. Clin Imaging. 37(3):427-39, 2013

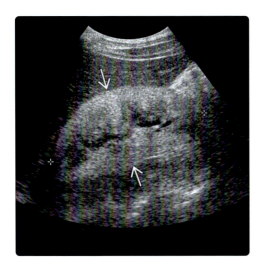

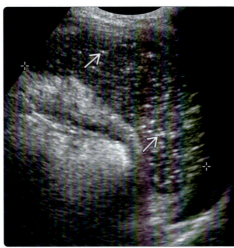

(Left) *Sagittal ultrasound demonstrates a normal-sized right kidney ➡, which is markedly echogenic, compatible with the patient's known HIV nephropathy. Unlike other forms of chronic renal failure, the kidneys in HIV nephropathy are often normal in size or enlarged.* (Right) *Transverse ultrasound demonstrates innumerable tiny calcifications ➡ (bright echogenic foci) in the spleen of an HIV patient, representing the sequelae of the patient's known prior Pneumocystis infection.*

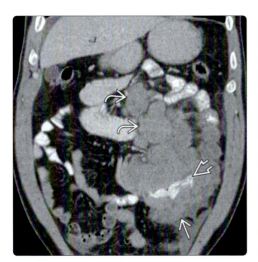

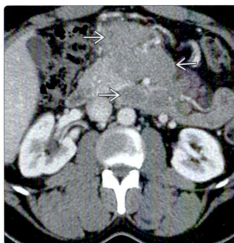

(Left) *Coronal CECT in an AIDS patient demonstrates diffuse mass-like wall thickening and aneurysmal dilatation of a loop of small bowel ➡ in the left lower quadrant with internal enteric contrast ➡. Note the extensive lymphadenopathy ➡ more superiorly. These findings are compatible with the patient's biopsy-proven AIDS-related non-Hodgkin lymphoma.* (Right) *Axial CECT in an AIDS patient demonstrates extensive mesenteric lymphadenopathy ➡ found to represent AIDS-related non-Hodgkin lymphoma.*

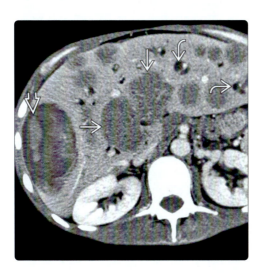

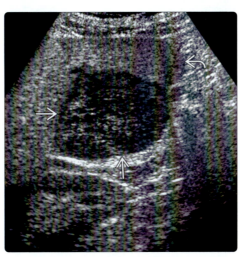

(Left) *Axial CECT in an AIDS patient illustrates multiple hepatic masses ➡, including a mass with internal hemorrhage ➡, which were proven to be non-Hodgkin lymphoma. An unusual feature in this case is the obstruction of the intrahepatic bile ducts ➡. (Right) Longitudinal ultrasound in a patient with AIDS demonstrates a large hypoechoic mass ➡ within the liver ➡. Biopsy revealed this to represent AIDS-related B-cell non-Hodgkin lymphoma.*

KEY FACTS

TERMINOLOGY

- Abbreviations & synonyms: IgG4-RD, IgG4-sclerosing disease, autoimmune pancreatitis
- Collection of disorders that share particular pathologic, serologic, imaging, and clinical features
- Tumor-like swelling of individual organs due to a fibroinflammatory process
- Can affect multiple organs, often simultaneously
- Pancreas, bile ducts, salivary glands, orbits, thyroid, retroperitoneum, kidneys, etc.

IMAGING

- Autoimmune pancreatitis
  - Most common abdominal manifestation of IgG4-RD
  - Focal or sausage-like enlargement of pancreas
  - Loss of normal fatty lobulation of pancreas
  - Hypodense halo, rim, capsule around pancreas
    - May show delayed enhancement
  - Strictures of pancreatic duct

- IgG4-related sclerosing cholangitis
  - 2nd most common abdominal site of IgG4-RD
  - Often (70-90%) occurs with autoimmune pancreatitis
  - Imaging features indistinguishable from primary sclerosing cholangitis
  - Multifocal strictures of intra- and extrahepatic bile ducts
- Best imaging tool: Contrast-enhanced CT or MR (with MRCP)

TOP DIFFERENTIAL DIAGNOSES

- Pancreatic ductal carcinoma
- Cholangiocarcinoma
- Chronic pancreatitis

PATHOLOGY

- Lymphoplasmacytic tissue infiltration by IgG4-positive plasma cells and lymphocytes
- Fibrosis with storiform features, obliterative phlebitis
- Strikingly similar in all tissues affected by IgG4-RD

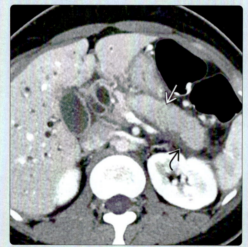
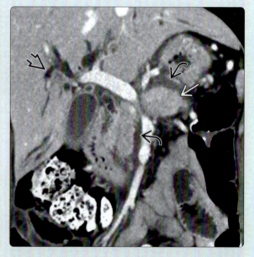

(Left) Axial CECT demonstrates a diffusely enlarged pancreas ➡ with a low-attenuation halo ⤢ around its margin, typical features of autoimmune pancreatitis. (Right) Coronal CECT from the same patient shows similar findings with a low-attenuation halo ⤢ around the enlarged pancreas ➡. Note the presence of biliary dilation ➲ in this patient with a history of biliary strictures. IgG4-RD commonly manifests as "autoimmune" pancreatitis and cholangitis.

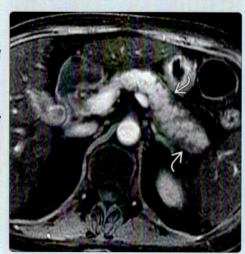
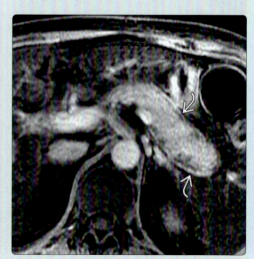

(Left) Axial T1 C+ MR in the arterial phase demonstrates diffuse pancreatic enlargement with a low-signal halo, rim, or capsule ➡ around the margin of the pancreas. (Right) Axial T1 C+ MR in a more delayed phase demonstrates that the capsule ➡ now shows avid delayed enhancement, a characteristic feature of autoimmune pancreatitis.

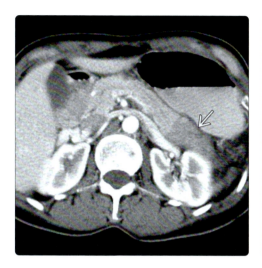
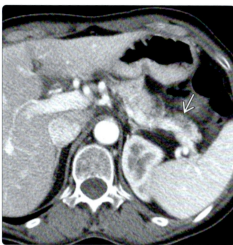

(Left) Initial axial CECT shows a focal, hypodense mass ➡ in the tail of the pancreas. Serologic testing (IgG4) suggested the diagnosis of autoimmune pancreatitis, and steroid therapy was started. (Right) Repeat axial CECT in the same patient 10 months later shows substantial decrease in size of the inflammatory mass ➡ and slight atrophy of the affected pancreatic tail segment.

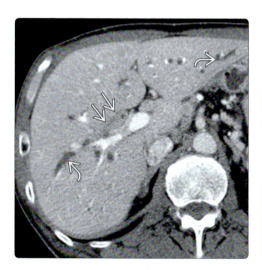
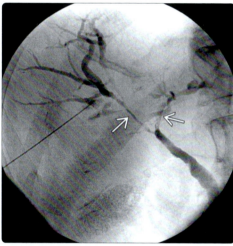

(Left) CECT of an elderly man with jaundice shows wall thickening of the proximal right and left hepatic ducts ➡ and dilation of the intrahepatic bile ducts ➡. (Right) Percutaneous transhepatic cholangiogram of the same patient shows strictures ➡ of the proximal right and left hepatic ducts. The patient's serum IgG4 was not elevated, but the strictures improved with steroid therapy. An elevated IgG4 is a sensitive and specific marker for IgG4-RD, though IgG4 levels may vary widely during the disease course.

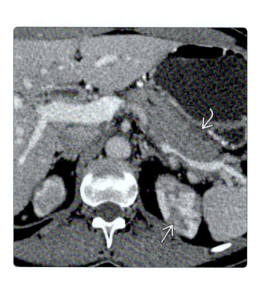
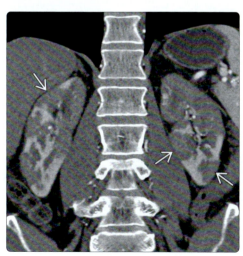

(Left) Axial CECT demonstrates mild enlargement of the pancreas with a subtle low-density capsule ➡ in a patient with an elevated IgG4, compatible with autoimmune pancreatitis. Note the low-density wedge-shaped lesions ➡ in the left kidney. (Right) Coronal CECT in the same patient better demonstrates the full extent of the wedge-shaped low-density lesions ➡ in both kidneys. Renal fibroinflammatory lesions are another abdominal manifestation of IgG4-RD.

KEY FACTS

TERMINOLOGY

- General term describing group of diseases characterized by inflammation and necrosis of blood vessels
- Classified by size of blood vessel involved
  - Large vessel: e.g., Takayasu arteritis
  - Medium vessel: e.g., polyarteritis nodosa
  - Small vessel: e.g., Henoch-Schönlein purpura, lupus, Behçet disease, Wegener granulomatosis

IMAGING

- **CT angiography is excellent, noninvasive imaging tool**
  - CT findings that cause or resemble bowel or renal ischemia in young person should raise concern for vasculitis
- **Takayasu arteritis**
  - Classically involves aortic arch
  - Wall thickening of vascular segment in acute phase
  - Chronic stenoses with poststenotic dilatation, aneurysms, occlusions, and collateral vessel formation

- **Polyarteritis nodosa**
  - Involves bifurcations of medium and small-sized arteries with branch-point aneurysms
  - Renal and mesenteric vessels most often involved
  - Renal infarction and atrophy with striated nephrograms
- **Henoch-Schönlein purpura (IgA vasculitis)**
  - GI tract often affected: Ischemia and hemorrhage
  - Bowel wall thickening, narrowing, and intussusceptions
- **Wegener granulomatosis (granulomatosis with polyangiitis)**
  - Kidneys are involved in 80% of cases
  - Microaneurysms with renal parenchymal scarring, hemorrhage, and bowel ischemia
- **Lupus vasculitis**
  - At risk for bowel complications/ischemia due to vasculitis and hypercoagulability (antiphospholipid syndrome)
- **Behçet disease**
  - Most often involves distal ileum and closely mimics Crohn's disease or malignancy

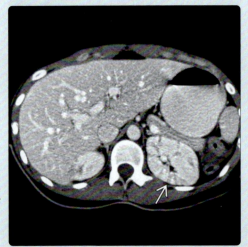
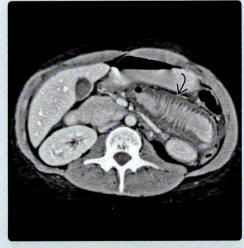

(Left) Axial CECT in a 21-year-old woman with severe abdominal pain shows wedge-shaped defects in the kidneys ➡ representing acute ischemic injury. (Right) Axial CECT in the same patient shows long-segment bowel wall thickening and submucosal edema ➡, findings compatible with enteric ischemia. Rheumatoid vasculitis was subsequently confirmed. Findings that suggest bowel or renal ischemia in a young patient, as in this case, should raise suspicion for vasculitis.

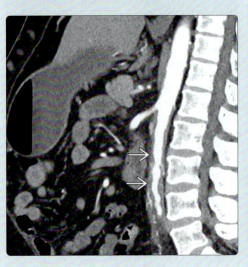
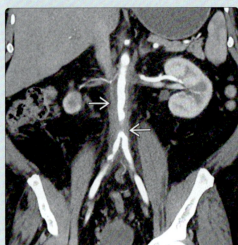

(Left) Sagittal CECT demonstrates diffuse narrowing of the abdominal aorta below the superior mesenteric artery with surrounding soft tissue thickening ➡. (Right) Coronal CECT in the same patient nicely demonstrates the narrowing and thickening ➡ of the abdominal aorta extending to involve the common iliac arteries. This is a common appearance for a large vessel vasculitis (giant cell vasculitis) with active inflammation.

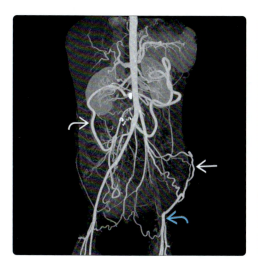

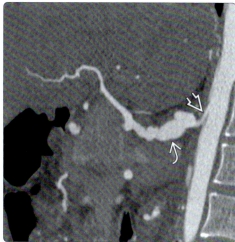

(Left) Coronal CT angiogram (CTA) in a young woman shows occlusion of the left common iliac artery with collateral vessels ➡ that reconstitute the left femoral artery ⬈. The superior mesenteric artery is also completely occluded with collaterals from an enlarged inferior mesenteric artery ➡. (Right) Sagittal CTA in the same patient shows that the origin of the celiac axis is markedly narrowed ➡ with alternating stenoses and aneurysms ➡ of the hepatic artery. These findings were due to Takayasu arteritis.

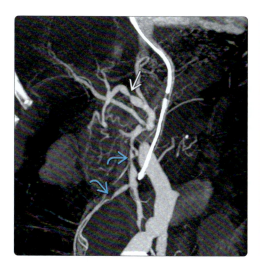

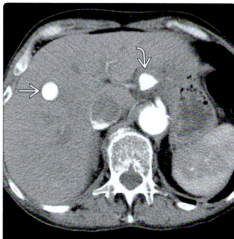

(Left) Coronal volume-rendered CTA shows diffuse beading ➡ and irregularity of the hepatic artery and its branches. Similar findings are seen in the superior mesenteric artery ⬈ and aorta. This was found to represent Takayasu arteritis, which more often affects the aortic arch. (Right) Axial CECT demonstrates large aneurysms arising from an intrahepatic branch of the hepatic artery ➡ and the origin of a replaced left hepatic artery ➡ in a patient with polyarteritis nodosa.

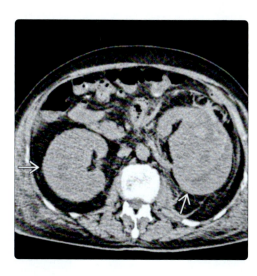

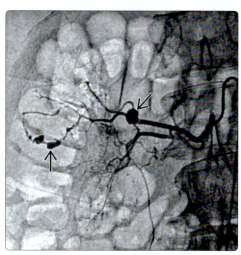

(Left) Axial NECT in a 46-year-old man with sudden bilateral flank pain shows bilateral renal and perirenal hemorrhage (high-attenuation fluid collections) ➡. (Right) Catheter angiography in the same patient shows multiple small renal aneurysms ⬈ that were the source of the bleeding. The diagnosis of Wegener arteritis was subsequently confirmed. Renal or perirenal hemorrhage is especially characteristic of Wegener vasculitis.

KEY FACTS

TERMINOLOGY

- Inflammatory disease of GI tract characterized by tissue eosinophilia that can involve all layers of wall
  - "Eosinophilic gastroenteritis" is misnomer; can affect any portion of GI tract
- Requires 4 criteria for diagnosis
  - Presence of GI symptoms
  - Biopsy proof of eosinophilic infiltration of 1 or more areas of GI tract
  - Absence of eosinophilic involvement of multiple organs outside GI tract
  - Absence of parasitic infestation

IMAGING

- Esophageal involvement (eosinophilic esophagitis)
  - Most characteristic findings: **Ringed esophagus (concentric, thin, web-like strictures)**
  - May coexist with longer strictures

- Strictures, webs, and spasm account for symptoms of food and pill impaction within esophagus
- GI involvement
  - Most common site of GI tract involvement
  - **Nonspecific fold thickening ± submucosal edema**
  - ± malabsorption pattern (dilution of barium, fluid distention of lumen)

TOP DIFFERENTIAL DIAGNOSES

- Intestinal parasites and infestation
- Other causes of esophagitis and stricture
- Esophageal webs

PATHOLOGY

- Most patients have history of food intolerance &/or multiple allergies

DIAGNOSTIC CHECKLIST

- Yield of imaging is probably highest in eosinophilic esophagitis

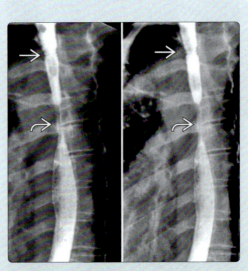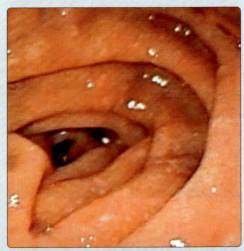

(Left) *Films from an esophagram in a 33-year-old woman complaining of food sticking in her esophagus demonstrate several ring-like strictures ➡ of the proximal esophagus as well as more distal and longer strictures ➡. These were persistent on multiple films.* (Right) *Endoscopic photograph in the same patient shows the same ring-like strictures likened to tracheal rings and considered characteristic of this disorder.*

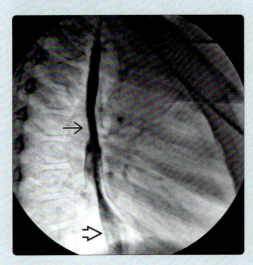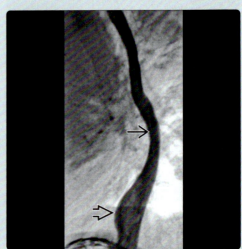

(Left) *Spot film from an esophagram in a 7-year-old girl shows a shortened esophagus pulling the stomach ➡ into the chest. A mild mid esophageal stricture ➡ is also noted. The appearance is diagnostic of esophagitis, but not the specific type.* (Right) *Oblique esophagram in the same patient shows the hiatal hernia ➡ and stricture ➡ again.*

Scleroderma and Related Disorders

KEY FACTS

TERMINOLOGY

- Multisystem disorder of small vessels and connective tissue of unknown etiology
  - Characterized by atrophy, fibrosis, and sclerosis of skin, vessels, and organs
  - GI tract involvement most common after cutaneous
- **CREST syndrome**: Minimal cutaneous and late visceral involvement
  - C: Calcinosis of skin
  - R: Raynaud phenomenon
  - E: Esophageal dysmotility
  - S: Sclerodactyly (involvement of fingers)
  - T: Telangiectasia

IMAGING

- Barium fluoroscopic exams and CT or MR enterography
- Esophagus
  - Atony of lower 2/3 (smooth muscle)
  - Mild to moderate dilatation of esophagus
  - Patulous lower esophageal sphincter (early disease)
  - Mucosal ulceration, distal peptic stricture, hiatal hernia
- Stomach
  - Dilation and delayed emptying
- Duodenum
  - Dilation with abrupt narrowing at midline
  - Often mimics superior mesenteric artery syndrome
- Small bowel
  - Dilated with thin, closely spaced transverse folds (hidebound pattern)
  - Wide-mouthed sacculations on antimesenteric border
  - ± pneumatosis intestinalis (due to steroid medications ± dilation of small bowel)
- Colon
  - Sacculations on antimesenteric border of colon
  - Marked dilatation (simulates Hirschsprung disease)
  - Stercoral ulceration (from retained fecal material)

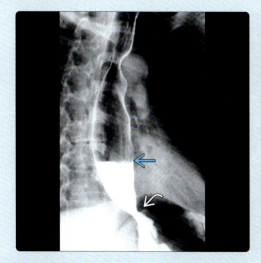

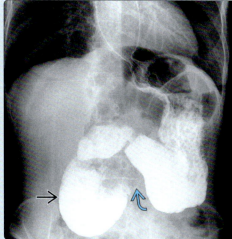

(Left) *Film from an esophagram in a young woman with dysphagia shows a dilated esophagus with a persistent air-fluid level ➡, indicating delayed emptying. There is stricture of the distal esophagus ➘.* (Right) *Subsequent film in the same patient shows a dilated duodenum ➡ with functional narrowing of its 3rd portion ➘. The duodenum is often dilated and atonic in patients with scleroderma.*

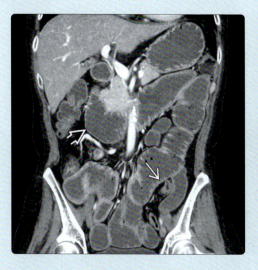

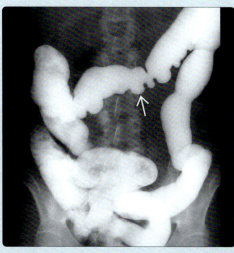

(Left) *Coronal CECT demonstrates a dilated small bowel with a hidebound appearance of thin folds ➡, particularly in the jejunum. Also note the dilation of the duodenum ➡, another common feature of scleroderma.* (Right) *Barium enema shows sacculation ➡ of the transverse colon and loss of a normal haustral pattern throughout most of the colon, all due to scleroderma.*

KEY FACTS

TERMINOLOGY

- Recessively inherited disorder of epithelial chloride transport caused by mutation of *CFTR* gene
- Cystic fibrosis (CF) is increasingly seen to affect GI tract due to improving life expectancy

IMAGING

- Most common sites of involvement are lungs, pancreas, bowel, liver, and exocrine glands
- Pancreas
  - Complete fatty infiltration and replacement of parenchyma (often by end of teenage years)
  - Pancreatic cysts: Usually small (< 3 mm), but can be larger and can completely replace pancreas (cystosis)
  - Repeated episodes of acute pancreatitis with development of chronic pancreatitis
- Liver
  - 30-50% develop hepatic steatosis ± hepatomegaly
  - Can develop multinodular cirrhosis in severe cases

- Biliary
  - Biliary abnormalities similar to primary sclerosing cholangitis (PSC)
- Bowel
  - Inspissated fecal material resulting in proximal obstruction, most often in infants (meconium ileus)
  - Obstruction can also occur in adults: **Distal intestinal obstruction syndrome (DIOS)**
  - Increased risk for intussusception
  - Chronically distended appendix may be difficult to distinguish from acute appendicitis

CLINICAL ISSUES

- Overall prognosis for CF has dramatically improved, with average life expectancy now 35-40 years
- Respiratory failure most common cause of mortality, with liver disease 2nd leading cause of death
- Pancreatic insufficiency most common (~ 85%) GI manifestation of CF

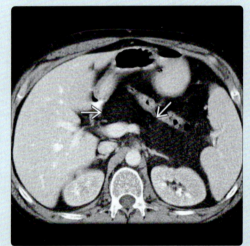
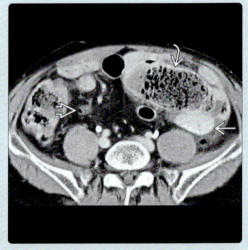

(Left) *Axial CECT shows the classic lipomatous replacement and pseudohypertrophy of the pancreas ➡ in a young adult patient with cystic fibrosis (CF).* (Right) *Axial CECT in the same patient shows dilated proximal small bowel ➡ and collapsed distal small bowel ➡. Just proximal to the point of transition is the classic small bowel feces sign ➡ associated with mechanical small-bowel obstruction, with the obstruction caused by inspissated enteric contents (distal intestinal obstruction syndrome or DIOS).*

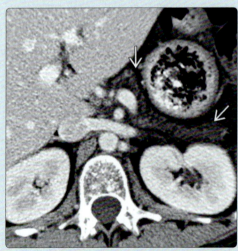
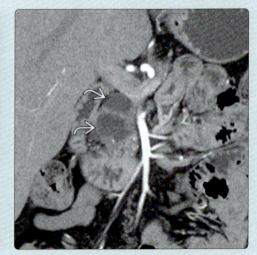

(Left) *Axial CECT demonstrates heterogeneous lipomatous replacement of the pancreatic parenchyma ➡ but less pseudohypertrophy. This 29-year-old woman had longstanding pancreatic exocrine dysfunction due to CF.* (Right) *Coronal CECT demonstrates simple-appearing cysts ➡ in the pancreatic head in a young patient with CF. While pancreatic cysts are often very small in CF patients, they can rarely be larger, as in this case.*

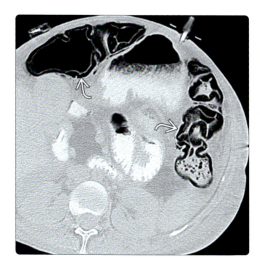
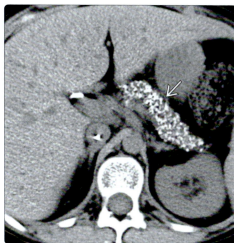

(Left) Axial CT shows diffuse pneumatosis ➡ of the transverse and left colon. The patient was completely asymptomatic, and this was felt to be benign pneumatosis due to gas dissecting from the chest into the bowel wall as a result of the patient's lung disease. (Right) Axial NECT in a 24-year-old woman with CF shows an unusually severe degree of pancreatic calcification ➡. Scattered, small calcifications are a more common finding in this disease.

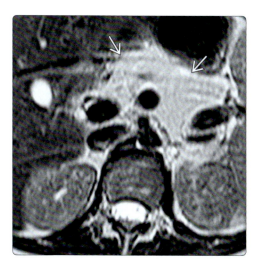
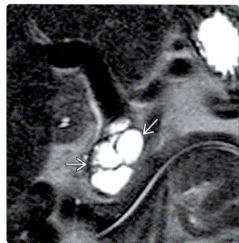

(Left) Axial T2WI MR in a 16-year-old girl with CF demonstrates complete fatty replacement ➡ of the body and tail of the pancreas, resulting in high T1WI signal. (Right) Coronal MRCP in the same patient shows a septate cystic mass in the pancreatic head ➡ that mimics a cystic neoplasm. However, pancreatic cysts of variable size are commonly encountered in patients with CF.

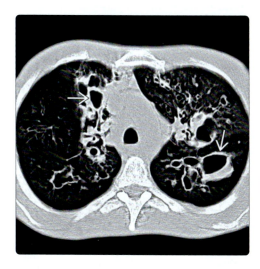
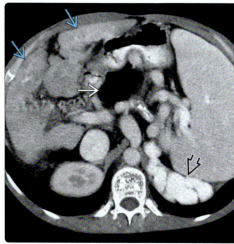

(Left) Axial CECT in a 31-year-old man shows classic cystic bronchiectasis ➡ in the lungs. Many patients are being kept alive longer with better medical care and even lung transplantation, resulting in an increased prevalence of extrapulmonary manifestations of CF. (Right) Axial CECT in the same patient shows that the liver ➡ is small and cirrhotic with obvious signs of portal hypertension, including splenomegaly and large varices ➡. The pancreas shows fatty replacement ➡.

KEY FACTS

IMAGING

- **Ingested foreign bodies**
  - Commonly affect children, developmentally challenged or psychiatric patients, and inebriated adults
  - Most ingested foreign bodies traverse GI tract without problem: < 1% cause obstruction or perforation
    - Elongated or sharp objects may impact at point of intestinal narrowing or sharp angulation
  - Foreign bodies vary in radiopacity and conspicuity on radiography vs. CT
  - For most nonsharp foreign bodies, begin with visual inspection of oropharynx and plain radiographs
  - For sharp objects at risk of complications, start with CT
- **Inserted foreign bodies**
  - Rectum, vagina, and urethra are common sites
  - Objects may be inserted during sexual practice, as result of assault, or to hide drugs
  - Perforation of rectosigmoid colon may occur with original insertion or during attempted removal

- **Retained surgical items**
  - Most common in abdominal surgery (especially emergent)
  - Most commonly woven cotton surgical sponge
    - Most have radiopaque stripe interwoven into fabric or as attached strip of cloth
    - **Gossypiboma**: Foreign body reaction to cotton fabric of sponge or towel producing inflammatory mass with sponge at center
      - Heterogeneous mass with internal low-density spongiform cotton center, with gas and linear radiopaque marker
- **Intentionally retained surgical material**
  - Oxidized regenerated cellulose (Gelfoam/Surgicel) deliberately left in place after surgery for hemostasis
  - Usually absorbed within 7-14 days
  - Tightly packed, swirled, or linear gas on CT
    - May be mistaken for abscess but contains very little fluid and never shows air-fluid level

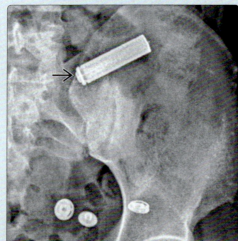
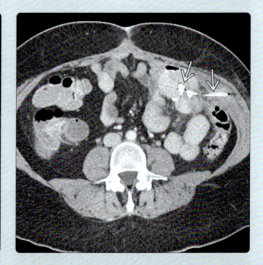

(Left) Plain film shows the appearance of a standard cylindrical-shaped battery ➡ after ingestion. Swallowing batteries is relatively common and can cause bowel perforation or obstruction as the acid in the battery may leak out. (Right) Axial CECT in a patient with a long psychiatric history demonstrates a linear metallic ingested foreign body ➡ in the small bowel, perforating the small bowel and extending into the abdominal wall.

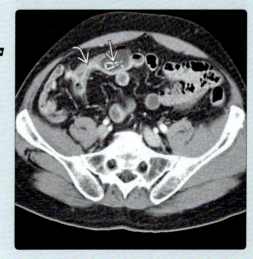
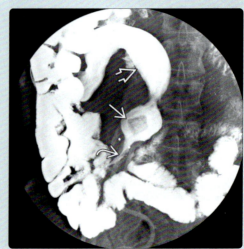

(Left) Axial CECT in a patient who had unintentionally swallowed a metallic clip demonstrates that the clip ➡ has caused an inflammatory stricture ➡ of the adjacent small bowel, which is thickened with mucosal hyperemia. (Right) Spot film from a small bowel follow-through in the same patient demonstrates a filling defect ➡ corresponding to the clip seen on CT. Note that the stricture ➡ in the immediately distal small bowel is causing mild obstruction with dilation of more proximal bowel ➡.

TERMINOLOGY

Abbreviations

- Foreign body (FB)

Definitions

- Ingestion or insertion of potentially injurious foreign objects into any site within body

IMAGING

Imaging Recommendations

- Best imaging tool
  - **Plain radiograph or CT, with CT usually more definitive**

Ingested Foreign Bodies

- Commonly affected patient groups
  - Children (vast majority of foreign body ingestions)
    - Often swallow coins, batteries, toys
  - Developmentally challenged or psychiatric patients
    - Common items include jewelry, batteries, silverware
  - Prisoners, criminals, and "drug mules"
    - Razor blades (often covered in radiolucent tape); drug packets
  - Edentulous, elderly, or inebriated adults
    - May swallow bones, toothpicks (common in martini drinkers)
    - Food bolus impaction in esophagus
- General principles
  - Most ingested FBs traverse GI tract without problem
    - < 1% cause obstruction or perforation of GI tract
  - Distinguish unintentional foreign bodies from medical devices (e.g., capsule endoscope, stents)
  - Elongated or sharp objects may impact at point of intestinal narrowing or sharp angulation
    - e.g., pylorus, duodenum, ileocecal valve, site of bowel stricture or adhesion
  - Common ingested foreign bodies and management
    - Longer objects > 6 cm in length (eating utensils, toothbrushes) are unlikely to traverse duodenum and should be retrieved endoscopically
    - Ingested disk (e.g., watch) batteries are caustic
      - □ Should be removed from esophagus or stomach if possible
      - □ Often can retrieve from esophagus with balloon-tipped rubber catheter, magnet, or endoscope
    - Sharp pointed objects (chicken/fish bones, paperclips, toothpicks, needles, etc.) have high risk of complications (1/3 of patients)
      - □ Should be endoscopically retrieved if in duodenum or stomach
    - Magnets
      - □ Can cause severe injury if multiple magnets are ingested, trapping bowel loops between 2 magnets' attractive force
      - □ Can lead to bowel wall necrosis, fistulas, bowel obstruction, etc.
      - □ All magnets should be retrieved immediately
  - Examine entire GI tract for additional FBs
    - For most nonsharp foreign bodies, begin with visual inspection of oropharynx and plain radiographs
    - For sharp objects at high risk of complications, start with CT

Inserted Foreign Bodies

- Any orifice may be involved; rectum, vagina, and urethra are common sites
- Objects may be inserted during sexual practice, as result of assault, to hide drugs and other illegal paraphernalia, or even sharp objects/weapons in prison setting
  - Majority of foreign bodies do not cause significant injury
  - Perforation of rectosigmoid colon may occur with original insertion or during attempted removal
  - Approach to removal (i.e., manual, endoscopic, surgical) will depend on type of FB, symptoms, perforation, etc.
- Any FB remaining in place within bladder or vagina will become encrusted with mineral salts, becoming progressively larger and more opaque
  - Bladder calculus of unusual shape, or in child, is likely encrusted FB

Retained Surgical Items

- Crucial to distinguish intentional or expected objects from unintended
  - Common intentional devices: Surgical drains, rubber retention sutures, metallic clips for wound closure, hemoclips, or intraarterial, intravenous, and intraintestinal catheters
  - Most common unintentional retained foreign body is woven cotton surgical sponge
    - Suggested by incorrect sponge count, although sponge counts are notoriously inaccurate
  - Retained needles or surgical instruments
    - Generally easy to recognize but may be misinterpreted on plain films as lying outside of patient
- Identification of retained surgical sponges or towels on imaging
  - Most have radiopaque stripe interwoven into fabric or as attached strip of cloth
    - Identified as curvilinear radiopaque line on radiographs or CT
  - Cotton fabric is invisible on radiographs but seen as swirled gas or soft tissue on CT scans
  - **Gossypiboma**: Foreign body reaction to cotton fabric of sponge or towel left inside patient; produces inflammatory mass with sponge at center
    - Heterogeneous mass with internal low-density spongiform cotton center, with gas and linear radiopaque marker

Intentionally Retained Surgical Material

- Oxidized regenerated cellulose (Gelfoam or Surgicel)
  - Upon contact with blood, fabric induces rapid hemostasis by inducing thrombus formation, and swells into gelatinous mass, trapping air (gas) within its interstices
  - Has radiographic and CT appearance of tightly packed, swirled, or linear gas bubbles without much fluid content
    - May be mistaken for abscess, but contains very little fluid and never shows air-fluid level

(Left) *In a psychiatric patient who complained of severe dysphagia, a spot film from an esophagram shows a comb ⇨ impacted within the esophagus. Endoscopic removal was successful.*
(Right) *In a man who "lost" a plastic dildo inserted into his rectum, a supine film shows a faintly opaque cylindrical object ⇨ in the expected position of the rectum. Following removal under anesthesia, a contrast enema should be considered to exclude perforation of the bowel.*

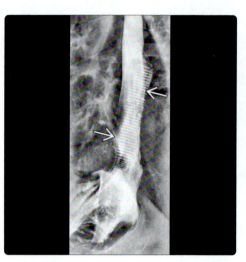
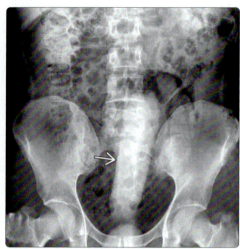

(Left) *In a patient who had inserted a penlight into his penis, neither physical exam nor plain films could localize its position. Axial NECT shows part of the foreign object ⇨ within the bladder.* **(Right)** *In the same patient, volume-rendered CT shows the position of the penlight ⇨ relative to the bony structures of the pelvis. The object was retrieved in the cystoscopy suite.*

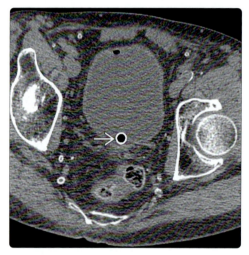
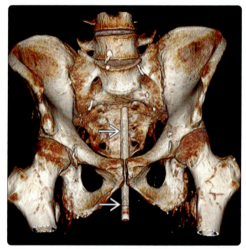

(Left) *Coronal CT scout view demonstrates a wavy radiopaque band ⇨ in the pelvis, typical of a retained surgical sponge. This radiopaque tag can be directly woven into the sponge or can be attached to it and makes these more apparent for plain film and CT detection.* **(Right)** *Axial CECT in the same patient demonstrates the radiopaque strip ⇨ and an inflammatory gas and fluid-containing mass ⇨ forming around the retained sponge, characteristic of a gossypiboma.*

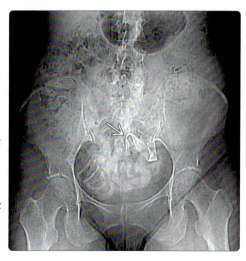
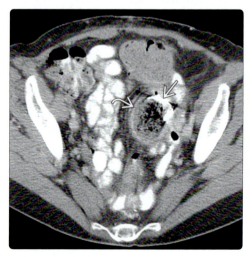

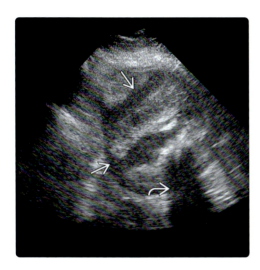

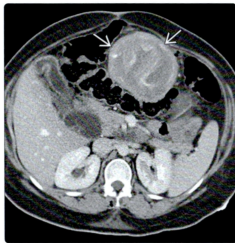

(Left) *In a patient with a palpable, tender abdominal mass, sonography shows a well-defined mass ➡ with internal alternating bands of hyper- and hypoechogenicity. Some of the hyperechoic bands with posterior acoustic shadowing ➡ may reflect gas within the mass.* (Right) *Axial CECT in the same patient shows a mass ➡ with the characteristic CT appearance of a chronic gossypiboma. Note the wavy, serpiginous pattern within the mass and the well-defined wall.*

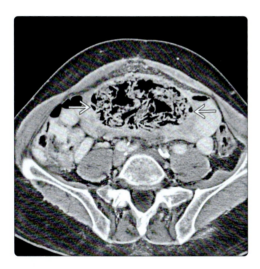

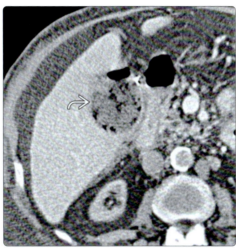

(Left) *Axial CECT in an elderly man with pain following aortic bypass surgery shows a large mass, a gossypiboma ➡, that was found to represent a surgical towel that had been left in the peritoneal cavity. Note the absence of a radiopaque marker.* (Right) *Axial CECT in a patient with abdominal pain and fever after cholecystectomy shows a collection of gas ➡ but little fluid in the cholecystectomy bed, mimicking an abscess. This represents retained oxidized cellulose (Surgicel), placed to control continued oozing of blood.*

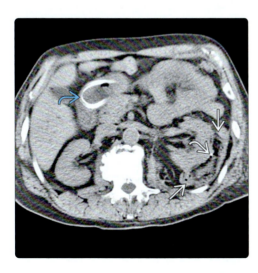

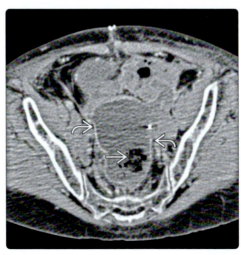

(Left) *Axial NECT in a patient with fever and pain following partial left nephrectomy shows a collection of gas and soft tissue density ➡ in the perirenal space. This represents Surgicel, not an abscess. Note the surgical clip ➡ at the site of resection, as well as a feeding tube ➡.* (Right) *Axial CECT in a patient with a postoperative abscess following partial colectomy shows a collection of gas representing Surgicel ➡, surrounded by a large collection of fluid with an enhancing capsule ➡, typical for an abscess.*

Barotrauma

KEY FACTS

TERMINOLOGY
- Alveolar rupture caused by elevated transalveolar pressure during mechanical ventilation

IMAGING
- **CT definitive test for presence & source of extraluminal gas**
  - Pleural spaces, mediastinum, subcutaneous, intra- and retroperitoneal, bowel wall
- Radiographic findings
  - Pneumothorax
    - Inferiorly displaced costophrenic angle on supine films (deep sulcus sign)
  - Pneumomediastinum
    - Radiolucent streaks outlining heart and trachea
  - Pneumoperitoneum
    - Best seen on upright and left decubitus films
    - Supine films: Air outlining bowel or falciform ligament
  - Subcutaneous emphysema
    - Radiolucent streaks outlining fat and muscles

TOP DIFFERENTIAL DIAGNOSES
- Perforated duodenal or gastric ulcer
- Iatrogenic introduction of ectopic gas
- Other causes of pneumothorax, pneumomediastinum, pneumoperitoneum, or pneumatosis
- Ischemic enteritis

PATHOLOGY
- Positive pressure ventilation → alveolar rupture → air leakage into pulmonary interstitium
- Interstitial air can dissect along perivascular sheaths into mediastinum
- Mediastinal and pleural air can leak into peritoneal and retroperitoneal cavities
- Primary risk factors include interstitial lung disease, asthma, acute respiratory distress syndrome (ARDS), and mechanical ventilation with high tidal volumes

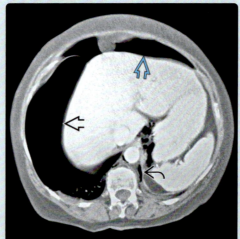
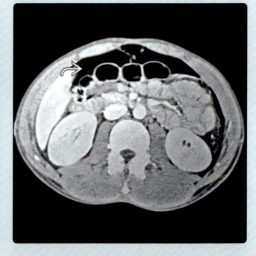

(Left) Axial CECT in a young man on a ventilator following a motor vehicle crash shows a tension pneumothorax ➡ on the right side and a smaller pneumothorax on the left ➡. Gas dissects under pressure along the peridiaphragmatic fat ➡. (Right) Axial CECT in the same patient shows the extraluminal air from the thorax dissecting into the peritoneal cavity ➡ to outline bowel loops. There was no intraabdominal injury.

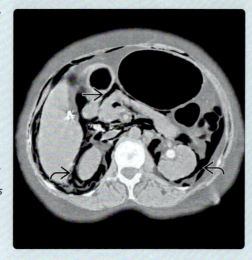
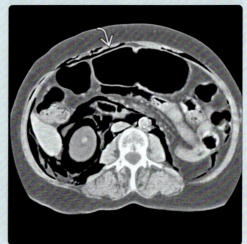

(Left) Axial CECT in an elderly man on positive pressure ventilation and with known large bilateral pneumothoraces and gas in the mediastinum shows the gas dissecting under pressure into the abdomen, including the retroperitoneum ➡ and mesentery ➡. (Right) Axial CECT in the same patient shows that in addition to the extensive retroperitoneal gas, intraperitoneal gas is also present ➡. In some cases, gas can dissect into the bowel wall, simulating pneumatosis from bowel ischemia.

Disorders Affecting Multiple Organs

Barotrauma

TERMINOLOGY

Definitions

- Alveolar rupture caused by elevated transalveolar pressure during mechanical ventilation

IMAGING

General Features

- Best diagnostic clue
  - Extraluminal air in patient treated with positive pressure ventilation
- Location
  - Ectopic gas in pleural space, mediastinum, subcutaneous soft tissues, intraperitoneal and retroperitoneal spaces, bowel wall

Radiographic Findings

- Radiography
  - Diagnosis is difficult because patient is usually supine and being ventilated
  - Pneumothorax
    - Radiolucent collection of gas between visceral and parietal pleura
    - Inferiorly displaced costophrenic angle on supine films (deep sulcus sign)
  - Pneumomediastinum
    - Radiolucent streaks outlining heart and trachea
  - Pneumoperitoneum
    - Best seen on upright and left decubitus films
    - Supine films: Air outlining bowel, falciform ligament
  - Subcutaneous emphysema
    - Radiolucent streaks outlining subcutaneous fat and muscles

CT Findings

- Free air in pleural and mediastinal spaces
- Free (extraluminal) gas in subcutaneous tissues and muscles, lung interstitium, retroperitoneum and mesentery, intraperitoneal spaces, and bowel wall (pneumatosis)

DIFFERENTIAL DIAGNOSIS

Perforated Duodenal or Gastric Ulcer

- Gas bubbles and infiltration of fat planes adjacent to duodenal bulb or in lesser sac (gastric ulcer)

Iatrogenic Introduction of Ectopic Gas

- Introduction of gas or air via surgery, catheterization, peritoneal lavage, or endoscopy

Other

- Multiple other causes of pneumothorax, pneumomediastinum, pneumoperitoneum, or pneumatosis (e.g., pneumoperitoneum due to bowel perforation, pneumothorax due to trauma)

Ischemic Enteritis

- Pneumatosis can result from ischemia, but also other causes, including medications and barotrauma
- Barotrauma is usually accompanied by pneumothorax and other sites of extraluminal air

PATHOLOGY

General Features

- Etiology
  - Positive pressure ventilation → alveolar rupture → air leakage into pulmonary interstitium
  - Interstitial air can dissect along perivascular sheaths into mediastinum
  - Mediastinal and pleural air can leak into peritoneal and retroperitoneal cavity
  - Rare complications include tension pneumothorax, bronchopleural fistula, subpleural air cyst, and air embolus

Staging, Grading, & Classification

- Risk factors
  - Interstitial lung disease; asthma
  - Acute respiratory distress syndrome (ARDS)

CLINICAL ISSUES

Presentation

- Most common signs/symptoms
  - Some patients may be asymptomatic
  - Tachypnea, tachycardia, hypertension or hypotension, oxygen desaturation
  - Abdominal distension, tenderness
  - Subcutaneous emphysema (crepitus on palpation)

Demographics

- Epidemiology
  - Older literature reported barotrauma seen in 3% of patients undergoing mechanical ventilation, but frequency has decreased due to low tidal volume ventilation becoming more common

Natural History & Prognosis

- Associated with ↑ morbidity and mortality

Treatment

- Conservative management
  - Close monitoring of pneumothorax for progression
  - Pneumomediastinum, pneumoperitoneum, and subcutaneous emphysema are self-limited
- Chest tube insertion for large pneumothorax
- Prevention: Maintaining plateau airway pressure < 30 cm H_2O

DIAGNOSTIC CHECKLIST

Consider

- Pneumoperitoneum and pneumatosis are rare complications of barotrauma, and abdominal source must be excluded

SELECTED REFERENCES

1. Santa Cruz R et al: High versus low positive end-expiratory pressure (PEEP) levels for mechanically ventilated adult patients with acute lung injury and acute respiratory distress syndrome. Cochrane Database Syst Rev, 2013

KEY FACTS

TERMINOLOGY

- Presence of intraperitoneal or body wall gas/fluid following surgery

IMAGING

- **Pneumoperitoneum** is common imaging finding after surgery on both plain radiographs and CT
  - CT has 2x sensitivity of plain films for detection of pneumoperitoneum
  - Pneumoperitoneum is seen on CT in 87% of patients following uncomplicated laparotomy at 3 days post surgery and 50% of patients at 6 days
  - No upper limit to normal persistence of pneumoperitoneum, but gas resolves in most patients within 1 week
  - Pneumoperitoneum more likely to persist in patients who have had prior surgery or peritonitis, have undergone open (rather than laparoscopic) surgery, or who have surgical drains
  - Volume of postoperative pneumoperitoneum is normally small (< 10 cc) in most patients
  - Large or massive pneumoperitoneum is **not** normal finding, even in immediate postoperative setting
    - Presence of massive pneumoperitoneum should raise concern for anastomotic leak or hollow viscus perforation
- **Free intraperitoneal fluid** is present in nearly all patients following open laparotomy or laparoscopy
  - Small, nonloculated collections without enhancing wall or mass effect are of little concern
  - Large volume free fluid or collection with mass effect, enhancing rim, or internal gas should raise concern for infected fluid collection or bowel/anastomotic leak
- **Extraperitoneal collections** (e.g., retroperitoneal and abdominal wall collections) of gas and fluid take longer to resolve than peritoneal air/fluid
  - Peritoneum is much better absorptive surface than granulation tissue, fat, or muscle

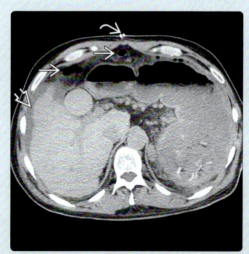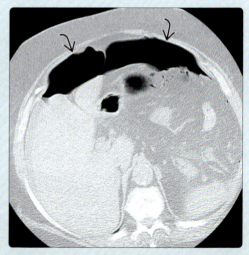

(Left) Axial NECT in a patient after surgery shows skin staples ➡ in the anterior abdominal wall with evidence of free air ➡ and perihepatic free fluid ➡. The patient was free of symptoms of infection or bowel leak and recovered without incident. (Right) Axial NECT in a patient after sigmoid colectomy demonstrates large amounts of free intraperitoneal gas ➡, much more than would be normally expected after surgery. Abundant free air after surgery must raise concern for an anastomotic leak or perforation.

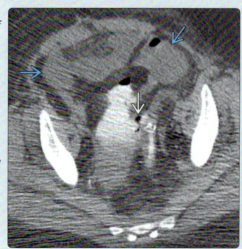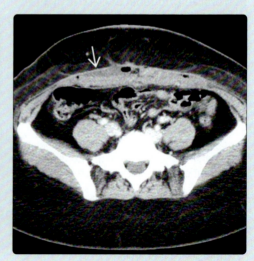

(Left) NECT in the same patient after administration of rectal enteric contrast demonstrates a leak of air & contrast media at the sigmoid anastomotic staple line ➡. Other collections of air & fluid ➡ are noted. (Right) Axial CECT in a patient with a recent hysterectomy shows a thin, encapsulated collection of gas and fluid ➡ in the abdominal wall musculofascial plane at the incision site. Needle aspiration of the collection revealed no evidence of infection, and the collection resolved.

TERMINOLOGY

Definitions

- Presence of intraperitoneal or body wall gas/fluid following surgery

IMAGING

General Features

- Patients who have had prior surgery or peritonitis seem to resorb free air and fluid less readily than those with normal peritoneal cavity
- Patients with surgical drains may have greater incidence of persistent free air (possibly introduced through drain)
- Persistent pneumoperitoneum is less likely after laparoscopic procedures compared to open procedures
  - Carbon dioxide is absorbed more readily than room air
  - Pig model showed persistent free air on CT at 2 days after laparoscopy and 6 days after open laparotomy
- Some older sources have suggested free air may resorb more quickly in obese patients, at least on plain films
  - More likely that plain films fail to detect small amounts of free air in obese patients
  - CT shows similar prevalence of persistent free air in both obese and thin patients

Imaging Recommendations

- Best imaging tool
  - CT

Radiographic Findings

- Plain radiographs may show evidence of **free intraperitoneal gas (air)**
  - Upright chest x-ray or left lateral decubitus position is most sensitive
  - Requires horizontal x-ray beam centered on most nondependent position of peritoneal cavity
    - Gas under diaphragm on upright chest film
    - Gas lateral to liver or medial to iliac crest on decubitus film
  - Requires minimum of several minutes for air to equilibrate (move into antidependent position)
  - Radiographically detectable pneumoperitoneum is seen in 30-77% of patients soon after surgery
    - Falls to average of 38% by day 3 and 17% by day 7

CT Findings

- CT detects free air with 2x sensitivity of plain films in studies comparing CT and plain films in same patients
  - Pneumoperitoneum was seen on CT in 87% of patients following uncomplicated laparotomy at 3 days post surgery and 50% of patients at 6 days
    - Plain film detection was 53% at 3 days and 18% (1 patient) at 6 days
  - No upper limit to normal persistence of pneumoperitoneum, but gas resolves in most patients within 1 week
    - CT evidence of persistent pneumoperitoneum in 44% up to 3 days post surgery and 30% between 4 and 18 days post surgery
    - Reports of persistent pneumoperitoneum 8 weeks after colectomy

- Frequent sites of collection on supine CT exam
  - Subphrenic spaces (right > left)
  - Abutting anterior abdominal wall
    - Between or along rectus muscles, which form concave recesses pointed downward
  - Between mesenteric leaves
- Most patients have < 10 mL of free air
  - Volumes up to 40 mL have been documented
- Large or massive pneumoperitoneum is **not** normal finding, even in immediate postoperative setting
  - Presence of massive pneumoperitoneum should raise concern for anastomotic leak or hollow viscus perforation
- **Free intraperitoneal fluid** is present in nearly all patients following open laparotomy or laparoscopy
  - Small, nonloculated collections without enhancing wall or mass effect are of little concern
  - Large volume free fluid collection or collections with mass effect, enhancing rim, or internal gas should raise concern for infected fluid collection or bowel/anastomotic leak
- Extraperitoneal collections (e.g., retroperitoneal and abdominal wall collections) of gas and fluid take longer to resolve
  - Fluid and gas may persist for many days (much longer than equivalent amount of intraperitoneal gas or fluid)
  - Peritoneum is much better absorptive surface than granulation tissue, fat, or muscle

Ultrasonographic Findings

- Has been shown to detect free air about as well as plain films but not as well as CT
  - Echogenic foci with ring-down artifact (dirty shadow)
  - Up against anterior abdominal wall in supine patient

CLINICAL ISSUES

Natural History & Prognosis

- Significance of persistent free intra- or extraperitoneal gas and fluid largely determined by clinical condition of patient
  - Persistent fever, leukocytosis, or signs of peritonitis increase likelihood of postoperative infection or clinically significant gas leak from bowel
  - Presence of large amounts of gas or fluid raises concern, especially if increasing over time after surgery
  - Presence of loculation, mass effect, or rim enhancement of fluid collection raises concern

DIAGNOSTIC CHECKLIST

Image Interpretation Pearls

- Presence of large or increasing pneumoperitoneum after surgery is abnormal finding that should raise concern for perforation or anastomotic leak

SELECTED REFERENCES

1. Peirce GS et al: Postoperative pneumoperitoneum on computed tomography: is the operation to blame? Am J Surg. ePub, 2014

Abdominal Incision and Injection Sites

IMAGING

- **Injection site fluid or gas collection**
  - Usually result from injection of subcutaneous heparin, self-injection of insulin, etc.
  - Low-density nodules associated with ectopic gas or fluid
- **Injection or incision site hematoma or seroma**
  - May be misinterpreted as neoplasm but should resolve over time
- **Injection or incision site abscess**
  - Suspicious imaging features include peripheral enhancement, surrounding soft tissue edema and stranding (i.e., cellulitis), and internal ectopic gas
- **Diabetic lipodystrophy**
  - Insulin-dependent diabetic patients may develop atrophy or hypertrophy of fat at injection sites
- **Keloid (hypertrophic scar)**
  - Benign fibrotic scar tissue or soft tissue overgrowth at site of healed skin injury (i.e., incisional scar)

- No clear distinguishing imaging features
- **Calcified or ossified scar**
  - Abdominal incision may develop cartilaginous, osseous, or myelogenous (bone marrow) elements
- **Endometrial implantation in abdominal incision**
  - Most often seen after cesarean section (80% of cases)
  - Cyclical pain at incision site with menstruation
  - Lesions appear solid and irregularly shaped/spiculated on CT or MR with moderate enhancement
- **Tumor implantation in incision sites**
  - Probably more common after laparoscopic surgery
  - Nonspecific imaging appearance, with soft tissue density mass near or within incision site
- **Injection granulomas**
  - Sequelae of subcutaneous injection of drugs resulting in local fat necrosis, scarring, and calcification
  - Usually rounded or linear soft tissue or calcific density lesion seen in subcutaneous fat of buttocks

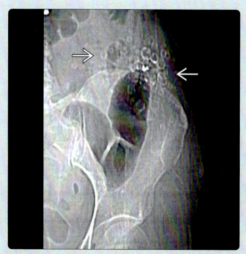

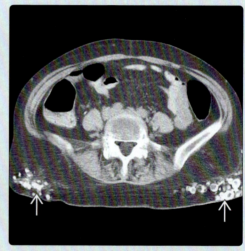

(Left) *Plain film radiograph shows rounded calcifications ➡ that overlap the lower abdomen. Some of these are lateral to the descending colon and close to the skin, establishing their extraabdominal location.* (Right) *Axial NECT in the same patient shows heavily calcified injection sites ➡ in the subcutaneous tissues over the buttocks. Renal failure may have contributed to the deposition of so much calcium in these lesions.*

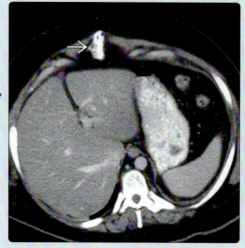

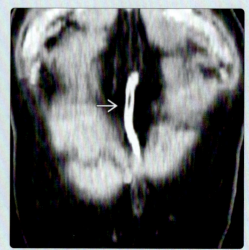

(Left) *Axial CECT shows a heavily calcified or ossified upper abdominal incision site ➡ immediately caudal to the xiphoid process.* (Right) *Coronal CECT in another patient shows a long ossification (over 10 cm) of the midline incision site ➡. The appearance is very similar to that of a rib, with both the cortex and medulla clearly seen.*

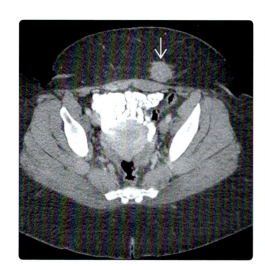

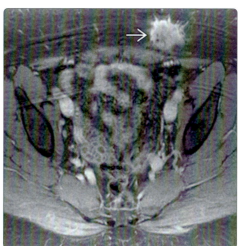

(Left) *Axial CECT in a young woman with history of cesarean section and cyclical anterior pelvic wall pain demonstrates a spiculated mass* ➡ *in the left anterior pelvic wall.* (Right) *Axial T1WI C+ MR in the same patient demonstrates the mass* ➡ *to be avidly enhancing. The location of the mass corresponded to the patient's cesarean section scar, and this was found to be an abdominal wall endometrioma at surgery.*

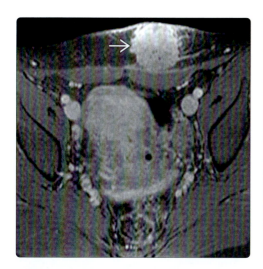

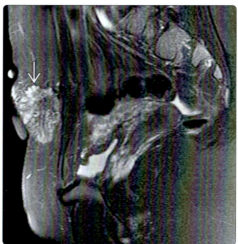

(Left) *Axial T1WI C+ MR in a young woman with cyclical abdominal wall pain at her cesarean section incision demonstrates an avidly enhancing mass* ➡, *found to be an abdominal wall endometrioma.* (Right) *Sagittal T2WI MR in the same patient shows the lesion* ➡ *to be T2 hyperintense, and the lesion was hypointense on T1WI (not shown). Abdominal wall endometriomas often look different from conventional endometriomas, appearing T1 hypointense, T2 hyperintense, and moderately enhancing.*

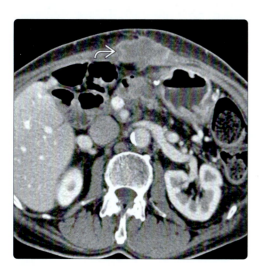

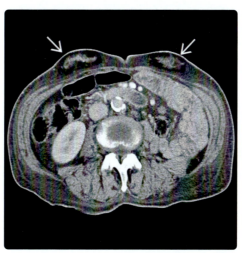

(Left) *Axial CECT in a patient status post Whipple surgery for pancreatic cancer demonstrates an irregularly shaped hypodense mass* ➡ *arising within the abdominal wall incision, found to be recurrent tumor at surgery.* (Right) *Diabetic lipohypertrophy in an elderly man shows fibrofatty masses* ➡ *present bilaterally in the subcutaneous tissues of the periumbilical region. This patient had been injecting insulin into these same 2 sites for many months.*

KEY FACTS

TERMINOLOGY

- Loculated fluid trapped within peritoneal adhesions, typically surrounding ovary

IMAGING

- Most often in pelvis (can rarely occur elsewhere)
- Ultrasound
  - Loculated cystic mass with "spiderweb" pattern due to peritoneal adhesions reflecting from ovary
  - Fine septations throughout collection
  - Normal ovary at center or lateral margin of cyst
  - No solid mural or septal nodule to suggest malignancy
  - Usually anechoic fluid, but can have internal echoes due to hemorrhagic or proteinaceous contents
- MR
  - Cystic mass with serous fluid (low signal on T1, high signal on T2) and thin internal septations
  - Margins of cyst outlined by other structures in pelvis (pelvic side walls, uterus, ovaries, loops of bowel)
  - Morphologically normal ovary at center of cyst

TOP DIFFERENTIAL DIAGNOSES

- Ovarian cancer
- Ovarian cyst or follicle
- Paraovarian cyst
- Hydrosalpinx

PATHOLOGY

- Most often in women with prior pelvic surgery or inflammatory disorders (endometriosis, pelvic inflammatory disease, inflammatory bowel disease)

CLINICAL ISSUES

- Primarily seen in women of reproductive age
- Can rarely occur in men or post-menopausal women

DIAGNOSTIC CHECKLIST

- Cystic ovarian neoplasm or malignancy if thick septations, solid component/mural nodularity, or large ascites

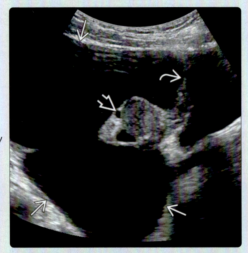
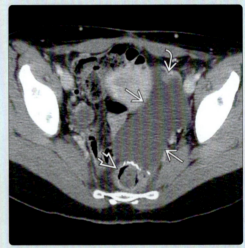

(Left) Transvaginal US in a patient with history of multiple prior surgeries for Crohn's disease shows an anechoic cyst ➡ with internal septations ⮞ enveloping a normal-appearing ovary ⮞, a classic appearance for peritoneal inclusion cyst. (Right) Axial CECT in a patient who had undergone colectomy with creation of a Hartmann pouch ⮞ shows a loculated, thin-walled pelvic fluid collection ➡ partially surrounding the left ovary ⮞, characteristic features of a peritoneal inclusion cyst.

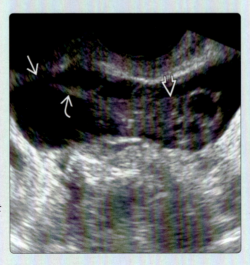
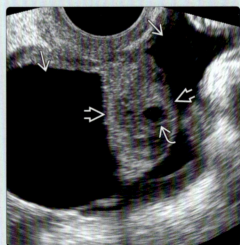

(Left) Longitudinal endovaginal US in a woman with 2-year history of pelvic pain and prior surgery for endometriosis demonstrates a complex fluid collection ➡ with internal septations ⮞ surrounding the left ovary ⮞, which contains normal follicles. Surgery revealed a peritoneal inclusion cyst and normal ovary. (Right) Transvaginal US shows the right ovary ⮞ enveloped by an anechoic fluid collection ➡. A normal follicle is present within the ovary ⮞. This is a typical appearance of a peritoneal inclusion cyst.

Peritoneal Inclusion Cyst

TERMINOLOGY

Definitions

- Loculated fluid trapped within peritoneal adhesions, typically surrounding ovary

IMAGING

General Features

- Best diagnostic clue
  - Loculated fluid collection surrounding ovary on endovaginal US with "spiderweb" pattern
- Location
  - Primarily arise in pelvis
  - Rarely in other locations (usually intraperitoneal)
- Size
  - 1-30 cm (large cysts can occupy entire pelvis)

Imaging Recommendations

- Best imaging tool
  - Ultrasound and MR

Ultrasonographic Findings

- Loculated cystic mass with "spiderweb" pattern due to peritoneal adhesions reflecting from ovary
  - Fine septations throughout collection
    - Rarely, low-resistance flow in vascularized septations
  - Normal ovary at center or lateral margin of inclusion cyst
  - No solid mural or septal nodule to suggest malignancy
  - Usually anechoic fluid, but can have internal echoes due to hemorrhagic or proteinaceous contents
  - Calcifications very uncommon
  - Only physiologic free fluid in pelvis (no frank ascites)

MR Findings

- Cystic mass with serous fluid (low signal on T1, high signal on T2), thin internal septations, and discrete wall
- Margins of cyst outlined by other structures in pelvis (pelvic side walls, uterus, ovaries, loops of bowel)
- Normal ovary often at center of cyst

CT Findings

- Loculated cyst in pelvis outlined by normal pelvic structures
- Ovary may be seen within cyst

DIFFERENTIAL DIAGNOSIS

Ovarian Cancer

- Mural or septal nodularity, thick septations, low resistance vascularity within septations or solid components, ascites, and lymphadenopathy raise suspicion for malignancy
- Normal ovary is not seen within cystic mass

Ovarian Cyst or Follicle

- Cyst located within ovary adjacent to normal ovarian stroma or follicles

Paraovarian Cyst

- Cyst in broad ligament adjacent to ovary
- Does not surround ovary like peritoneal inclusion cyst

Hydrosalpinx

- Oblong, tubular cystic mass with "cog wheel" appearance
- Ovary separate from dilated tube

Lymphocele

- Prior history of lymph node dissection
- Rounded cysts along pelvic side wall

PATHOLOGY

General Features

- Etiology
  - Most often found in women with history of prior pelvic surgery or inflammatory disorder of abdomen/pelvis
    - Most often after gynecologic surgery
    - Inflammatory causes include endometriosis, pelvic inflammatory disease, inflammatory bowel disease
  - Active ovarian function exudates fluid that then becomes trapped by adhesions

CLINICAL ISSUES

Presentation

- Most common signs/symptoms
  - Pelvic pain, abdominal distension
- Other signs/symptoms
  - Bowel or urinary symptoms due to mass effect
  - Can cause infertility
  - 10% are incidental findings on imaging or pelvic surgery
  - Laboratory markers: Cancer antigen 125 (CA-125) normal

Demographics

- Age
  - 16-45
- Gender
  - Primarily women of reproductive age
  - Can rarely occur in post-menopausal women and men with extensive surgical history

Natural History & Prognosis

- May be stable for many years
- May decrease in size or resolve during menopause

Treatment

- No treatment for asymptomatic cysts if cyst can be confidently distinguished from malignancy
- Oral contraceptives can decrease cyst size by reducing ovarian fluid from ovulation
- Cyst aspiration may provide short term symptom relief
  - Temporary solution, as fluid usually reaccumulates
- Image-guided sclerotherapy may be an option
- Surgery for symptomatic patients or if malignancy cannot be confidently excluded based on imaging and CA-125
  - Cysts recur in 30-50% of patients undergoing surgery

DIAGNOSTIC CHECKLIST

Consider

- Cystic ovarian neoplasm or malignancy if thick septations, solid component/mural nodularity, or large ascites

SELECTED REFERENCES

1. Veldhuis WB et al: Peritoneal inclusion cysts: clinical characteristics and imaging features. Eur Radiol. 23(4):1167-74, 2013

TERMINOLOGY

- Heterogeneous group of hematologic malignancies of lymphoid or myeloid origin

IMAGING

- **Gastrointestinal tract**
  - Circumferential wall thickening, large cavitary lesion, polypoid mass, or multiple discrete submucosal nodules
- **Spleen**
  - Diffuse splenomegaly without discrete masses
  - Multiple small, hypodense splenic lesions
  - Solitary dominant splenic mass
- **Liver**
  - Solitary mass, multiple masses, or diffuse infiltration
- **Pancreas**
  - Can present as discrete mass or diffuse infiltration
  - No ductal dilatation, glandular atrophy, or biliary obstruction
- **Kidneys**

- Solitary, dominant mass or bilateral nodules
- Nephromegaly with diffuse tumor infiltration of kidney
- Perinephric soft tissue "rind" encasing kidney
- **Peritoneum and omentum (lymphomatosis)**
  - Can be indistinguishable from peritoneal carcinomatosis
- **Lymph nodes**
  - Enlargement is most common, though nonspecific sign of involvement
    - Size criteria not reliable and vary by region
- **Testicles**
  - Solitary or multifocal hypoechoic masses on ultrasound
  - Involved sites show increased color flow vascularity

TOP DIFFERENTIAL DIAGNOSES

- Metastatic lymphadenopathy
- Sarcoidosis
- Infections
- Primary visceral organ malignancies
- Metastatic disease

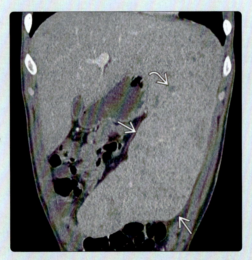
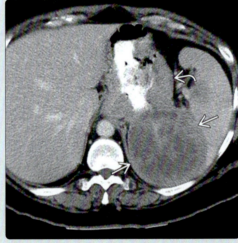

(Left) Coronal CECT in a patient with lymphoma demonstrates massive enlargement of the spleen ➡ with innumerable tiny hypodense foci ➤ within the splenic parenchyma, in keeping with diffuse splenic lymphomatous involvement. (Right) Axial CECT demonstrates a large mass ➡ centered in the spleen extending medially to involve the stomach, which also appears thickened along the greater curvature ➤. These findings were found to be manifestations of non-Hodgkin lymphoma (NHL).

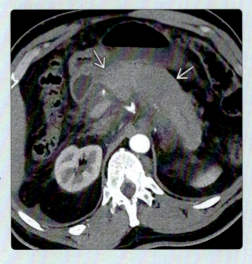
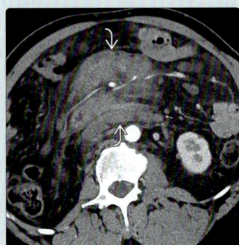

(Left) Axial CECT demonstrates diffuse enlargement and infiltration of the pancreas ➡, superficially resembling pancreatitis. (Right) Axial CECT in the same patient demonstrates extensive adenopathy ➤ in the mesentery inferior to the pancreas. Notice the manner in which the lymph nodes surround the mesenteric vessels, often described as the sandwich sign. These findings, including the enlargement of the pancreas, were found to represent NHL.

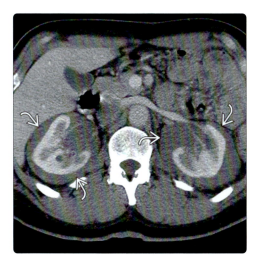
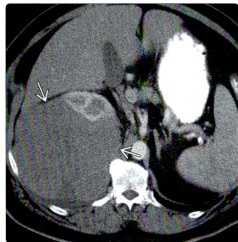

(Left) Axial CECT demonstrates a "rind" of hypodense soft tissue ⮕ encasing both kidneys, a classic appearance of perirenal lymphoma. (Right) Axial CECT demonstrates a large soft tissue mass ⮕ surrounding the right kidney, representing a manifestation of perirenal NHL.

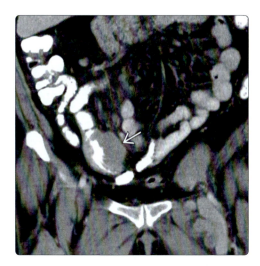
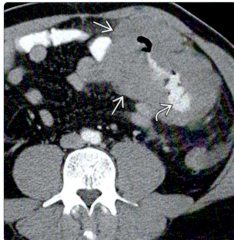

(Left) Coronal CECT demonstrates mass-like soft tissue thickening ⮕ of a loop of ileum. Note the lack of bowel obstruction despite significant bowel involvement, a characteristic feature of lymphoma. (Right) Axial CECT in an HIV-positive patient demonstrates a large, ulcerated mass ⮕ containing enteric contrast ⮕ arising from the small bowel. Note the classic aneurysmal dilatation of the involved bowel due to tumor infiltration, a common manifestation of bowel lymphoma.

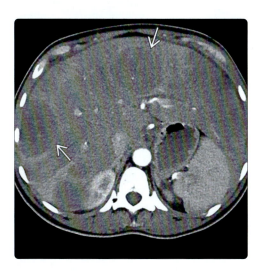
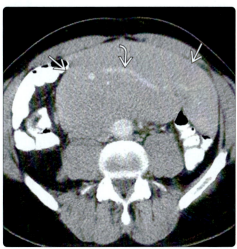

(Left) Axial CECT demonstrates multiple discrete hypodense masses ⮕ in the liver as well as more diffuse hypodense infiltration of much of the remaining liver parenchyma. This was all found to represent lymphomatous infiltration of the liver on biopsy. (Right) Axial CECT demonstrates a large conglomerate nodal mass ⮕ in the mesentery. Note the encasement of mesenteric vessels ⮕, which course through the mass but remain patent, characteristic of lymphoma.

TERMINOLOGY

- Submucosal tumor of gastrointestinal (GI) tract derived from interstitial cells of Cajal
- Gastrointestinal stromal tumor (GIST)

IMAGING

- **Multiplanar, multiphasic CT, PET are best imaging tools**
  - CT (& MR) accurately detect & characterize GISTs
    - Sensitivity: 93%; specificity: 100%
- Hypo- or hypervascular, well-circumscribed, submucosal mass on arterial phase images
  - Often exophytic; sometimes hemorrhagic
  - Ulceration and necrosis are common
  - Calcifications are present in 25% of cases
- PET is superior to CT in predicting early response to Gleevec (imatinib)
  - Hypermetabolic foci for both primary tumor and metastases
  - Sensitivity: 86%; specificity: 98%

PATHOLOGY

- Distinct, not synonymous with leiomyoma/sarcoma
  - May not be diagnosed by light microscopy alone
- Can be benign or malignant
- Stomach is most common site (2/3 of cases)
  - Duodenum is 2nd most common site
  - Can occur anywhere along GI tract

CLINICAL ISSUES

- Most common mesenchymal tumor of GI tract
- Symptoms: Nausea, vomiting, weight loss
  - Mass effect from bulky tumor
  - GI bleeding when ulcerated
- Excellent prognosis for completely resected benign lesions
- Good response to chemotherapy (imatinib) in patients with metastatic disease and *c-KIT* mutation
- Prognosis often depends on tumor size
  - Poor if > 5 cm

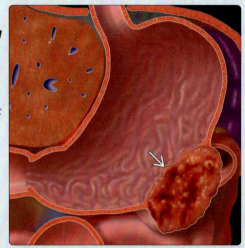
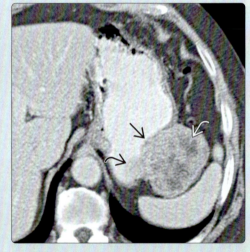

(Left) Anatomic depiction of a gastric GIST shows an exophytic submucosal mass ➡ with internal necrosis. (Right) Axial CECT shows a soft tissue density LUQ mass ➡ that is solid with foci of central necrosis ➡, typical of GIST. The origin of the mass may not be evident, except for a small projection ➡ into the gastric lumen.

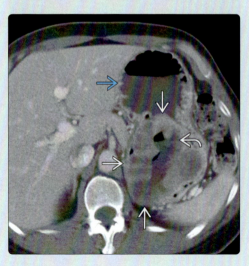
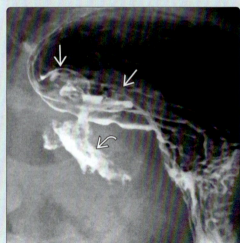

(Left) Axial CECT shows a large LUQ mass ➡. The stomach ➡ appears almost normal except for being indented along its dorsal surface by the mass, which is necrotic in its center and contains a gas-fluid level ➡ due to communication with the gastric lumen. (Right) A spot film from an upper GI series in the same case shows the mass effect on the stomach ➡ and extravasation of barium into the cavitated center of the gastric GIST ➡.

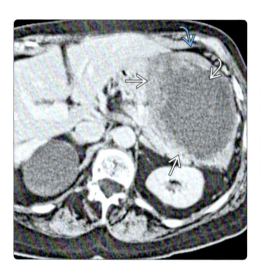
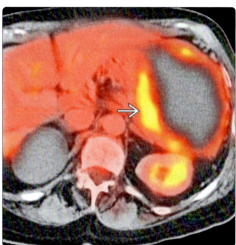

(Left) *Axial CECT shows a large, exophytic GIST arising from the greater curve of the stomach ⇥. It has a thick, mildly enhancing wall ➡ and a necrotic center ⬂.* (Right) *Axial fused PET/CT in the same case shows FDG uptake ➡ within the solid portion of this mass. FDG PET will show activity in the primary tumor and aids in the detection of metastatic disease. It can also detect early response to therapy before morphologic changes are seen in the tumor.*

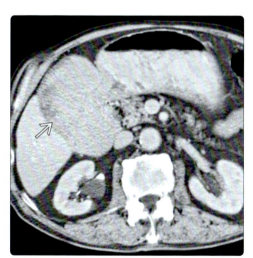
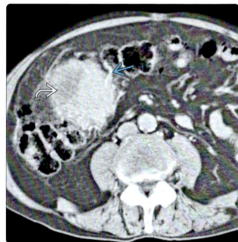

(Left) *Axial CECT shows an exophytic soft tissue-density mass ➡ distorting the distal stomach and duodenum.* (Right) *Axial CECT in the same patient shows brisk enhancement of this mass with areas of necrosis ➡ as well as prominent feeding vessels ⇥. These are typical findings for GIST.*

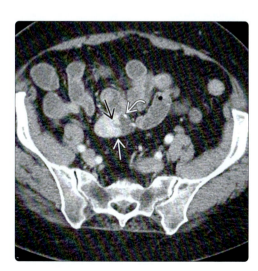
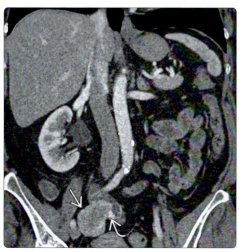

(Left) *A 71-year-old woman presented with hematochezia. CT enterography shows a brightly enhancing mass ➡ that is mostly exophytic and does not obstruct the bowel lumen. Ulceration ⇥ of the surface of the mass is suggested. Active bleeding into the bowel lumen is seen as a brightly enhancing focus ⬂.* (Right) *Coronal CT in the same patient clearly shows the exophytic nature of the mass ➡ and also the active bleeding ➡ into the bowel lumen. A GIST was excised from the small bowel.*

KEY FACTS

TERMINOLOGY

- Terms such as carcinoid and islet cell tumor are decreasing in use, in favor of well-differentiated (low-grade) or poorly differentiated (high-grade) NETs
- GI tract: Most common primary site (74%), followed by bronchopulmonary (24%)
  - Small bowel most common (~ 60%); ileum in majority
  - Pancreas: < 1% of all NETs

IMAGING

- Patients with known or suspected NET require multimodality imaging approach, combining anatomic (morphologic) and functional (physiologic) imaging tests
- Multiphasic, multiplanar CT is preferred initial test, allowing for comprehensive evaluation of chest, abdomen, and pelvis
  - Multiphasic, multiplanar CT is mandatory
  - Primary tumors and metastases are typically hypervascular and best seen on arterial phase

- MR has greater sensitivity and specificity than CT for pancreatic NETs (PNETs) and for liver involvement
  - Liver metastases are often very bright on T2WI, may mimic hemangioma or cyst, though distinction is possible
- Functional imaging with somatostatin analogs is recommended for most patients
  - Can detect tumor sites missed on CT and MR
  - Uptake of radiolabelled somatostatin analogs is predictive of clinical response to therapy with somatostatin analogs and peptide receptor radionuclide therapy
  - Indium-111 octreotide scintigraphy is most widely available
  - Gallium-68 octreotate (DOTATATE) PET/CT is now preferred due to faster scan time, lower radiation dose, and improved spatial resolution
- Endoscopic or intraoperative US
  - Can detect small PNETs with greater sensitivity than CT or MR

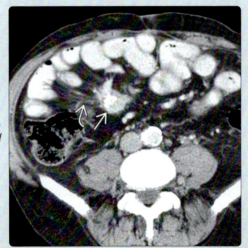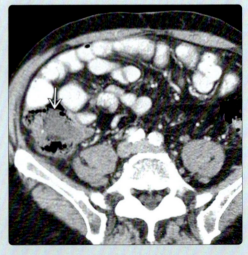

(Left) Axial CECT in a man with abdominal pain shows a hypervascular mesenteric mass ➡ with central calcification. Mesenteric vessels are engorged ➡ and small bowel (SB) loops appear tethered. (Right) Venous-phase CT in the same patient shows an equivocal mass ➡ in the ileocecal area, a confirmed neuroendocrine tumor (NET, "carcinoid") at surgery. The mesenteric metastasis was more evident on CT than the primary tumor, due in part to dense contrast media within bowel and lack of arterial-phase imaging.

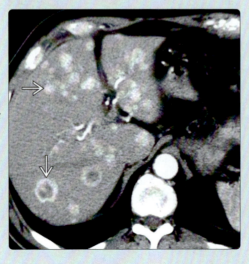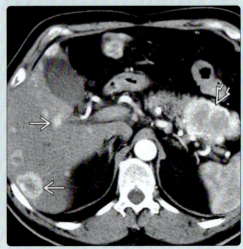

(Left) Axial CECT in the arterial phase of a patient with a metastatic nonsyndromic NET shows innumerable hypervascular liver lesions ➡, some of which have ring-shaped enhancement patterns. (Right) Axial CECT in the same patient shows a large, hypervascular pancreatic mass ➡ and additional hepatic metastases ➡. This constellation of findings is typical of a malignant NET of the pancreas, a glucagonoma in this case. Glucagonomas are more commonly malignant than insulinomas.

TERMINOLOGY

Abbreviations

- Neuroendocrine tumor (NET); pancreatic NET (PNET)
- Carcinoid syndrome
  - Symptoms: Flushing, diarrhea, palpitations
    - Usually indicates liver metastases from gastrointestinal (GI) or bronchopulmonary NET

Synonyms

- Tumors arising from enterochromografin cells
- **Terms such as carcinoid and islet cell tumor are decreasing in use, in favor of more specific terminology [World Health Organization (WHO) and European NET Society (ENETS) 2010 classification]**
  - Islet cell tumor (PNET)
  - Carcinoid tumor (relatively well-differentiated NET)
- General concepts
  - Divided into well-differentiated (low-grade) or poorly differentiated (high-grade) NETs based on WHO/ENETS classification
  - No longer divided into functioning or nonfunctioning, as all NETs are now considered hormonally active
  - May be classified also into syndromic (produce clinical syndrome with abnormal lab findings) or nonsyndromic
    - Syndromic tumors: Secrete multiple pancreatic hormones, but patients often have dominant clinical syndrome (e.g., hypoglycemia: Insulinoma)
      - Insulinoma, glucagonoma, gastrinoma, somatostatinoma, VIPoma (vasoactive intestinal polypeptide)
    - Nonsyndromic tumors: Hypofunctioning or clinically silent tumors
      - Larger than syndromic tumors at diagnosis due to lack of symptoms or laboratory abnormalities

Associated Syndromes

- Multiple endocrine neoplasia type 1, von Hippel-Lindau, neurofibromatosis type 1, tuberous sclerosis
- Zollinger-Ellison syndrome: Gastrinoma
- May have or develop other malignant tumors (colorectal > prostate, cervical)

IMAGING

General Features

- Location
  - Can arise in virtually any organ in body
    - GI tract: Most common primary site (74%), followed by bronchopulmonary (24%)
      - Small bowel (SB) most common (~ 60%); ileum in majority
      - Can be multifocal throughout SB
      - Duodenal: 2-8%
      - Colorectal; rectum most common (~ 20%)
      - Appendix: Usually incidental finding at appendectomy
      - Stomach: ~ 5%; more often in Zollinger-Ellison syndrome
    - Pancreas: < 1% of all NETs
      - Comprise ~ 3% of all pancreatic neoplasms
      - Gastrinomas usually (90%) arise in gastrinoma triangle (pancreatic head and duodenum)

Protocol Advice

- Patients with known or suspected NET require multimodality imaging approach, combining anatomic (morphologic) and functional (physiologic) imaging tests
- **Multiphasic, multiplanar CT** is preferred initial test, allowing for comprehensive evaluation of chest, abdomen, and pelvis
- **MR** has greater sensitivity and specificity than CT for PNETs and for liver involvement
- **Functional imaging** with somatostatin analogs is recommended for most patients
  - Uptake of radiolabelled somatostatin analogs is predictive of clinical response to therapy with somatostatin analogs and peptide receptor radionuclide therapy
  - Can detect tumor sites missed on CT and MR
  - Indium-111 octreotide scintigraphy is more widely available
  - **Gallium-68 octreotate (DOTATATE) PET/CT** is now preferred due to faster scan time, lower radiation dose, and improved spatial resolution
- **Endoscopic or intraoperative US**
  - Can detect small PNETs with greater sensitivity than CT or MR
  - Especially valuable in detecting gastrinomas that arise in duodenal region

CT Findings

- Multiphasic, multiplanar CT is mandatory
  - Arterial, venous, and delayed phases; viewed in axial and coronal planes
  - Primary tumors and metastases are usually more evident on arterial-phase imaging
  - Coronal plane imaging allows better visualization of bowel and mesenteric disease and easier correlation with coronal plane of PET imaging
  - Do not give "positive" (opaque) oral contrast media; give water instead
- **GI NETs**
  - Solitary or multiple intramural mass(es)
  - 80-95% are hypervascular, best detected on arterial-phase imaging
    - Primary site and metastases (nodal, mesenteric, hepatic, peritoneal)
    - Metastatic foci are often larger and more apparent than primary tumor site
  - SB NETs usually secrete serotonin with visible effects on mesentery and regional bowel
    - Infiltration; kinking; tethering; occasional SB obstruction
    - Most evident on coronal plane imaging
    - Mesenteric veins and lymphatics may be occluded (leads to vessel engorgement and SB wall thickening)
  - Calcification is present in ~ 70% of primary and mesenteric metastatic foci
- **PNETs**
  - Well-circumscribed pancreatic mass with noninfiltrative margins that is usually (but not always) hypervascular and most conspicuous on arterial phase

ENETS/WHO Nomenclature and Classification for Digestive System Neuroendocrine Tumors

Differentiation	Grade	Mitotic Count*	Ki-67 Index	Traditional	ENETS, WHO
Well differentiated	Low grade (G1)	< 2 per 10 HPF	< 3%	Carcinoid, islet cell, pancreatic (neuro)endocrine tumor	Neuroendocrine tumor, grade 1
	Intermediate grade (G2)	2-20 per 10 HPF	3-20%	Carcinoid, atypical carcinoid, islet cell, pancreatic (neuro)endocrine tumor	Neuroendocrine tumor, grade 2
Poorly differentiated	High grade (G3)	> 20 per 10 HPF	> 20%	Small cell carcinoma	Neuroendocrine carcinoma, grade 3, small cell
				Large cell neuroendocrine carcinoma	Neuroendocrine carcinoma, grade 3, large cell

WHO = World Health Organization, ENETS = European Neuroendocrine Tumors Society.

- – Lesions usually hyperenhance to lesser degree on venous phase, making smaller lesions difficult to detect
  - □ Rarely can be most conspicuous on venous phase
- – Syndromic tumors tend to be smaller at presentation (usually < 3 cm with insulinomas < 2 cm)
- – Nonsyndromic tumors are typically much larger at presentation (average > 5 cm)
  - □ Usually hypervascular but less so than syndromic
  - □ Large tumors are more likely to demonstrate central necrosis, cystic change, and calcification
- o Lesions often demonstrate calcification (central or diffuse)
- o Usually no biliary or pancreatic duct obstruction (unless large) or upstream pancreatic atrophy
  - – Some small tumors may rarely secrete serotonin that can cause fibrosis and obstruction of pancreatic duct
- o Invasion (rather than encasement) by tumor of splenic or superior mesenteric vein
- o Cystic NET can mimic other pancreatic cystic lesions
  - – Presence of peripheral enhancement or nodularity on arterial phase should strongly suggest diagnosis
- o Metastases demonstrate similar characteristics to primary tumor: Hypervascular lymph node and liver metastases
  - – Most common sites of metastases include liver, local lymph nodes, and bone (sclerotic lesions)
  - – Fluid-fluid levels within neuroendocrine liver metastases are described as specific feature
- o Zollinger-Ellison syndrome (gastrinoma): Avid enhancement and wall thickening of gastric wall

MR Findings

- NETs tend to be hypointense (relative to normal pancreas) on T1WI, hyperintense on T2WI, and enhance similarly to CECT on T1WI C+
  - o Homogeneous enhancement for small tumors < 2 cm
  - o Heterogeneous enhancement with areas of necrosis for larger lesions
- Liver metastases are typically very hyperintense on T2WI and mimic hemangiomas or cysts
  - o Fluid-fluid levels may be visualized within liver metastases, particularly on T2WI
  - o Liver metastases usually T1WI hypointense but may show hyperintensity due to intratumoral hemorrhage

- DWI: Lesions show variable ADC values, but DWI can help identify tiny lesions that are otherwise occult

Ultrasonographic Findings

- Endoscopic US: Sensitivity and specificity > 90% for PNETs
  - o Can be helpful to identify small NET that may be missed on CT/MR in patients with high clinical suspicion
  - o Can "tattoo" lesion to guide laparoscopic surgery
  - o No specific imaging features, as lesions tend to be hypoechoic or isoechoic to surrounding pancreas
- Intraoperative US: Can detect small nonpalpable lesions and help guide surgical resection

Nuclear Medicine Findings

- Gallium-68 DOTATATE PET/CT
  - o Key imaging technique for detection and characterization of NETs
  - o Allows whole-body detection and characterization of NETs that secrete somatostatin (well-differentiated GI and PNETs)
  - o May detect tumor sites missed by CT or MR
  - o Can exclude distant metastases in patients being considered for surgical intervention
- FDG PET/CT
  - o Complementary role to DOTATATE PET/CT
  - o Detects poorly differentiated NETs better than Ga-DOTATATE PET/CT
    - – Detects tumors that are metabolically active, high-grade tumors that do not secrete somatostatin
- Indium-111 DTPA octreotide (Octreoscan)
  - o Overall sensitivity of 75-90%; 50-60% for insulinomas
  - o Combined with SPECT or SPECT/CT for better anatomical localization
  - o Most widely available scintigraphic study for NETs
  - o Overall accuracy is not as good as that of DOTATATE PET/CT

SELECTED REFERENCES

1. Maxwell JE et al: Imaging in neuroendocrine tumors: an update for the clinician. Int J Endocr Oncol. 2(2):159-168, 2015
2. Haug AR et al: Neuroendocrine tumor recurrence: diagnosis with 68Ga-DOTATATE PET/CT. Radiology. 270(2):517-25, 2014

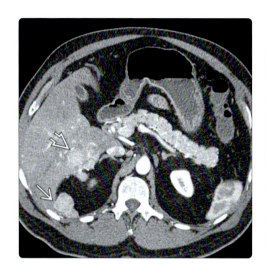

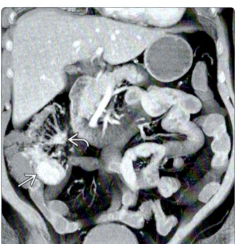

(Left) *This 54-year-old man had crampy abdominal pain and flushing. Axial CT shows hypervascular hepatic ⇒ and peritoneal metastases ⇒ from an ileal NET (carcinoid).* (Right) *Coronal reformatted CT in the same patient shows a hypervascular mass ⇒ in the terminal ileum (the primary NET) with mesenteric metastases ⇒ having a desmoplastic effect on the ileal mesentery. These are classic clinical and imaging features of "carcinoid syndrome."*

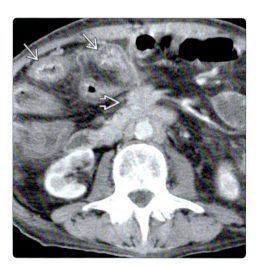

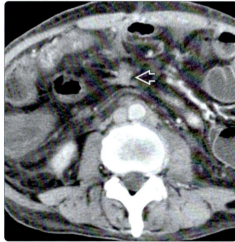

(Left) *Axial CT of the same patient shows a mesenteric mass ⇒ and paraaortic tissue, representing metastases. Note the tethered appearance and submucosal edema ⇒ of the distal SB, due to the desmoplastic effect on the mesentery and constriction of mesenteric lymphatics and veins that are characteristic of a carcinoid tumor (NET).* (Right) *Axial CECT in the same patient shows a more discrete mass ⇒ at the base of the mesentery, which has the typical spiculated appearance of a carcinoid (NET) metastasis.*

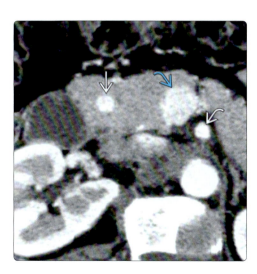

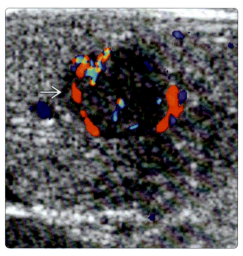

(Left) *Axial CECT in a patient suspected to have an insulinoma based on clinical symptoms shows a small (6 mm) hypervascular mass ⇒ in the head of the pancreas. The SMA ⇒ and SMV ⇒ are marked.* (Right) *Intraoperative US in the same patient demonstrates a hypervascular, hypoechoic lesion ⇒ that was not palpable. The patient underwent a Whipple resection, and an insulinoma was found at pathology. Intraoperative US is extremely valuable to localize lesions and to guide surgical resection of small NETs.*

(Left) *Arterial-phase CECT demonstrates an avidly enhancing pancreatic neck mass ➡ in keeping with a pancreatic NET. In this case, the upstream pancreas is markedly atrophic ➡, an atypical feature for NETs, which do not typically obstruct the pancreatic duct or cause parenchymal atrophy.* **(Right)** *While the mass ➡ is still enhancing on this axial venous-phase CECT from the same patient, note that the mass demonstrates a much lesser degree of enhancement compared to the arterial-phase image.*

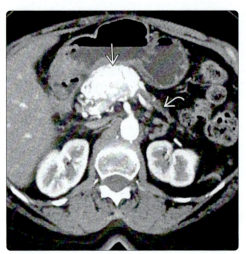
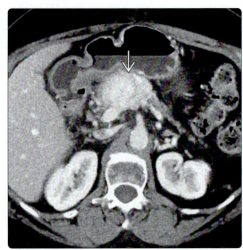

(Left) *Axial CECT demonstrates a cystic lesion ➡ in the pancreatic tail. While IPMN or mucinous cystic neoplasm are possibilities, the peripheral enhancing soft tissue ➡ should suggest the correct diagnosis of cystic NET.* **(Right)** *Coronal CECT shows a hypovascular mass ➡ in the pancreatic uncinate with multiple liver metastases ➡. Note that the lesion is invading the SMV ➡, a feature uncommon with adenocarcinoma and more common with NET. This was found to be a NET at resection.*

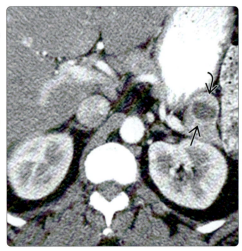
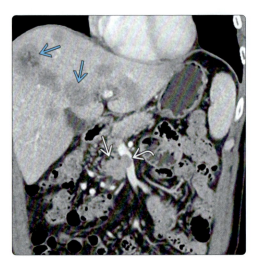

(Left) *Axial arterial-phase CECT demonstrates a massive hypervascular NET ➡ replacing nearly the entirety of the pancreas. Nonsyndromic tumors, as in this case, are often larger at presentation.* **(Right)** *Axial T2WI MR in the same patient demonstrates several hyperintense liver lesions ➡. While these lesions could easily be mistaken for cysts or hemangiomas, NET metastases to the liver are well known for being very T2 hyperintense.*

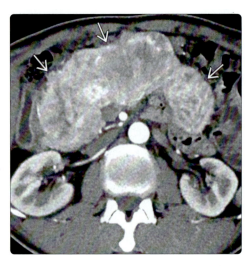
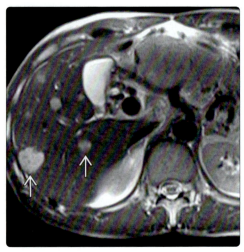

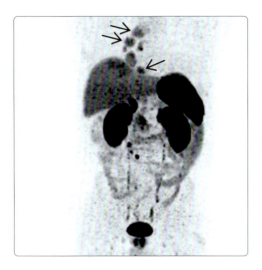

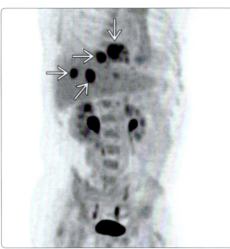

(Left) *In this 70-year-old woman, a coronal DOTATATE PET shows more obvious uptake in the thoracic lesions (well-differentiated NET)* ➡ *than in the liver lesions, where poorly differentiated NET was biopsy confirmed.* **(Right)** *In the same patient, coronal oblique FDG PET shows multiple sites of FDG-avid tumor in the chest and liver* ➡. *The fused PET/CT images are not shown. Sites of high-grade (poorly differentiated) NETs often are better shown on FDG PET/CT scans.*

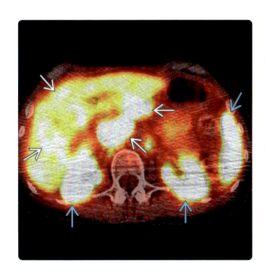

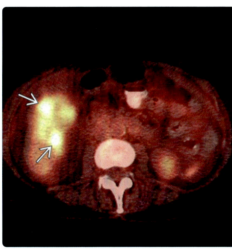

(Left) *In this 65-year-old woman, a fused axial DOTATATE PET/CT shows avid uptake* ➡ *in porta hepatis nodes and hepatic masses along with physiologic uptake in the kidneys and spleen* ➡. **(Right)** *In the same patient, a fused FDG PET/CT shows only the hepatic lesions* ➡ *as being FDG avid, probably indicating foci of higher grade NET.*

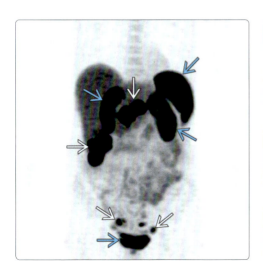

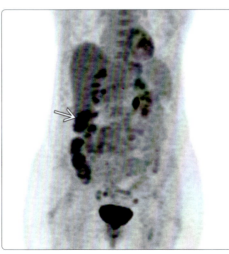

(Left) *Coronal MIP from the DOTATATE PET/CT study in the same patient shows uptake* ➡ *in the liver and pelvic metastases and porta hepatis nodes along with normal physiologic uptake in the kidneys, spleen, and bladder* ➡. **(Right)** *Coronal FDG PET/CT in the same patient shows only the liver metastases* ➡ *along with numerous foci of normal physiologic uptake. Well-differentiated NETs may not be FDG avid.*

SECTION 3

Abdominal Wall, Mesentery, and Peritoneal Cavity

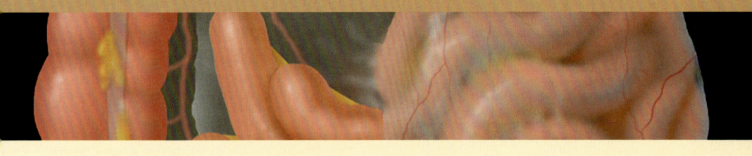

Embryology and Relevant Anatomy

The fetal gut is suspended between the anterior and posterior abdominal walls by the ventral and dorsal mesenteries, which separate to enclose the developing alimentary tube. Important viscera develop within the mesentery of the caudal part of the foregut, such as the liver, pancreas, spleen, and biliary tree. The various mesenteries either regress or elongate. The dorsal mesentery lengthens with the progressive elongation of the small intestine. The ventral mesentery resorbs, which allows communication between the right and left sides of the peritoneal cavity in adults.

Variations in the complex rotation, fusion, growth, and resorption of mesenteries and the viscera that develop within them result in common variations in peritoneal and retroperitoneal spaces in adults with clinical manifestations, such as internal hernias. All **peritoneal recesses** potentially communicate, although adhesions and other pathologic processes may seal off loculated collections of fluid, such as infected or malignant ascites.

Peritoneal Cavity

The **abdominal cavity** contains all of the abdominal viscera, both intra- and retroperitoneal, and is not synonymous with the peritoneal cavity. The abdominal cavity is limited by abdominal wall muscles, diaphragm, and pelvic brim.

The **peritoneal cavity** is a potential space within the abdomen that lies between the visceral and parietal peritoneum. It usually contains only a small amount of fluid (for lubrication).

The peritoneal cavity is composed mostly of the **greater sac** (or general peritoneal cavity). The **lesser sac** (omental bursa) communicates with the greater sac through the epiploic foramen (of Winslow) and is bounded in front by the caudate lobe, stomach, and greater omentum and in back by the pancreas and left kidney. To the left, the lesser sac is bound by the splenorenal and gastrosplenic ligaments and on the right by the lesser omentum and epiploic foramen.

While the lesser sac is in communication with the rest of the peritoneal cavity, ascites usually does not enter into it readily. Lesser sac fluid collections usually result from a local source (e.g., pancreatitis or perforated gastric ulcer) or from generalized infection or tumor (e.g., infectious or malignant ascites).

Peritoneum

The peritoneum is a thin serous membrane consisting of a single layer of squamous epithelium (mesothelium). The **parietal peritoneum** lines the abdominal wall and contains nerves to the adjacent abdominal wall, making it sensitive to pain with sharp localization. Intraabdominal disease processes that result in sharply localized pain or tenderness have generally progressed to perforation or other sources of peritoneal irritation. The **visceral peritoneum** (**serosa**) lines the abdominal organs. Its pain receptors are sensitive only to stretching (e.g., from distended bowel) and result in poor localization of the source of pain.

Mesentery

Each mesentery is a double layer of peritoneum that encloses an organ and connects it to the abdominal wall. These include the small bowel mesentery and the transverse and sigmoid mesocolons. The mesentery is covered on both sides by mesothelium and has a core of loose connective tissue containing fat, lymph nodes, blood vessels, and nerves, which pass to and from viscera.

Most mobile parts of the gut have a mesentery, while the ascending and descending colon and some parts of the duodenum are considered retroperitoneal, as they are covered only on their anterior surfaces. The root of the mesentery attaches to the posterior abdominal wall. Processes that originate in retroperitoneal organs, such as pancreatitis, may involve intraperitoneal organs by easily spreading through the "subperitoneal space" via the mesenteries.

Omentum

An omentum is a multilayered fold of peritoneum that extends from the stomach to adjacent organs. The **lesser omentum** joins the lesser curve of the stomach and proximal duodenum to the liver. The hepatogastric and hepatoduodenal ligaments form the lesser omentum and carry or contain the bile duct, portal vein, hepatic artery, and important lymph nodes.

The **greater omentum** is a 4-layered fold of peritoneum that hangs from the greater curve of the stomach like an apron covering the transverse colon and much of the small intestine. The greater omentum contains variable amounts of fat and abundant lymph nodes. It is mobile and can fill gaps between viscera, acting as a barrier to generalized spread of intraperitoneal infection or tumor, hence the nickname "nature's Band-Aid."

Ligaments

All double-layered folds of peritoneum, other than the mesentery and omentum, are called peritoneal ligaments. Ligaments connect 1 viscus to another (e.g., the splenorenal ligament) or a viscus to the abdominal wall (e.g., the falciform ligament) and contain blood vessels or remnants of fetal vessels.

Peritoneal Recesses

Recesses are the dependent pouches formed by reflections of peritoneum. Due to their clinical importance, these often are known by eponyms, such as the **Morison pouch** (posterior subhepatic or hepatorenal fossa) or the **pouch of Douglas** (rectouterine fossa or recess).

Clinical Implications

The peritoneal cavity and its various mesenteries and recesses are usually not apparent on imaging studies unless they are distended or outlined by intraperitoneal fluid or air. Peritoneum that is evident on imaging is thickened due to inflammation, infection, or tumor. Nodular thickening is a sign of malignancy (**peritoneal carcinomatosis**). **Peritoneal recesses** are common sites for accumulation of peritoneal fluid (ascites), pus, and peritoneal tumor implants.

Abdominal Wall

Musculature

The muscles of the anterior abdominal wall and their aponeuroses (sheet-like tendons) act as a corset to confine and protect the abdominal viscera. These muscles help to flex and twist the trunk and maintain posture. They increase intraabdominal pressure voluntarily, assisting in defecation, micturition, and childbirth.

The **rectus sheath** is formed by interlacing fibers of the aponeuroses of the oblique and transverse abdominal muscles. The sheath contains the rectus muscles and the superior and inferior epigastric vessels.

The muscles of the posterior abdominal wall are the psoas, iliacus, and quadratus lumborum. These help maintain posture, flex and extend the trunk, and flex the thigh.

Clinical Implications
The rectus and iliopsoas compartments are common sites for spontaneous bleeding in patients with coagulopathy (e.g., heparin therapy). The rectus sheath is incomplete caudally, allowing rectus sheath bleeding to extend into the pelvic extraperitoneal spaces.

Obesity and lack of exercise result in atrophy of the abdominal wall muscles. A pannus is a lax abdominal wall with excessive subcutaneous fat that may simulate a ventral hernia on clinical exam and imaging.

Hernias may be postsurgical or occur at congenital points of weakness in aponeuroses. For example, a ventral hernia occurs through the linea alba in the midline. A spigelian hernia occurs lateral to the rectus muscle, below the umbilicus through a defect in the aponeurosis of the internal oblique and transverse abdominal muscles. Lumbar hernias occur at a congenital point of deficiency just above the iliac crest at what is known as the inferior lumbar triangle (of Petit).

Abdominal wall hernias often do not come to clinical attention until adulthood when a general weakening and thinning of the musculofascial plane allows abdominal contents to herniate through the congenital defect.

Differential Diagnosis

Mesenteric or Omental Mass (Solid)
Common
- Lymphoma
- Lymphadenopathy, mesenteric
- Peritoneal metastases
- Pancreatitis, acute
- Diaphragm insertions (mimic)
- Mesenteric hematoma

Less Common
- Mesothelioma
- Desmoid
- Sclerosing mesenteritis
- Tuberculous peritonitis
- Carcinoid tumor
- Splenosis

Rare but Important
- Papillary serous carcinoma of mesentery
- Small bowel stromal tumor (GI stromal tumor)
- Sarcoma of mesentery or retroperitoneum
- Weber-Christian disease
- Inflammatory pseudotumor
- Solitary fibrous tumor
- Desmoplastic small round cell tumor
- Benign mesenchymal tumors
- Leukemic peritoneal implants

Mesenteric Lymphadenopathy
Common
- Lymphoma
- Metastases: Colon carcinoma, pancreatic ductal carcinoma, carcinoid tumor, small bowel carcinoma
- Appendicitis
- Mesenteric adenitis

- Crohn's disease
- Sclerosing mesenteritis
- Mononucleosis
- Kaposi sarcoma, mycobacterial infection (intestinal)
- Sarcoidosis, abdominal signs

Less Common
- Ulcerative colitis
- Diverticulitis
- Scleroderma, intestinal
- Mastocytosis
- Celiac-sprue, Whipple, or Castleman disease

Pneumoperitoneum
Common
- Duodenal or gastric ulcer
- Diverticulitis
- Intestinal trauma
- Iatrogenic injury, postoperative, bowel anastomotic leak
- Pneumothorax, atelectasis (subsegmental), cystic lung disease, barotrauma (mimics)
- Colonic interposition (mimic)
- Subphrenic fat (mimic)

Less Common
- Perforated colon
- Peritonitis
- Abdominal abscess
- Pneumatosis of intestine
- From female genital tract
- Small bowel diverticula
- Foreign body perforation

Hemoperitoneum
Common
- Splenic, hepatic, intestinal, or mesenteric trauma
- Complication of surgery
- Coagulopathic hemorrhage
- Ruptured ovarian cyst, corpus luteum, or ectopic pregnancy, HELLP
- Bladder trauma (mimic)
- Ruptured aneurysm

Less Common
- Neoplastic hemorrhage: Hepatic adenoma, hepatocellular carcinoma, hepatic metastases and lymphoma
- Ruptured spleen: Mononucleosis, lymphoma

Abdominal Wall Mass
Common
- Hernia (e.g., ventral or umbilical)
- Abdominal wall abscess
- Sebaceous cyst
- Lipoma
- Keloid
- Hematoma
- Paraumbilical varices
- Muscle asymmetry
- Injection site

Less Common
- Endometriosis
- Calcinosis syndromes
- Metastases
- Lymphoma and leukemia
- Desmoid
- Sarcoma

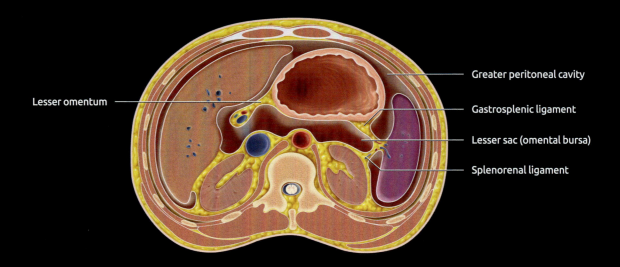

Lesser omentum

Greater peritoneal cavity

Gastrosplenic ligament

Lesser sac (omental bursa)

Splenorenal ligament

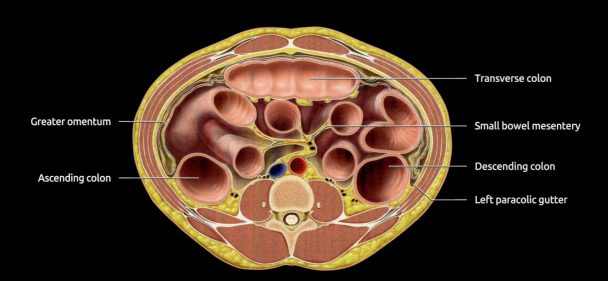

Greater omentum

Ascending colon

Transverse colon

Small bowel mesentery

Descending colon

Left paracolic gutter

(Top) *The borders of the lesser sac (omental bursa) include the lesser omentum, which conveys the common bile duct and hepatic and gastric vessels. The left borders include the gastrosplenic ligament (with short gastric vessels) and the splenorenal ligament (with splenic vessels).* **(Bottom)** *The paracolic gutters are formed by reflections of peritoneum covering the ascending and descending colon and the lateral abdominal wall. Note the innumerable potential peritoneal recesses lying between the bowel loops and their mesenteric leaves, accounting for the polygonal shape of many interloop or mesenteric fluid collections. The greater omentum covers much of the bowel like an apron.*

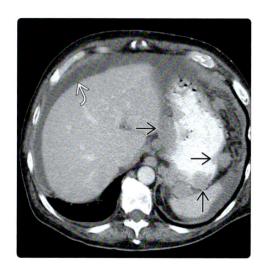
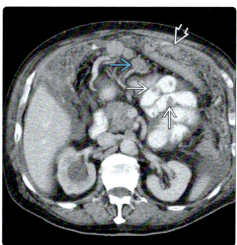

(Left) Axial CT in a man with metastatic melanoma shows nodular metastases on the serosal surface of the stomach ⬌ and ascites ➡. (Right) CT in the same patient shows nodular metastases to the omentum ➡, mesentery ➡, and serosal surface of the small bowel ➡. Note the clustered adherence of the small bowel segments due to the serosal metastases, often resulting in a functional small bowel obstruction.

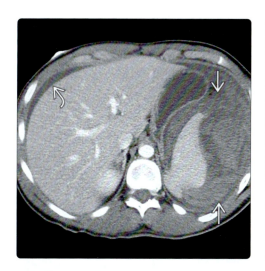
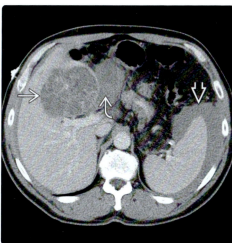

(Left) In this trauma case, CT shows extensive, heterogeneous, clotted blood ➡ surrounding the spleen and lower density, more homogeneous blood in the right subphrenic space ➡. This sentinel clot sign helped to identify the spleen as the source of hemorrhage. (Right) Axial CT in a man with melanoma and acute abdominal pain shows a metastasis ➡ to the liver with an adjacent sentinel clot ➡, indicating capsular rupture and bleeding. Lower density hemoperitoneum is also seen ➡.

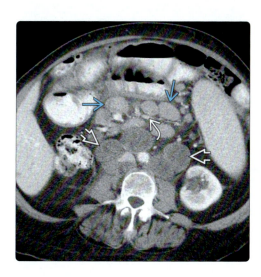
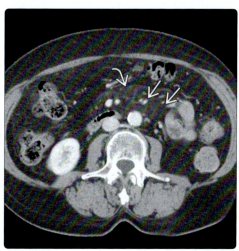

(Left) Axial CT in a 64-year-old woman with non-Hodgkin lymphoma shows splenomegaly and massive diffuse lymphadenopathy, including mesenteric ➡, "sandwiching" the superior mesenteric vessels ➡. Some retroperitoneal nodes ➡ are unusually low in density, a finding that can also be seen in tuberculosis and Whipple disease. (Right) Axial CECT illustrates typical features of mesenteritis, including involvement of the jejunal mesentery, cluster of enlarged nodes ➡, thin capsule ➡, and perivascular halo of sparing.

KEY FACTS

TERMINOLOGY

- Infectious or inflammatory process involving peritoneum or peritoneal cavity

IMAGING

- **Contrast-enhanced, multiplanar CT is 1st-line imaging**
- Ascites ± loculated fluid collections or discrete abscess
  - Ascites may be slightly higher in attenuation (15-30 HU) on CT than simple ascites (~ 0 HU)
  - Internal complexity within ascites fluid (septations, debris) is common and easier to appreciate on MR or US
- Smooth thickening and hyperenhancement of peritoneum
- Infiltration and fat stranding within mesentery and omentum
- Presence of ectopic gas suggests either hollow viscus perforation or gas-forming infection
- Other imaging findings may reveal cause of peritonitis (e.g., diverticulitis, appendicitis, low-density mesenteric nodes in tuberculosis)

- In chronic setting, peritoneal lining may be thickened with smooth, curvilinear calcification of parietal and visceral peritoneum
  - Most common cause is chronic peritoneal dialysis; may result in "peritoneal cocoon" with functional small bowel obstruction, chronic pain

TOP DIFFERENTIAL DIAGNOSES

- Peritoneal carcinomatosis
- "Benign" (transudative) ascites
- Pseudomyxoma peritonei

CLINICAL ISSUES

- Asymptomatic or abdominal pain & rigidity; fever; encephalopathy
- Many causes, including spontaneous bacterial & fungal peritonitis in cirrhotic patients, bowel perforation, gastrointestinal infections, bile leak, tuberculosis, etc.
- Sterile peritonitis is also possible (e.g., from bile leak or perforated ulcer)

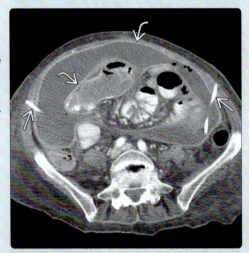 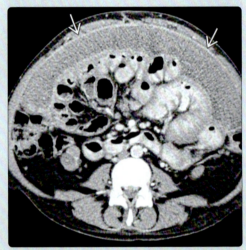

(Left) Axial CECT in a cirrhotic patient with spontaneous bacterial peritonitis demonstrates loculated ascites with enhancement and thickening of the parietal and visceral peritoneum (serosa) ➿. There are bilateral drains ➡ in place. (Right) Axial CECT in a patient on chronic peritoneal dialysis with constant symptoms of bowel obstruction shows loculated ascites ➡ with thickened, enhancing parietal and visceral peritoneum encasing the small bowel and creating functional small bowel obstruction.

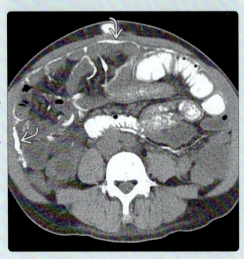 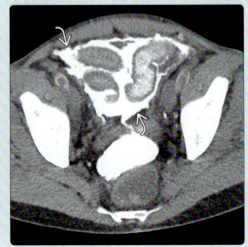

(Left) Axial NECT in a patient with a history of peritoneal dialysis demonstrates extensive calcifications ➡ and thickening of the peritoneal lining, forming a peritoneal or abdominal "cocoon." (Right) Axial NECT in the same patient demonstrates even more dramatic calcification ➡ surrounding bowel loops in the pelvis. These findings are classic for sclerosing peritonitis, most typically seen in patients on chronic peritoneal dialysis.

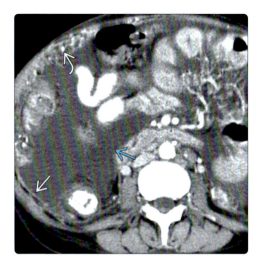

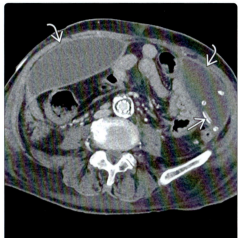

(Left) *Axial CECT of tuberculosis peritonitis shows ascites* ⇥*, enhancement and thickening of the parietal peritoneum* ⇥*, and calcification* ⇗ *within a thickened omentum. Carcinomatosis could have a similar appearance.* (Right) *Axial CECT in a patient with peritonitis after necrotizing pancreatitis demonstrates large loculated fluid collections with prominent thickening and enhancement of the adjacent peritoneal lining* ⇗*. A percutaneously placed drain* ⇥ *is in place.*

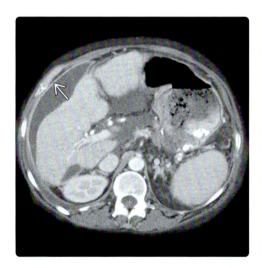

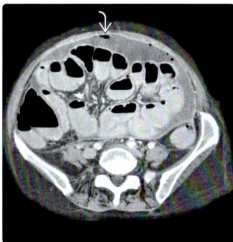

(Left) *Axial CECT in a patient who presented with alcoholic cirrhosis and abdominal pain demonstrates a nodular liver and splenomegaly with ascites, findings consistent with the patient's diagnosis of cirrhosis. Note the loculated ascites and thickened, enhancing parietal peritoneum* ⇗*, suggesting the correct diagnosis of spontaneous bacterial peritonitis.* (Right) *Axial CECT in the same patient reveals a few foci of ectopic gas* ⇗ *within the ascites fluid, a classic imaging finding of bacterial peritonitis.*

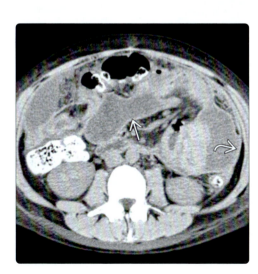

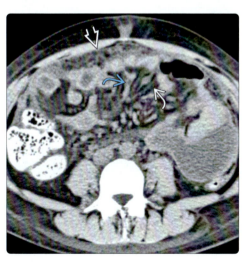

(Left) *Axial NECT in a patient with Crohn's disease and bacterial peritonitis shows loculations of ascites throughout the abdomen, including thick-walled collections between bowel loops in the mesentery* ⇗*. The thickened parietal peritoneum* ⇗ *is evidence of an inflammatory or exudative etiology.* (Right) *Axial NECT in the same patient shows infiltration of the omental* ⇥ *and mesenteric fat* ⇗*, plus mesenteric vessel engorgement* ⇗ *due to the generalized inflammatory process and peritonitis.*

KEY FACTS

TERMINOLOGY

- Inflammatory and fibrotic disorder affecting mesentery

IMAGING

- **Multiplanar CT is diagnostic procedure of choice**
- Acute mesenteritis
  - Located in left upper quadrant (jejunal) mesentery
  - "Misty mesentery": Increased attenuation of mesentery with fat stranding and induration
  - Thin pseudocapsule encasing inflamed mesentery
  - Cluster of mildly enlarged (5- to 9-mm) mesenteric nodes
  - Mesenteric vessels and nodes have halo of spared fat (fat ring or fat halo sign)
- Chronic phase
  - Discrete fibrotic soft tissue mass with desmoplastic reaction
  - Stellate appearance ± calcification within mass
  - Encasement and obstruction of mesenteric veins and lymphatics

- — → small bowel wall edema and mucosal hyperemia
  - Tethering of bowel loops can lead to bowel obstruction
- **MR**: Variable signal intensity due to varying elements of inflammation, fat necrosis, calcification, and fibrosis
- **PET/CT**: May be FDG-avid and mistaken for malignancy

TOP DIFFERENTIAL DIAGNOSES

- Non-Hodgkin lymphoma
  - **Treated** mesenteric lymphoma can look identical
- Carcinoid tumor
  - Usually involves ileal mesentery in right lower quadrant
  - Mesenteric metastases and primary tumor are hypervascular (unlike mesenteritis)

CLINICAL ISSUES

- Has been reported with other IgG4-related inflammatory and fibrotic disorders
- Natural history or frequency of progression to chronic fibrotic phase not well understood

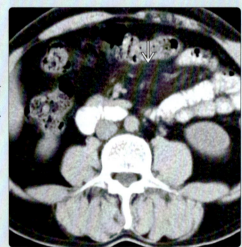
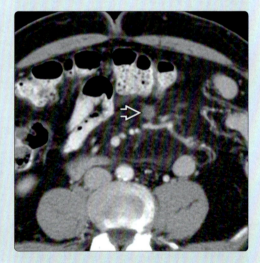

(Left) Initial CECT evaluation in an elderly man with abdominal pain shows infiltration of the jejunal mesentery marked by a pseudocapsule ➡. (Right) Axial CECT in the same patient shows clusters of mildly enlarged mesenteric nodes ➡. No diagnosis was made at this time, and the patient was not given treatment.

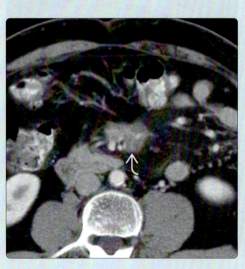
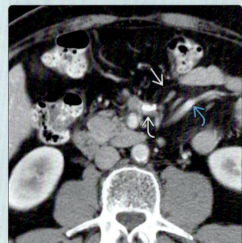

(Left) The same patient returned for evaluation 5 years later, having had chronic pain intermittently for the entire time without a diagnosis being made. Axial CECT shows a soft tissue mass ➡ in the mesentery that encases the mesenteric vessels. (Right) Axial CECT in a 2nd study of the same patient shows calcification ➡ within the fibrotic mesenteric mass and engorged mesenteric veins ➡. The infiltrated mesentery and pseudocapsule ➡ are still evident. This case illustrates progression of the disease over time.

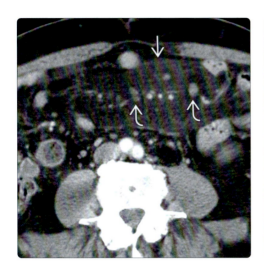

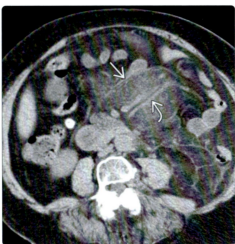

(Left) Axial CECT in a patient with pain and fever shows infiltration of the jejunal mesentery, demarcated by a pseudocapsule ➡. Multiple prominent mesenteric nodes are present ➡ with a fat halo. PET showed no increased activity, and symptoms improved with steroids. (Right) Axial NECT in a patient with chronic pain shows infiltration of the jejunal mesentery with a pseudocapsule ➡. The mesenteric vessels ➡ are encased but not obstructed. This was found to represent sclerosing mesenteritis.

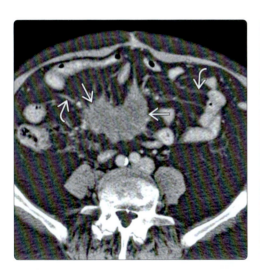

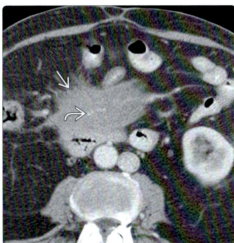

(Left) Axial CECT shows an infiltrative mesenteric mass ➡ that encases blood vessels. Note the engorgement of the mesenteric veins ➡. This was found to represent sclerosing mesenteritis. (Right) Axial CECT in an elderly woman with chronic pain and diarrhea shows a soft tissue mass ➡ at the base of the small bowel mesentery, encasing and narrowing the mesenteric vessels ➡. This was found to represent fibrosing mesenteritis at biopsy.

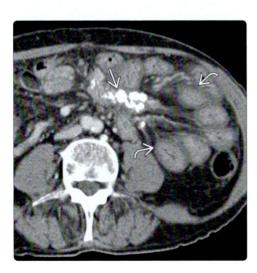

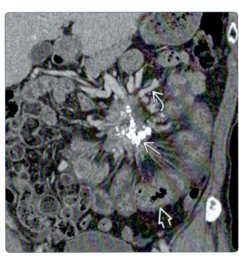

(Left) Axial CECT demonstrates a partially calcified mass ➡ in the jejunal mesentery with tethering of adjacent bowel loops ➡. (Right) Coronal CECT in the same patient demonstrates the partially calcified mass ➡. Note the venous collaterals ➡ due to obstruction of the superior mesenteric vein as well as diffuse small bowel wall thickening ➡ due to venous/lymphatic obstruction. This was biopsy-proven retractile mesenteritis.

KEY FACTS

TERMINOLOGY

- Pathologic accumulation of fluid within peritoneal cavity

IMAGING

- **Transudative ascites**: Usually has density of 0-15 Hounsfield units (HU) on CT and appears free flowing
  - Free-flowing ascites conforms to shape of surrounding structures and flows to dependent recesses
  - Simple fluid signal on T1WI (hypointense, "dark") and T2WI (hyperintense, "bright") MR
  - No appreciable complexity within ascites fluid
- **Exudative ascites**: Typically demonstrates increasing density of fluid with increasing protein content
  - Often mildly hyperdense on CT (15-30 HU) relative to transudative ascites
  - May demonstrate complexity, including septations, peritoneal thickening/enhancement, and loculation
  - Loculated ascites fluid exerts mass effect and displaces adjacent structures (such as bowel loops)

- Usually simple fluid signal on T1WI and T2WI MR, but internal complexity and protein can result in intermediate T1 and T2 signal
- Chylous ascites can measure < 0 HU or demonstrate fat-fluid levels

PATHOLOGY

- Ascites is typically divided into 2 types
  - **Transudative** ascites is caused by high portal venous pressures and is characterized by low protein, low lactate dehydrogenase, normal glucose, and low specific gravity
    - Transudative ascites is simple ascites fluid most often caused by cirrhosis, hepatitis, heart failure, renal failure, hypoproteinemia, etc.
  - **Exudative** ascites is characterized by high protein and high specific gravity
    - Exudative ascites related to multiple causes, such as infection, ischemia, peritoneal carcinomatosis, peritonitis, or pancreatitis

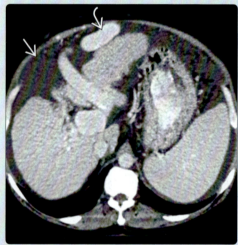
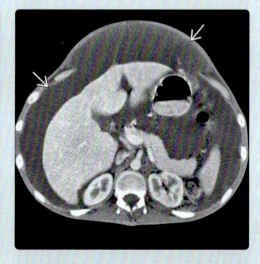

(Left) Axial CECT shows ascites ➡ due to hepatic cirrhosis with large varices ➡ and splenomegaly. Notice the relatively simple, uncomplicated appearance of this transudative ascites. (Right) Axial CECT shows massive ascites ➡ due to right heart failure. Like other forms of transudative ascites, note that the fluid appears simple without evidence of complexity, nodularity, or adjacent peritoneal thickening/enhancement.

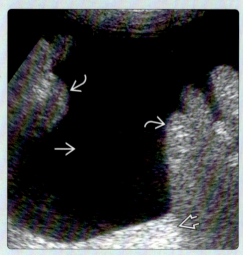
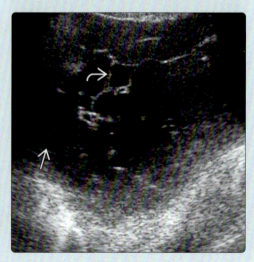

(Left) Ultrasound shows a large collection of anechoic ascites ➡ in the lower abdomen displacing bowel loops ➡ in a patient with cirrhosis. As in this case, simple transudative ascites is classically anechoic, freely mobile, and shows posterior acoustic enhancement ➡. (Right) Ultrasound shows complicated ascites ➡ in a cirrhotic patient. The fluid was nonmobile and loculated on real-time scanning, and there are multiple internal septations ➡ suggesting this is exudative ascites. The fluid was found to be infected.

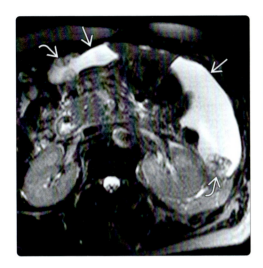
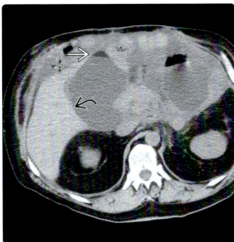

(Left) *Axial T2 fat-suppressed MR demonstrates loculated T2-hyperintense ascites* ➡. *Notice the presence of discrete nodules* ➡ *within the ascites fluid, indicating that this is malignant ascites in a patient with peritoneal carcinomatosis from appendiceal cancer.* (Right) *Axial NECT in a patient after small bowel transplantation demonstrates fat-fluid levels* ➡ *within fluid collections that indicate the chylous nature of the fluid and that it represents leakage from small bowel lymphatics. The liver is marked* ➡ *for comparison.*

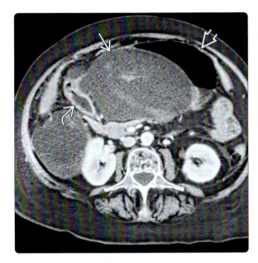
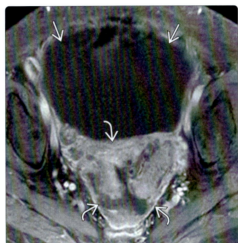

(Left) *Axial CECT shows complex, loculated ascites* ➡ *from bile peritonitis due to a biliary injury. Lesser sac ascites, which displaces the stomach* ➡ *and duodenum* ➡, *as in this case, is usually due to a local source (e.g., pancreatitis, gastric ulcer), peritonitis, or carcinomatosis.* (Right) *Axial T1 contrast-enhanced MR demonstrates loculated ascites* ➡ *in the pelvis. Notice the extensive peritoneal thickening* ➡ *and hyperenhancement in the pelvis, consistent with this patient's malignant ascites and peritoneal carcinomatosis.*

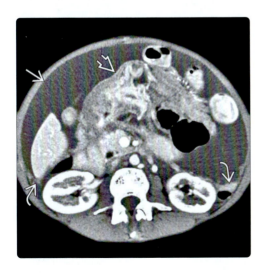
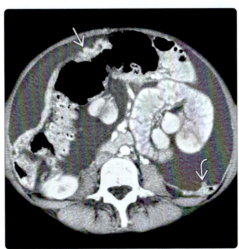

(Left) *Axial CECT shows marked thickening of the distal stomach wall* ➡ *compatible with malignancy. Extensive ascites* ➡ *is present with nodular thickening of the parietal peritoneum* ➡, *indicating malignant ascites from gastric carcinoma.* (Right) *Axial CECT in the same patient shows the tumor extending along the gastrocolic ligament to involve the transverse colon* ➡. *Note the nodular thickening of the parietal peritoneum* ➡. *Primary GI malignancy is the most common source of malignant ascites in men.*

KEY FACTS

TERMINOLOGY

- Fat necrosis caused by interruption of arterial blood supply to part of omentum

IMAGING

- **Multiplanar CT is definitive in most cases**
  - Primary (idiopathic) type: "Big ball of dirty fat," (3-15 cm) between ascending colon & abdominal wall
  - Secondary type is located near site of prior surgery
  - Usually circumscribed with peripheral thin rim
    - May appear ill defined as poorly marginated fat stranding without discrete mass in earliest stages
  - No central dot sign (unlike epiploic appendagitis, which is "small ball of dirty fat")
  - Whorled pattern of vessels within or leading to infarct may reflect torsion of vessels feeding omentum (unusual cause for omental infarction)
  - Only rarely causes reactive colonic wall thickening
- **Ultrasound appearance**

- Hyperechoic, nonmobile, noncompressible fixed mass
  - Decreased or absent flow within echogenic mass
- Focal tenderness with graded compression

CLINICAL ISSUES

- Can affect any age group, though elderly & obese have greatest prevalence
- Clinical presentation may mimic acute appendicitis
  - Right-sided pain & tenderness in > 90% of cases
    - Other sites of involvement are usually due to surgical complication
  - Usually normal WBC & lack of nausea, vomiting, diarrhea, or constitutional symptoms
- Usually self-limiting process that resolves spontaneously & should be treated only with pain management
- If diagnosed prospectively on CT, surgery **should not be performed**
  - Unless there is unusual complication, such as secondary infection

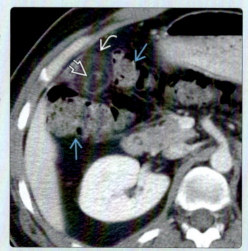
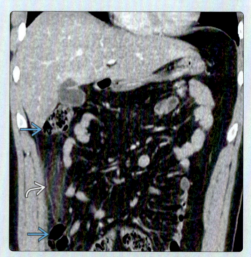

(Left) Axial CECT in a patient with RLQ pain shows a classic "primary" omental infarct as a fatty mass ⮑ adjacent to the ascending colon ➡. Note the swirled appearance of an omental vessel ⮎ within the infarcted omentum, indicating twisting of the omental pedicle. (Right) Coronal CECT in a patient with RLQ pain shows an encapsulated fatty mass ⮑ in the RLQ omentum, adjacent to ascending colon, ➡ with surrounding fat stranding, characteristic of an idiopathic (primary) omental infarct.

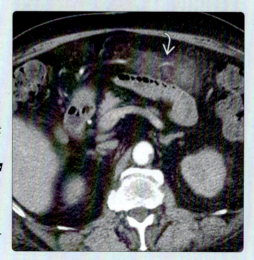
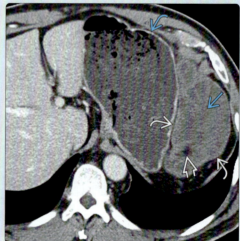

(Left) Axial CECT in a patient with polyarteritis nodosa and abdominal pain shows focal fat stranding ⮑ in the anterior omentum, corresponding to the site of the patient's pain. This represents an omental infarct likely related to the vasculitis. (Right) Axial CECT in a patient who had recently undergone distal pancreatectomy shows a large circumscribed mass ⮑ adjacent to stomach ➡. Note the presence of internal fat density ⮎ and liquified necrosis ➡ in this secondary (postsurgical) omental infarct.

Inguinal Hernia

KEY FACTS

IMAGING

- **US is 1st-line study**: Can scan patient either with Valsalva maneuver or in upright position to precipitate hernia
  - US can determine reducibility of hernia (unlike CT) and identify reducible hernias that may not be seen on CT
- **CT**: Useful when strangulation or bowel obstruction is suspected
- **Direct inguinal hernia**: Hernia passes through Hesselbach triangle (bounded by inguinal ligament, lateral margin of rectus abdominis, and inferior epigastric artery)
  - CT: Arises **anteromedial** to origin of inferior epigastric artery and extends through anterior abdominal wall lateral to rectus muscle
    - Contents of inguinal canal (testicular vessels, vas deferens) can be seen as crescent of density along lateral aspect of hernia as it protrudes
    - No compression of femoral artery/vein

- **Indirect inguinal hernia**: Hernia passes through internal inguinal ring, down inguinal canal, and emerges at external ring
  - CT: Arises **superolateral** to inferior epigastric vessels and extends lateral to medial within inguinal canal
  - Lateral crescent sign not present with indirect hernias

PATHOLOGY

- Indirect inguinal hernia is usually congenital defect due to patency of processus vaginalis, while direct hernias are acquired due to abdominal wall weakness

CLINICAL ISSUES

- Much more common in men than women, especially indirect hernias
- Complications: Incarceration and strangulation (much more common with indirect than direct inguinal hernia)
- Symptomatic hernias are usually surgically repaired on elective basis, although conservative management possible in some asymptomatic or minimally symptomatic patients

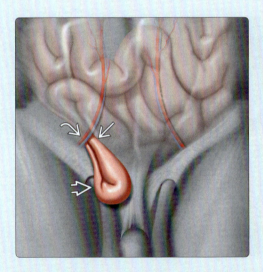
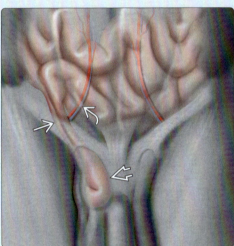

(Left) Illustration demonstrates a direct inguinal hernia ➡ with the hernia neck ➡ located medial to the inferior epigastric artery and vein ➡. (Right) Illustration demonstrates an indirect inguinal hernia ➡ with the hernia neck ➡ located lateral to the inferior epigastric artery and vein ➡. The inferior epigastric vessels serve as the key landmark in distinguishing direct and indirect inguinal hernias. Note extension into the scrotum.

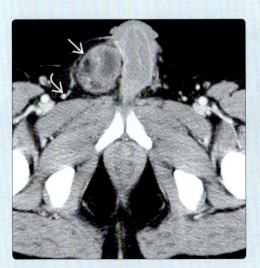
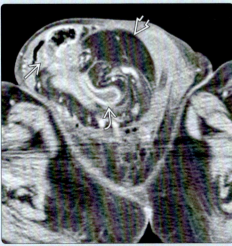

(Left) Axial CECT in an elderly man who presented with groin pain and a palpable mass demonstrates a right inguinal hernia. Note that the hernia sac is in the right inguinal canal ➡ and medial to the inferior epigastric vessels ➡, identifying it as a direct inguinal hernia. (Right) Axial CECT in an elderly man who presented with a large groin mass and a small bowel obstruction demonstrates a large right inguinal hernia containing sections of the small bowel ➡, colon ➡, and omentum ➡.

KEY FACTS

TERMINOLOGY

- Protrusion of abdominal contents through femoral ring into femoral canal

IMAGING

- **Multiplanar, contrast-enhanced CT is 1st-line test**
  - US may be diagnostic, but is more operator dependent
- Omental fat or bowel herniating into femoral canal **medial to femoral vein** and **inferior to inferior epigastric vessels**
- Femoral vein often indented or compressed by hernia sac
- Hernia sac located posterior and lateral to pubic tubercle
- Narrow, funnel-shaped neck
- Twice as common on right side compared to left

TOP DIFFERENTIAL DIAGNOSES

- Inguinal hernia
  - Seen **anterior** to horizontal plane of pubic tubercle
  - Abdominal contents within inguinal canal **anteromedial** to femoral vessels with extension into scrotum

- Lymphadenopathy

CLINICAL ISSUES

- Primarily occur in elderly women with 36% occurring in patients > 80 years old
- Relatively uncommon, representing only 2-4% of groin hernias in adults
  - ~ 1/10 as common as inguinal hernias
  - ~ 1/3 of groin hernias occur in women
- Highest risk of incarceration/strangulation (25-40%) among all groin hernias
  - 8-12x more prone to incarceration/strangulation than inguinal hernias
- Significant risk of mortality, primarily related to incarceration and intestinal obstruction
  - Mortality: 1% in 70-79 age group; 5% in 80-90 age group
- Symptomatic hernia (or newly discovered asymptomatic hernia) should undergo immediate surgical repair

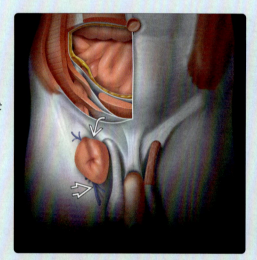
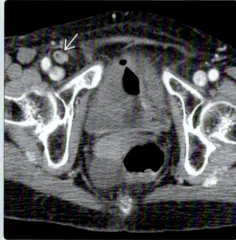

(Left) *Graphic of a femoral hernia demonstrates a characteristic "knuckle" of small bowel ➡ closely associated with the femoral vein ➡. Femoral hernias are usually found medial to the femoral vessels with frequent compression of the femoral vein.* (Right) *Axial CECT demonstrates a herniated small bowel loop ➡ lying within the femoral canal, compressing the femoral vessels, compatible with a femoral hernia.*

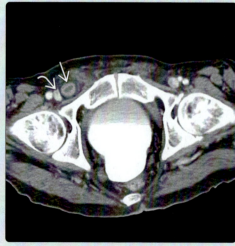
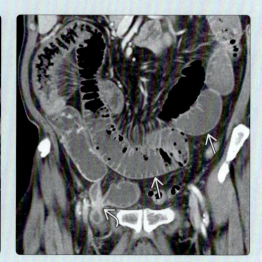

(Left) *Axial CECT shows a loop of thickened, hyperemic bowel ➡ herniating into the right groin medial to the femoral vessels. Notice that the femoral vein ➡ is being compressed, and the herniated bowel lies posterolateral to the pubic tubercle.* (Right) *Coronal CECT in the same patient shows multiple dilated small-bowel loops ➡ with a transition point ➡ within the hernia. This thickened, hyperenhancing bowel within the hernia sac was found to be ischemic at surgery. Femoral hernias are at high risk for strangulation and obstruction.*

Ventral Hernia

KEY FACTS

TERMINOLOGY

- Ventral hernia is generic term encompassing variety of hernias through anterior and lateral abdominal wall

IMAGING

- **Epigastric** and **hypogastric** hernias occur at midline through linea alba
  - Epigastric hernias arise above umbilicus and below xiphoid process
  - Hypogastric hernias arise below umbilicus
- **Incisional** hernias develop at prior abdominal wall incision
- **CT: Most accurate test for detection** of ventral hernias
  - Defect in musculofascial layers of abdominal wall through which omentum ± bowel protrude anteriorly

PATHOLOGY

- Depending on hernia type, ventral hernias may be due to either acquired or congenital factors

- Incisional hernias: Acquired hernias at site of prior surgery, incision, or abdominal wall injury
  - May be related to previous abdominal surgery, laparoscopy, peritoneal dialysis, or stab wound
- Epigastric and hypogastric hernias: Possible congenital predisposition due to weakness of linea alba
  - Acquired risk factors include wound infection, obesity, increased intraabdominal pressures, and abdominal wall strains

CLINICAL ISSUES

- Incisional hernias usually occur during first 4 months after surgery but can develop many years later
- Ventral hernias do not close spontaneously and almost always enlarge over time
- Bowel incarceration and strangulation are common
- Surgical closure is usually recommended due to risk of incarceration and strangulation
  - Tension-free mesh repair is now gold standard

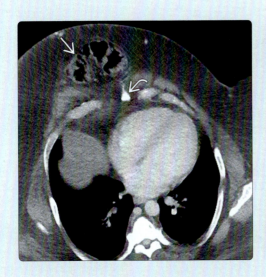
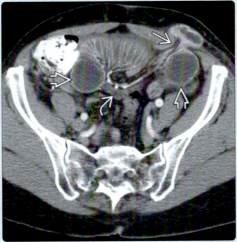

(Left) Axial CECT demonstrates a hernia ⟹ containing bowel arising in the midline above the umbilicus and below the xiphoid ⟹, characteristic of an epigastric hernia. (Right) Axial CECT in a younger woman with nausea and vomiting due to a strangulated hernia shows herniation of small bowel through a laparoscopy port ⟹ with bowel obstruction. Bowel proximal to the hernia is dilated ⟹; bowel distal to the hernia is collapsed ⟹.

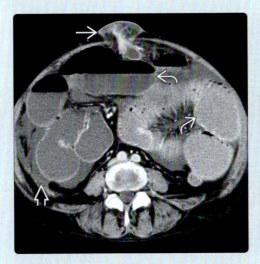
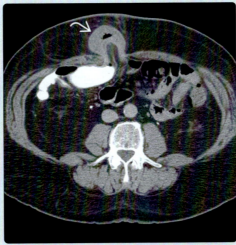

(Left) Axial CECT in a middle-aged woman with nausea and vomiting shows a ventral hernia ⟹ with dilated, strangulated, obstructed small bowel ⟹ as well as ascites ⟹, suggesting bowel ischemia. (Right) Axial CECT demonstrates a ventral hernia containing a markedly thickened, hypoenhancing loop of small bowel ⟹. The hernia was not reducible at clinical examination, and the bowel loop within the hernia sac was found to be ischemic at surgery.

KEY FACTS

TERMINOLOGY

- Protrusion of abdominal contents (omental fat ± bowel) into or through anterior abdominal wall via umbilical ring

IMAGING

- Hernia sac located at midline (usually upper 1/2 of umbilicus) with protrusion of omental fat ± bowel loops
- Fat stranding/fluid within hernia sac (in absence of abnormal bowel) suggests fat necrosis due to incarceration
- Findings of bowel ischemia include evidence of bowel obstruction, bowel wall thickening, fat stranding, etc.

TOP DIFFERENTIAL DIAGNOSES

- Omphalocele
- Ventral hernia
- Spigelian hernia

PATHOLOGY

- Congenital: Due to incomplete closure of umbilical ring

- More likely in children with Down syndrome, trisomy 18, mucopolysaccharidoses, Ehlers-Danlos syndrome, and Beckwith-Wiedemann syndrome
- Acquired: Results from weakening of cicatricial tissue that normally closes umbilical ring
  - Usually secondary to ↑ intraabdominal pressure (e.g., obesity, multiple pregnancies, tense ascites, etc.)

CLINICAL ISSUES

- Congenital type: Diagnosed in infancy
  - Congenital type 8x more common in African Americans
  - 80% close spontaneously within 4-6 years
  - Treatment only if hernia is large, symptomatic, or persistent (> 5 years of age)
- Acquired type: Develops in later life (usually middle age)
  - Acquired type more common in women (M:F = 1:3)
  - Small and asymptomatic hernias do not undergo repair
  - Symptoms, large hernia size, and incarceration all necessitate surgical repair

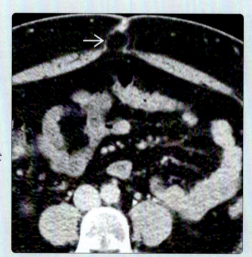
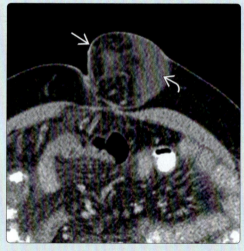

(Left) Axial CECT shows herniation of omental fat ➡ into the umbilicus between the rectus sheaths, a characteristic appearance for a small umbilical hernia. (Right) Axial CECT demonstrates an umbilical hernia ➡ with internal fluid ➡ and fat stranding in a patient with intense pain at this site. Extensive internal fat necrosis due to strangulation was found within the hernia sac at surgery. Incarcerated umbilical hernias with fat necrosis can be very painful but do not necessitate emergent surgery.

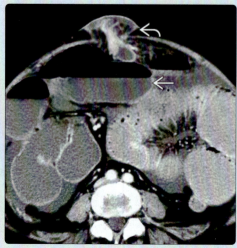
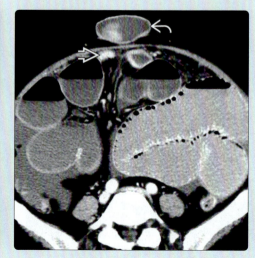

(Left) Axial CECT in a middle-aged man with cirrhosis shows ascites, dilated small bowel ➡, and an umbilical hernia ➡ containing ascites and small bowel. (Right) Axial CECT in the same patient again demonstrates the umbilical hernia ➡. Note the collapsed loop of small bowel ➡ leaving the hernia sac, confirming the hernia as the cause of the small bowel obstruction. Umbilical hernias are common among patients with cirrhosis and ascites due to thin abdominal wall musculature and chronically increased intraabdominal pressure.

Obturator Hernia

KEY FACTS

IMAGING

- **Multiplanar, contrast-enhanced CT**
- Loop of bowel protruding through obturator foramen
  - Hernia most commonly contains loop of Ileum, although can rarely involve other pelvic viscera (e.g., bladder)
  - Most often trapped between obturator externus and pectineus muscles
  - May also be located between superior and middle fasciculi of obturator externus or between internal and external obturator muscles
- Hernia sac exits pelvis near obturator vessels and nerve
- Right side more common

TOP DIFFERENTIAL DIAGNOSES

- Inguinal hernia
- Sciatic hernia
- Perineal hernia
- Femoral hernia

PATHOLOGY

- Defect in pelvic floor or laxity of pelvic muscles and fascia
- Made worse by any chronic increase in abdominal pressure (COPD, constipation, pregnancy, etc.)
- More common in thin or emaciated patients, as preperitoneal fat usually supports obturator canal

CLINICAL ISSUES

- Accounts for < 1% of all hernias
- **> 90% occur in elderly women** (mean age 82)
- Acute or recurrent small bowel obstruction, partial > complete
  - 80% of patients present with symptoms of bowel obstruction
  - Majority require resection of strangulated small bowel
- Rare occurrence and nonspecific signs often lead to late diagnosis
  - Correct clinical diagnosis in only 10-30% of cases
  - Diagnosis best made by CT/MR rather than clinical exam

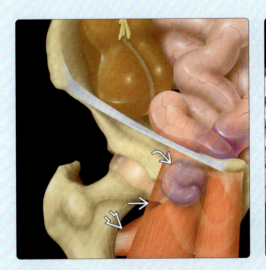
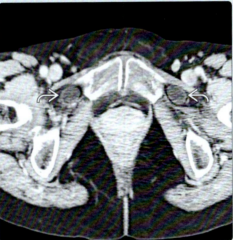

(Left) *Graphic shows a bowel obstruction caused by an obturator hernia. Strangulated bowel ➜ lies deep to the pectineus muscle ➜ and superficial to the obturator externus muscle ➔.* (Right) *Axial CECT in a 73-year-old woman shows a protrusion of portions of the bladder into bilateral obturator hernias ➜. Obturator hernias most commonly contain herniated ileum, but other pelvic viscera can also herniate, as in this case.*

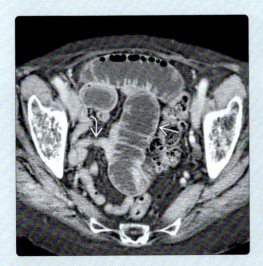
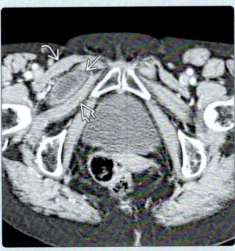

(Left) *Axial CECT in a 90-year-old woman with bowel obstruction shows dilated proximal small bowel loops ➜ and collapsed distal bowel ➔.* (Right) *Axial CECT in the same patient shows the herniated and strangulated segment of the ileum ➜ trapped between the obturator externus ➔ and the pectineus ➜ muscles. These are the classic clinical and imaging features of an obturator hernia.*

Abdominal Wall, Mesentery, and Peritoneal Cavity

TERMINOLOGY

- Hernia through defect in aponeurosis of internal oblique and transverse abdominal muscles

IMAGING

- Hernia occurs along lateral border of rectus abdominis muscles, inferior/lateral to umbilicus, at level of arcuate line
  - Lies deep to external oblique aponeurosis and muscle
  - 90% within spigelian belt of Spangen, 6-cm transverse band above line joining anterior superior iliac spines
- Most often contains portions of greater omentum, small bowel, or colon
  - Rarely can involve appendix, bladder, and other abdominal/pelvic structures
- Defect size is small (usually < 2 cm in size) resulting in narrow hernia neck and high risk of strangulation

TOP DIFFERENTIAL DIAGNOSES

- Ventral hernia

- Umbilical hernia
- Hernia through laparoscopy port

PATHOLOGY

- Probably multifactorial etiology, including congenital weakness of spigelian fascia
  - Usually congenital defect in children and acquired in adults
  - Prior history of abdominal surgery and obesity are biggest risk factors in adults
  - Other risk factors include multiple pregnancies, rapid weight loss, COPD, and trauma

CLINICAL ISSUES

- Rare hernia; accounts for 1-2% of anterior abdominal hernias
- Difficult to diagnose clinically due to deep anatomic location, especially in obese patients
- Surgical treatment indicated in virtually all patients due to high risk of strangulation and incarceration

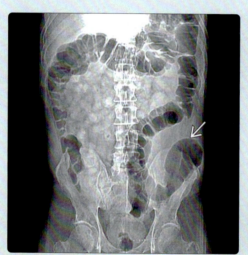
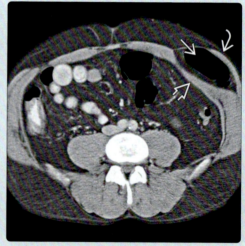

(Left) *Radiograph in a 52-year-old man with a palpable, tender abdominal mass shows a partial colonic obstruction due to herniation of the descending colon ➡ through a spigelian hernia (SH).* (Right) *Axial CECT in the same patient shows herniation of the colon ➡ into an intermuscular space between the internal oblique and transverse abdominal muscles ➡ (deep) and the external oblique muscle and fascia ➡ (superficially).*

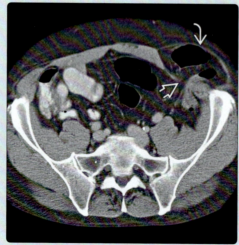
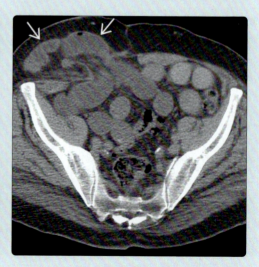

(Left) *Axial CECT, more caudal, in the same patient shows the defect ➡ in the spigelian aponeurosis (that of the internal oblique and transverse abdominal muscles). Note the hernia sac covered by intact aponeurosis of external oblique muscle ➡ and the hernia caudal to the umbilicus and just lateral to the rectus sheath.* (Right) *Axial CT shows a small bowel obstruction and an SH ➡. The hernia is evident just lateral to the rectus muscle. A segment of small bowel herniates through the defect, resulting in partial obstruction.*

Lumbar Hernia

TERMINOLOGY

- Lumbar hernia: Protrusion of abdominal contents through defect in lumbar region
  - Can occur in either superior lumbar triangle of Grynfeltt-Lesshaft or inferior lumbar triangle of Petit
    - Superior lumbar triangle of Grynfeltt-Lesshaft defined by 12th rib superiorly, superior border of internal oblique inferiorly, and erector spinae medially
    - Inferior lumbar triangle of Petit defined by latissimus dorsi muscle medially, iliac crest inferiorly, and free border of external oblique muscle laterally
  - Overall, hernias are more common in superior triangle

IMAGING

- Disruption of thoracolumbar fascia at insertion of aponeurosis of internal oblique and transverse abdominal muscles
- Hernia may contain extraperitoneal fat, colon, kidney, or intraperitoneal structures (small bowel, ascites)

- Most commonly involved are colon and small bowel

PATHOLOGY

- 80% of lumbar hernias are acquired
  - Can be spontaneous (especially in older patients and patients with excessive weight loss) or secondary to trauma, infection, or previous surgery in flank
  - Most commonly occurs following flank incision for renal surgery or iliac crest bone harvesting
- 20% of lumbar hernias are congenital

CLINICAL ISSUES

- Very difficult to detect (and often missed) on physical examination and more likely to be diagnosed on CT
- Incarceration and strangulation are uncommon because of large size of opening into hernia
  - Incarceration more common with acute traumatic lumbar hernias (8-10%)
- Treatment: Early surgical repair because repair becomes technically more difficult as hernia enlarges

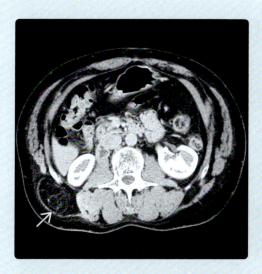

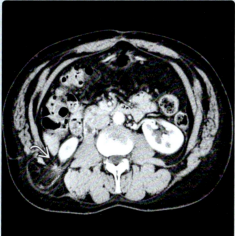

(Left) Axial CECT shows herniation of retroperitoneal fat that is covered only by the thinned latissimus dorsi muscle ➡ in a patient with right flank discomfort. (Right) Axial CECT in the same patient shows the site of herniation immediately above the iliac crest. The lumbar hernia is a defect ➡ in the aponeurosis of the internal oblique and transverse abdominal muscles, which should insert on the thoracoabdominal fascia that envelops the quadratus lumborum and erector spinae muscles.

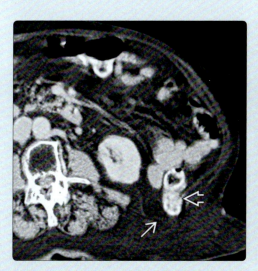

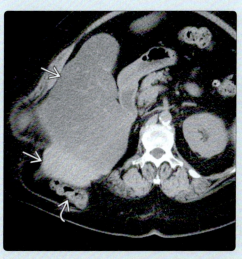

(Left) Axial CECT in an elderly woman shows a defect ➡ in the left thoracolumbar fascia through which the descending colon ➡ herniates dorsally. The thoracolumbar fascia should be a strong sheet of tissue that inserts on the iliac crest. (Right) Axial NECT demonstrates a fascial defect in the right lumbar region with herniation of the liver ➡ and colon ➡. Notice that while the liver is diffusely steatotic, the liver within the lumbar hernia is higher in density, probably as a result of differential perfusion due to entrapment in the hernia.

Abdominal Wall, Mesentery, and Peritoneal Cavity

KEY FACTS

TERMINOLOGY

- Congenital internal hernia resulting from protrusion of bowel loops through abdominal mesenteric defect

IMAGING

- Paraduodenal hernias may be located either on left or right
  - Left (75%): Protrusion of small bowel through paraduodenal mesenteric **fossa of Landzert**
  - Right (25%): Protrusion of small bowel through jejunal mesentericoparietal **fossa of Waldeyer**
- CT features
  - Left paraduodenal hernia
    - Encapsulated "cluster" or sac-like mass of small bowel loops located between pancreatic body/tail and stomach to left of ligament of Treitz
    - Crowded, engorged mesenteric vessels supplying bowel loops within hernia sac
  - Right paraduodenal hernia
    - Clustered, encapsulated small bowel in right upper abdomen lateral/inferior to descending duodenum
    - Unusual "looping" course of superior mesenteric artery and superior mesenteric vein to supply bowel in hernia sac
- **Small bowel follow-through**
  - Abnormally crowded, clustered bowel loops to left or right side of colon
  - Fixation, stasis, and delayed flow of contrast seen in bowel within hernia sac

CLINICAL ISSUES

- Most often occurs in men during 4th-6th decades of life
- Smaller hernias are clinically silent and reduce spontaneously
- Larger hernias are more commonly symptomatic (e.g., vague discomfort, abdominal distension, postprandial pain)
  - Very high (~ 50%) lifetime risk of strangulation or incarceration

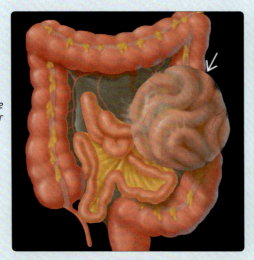
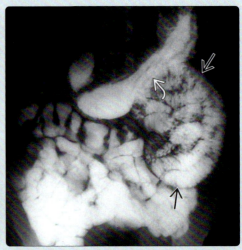

(Left) Graphic shows a left paraduodenal hernia ➡ containing dilated proximal jejunal loops in a peritoneal sac. (Right) Small bowel follow-through demonstrates an ovoid cluster ➡ of mildly dilated jejunal segments in the left upper quadrant. The outer confines of the hernia sac are well defined. The herniated bowel exerts mass effect on the greater curvature of the stomach ➡, characteristic of a left paraduodenal hernia.

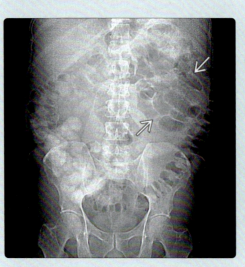
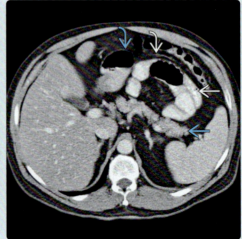

(Left) Abdominal radiograph shows an unusual cluster of dilated jejunal small bowel loops ➡ in the left upper quadrant. (Right) Axial CECT in the same patient shows the same cluster of dilated bowel ➡ interposed between the pancreas ➡ and stomach ➡. Note the displaced inferior mesenteric vein ➡ that runs along the anterior edge of the hernia sac. This constellation of findings is characteristic of a left paraduodenal hernia.

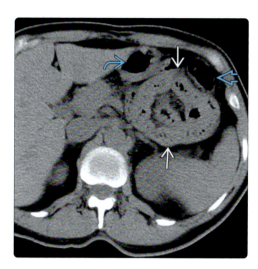

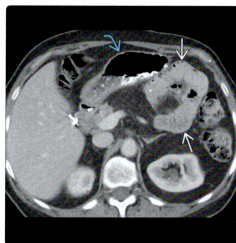

(Left) *Axial NECT demonstrates a cluster of encapsulated small bowel* ➡️ *in the left abdomen. Notice the location of these loops, immediately adjacent to the distal duodenum, posterior wall of the stomach* ➡️*, and colon* ➡️*, in keeping with a paraduodenal hernia.* (Right) *Axial CECT demonstrates a cluster of mildly dilated small bowel loops* ➡️ *in the left upper quadrant, displacing the stomach* ➡️*forward. Mesenteric vessels supplying the herniated bowel segments converge toward the center of the cluster.*

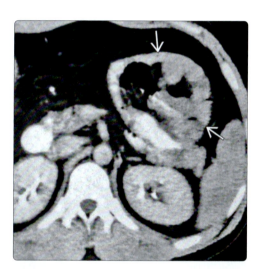

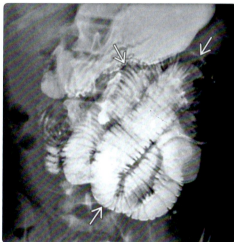

(Left) *Axial CECT shows an oval cluster of jejunum* ➡️ *in the left upper quadrant. Note the sharply defined outer margin of the peritoneal sac around the herniated bowel, and the mesenteric vessels converging toward the sac center, compatible with a left paraduodenal hernia.* (Right) *Delayed film from an upper GI series in the same patient shows a tight cluster of dilated jejunum* ➡️ *and delayed passage of contrast to the normal caliber distal small bowel.*

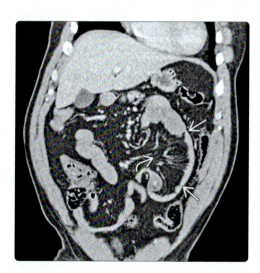

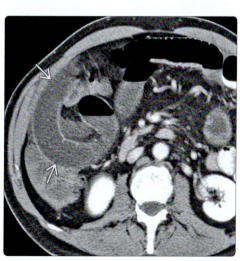

(Left) *Coronal CECT demonstrates the characteristic encapsulated morphology of a left paraduodenal hernia* ➡️*. Note the engorged mesenteric vessels* ➡️ *extending directly into the hernia sac.* (Right) *Axial CECT shows a right paraduodenal hernia causing small bowel obstruction. Note the U-shaped configuration of the bowel loop within the right paraduodenal hernia sac* ➡️*.*

TERMINOLOGY

- Protrusion of bowel loops through acquired or congenital abdominal mesenteric defect

IMAGING

- **Multiplanar, contrast-enhanced CT is imaging tool of choice**
- Displacement or twisting of superior mesenteric vessels in ~ all cases
- Whirl sign [small bowel (SB) volvulus with twisting of mesenteric vessels around central point]
  - Mesenteric vessels appear engorged, crowded, or twisted
- SB obstruction with dilated bowel loops and discrete transition point from dilated to nondilated bowel
- Thickened bowel wall and ascites, particularly in cases with bowel ischemia
- SB mesenteric fat is infiltrated

- In patients with Roux-en-Y gastric bypass, jejunal anastomotic line is displaced from expected left mid abdominal position

TOP DIFFERENTIAL DIAGNOSES

- Closed loop bowel obstruction (other etiology)
- Paraduodenal or pericecal internal hernia with obstruction

CLINICAL ISSUES

- **Usually related to prior abdominal surgery in adults**
  - Most commonly **Roux-en-Y gastric bypass and liver transplantation**
- Onset usually months after original surgery
- High risk of volvulus (~ 30%) and ischemia (~ 40%)
- Symptoms are more likely to be acute compared to other types of internal hernias
- Treatment: Laparotomy or laparoscopy with bowel decompression and surgical correction of mesenteric defect

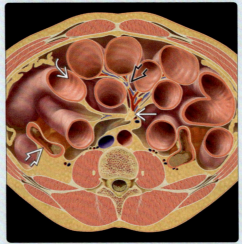
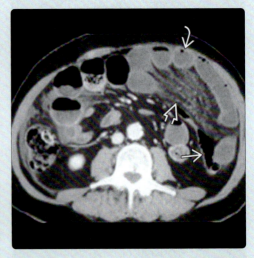

(Left) Axial graphic shows dilated small bowel (SB) herniating through a mesenteric defect ➡. Note the peripheral position of the SB ➡, medial displacement of the colon ➡, and the displaced mesenteric vessels ➡. (Right) Axial CECT in a patient with prior colonic resection shows a cluster of dilated SB ➡ in the left abdomen. These loops lie ventral to the transverse colon ➡, and the mesenteric vessels ➡ are distorted and congested. These findings are typical of a transmesenteric hernia.

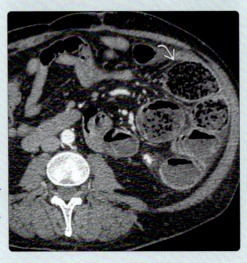
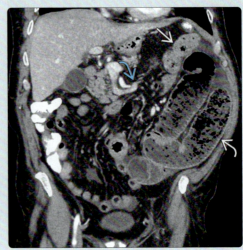

(Left) Axial CECT in a patient with a history of prior abdominal surgery demonstrates multiple dilated, fecalized loops of SB ➡ in the left abdomen, indicating a SB obstruction. (Right) Coronal CT in the same patient shows that these bowel loops ➡ are clustered in the lateral aspect of the abdomen, directly abutting the abdominal wall, and displacing the colon ➡. Mesenteric vessels ➡ are distorted. This constellation of findings is classic for a postoperative transmesenteric hernia.

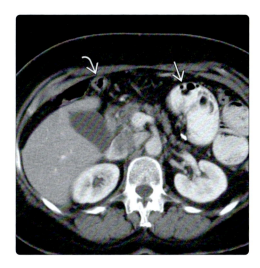
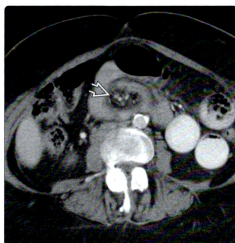

(Left) Axial CECT in a patient status post gastric bypass procedure shows that the Roux limb and proximal SB ⮕ are dilated, while the distal SB and colon ⮢ are collapsed. (Right) Axial CECT in the same patient demonstrates the twisting of the SB mesenteric root (whirl sign) ⮕ and the engorgement of the mesenteric veins draining the herniated and obstructed segments. This was found to be a transmesenteric internal hernia with volvulus.

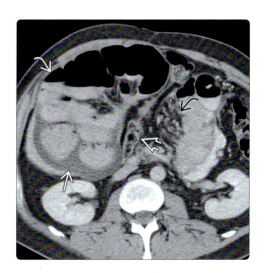
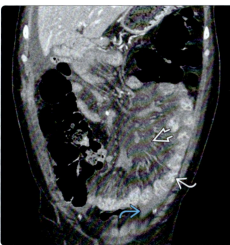

(Left) Axial CECT shows a cluster of dilated SB ⮕ lateral to and displacing the colon ⮕ as well as focal ascites ⮕ and engorged vessels ⮢, typical of a transmesenteric hernia. (Right) Coronal CECT in a patient with prior Whipple surgery demonstrates the jejunum ⮕ to be abnormally lying against the abdominal wall with thickened walls, engorged mesenteric vessels, mesenteric infiltration ⮕, and ascites ⮢. This was a postsurgical transmesenteric hernia causing bowel ischemia.

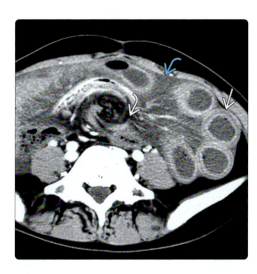
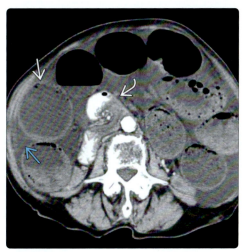

(Left) Axial CT shows SB herniation through a defect in the sigmoid mesentery and twisting of the mesenteric vasculature ⮕ at the herniation site (whirl sign). The herniated bowel is dilated and thick-walled ⮕ with ascites and infiltrated mesenteric fat ⮢. (Right) Axial CT in a patient with severe pain demonstrates dilated bowel ⮕, ascites ⮢, and the whirl sign ⮕ with twisting of the SB and mesenteric vessels around their axes. SB was herniated through a mesenteric defect and ischemic.

KEY FACTS

TERMINOLOGY

- Type of congenital diaphragmatic hernia resulting in protrusion of abdominal contents through defect in posterolateral portion of diaphragm

IMAGING

- **Multiplanar CT is imaging tool of choice**
- More common on **left side** (~ 80%)
- Defect in posterolateral diaphragm usually containing just retroperitoneal fat
  o Larger hernias may contain kidney, bowel, stomach, spleen, or liver
- Radiographic findings
  o Soft tissue, fat, or air density at base of lung
  o Located posteriorly on lateral chest film
- CT findings
  o Air, fat, or soft tissue density within hernia in chest
  o Coronal/sagittal reformats helpful for delineating defect

o CECT is helpful for assessment of complications (incarceration, strangulation)

TOP DIFFERENTIAL DIAGNOSES

- Diaphragmatic eventration
- Mediastinal and thoracic masses
  o Mediastinal lipoma/liposarcoma, diaphragm tumors, etc.
- Pulmonary and pleural lesions
  o Atelectasis, pneumonia, abscess, pleural effusion, etc.

PATHOLOGY

- Congenital defect in posterolateral diaphragm due to failure in closure of pleuropulmonary canal
- Rare secondary causes in adults include pregnancy (most common), trauma, obesity, coughing, and COPD

CLINICAL ISSUES

- Usually incidental finding in asymptomatic adults
- Can be associated with severe morbidity and mortality in neonates (particularly when large)

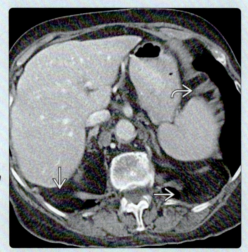
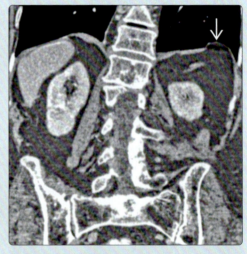

(Left) Axial CECT in an 88-year-old man shows bilateral defects in the posterior diaphragm ➡ with herniation of fat into the thorax. Also note the finger-like "slips" of diaphragm ➡ that might be mistaken for peritoneal nodules on an individual axial section. (Right) Coronal CECT in the same patient shows the left-sided Bochdalek hernia ➡. These are common and usually insignificant findings in elderly patients, especially those with chronic obstructive lung disease.

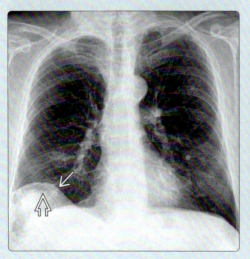
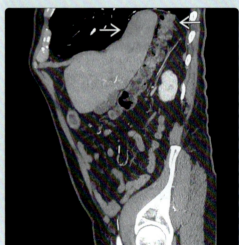

(Left) Frontal radiograph shows focal elevation and an abnormal contour of the right hemidiaphragm ➡. There is a small gas collection ➡ within this bulge in the diaphragm. (Right) Sagittal CECT in the same patient shows the liver and colon extending through a defect in the diaphragm ➡, corresponding to the findings on the radiographs, which are diagnostic of a Bochdalek hernia.

Morgagni Hernia

KEY FACTS

TERMINOLOGY

- Protrusion of abdominal cavity contents through retrosternal defect in diaphragm
- 90% are located on **right side** (8% bilateral, 2% on left)

IMAGING

- **Radiographic findings**
  - Soft tissue, fat, or air density along heart border
  - Usually located in right cardiophrenic angle and anterior to heart on lateral view
  - Smoothly marginated with silhouetting of heart border
- **CT and MR findings**
  - Defect in retrosternal part of diaphragm with hernia sac extending upward **anterior** to heart
  - Hernia sac most often contains only omental fat
  - Can also contain: Transverse colon > liver > small bowel > stomach
  - Hernias in adults usually contain omental fat; involvement of bowel or liver more likely in children

- With pericardial defect, hernia sac may protrude into pericardial cavity, or heart may protrude downward

TOP DIFFERENTIAL DIAGNOSES

- Pericardial fat pad
- Mediastinal and thoracic masses
- Pulmonary parenchymal lesions

CLINICAL ISSUES

- Rare, 3-4% of all diaphragmatic hernias
- Most cases are diagnosed in adults
- Often asymptomatic in adults and more likely symptomatic in children
  - Symptoms often include chronic GI complaints
  - Rarely acute symptoms due to incarceration, strangulation, obstruction, or volvulus
- Surgical repair in symptomatic patients via thoracotomy, laparotomy, or laparoscopic approach
- Surgical repair in asymptomatic patients more controversial

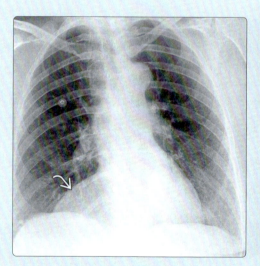
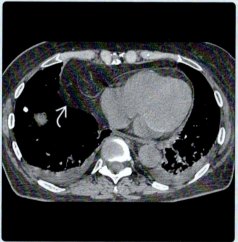

(Left) Frontal radiograph shows a large, relatively lucent mass ⇗ in the right costophrenic angle. (Right) Axial NECT in the same patient shows that the opacity on the radiograph corresponds to a fat-containing mass ⇗ in the right cardiophrenic angle.

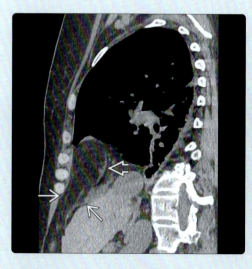
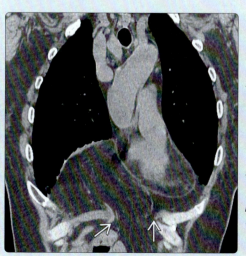

(Left) Sagittal NECT in the same patient shows that the previously visualized fatty mass actually represents a Morgagni hernia with omental fat herniating into the chest. Notice the discrete defect ⇨ in the diaphragm and the numerous small omental vessels ⇨ extending upward into the hernia sac. (Right) Coronal NECT in the same patient again demonstrates the Morgagni hernia with a discrete diaphragmatic defect ⇨ and omental fat herniating into the chest.

Traumatic Abdominal Wall Hernia

KEY FACTS

TERMINOLOGY

- Traumatic disruption of musculature and fascia of anterior abdominal wall due to blunt trauma

IMAGING

- **Contrast-enhanced, multiplanar CT**
- Common locations include iliac crest region in seat belt injuries and lower abdomen (lateral to rectus sheath or inguinal region)

PATHOLOGY

- Most hernias develop due to combination of sudden increase in intraabdominal pressure, direct force of traumatic impact, acceleration-deceleration shear injury, and compressive force of seat belt
  - High-energy injuries: Motor vehicle accidents constitute ~ 50% of cases, with seat belt use increasing risk
    - "High-riding" seat belt incorrectly placed over abdomen increases risk (muscle avulsion from iliac crest)

- Other traumatic injuries are common (~ 80%), with up to 50% of patients suffering other abdominal injuries requiring surgery
  - Low-energy injuries (most common in children): Impact by small blunt object (such as bicycle handlebar, i.e., handlebar hernia)

CLINICAL ISSUES

- May be overlooked clinically at time of injury and often diagnosed due to hernia-related complications
  - Complications: Incarceration; bowel strangulation, perforation, and ischemia
- Peak incidence in children < 10 years of ag,e due to handlebar injuries
  - 2nd most common age group is 20-50 years, due to motor vehicle accidents
- Treatment: Delayed repair of hernia usually performed 6-8 weeks following high-energy injuries to allow primary tissue damage to subside

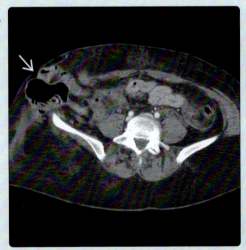
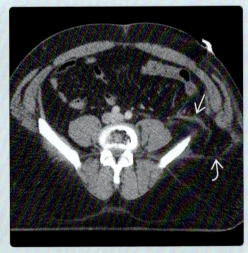

(Left) Axial CECT demonstrates small bowel and colon ➡ herniating through a traumatic abdominal wall defect. At surgery, several segments of small bowel had serosal tears and avulsions, requiring resection. (Right) Axial CECT demonstrates a traumatic lumbar hernia, with herniated abdominal fat covered only by the latissimus dorsi muscle ➡. Also noted is infiltration of the intraabdominal fat ➡ adjacent to the hernia. At surgery, a serosal tear of the descending colon was identified.

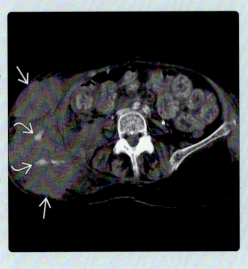
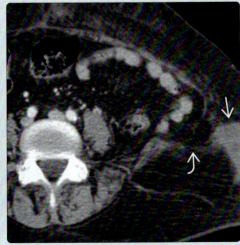

(Left) Axial CECT demonstrates a large amount of hypoenhancing small bowel ➡ herniated through a traumatic hernia of the right abdominal wall. Active arterial bleeding ➡ is evident. Much of the herniated bowel was not viable at the time of surgery. (Right) Axial CECT shows disruption of the abdominal wall muscles ➡ in the left lower quadrant, with the muscles avulsed from their attachment to the iliac crest. Note the presence of adjacent subcutaneous hematoma ➡. This is a typical example of a seat belt injury.

Traumatic Abdominal Wall Hernia

TERMINOLOGY

Abbreviations

- Traumatic abdominal wall hernia (TAWH)

Definitions

- Traumatic disruption of musculature and fascia of anterior abdominal wall due to blunt trauma (in absence of penetrating injury) ± herniation of bowel or visceral organs into subcutaneous space
- Handlebar hernia: Localized abdominal wall hernia caused by handlebar (or similar) injury

IMAGING

General Features

- Best diagnostic clue
  - Development of new abdominal wall hernia in patient with recent blunt trauma (without penetrating injury)
- Location
  - Roughly 75% occur in lower abdomen
    - May reflect inherent weakness of lower abdomen due to natural orifices (such as inguinal canals) and susceptibility to increased intraabdominal pressures
  - Equally common in right and left sides of abdomen
  - Common locations include
    - Region of iliac crest in seat belt injury (site of lap and shoulder strap junction)
    - Focal hernias often occur in lower abdomen lateral to rectus sheath or inguinal region
    - Larger abdominal wall defects most often sustained in motor vehicle accidents
- Size
  - Anatomical defects vary from small defects (few centimeters) to large disruptions
- Morphology
  - All layers of muscle and fascia are usually involved, while skin remains intact

CT Findings

- Contrast-enhanced, multiplanar
- Best modality to demonstrate size of defect, contents of hernia, and concomitant visceral organ injuries

DIFFERENTIAL DIAGNOSIS

Other Nontraumatic Hernias

- Post-traumatic hernias may have identical appearance to other types of nontraumatic hernias, and key to distinction is clinical history of trauma

PATHOLOGY

General Features

- Etiology
  - Most hernias develop due to combination of sudden increase in intraabdominal pressure, direct force of traumatic impact, acceleration-deceleration shear injury, and compressive force of seat belt
    - Force is insufficient to penetrate skin but strong enough to disrupt muscle and fascia
  - High-energy injuries: ~ 50% of cases result from motor vehicle accidents, with seat belt use increasing the risk

- Shearing force applied across bony prominences (e.g., iliac crest)
  - "High-riding" seat belt incorrectly placed over abdomen (rather than bony pelvis) increases risk of TAWH (particularly muscle avulsion from iliac crest)
    - Obese patients at higher risk for this mechanism
  - Low-energy injuries: Impact by small blunt object
    - e.g., impaction of bicycle handlebar on abdominal wall (handlebar hernia)
    - Hernias can develop after relatively minor trauma in children
- Associated abnormalities
  - Other traumatic injuries are common (~ 80% of cases), with up to 50% of patients suffering other intraabdominal injuries requiring surgery and 1/3 of patients suffering bone injuries

CLINICAL ISSUES

Presentation

- Abdominal skin ecchymosis or abrasions ("seat belt" ecchymosis)

Demographics

- Age
  - Peak incidence < 10 years, due to handlebar injuries
  - 2nd most common 20-50 years, due to motor vehicle accidents
- Epidemiology
  - Uncommon (< 1% of blunt abdominal trauma)

Natural History & Prognosis

- May be overlooked at time of injury due to attention focused on concomitant injuries, and often diagnosed due to development of hernia-related complications
  - Only 22% of TAWH patients in 1 series were diagnosed clinically, making CT essential to diagnosis
- Complications: Incarceration, bowel strangulation, bowel perforation, and bowel ischemia

Treatment

- High-energy injuries: Immediate exploratory laparotomy to treat visceral injuries
  - Delayed repair of hernia can be performed 6-8 weeks following injury to allow primary tissue damage to subside
  - In rare cases, stable patients with only mild intraabdominal injuries may undergo simultaneous repair of hernia during initial exploratory laparotomy
- Low-energy injuries: Surgical options include local exploration, incision overlying defect, laparoscopic repair, and open repair

DIAGNOSTIC CHECKLIST

Consider

- TAWH can be easily missed both on clinical examination and imaging due to presence of concomitant major injuries

SELECTED REFERENCES

1. Matalon SA et al: Don't Forget the Abdominal Wall: Imaging Spectrum of Abdominal Wall Injuries after Nonpenetrating Trauma. Radiographics. 37(4):1218-1235, 2017

KEY FACTS

IMAGING

- 90-98% occur on left side (usually posterolateral diaphragm)
- Multiple different CT signs of diaphragmatic injury, each with variable sensitivity and specificity
  - Discontinuity of hemidiaphragm with focal defect (segmental diaphragmatic defect)
  - Dangling diaphragm sign: Free edge of torn diaphragm curls inward on axial images rather than continuing its normal course parallel to chest wall
  - Absent diaphragm sign: Absence of diaphragm in expected location without visualization of discrete tear
  - Herniation of abdominal contents through discrete diaphragmatic defect
  - Collar sign: Waist-like narrowing of herniated structure as it extends through diaphragmatic tear
  - Fallen or dependent viscus sign: Herniated viscus abuts posterior ribs and thoracic wall without intervening lung

- Secondary signs of injury include simultaneous presence of pneumothorax and pneumoperitoneum or hemothorax and hemoperitoneum, active extravasation of contrast in or near diaphragm, or injuries to organs lying near diaphragm

PATHOLOGY

- 75% of cases caused by blunt trauma, and 25% caused by penetrating trauma
- Strong association with polytrauma and other major traumatic injuries

CLINICAL ISSUES

- 1-5% of all patients with substantial blunt abdominal or thoracic trauma
- True incidence is likely underestimated, as these injuries may be frequently missed on imaging
- Surgical repair of diaphragm indicated for all diaphragmatic injuries, even when small

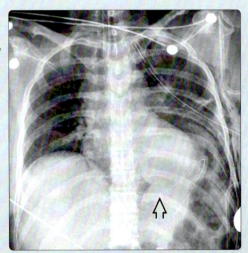
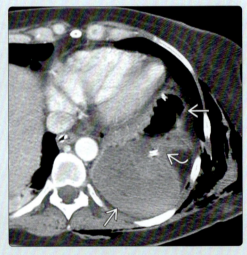

(Left) Chest x-ray in a young man following a motor vehicle crash shows a pneumothorax, chest tube, and an NG tube ➡ that is curved up toward the chest. (Right) Axial CT in the same patient shows the typical signs of diaphragmatic injury, including the fallen viscus sign. The stomach ➡ lies in the chest. Note that it has "fallen" medially and posteriorly to lie against the posteromedial chest wall. The stomach appears pinched ➡ as it traverses the defect in the diaphragm (collar sign).

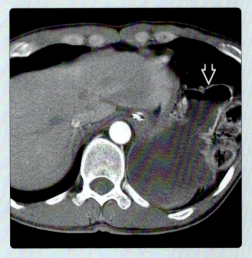
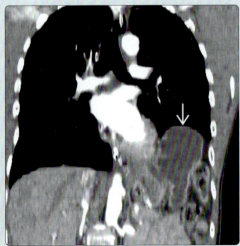

(Left) Axial CECT shows the stomach in the thorax, and it has "fallen" through the diaphragmatic defect to lie against the posteromedial chest wall. The anterior wall of the stomach ➡ directly abuts the lung and is not confined by the diaphragm. (Right) Coronal CECT in the same patient demonstrates the stomach ➡ extending upward through a diaphragmatic defect.

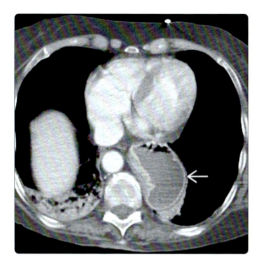
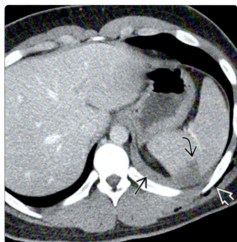

(Left) *Axial CECT in a patient following MVC shows the stomach* ➡ *lying too far medial, posterior, and superior, indicating herniation through the diaphragm. This is the fallen viscus sign.* (Right) *Axial CECT in a patient after a stab wound demonstrates a splenic laceration* ➡ *with hematoma, left hemothorax* ➡*, and subcutaneous emphysema* ➡*. The presence of hematoma above and below the left diaphragm was concerning for diaphragmatic injury, subsequently confirmed at surgery.*

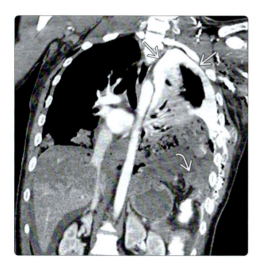
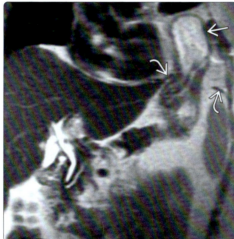

(Left) *Coronal CECT in a trauma patient demonstrates a gap in the left hemidiaphragm with the colon* ➡ *protruding into the thorax. Note the extensive enteric contrast material* ➡ *throughout the left thorax due to colonic perforation.* (Right) *Coronal T2 MR demonstrates diaphragmatic injury due to surgical error. A tear is seen in the left hemidiaphragm with the stomach* ➡ *herniating into the chest. The diaphragm is identified as a low-signal curvilinear structure* ➡ *with a central gap.*

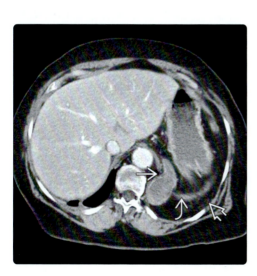
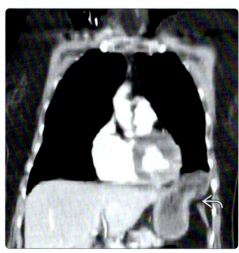

(Left) *Axial CECT in a trauma patient demonstrates that the stomach is "pinched"* ➡ *as it traverses a defect in the left diaphragm. Another sign of diaphragmatic rupture is the presence of abdominal fat* ➡ *outside the confines of the diaphragm* ➡ *(therefore, in the thorax).* (Right) *Coronal CECT in the same patient demonstrates how coronal reformations help to visualize the diaphragmatic defect* ➡*.*

Lymphangioma (Mesenteric Cyst)

TERMINOLOGY

- Rare benign malformation of lymphatic system due to failure of embryologic lymphatic development
- Generic descriptive term for benign congenital cystic mass arising in mesentery or omentum

IMAGING

- **Multiplanar CT or MR is definitive modality**
- **Contrast-enhanced CT**
  - Circumscribed cystic mass with variable density
    - Typically water density (near 0 HU) or chylous (< -20 HU), and only rarely hemorrhagic
    - No enhancement of fluid contents
    - Usually multiloculated (± septations) with feathery appearance
    - Septa may have focal calcifications
    - Soft lesions with minimal mass effect
      - Easily indented by surrounding structures, such as mesenteric vessels/bowel

- **MR**
  - Multiloculated cyst, usually hypointense on T1WI and hyperintense on T2WI
  - Fluid-filled cystic structure with thin, internal septa
  - Can be T1 hyperintense due to internal fat/chyle
- **Ultrasonography**
  - Very thin-walled cyst or "loculated fluid collection"
  - ± internal echoes due to debris, hemorrhage, or infection

TOP DIFFERENTIAL DIAGNOSES

- Loculated ascites
- Gastrointestinal duplication cyst
- Peritoneal inclusion cyst
- Cyst or cystic tumor arising from visceral organ

DIAGNOSTIC CHECKLIST

- Differentiate from cystic tumors of pancreas or other viscera
- **Do not mistake for cystic pancreatic mass**

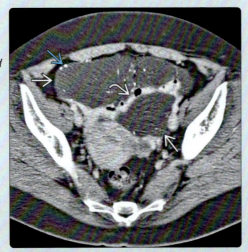 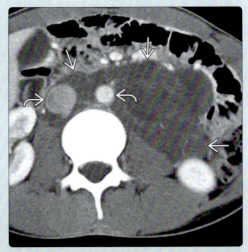

(Left) Axial CECT shows a complex cystic mass ➡ in the mesentery sandwiching a small bowel segment ➡. The mass is near-water density and has small foci of calcification ➡ in its septa and peripheral walls. The soft nature of the mass is indicated by the absence of bowel obstruction. (Right) Axial CECT demonstrates a large, multiseptate mass or multiple low-density cystic masses ➡ throughout the retroperitoneum. The lesion(s) surround the major vessels ➡ with minimal mass effect and no compression.

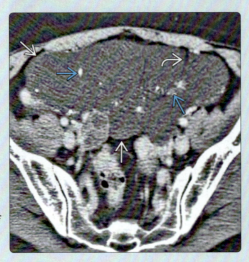 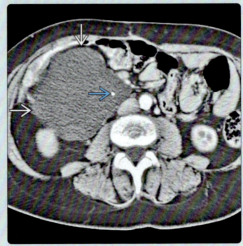

(Left) Axial CECT in a young woman shows a large cystic mass ➡ with multiple septations ➡ filling much of the lower abdomen. Note the calcifications ➡ in the septa and the peripheral walls. (Right) Axial CECT in a young woman shows a cystic retroperitoneal mass ➡ with subtle septa and a small focus of calcification ➡. The mass was resected and found to contain chylous fluid (typical of a lymphangioma) and an epithelial lining, features that help account for the variety of names for this tumor.

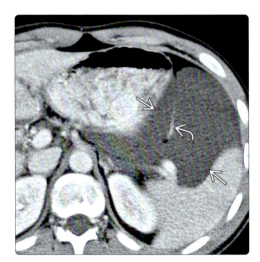
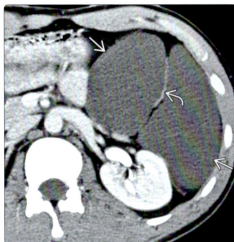

(Left) *Axial CECT shows a thin-walled mass* ➡ *of water density, indented by a mesenteric vessel* ➡ *in this patient with cystic lymphangioma.* **(Right)** *Axial CECT shows another view of the water-density, thin-walled mass* ➡ *being indented by a mesenteric vessel* ➡. *Note the absence of occlusion of the mesenteric vessel, indicating the soft, noninvasive nature of lymphangiomas.*

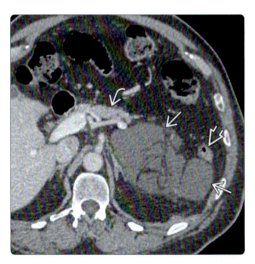
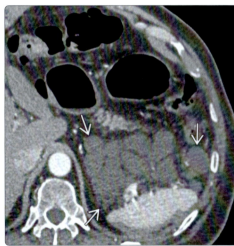

(Left) *Axial CECT demonstrates a cystic mass* ➡ *in the left retroperitoneum. The lesion abuts the pancreatic body* ➡ *and left colon* ➡ *without appreciable mass effect.* **(Right)** *Axial CECT in the same patient demonstrates the multiloculated, feathery morphology of the lesion* ➡. *This appearance is quite common with lymphangiomas, which frequently appear to have multiple internal discrete components or locules.*

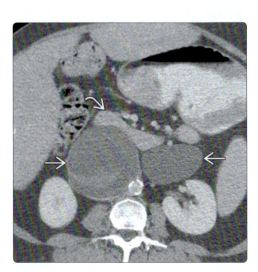
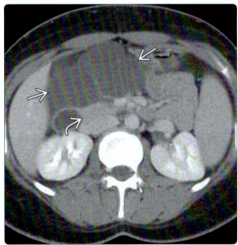

(Left) *Axial CECT shows a near-water-density, bilobed cystic mass* ➡ *in the retroperitoneum, a lymphangioma. Note the ventral displacement of the duodenum* ➡. **(Right)** *Axial CECT shows a complex, water-density, septate mass* ➡ *in the mesentery, immediately adjacent to the pancreas* ➡, *a lymphangioma. Since the mass was adjacent to the pancreas, a pancreatic cystic mass was considered in the differential diagnosis.*

Desmoid

TERMINOLOGY

- Rare, benign, locally aggressive, nonencapsulated mesenchymal neoplasms of connective or fibrous tissue

IMAGING

- **Contrast-enhanced CT or MR is best for evaluation**
- Can be intra- or extraabdominal (including abdominal wall)
  - Often involve rectus or oblique muscles, frequently at incision sites
  - May retract or compress adjacent bowel loops ± small bowel obstruction
- Usually solid with well-defined margins (but can be infiltrative in appearance)
- CT: Hyperdense to muscle on NECT and usually hypoenhancing on CECT (but rarely avidly enhancing)
- MR: Classically thought to be low signal on all MR pulse sequences due to fibrous content, but this is unreliable
  - Usually heterogeneously high signal on T2WI and STIR
  - Usually homogeneously isointense/hypointense on T1WI

- Bands of internal low signal on all pulse sequences

TOP DIFFERENTIAL DIAGNOSES

- Soft tissue sarcoma
- Leukemia and lymphoma
- Primary small bowel tumors extending into mesentery

PATHOLOGY

- Strong associations with Gardner syndrome and familial adenomatous polyposis, especially for abdominal desmoids
- Other major risk factors include previous abdominal surgery (75% of cases), trauma, or oral contraceptives

CLINICAL ISSUES

- Complications arise from locally aggressive growth pattern with compression and invasion of adjacent structures
- Surgical resection is difficult in many cases as result of involvement of adjacent critical structures
- Recurrence after surgery is very common in patients with Gardner syndrome

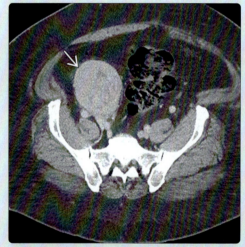
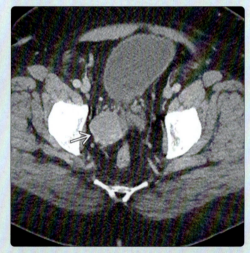

(Left) Axial CECT demonstrates a relatively homogeneous, enhancing, well-circumscribed mass ➡ in the right anterior pelvis. (Right) Axial CECT in the same patient demonstrates a very similar-appearing smaller mass ➡ in the more inferior pelvis. This was a patient with Gardner syndrome, and both of these lesions were found to represent desmoid tumors.

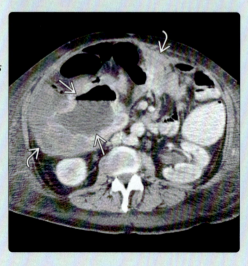
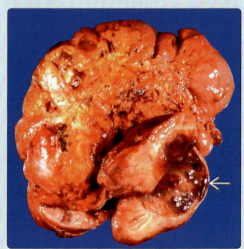

(Left) Axial CECT in a 43-year-old man with Gardner syndrome shows a huge mesenteric mass ➡ that encases and partially obstructs the small bowel. A portion of the mass has central cavitation ➡ and an air-fluid level that might be misinterpreted as aneurysmal dilation of the bowel lumen. (Right) Gross pathology of the resected mass from the same patient shows encasement of the small bowel. A portion of the mass is necrotic ➡ and communicates with the bowel lumen, accounting for the air-fluid level on CT.

Desmoid

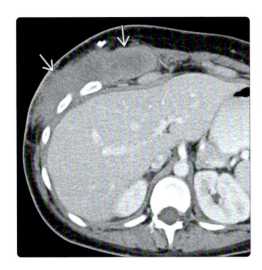
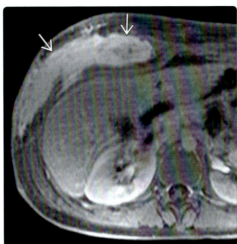

(Left) Axial CECT demonstrates an infiltrative, hypoenhancing mass ➡ in the right anterior abdominal wall musculature at the site of a prior surgical incision. (Right) Axial T1WI C+ FS MR in the same patient demonstrates relatively avid enhancement of the mass ➡, which is once again noted to be quite infiltrative and poorly marginated. In cases like this, only histologic confirmation can differentiate a desmoid from other soft tissue malignancies, such as sarcomas.

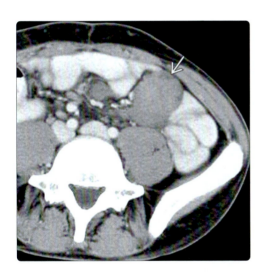
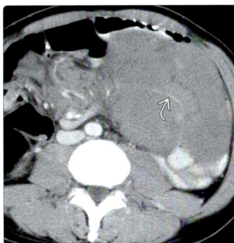

(Left) Axial CECT in a patient with Gardner syndrome shows a small soft tissue density mesenteric mass ➡, a typical desmoid in this setting. This caused no symptoms and was not resected. (Right) Axial CECT in the same patient 8 months later shows the mesenteric desmoid to have dramatically grown and now encases mesenteric vessels ➡ and the bowel. The patient was treated with complete resection of the small bowel and mesentery followed by small bowel transplantation.

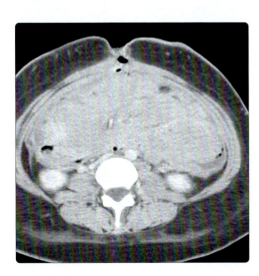
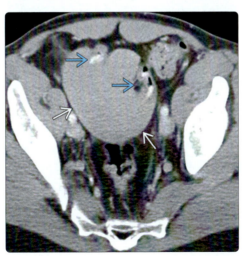

(Left) Axial CECT in a young woman with Gardner syndrome 2 years after total colectomy shows mesenteric fibromatosis (desmoids) encasing the entire small bowel mesentery, filling the abdominal cavity. (Right) Axial CECT demonstrates a very homogeneous, hypoenhancing mass ➡ in the pelvis encasing loops of adjacent bowel ➡. This was found to be a desmoid tumor. Desmoids with extensive involvement of the bowel can be very difficult to resect.

KEY FACTS

TERMINOLOGY

- Lymphoma deposits or metastatic disease to omentum, peritoneal surface, peritoneal ligaments, or mesentery

IMAGING

- **CT**: Poor sensitivity for implants < 1 cm (7-50%)
  - **Micronodular** pattern: Earliest findings may be subtle peritoneal thickening and hyperenhancement
    - Stranding and nodularity in mesentery may result in pleated or stellate appearance
  - **Nodular** pattern: More discrete nodules may be present
    - Measuring > 5 mm in size
  - **Omental caking**: Discrete omental masses coalesce into larger conglomerate omental masses
  - Thickening and nodularity along surface of bowel may reflect tumor implants on serosal surface
  - Ascites (often loculated) may be present
- **MR**: Sensitivity of MR is comparable to, or better than, CT for implants > 1 cm but limited for small implants

- Diffusion-weighted imaging (DWI) may ↑ sensitivity
- Tumor implants typically T1WI hypointense, intermediate signal on T2WI, and variable enhancement on T1WI C+ images depending on type of tumor

TOP DIFFERENTIAL DIAGNOSES

- Tuberculous peritonitis
- Abdominal mesothelioma
- Primary peritoneal serous papillary carcinoma
- Pseudomyxoma peritonei

PATHOLOGY

- Usually due to peritoneal spread of surface epithelium tumors, although hematogenous spread also possible
- Most common: Ovarian and GI adenocarcinomas (gastric, colorectal, pancreas, appendix, gallbladder)

CLINICAL ISSUES

- Common complications: Bowel and ureteral obstruction

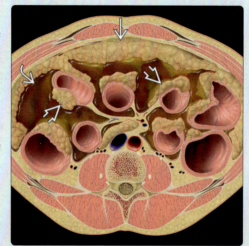
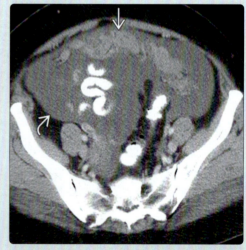

(Left) *Axial anatomic rendering of peritoneal metastases. Note the anterior omental cake ➡ and serosal implants ⇨ with ascites ➡.* (Right) *Axial CECT demonstrates extensive omental caking ➡ in the pelvic omentum, compatible with carcinomatosis. Notice the presence of ascites ➡, which is commonly associated with carcinomatosis.*

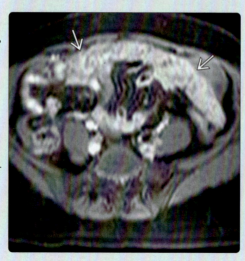
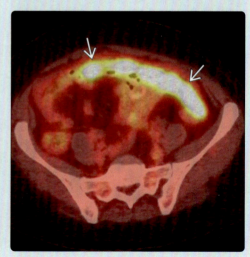

(Left) *Axial T1 C+ FS MR in the same patient demonstrates enhancing soft tissue ➡ in the omentum. Although debatable, some sources suggest that MR may have slightly increased sensitivity for carcinomatosis compared to CT.* (Right) *Axial PET/CT in the same patient demonstrates that the omental caking ➡ shows avid FDG uptake. No primary tumor was discovered in this case, and this was found to be primary peritoneal serous papillary carcinoma.*

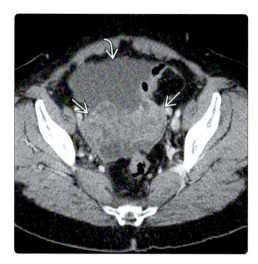
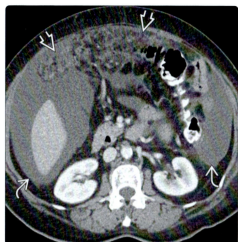

(Left) Axial CECT demonstrates a large mixed cystic/solid mass ➡ in the pelvis with adjacent ascites ➡, ultimately found to be a primary ovarian cancer. (Right) Axial CECT in the same patient demonstrates a micronodular pattern of carcinomatosis with ill-defined soft tissue induration ➡ studding the omentum with ascites ➡.

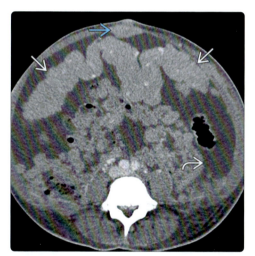
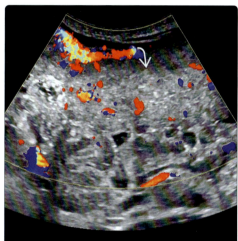

(Left) Axial CECT in a patient with ocular melanoma demonstrates extensive confluent soft tissue ➡ in the omentum (omental cake), ascites ➡, and a parietal peritoneal metastasis ➡. (Right) Color Doppler ultrasound in the same patient demonstrates extensive soft tissue ➡ throughout the omentum with internal color flow vascularity, in keeping with carcinomatosis.

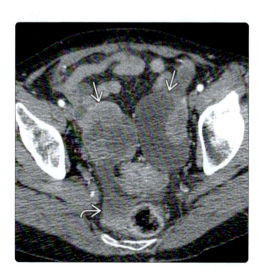
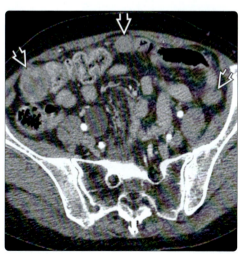

(Left) Axial CECT in an elderly woman demonstrates bilateral cystic and solid adnexal masses ➡ with adjacent ascites ➡, ultimately found to represent primary ovarian cancer. (Right) Axial CECT in the same patient demonstrates several discrete nodular soft tissue tumor implants ➡ in the omentum and parietal peritoneum, consistent with carcinomatosis.

Abdominal Mesothelioma

TERMINOLOGY

- Primary malignant neoplasm arising from peritoneum

IMAGING

- Malignant mesothelioma can arise from any serosal membrane (pleura, peritoneum, pericardium, tunica vaginalis)
  - 20-30% of malignant mesotheliomas arise in peritoneum
- **CT (test of choice)**: Omental and peritoneal stranding, nodularity, and discrete masses
  - Stellate, thickened (pleated) mesentery secondary to encasement and straightening of mesenteric vessels
  - Tumor spreads along serosal surfaces and can directly invade adjacent viscera, especially colon and liver
  - Can spread across diaphragm into pleural cavity
  - Usually less ascites than in peritoneal carcinomatosis
  - Calcified pleural plaques may be clue to diagnosis (but rarely present)

- MR: Low to intermediate T1 and intermediate to high T2 signal intensity of omental and peritoneal masses
- Typically no distant metastatic disease or lymphadenopathy

TOP DIFFERENTIAL DIAGNOSES

- Peritoneal carcinomatosis
- Lymphomatosis
- Pseudomyxoma peritonei
- Tuberculous peritonitis
- Sclerosing mesenteritis

PATHOLOGY

- Peritoneal mesothelioma generally requires much higher exposure to asbestos than pleural mesothelioma

CLINICAL ISSUES

- Rare tumor (1-2 cases per 1 million) with extremely poor prognosis (most patients die within 1 year)
- M:F > 4:1; usually 6th-7th decades

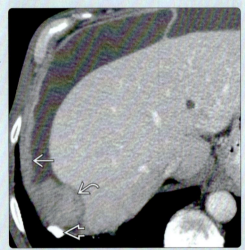
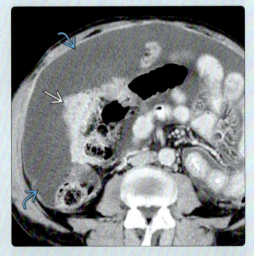

(Left) Axial CECT in an elderly man with abdominal distention shows a calcified pleural asbestos plaque ➡. The parietal peritoneum under the diaphragm is diffusely thickened ➡ with a discrete mass ➡. (Right) Axial CECT in the same patient shows an omental mass ➡ with loculated ascites ➡. The abdominal findings are indistinguishable from peritoneal carcinomatosis, but the asbestos plaque is an important clue to the diagnosis of mesothelioma.

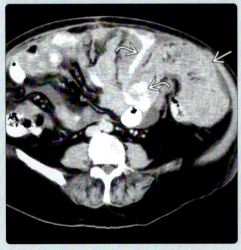
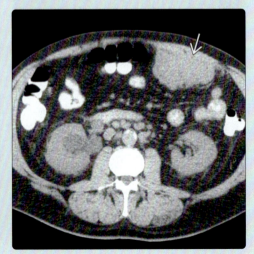

(Left) Axial CECT in an elderly man with abdominal pain shows marked mass-like omental thickening ➡ and encasement of bowel loops ➡. Open biopsy confirmed malignant mesothelioma. Note very little ascites. (Right) Axial NECT in a patient with renal insufficiency shows a lobulated mass ➡ in the omentum abutting the anterior abdominal wall. Surgical biopsy confirmed malignant mesothelioma. Such an isolated mass is an unusual manifestation of the disease, which is usually widespread at the time of diagnosis.

Pseudomyxoma Peritonei

KEY FACTS

TERMINOLOGY

- Diffuse intraperitoneal accumulation of gelatinous mucinous implants due to rupture of appendiceal mucinous neoplasm
- Some authors also use term pseudomyxoma peritonei (PMP) for mucinous dissemination after rupture of mucin-producing tumors at other sites (e.g., colon, ovary, etc.)
- Some authors use term disseminated peritoneal adenomucinosis rather than PMP

IMAGING

- **CT**: Low-attenuation masses (usually < 20 HU) scattered throughout peritoneum
  - Frequently associated with loculated ascites of similar attenuation to individual implants
  - Implants cause mass effect on liver and spleen, producing characteristic scalloped appearance
  - Implants may demonstrate curvilinear calcification
  - Dominant cystic or solid mass often present in right lower quadrant (in expected location of appendix)
  - Metastases to ovary are common, so cystic masses in ovaries may not represent primary ovarian neoplasm
  - Imaging findings of bowel obstruction
- **MR**: Implants usually low signal on T1WI and high signal on T2WI with possible internal enhancement on T1WI C+

PATHOLOGY

- Mucin-producing neoplasm of appendix causes appendiceal distension and subsequent perforation with diffuse intraperitoneal spread of mucinous implants

CLINICAL ISSUES

- Slowly progressive process with accumulation of implants and development of multiple bowel obstructions
- Primary treatment is cytoreductive surgery and infusion of heated intraperitoneal chemotherapy

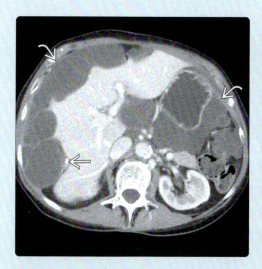
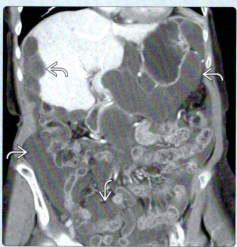

(Left) Axial CECT in a patient with a ruptured appendiceal tumor demonstrates large, low-density mucinous implants ⊒ with "scalloping" of the border of the liver, a characteristic appearance of pseudomyxoma peritonei (PMP). At least 1 implant demonstrates peripheral calcification ⊒. (Right) Coronal volume-rendered CECT in the same patient demonstrates the full extent of this patient's extensive pseudomyxoma with implants ⊒ surrounding the liver and stomach as well as extending into the pelvis.

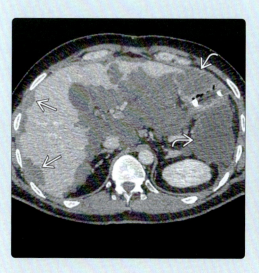
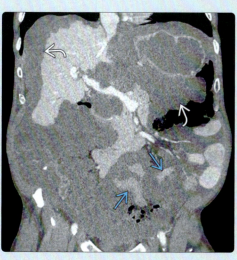

(Left) Axial CECT demonstrates characteristic "scalloping" of the liver by small perihepatic implants ⊒. These and other implants ⊒ are low density but slightly higher in attenuation (~ 20 HU) than simple fluid. (Right) Coronal CECT in the same patient demonstrates extensive low-density implants ⊒ occupying a substantial portion of the abdomen and pelvis. Not surprisingly, the patient suffered from frequent bouts of small bowel obstruction, as the small bowel ⊒ is encased by the mucinous implants.

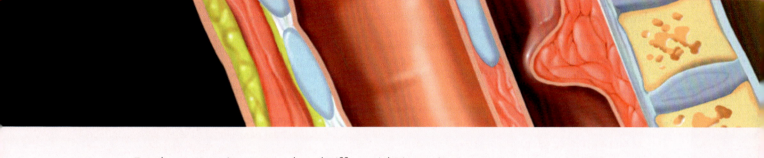

Esophageal Anatomy and Terminology

The esophagus is a fibromuscular tube ~ 25 cm long extending from the pharynx to the stomach. It begins at the upper esophageal sphincter, which is formed primarily by the cricopharyngeus muscle.

The **lower esophageal sphincter** (LES) is also known as the phrenic ampulla or the esophageal vestibule and is further defined as the zone of higher resting tone or pressure. The LES is occasionally recognized radiographically as a 2-4 cm long luminal dilation between the esophageal "A" and "B" rings.

The "A" ring is a sporadically imaged indentation of the esophageal lumen at the cephalic end of the LES.

The **"B" ring** is a transverse mucosal fold that marks the gastroesophageal (GE) junction and often corresponds to the mucosal junction between the epithelium of the esophagus and that of the stomach. The endoscopist often recognizes a "Z" line at this junction with the esophageal mucosa appearing pearly pink in color and texture, while the gastric mucosa is more textured and deeper in color.

Pharynx

The pharynx is essential for effective speech, respiration, and swallowing. The nasopharynx extends from the skull base to the top of the soft palate and lies posterior to the nasal cavity. The oro (mesopharynx) lies between the soft palate and the hyoid bone. It lies posterior to the oral cavity. The hypo (laryngopharynx) extends from the hyoid to the cricopharyngeus muscle. It lies posterior and lateral to the larynx.

Mural Anatomy

The esophagus has an internal circular and an outer longitudinal layer of muscle. The upper 1/3 of the esophagus (to ~ the level of the aortic arch) is composed of striated ("voluntary") muscle, while the lower 2/3 is smooth muscle. The esophagus lacks a serosal coat and is lined by stratified columnar epithelium.

The GE junction is attached to the diaphragm by the phrenicoesophageal ligaments (collagenous bands), which tend to weaken and elongate with age, predisposing to hiatal hernia and reflux.

The venous drainage of the esophagus is through the azygous system (systemic) and left gastric (portal).

Lymphatic drainage is variable, but the upper 2/3 usually drain primarily to the posterior mediastinal nodes, while the lower 1/3 drains to the left gastric and celiac nodes. Overlaps and variations of these patterns are common.

Imaging Protocols

Imaging should be tailored to the specific symptom complex.

- **For dysphagia, choking, aspiration pneumonitis, dysphonia**: Modified barium swallow is optimal to evaluate motility or plan therapy (usually performed with a speech pathologist); varying consistencies of barium are given by mouth with a recording of swallowing
- **For odynophagia, evaluation for Barrett esophagus or early cancer**: Air-contrast barium esophagram can be performed using gas-forming crystals to distend esophagus and heavy barium to coat the mucosa;

procedure is complementary to, or competitive with, endoscopy
- **For stricture or suspected mass lesion ("food sticking in esophagus")**: Single-contrast barium esophagram using no gas distention and lighter weight barium (complementary to endoscopy)
- **For suspected reflux [GE reflux disease (GERD)]**: Barium esophagram using provocative maneuvers to elicit reflux plus pH testing by esophageal probe or capsule
- **For dysphagia or chest pain possibly related to esophageal dysmotility**: Single-contrast esophagram (complementary to esophageal manometry)
- **For symptoms of dyspepsia, early satiety, abdominal &/or chest pain**: Upper GI series with esophageal evaluation (complementary to endoscopy and CT)
- **For evaluation of depth of esophageal tumor invasion**: Endoscopic ultrasonography
- **For staging known esophageal cancer**: PET/CT

Anatomy-Based Imaging Issues

Pharyngeal dysfunction is extremely common. Etiologies include cerebrovascular accident, deconditioning, prior surgery, etc.

Barium fluoroscopic examinations of the pharynx and esophagus are critical to diagnosing the source of the problem and identifying possible therapeutic endeavors (e.g., modified diet).

GE reflux is very common and accounts for the epidemic of GERD and the increasing prevalence of Barrett esophagus with its attendant risk of adenocarcinoma.

Hiatal hernia may result from or cause GERD. Reflux irritates the esophageal mucosa and may interrupt motility with spasm of the longitudinal muscle layer. This leads to a foreshortened esophagus with the gastric cardia pulled into the thorax (type 1 hernia).

Paraesophageal hernias are becoming more common, especially type 3. These are often quite symptomatic and require surgical repair, often involving repair of the large diaphragmatic defect as well as fundoplication.

Even with the widespread use of proton-pump inhibitors and other antacids, many patients elect to have surgical intervention for GERD with fundoplications of various types the most common approach. It is important for radiologists to understand the expected appearance of the esophagus and stomach following **fundoplication** and to recognize the imaging signs of operative complications.

Esophageal cancer is also becoming more common, with a shift in its epidemiology, with adenocarcinoma becoming more prevalent as a direct result of GERD and development of Barrett metaplasia of the esophagus. The lack of a serosal coat allows esophageal cancer to invade adjacent mediastinal structures, and the rich and varied lymphatic and venous drainage predispose to widespread metastases. Accurate staging may require a combination of modalities, including endoscopic sonography (for depth of wall invasion), thoracoabdominal CT, &/or PET/CT.

The most common treatment for esophageal carcinoma has become **esophagectomy** with some form of **gastric interposition** (Ivor-Lewis or other modification). Once again, familiarity with the expected postoperative findings, as well as its complications, is essential.

Esophageal dysmotility has also become more prevalent with the aging population, and imaging plays a major role in its evaluation, being complementary to manometry. Proper characterization of the type and degree of dysmotility helps in planning effective therapy, such as a Heller myotomy for achalasia or a modified fundoplication for scleroderma of the esophagus.

Esophageal dysmotility accounts for nearly all **pulsion diverticula** of the pharynx or esophagus. Effective therapy often depends on recognition and intervention for the underlying motility disorder.

Differential Diagnosis

Esophageal Strictures

Common
- Reflux esophagitis
- Barrett esophagus
- Esophageal carcinoma
- Scleroderma, esophagus

Less Common
- Esophageal metastases and lymphoma
- Radiation esophagitis
- Caustic esophagitis
- Drug-induced esophagitis
- Candida esophagitis
- Nasogastric intubation
- Crohn's disease
- Esophagitis, eosinophilic
- Graft-vs.-host disease
- Glutaraldehyde-induced injury
- Epidermolysis and pemphigoid

Dilated Esophagus

Common
- Achalasia, esophagus
- Scleroderma, esophagus
- Postvagotomy state
- Fundoplication complications
- Reflux esophagitis
- Esophageal carcinoma

- Hiatal hernia (mimic)
- Postesophagectomy (mimic)

Less Common
- Gastric carcinoma
- Metastases and lymphoma, esophageal
- Chagas disease

Esophageal Outpouchings (Diverticula)

Common
- Zenker diverticulum (pharyngoesophageal)
- Traction diverticulum (midesophageal)
- Pulsion diverticulum (usually distal esophageal)
- Hiatal hernia (mimic)
- Postesophagectomy (mimic)
- Fundoplication complications (mimic)

Less Common
- Killian-Jamieson diverticulum
- Intramural pseudodiverticulosis
- Boerhaave syndrome (mimic)

Esophageal Dysmotility

Common
- Presbyesophagus
- Diffuse esophageal spasm
- Achalasia, esophagus
- Scleroderma, esophagus
- Reflux esophagitis
- Fundoplication complications
- Postvagotomy state

Less Common
- Neuromuscular disorders
- Esophageal carcinoma
- Gastric carcinoma

Selected References

1. Flanagan JC et al: Esophagectomy and gastric pull-through procedures: surgical techniques, imaging features, and potential complications. Radiographics. 36(1):107-21, 2016
2. Carucci LR et al: Dysphagia revisited: common and unusual causes. Radiographics. 35(1):105-22, 2015
3. Godoy MC et al: Multidetector CT evaluation of airway stents: what the radiologist should know. Radiographics. 34(7):1793-806, 2014
4. Goldberg MF et al: Diffuse esophageal spasm: CT findings in seven patients. AJR Am J Roentgenol. 191(3):758-63, 2008

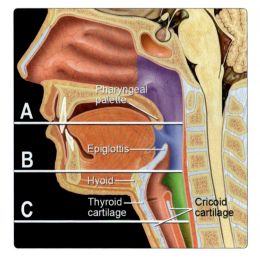

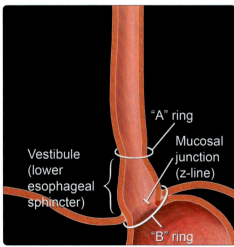

(Left) Graphic shows the nasopharynx (A, purple, base of skull to palate), oropharynx (B, blue, palate to base of epiglottis), hypopharynx, (C, green, epiglottis to cricopharyngeus), and esophagus (D, below cricopharyngeus muscle). The cricopharyngeal muscle usually lies at the C5-C6 level. (Right) Graphic shows normal esophageal landmarks and anatomy. The lower esophageal sphincter extends from the "A" to the "B" ring and is sometimes referred to as the phrenic ampulla or vestibule.

Esophagus

(Left) *This woman had dysphagia with food sticking in her throat. A film from a rapid sequence filming of the pharynx during swallowing shows prominence and spasm of the cricopharyngeal muscle ➡️ at the level of the C5-C6 vertebral disk space.* **(Right)** *Film of the lower esophagus in the same patient shows a type 1 hiatal hernia ➡️, a patulous GE junction ➡️, and free reflux. In this patient, cricopharyngeal achalasia is probably related to reflux esophagitis and the dysmotility that often accompanies GERD.*

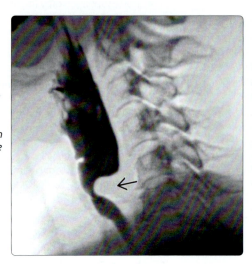
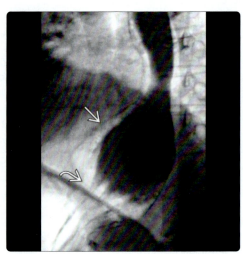

(Left) *Spot film from an upper GI series demonstrates a type 3 paraesophageal hernia in which the GE junction ➡️ and fundus ➡️ lie within the thorax. The herniated stomach is pinched at the esophageal hiatus ➡️.* **(Right)** *Two views from an esophagram in an elderly man with dysphagia show deep, nonpropulsive contractions ➡️, imparting a corkscrew appearance to the esophagus. There is a persistent, large outpouching from the mid esophagus ➡️ representing a pulsion diverticulum. The diaphragm ➡️ is marked.*

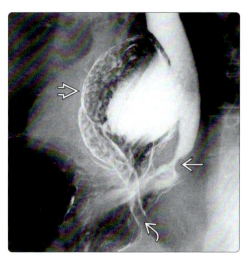
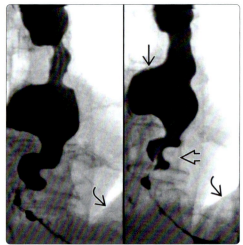

(Left) *Spot film from a barium esophagram shows a shortened and strictured esophagus ➡️ with the proximal stomach ➡️ pulled into the chest. This benign-appearing stricture was due to caustic ingestion.* **(Right)** *Spot film from an esophagram shows an "apple core" lesion of the distal esophagus ➡️ representing carcinoma. There is an abrupt transition, or shoulder, at the proximal end of the tumor as it abuts the normal esophagus.*

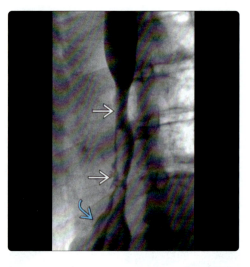
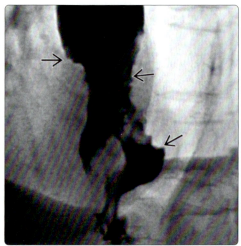

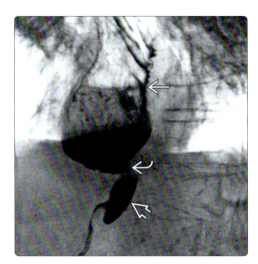

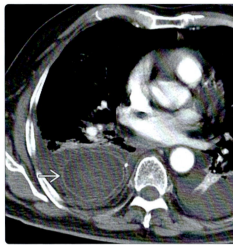

(Left) *This patient had a partial esophagectomy with gastric pull through for esophageal carcinoma. An upright film from an esophagram shows a dilated gastric conduit with barium-fluid-air levels ➡ indicating delayed emptying. The stomach is narrowed as it traverses the diaphragm ➡. The abdominal portion of the stomach ➡ is normal.* (Right) *CT in a similar patient shows a dilated, fluid-distended gastric conduit ➡ along with bilateral pleural effusions and airspace consolidation due to aspiration pneumonia.*

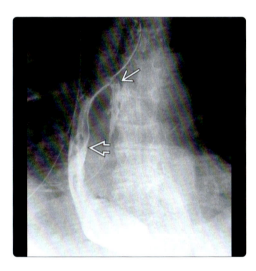

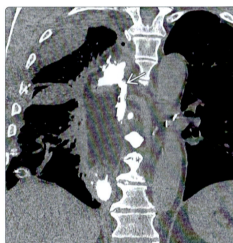

(Left) *This elderly man had a recent esophagectomy for carcinoma. Spot film from an esophagram shows displacement of the gastric conduit ➡ to the right and a leak of contrast from the esophagogastric anastomosis ➡.* (Right) *Coronal CT in the same patient shows the leak ➡ extending into the mediastinum.*

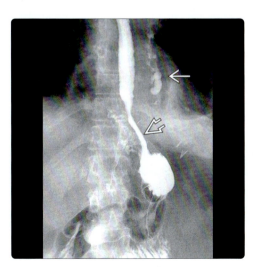

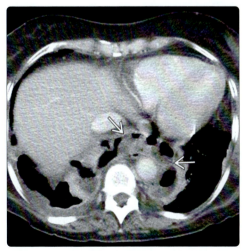

(Left) *Following a recent fundoplication, this patient was evaluated by esophagography. Spot film shows the expected compression ➡ by an intact fundal wrap but also shows extravasated gas and contrast material ➡ into the mediastinum.* (Right) *CT in the same patient shows mediastinal gas and fluid ➡ due to perforation of the wrap or distal esophagus.*

TERMINOLOGY

- Inflammation of esophageal mucosa due to gastroesophageal (GE) reflux

IMAGING

- Irregular ulcerated mucosa of distal esophagus
- Foreshortening of esophagus: Due to muscle spasm
- Inflammatory esophagogastric polyps: Smooth, ovoid elevations
- Hiatal hernia in > 95% of patients with stricture
  - Probably is result, not cause, of reflux
- Peptic stricture (1- to 4-cm length): Concentric, smooth, tapered narrowing of distal esophagus

TOP DIFFERENTIAL DIAGNOSES

- Scleroderma
- Drug-induced esophagitis
- Infectious esophagitis
- Eosinophilic esophagitis

- Caustic esophagitis

PATHOLOGY

- Lower esophageal sphincter: Decreased tone leads to increased reflux
- Hydrochloric acid and pepsin: Synergistic effect

CLINICAL ISSUES

- 15-20% of Americans commonly have heartburn due to reflux; ~ 30% fail to respond to standard-dose medical therapy
  - Prevalence of GE reflux disease has increased sharply with obesity epidemic
- Symptoms: Heartburn, regurgitation, angina-like pain
  - Dysphagia, odynophagia
- Confirmatory testing: Manometric/ambulatory pH-monitoring techniques
  - Endoscopy, biopsy

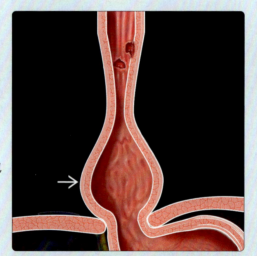
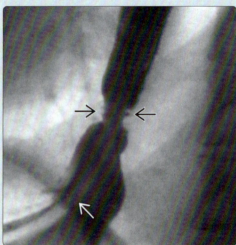

(Left) *Graphic shows a small type 1 (sliding) hiatal hernia* ➡ *associated with foreshortening of the esophagus, ulceration of the mucosa, and a tapered stricture of the distal esophagus.* (Right) *Spot film from an esophagram shows a small hiatal hernia with gastric folds* ➡ *extending above the diaphragm. The esophagus appears shortened, presumably due to spasm of its longitudinal muscles. A stricture is present at the GE junction and persistent collections of barium* ➡ *indicate mucosal ulceration.*

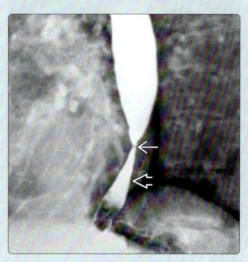
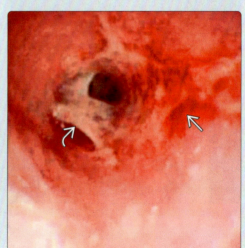

(Left) *Prone film from an esophagram shows a tight stricture* ➡ *just above the GE junction with upstream dilation of the esophagus. The herniated stomach* ➡ *is pulled taut as a result of the foreshortening of the esophagus, a common and important sign of reflux esophagitis.* (Right) *Endoscopic image of the distal esophagus in the same patient demonstrates pseudomembranes* ➡, *mucosal ulceration* ➡, *nodularity, and stricture.*

Barrett Esophagus

TERMINOLOGY

- Metaplasia of distal esophageal squamous epithelium to columnar (intestinal) epithelium
- Long segment: Columnar epithelium > 3 cm above gastroesophageal (GE) junction
  - Due to more severe reflux disease
  - Hiatal hernia in almost all patients
  - Midesophageal mucosal irregularity, stricture, deep ulceration
  - Risk of cancer is higher
- Short segment: Columnar epithelium ≤ 3 cm above GE junction
  - More common than long segment (reported in 2-12% of patients with chronic reflux at endoscopy)
  - Due to less severe reflux disease

IMAGING

- **Double- or single-contrast esophagram: Can suggest Dx**
  - Midesophageal stricture with hiatal hernia and reflux is highly suggestive
  - Distal esophageal reticular mucosa, ± stricture, ± shallow ulceration may be seen on double-contrast barium esophagram
- **CT or PET/CT**
  - Useful in diagnosis and staging
  - **When esophageal cancer is diagnosed or suspected**

TOP DIFFERENTIAL DIAGNOSES

- Esophageal carcinoma
  - Raised plaque; irregular stricture; polypoid mass
- Reflux esophagitis
  - May cause ulceration and stricture similar to Barrett esophagus

CLINICAL ISSUES

- Diagnosis: Endoscopy with biopsy

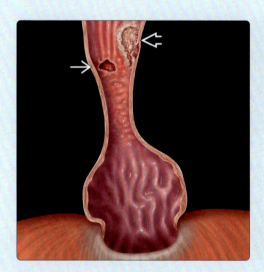

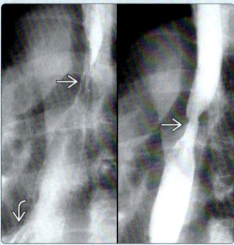

(Left) Graphic shows a type 1 hiatal hernia, distal esophageal stricture, and nodular mucosal surface. Note the discrete ulcer ➡ and an adenocarcinoma ➡ represented by a raised sessile lesion with an irregular surface. (Right) Two views from an esophagram show a mid-esophageal stricture ➡ and ulcer in a patient with a small hernia ➡ and reflux.

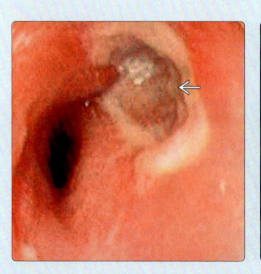

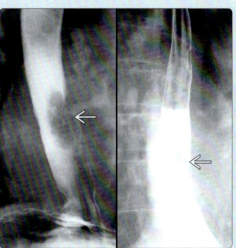

(Left) Endoscopic image shows a large ulcer ➡ with the velvet texture of Barrett mucosa and stricture. Normal esophageal mucosa has a shiny, smooth, pink surface. (Right) Two views from an esophagram show a polypoid mass ➡ that represents an adenocarcinoma arising in Barrett mucosa.

TERMINOLOGY

- Esophageal injury due to ingestion of strong alkali or acid
  - Causes mild to severe injury to upper GI tract
    - Esophagus > stomach > duodenum

IMAGING

- **Imaging evaluation: CT for acute injury; barium esophagram for chronic**
  - If esophagram is performed in acute phase, use nonionic, water-soluble agent (e.g., Omnipaque)
- Fluoroscopic: Esophagram
  - Stage 1: Acute severe phase (1-4 days)
    - Narrowed lumen with irregular contour/ulcerations
    - May have signs of perforation (extraluminal gas and contrast medium)
  - Stage 2: Ulcer granulation phase (5-28 days)
    - More defined ulcers; spasm
  - Stage 3: Cicatrization and scarring (3-4 weeks)

- Strictures, usually long and smooth, can be irregular and eccentric
- Sacculations, pseudodiverticula
- Stomach is often pulled up into chest by esophageal shortening
- CT findings
  - Acute phase
    - Target sign: Mucosal enhancement and hypodense submucosa
    - Esophageal perforation: Pneumomediastinum, pleural effusion
  - Chronic phase: Luminal irregularity & narrowing; wall thickening
    - Similar findings in stomach ± duodenum

CLINICAL ISSUES

- Complications: Perforation, mediastinitis, peritonitis, fistulas, shock

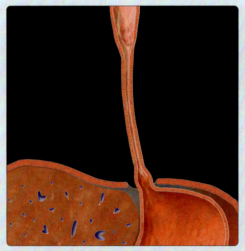
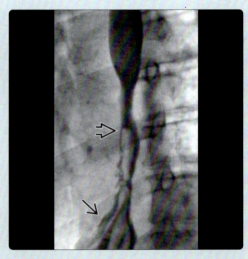

(Left) *Graphic shows a long stricture of the esophagus and ulceration of the mucosa. The stomach is pulled up into the chest due to foreshortening of the esophagus by fibrosis &/or spasm.* (Right) *Spot film from a barium esophagram in a patient with a chronic stricture ⊟ from caustic ingestion shows a shortened and strictured esophagus with the proximal stomach ⊟ pulled into the chest. This stricture has been treated repeatedly by balloon dilation, and the patient has not required surgery.*

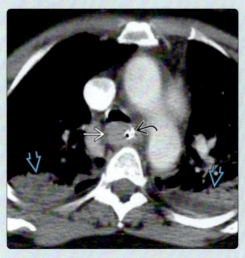
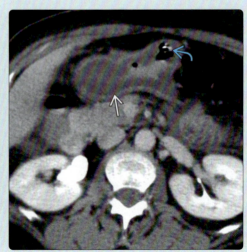

(Left) *Axial CECT of a patient 2 hours after caustic ingestion shows marked thickening of the esophageal wall ⊟ and bilateral aspiration pneumonitis ⊟. A nasogastric tube ⊟ is present in the esophagus.* (Right) *Axial CECT in the same patient shows marked thickening of the gastric wall with submucosal edema ⊟, indicating corrosive gastritis. The nasogastric tube ⊟ is again noted.*

Drug-Induced Esophagitis

KEY FACTS

TERMINOLOGY

- Esophageal injury induced by direct contact with oral medications

IMAGING

- **Barium esophagography is imaging procedure of choice**
- Ulcers and spasm or stricture occur at sites of esophageal narrowing
  - Aortic arch, left main bronchus, retrocardiac
- Findings on esophagram (double contrast)
  - Solitary or localized cluster of tiny ulcers distributed circumferentially on normal background mucosa
  - Punctate, linear, stellate, serpiginous, or ovoid; collections of barium on esophageal surface
  - Longer areas of ulceration with potassium chloride, quinidine, biphosphonates, and in patients with cardiomegaly
  - Mass effect surrounding ulcer due to edema and inflammation; can mimic ulcerated carcinoma

- Superficial ulceration
  - Giant, flat ulcers are uncommonly seen

TOP DIFFERENTIAL DIAGNOSES

- Reflux esophagitis
- Viral esophagitis
- Esophageal carcinoma
- Barrett esophagus

CLINICAL ISSUES

- Patient wakes up with severe odynophagia in morning after taking medications at bedtime with insufficient water
  - Usually resolves spontaneously
- Main classes of medications at fault
  - Antibiotics (especially tetracyclines)
  - Antiinflammatories (aspirin, NSAIDs, etc.)
  - "Cardiac" drugs (quinidine, potassium chloride, etc.)
  - Biphosphonates (to prevent bone loss; can cause severe, longer segment esophageal ulceration)

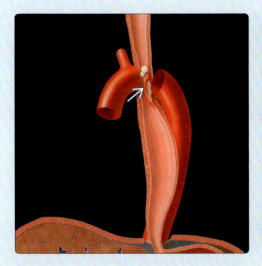
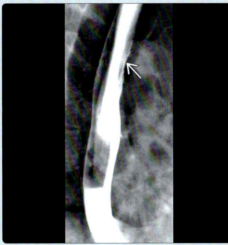

(Left) *Graphic shows medication pills stuck at the level of the aortic arch with focal spasm and ulceration* ➡. (Right) *Esophagram shows broad, shallow ulceration* ➡ *at the aortic arch level. The patient had odynophagia and recent tetracycline ingestion, and the symptoms resolved spontaneously. Physiological points of esophageal narrowing, such as at the aortic arch and the retrocardiac portion of the esophagus, are the most commonly cited for pill-induced esophagitis.*

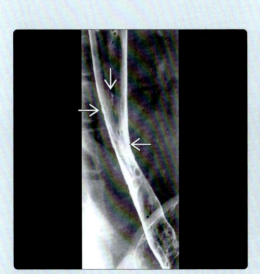
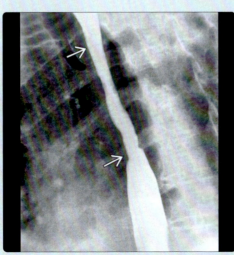

(Left) *Double-contrast barium esophagram in a 50-year-old woman with odynophagia while taking tetracycline shows multiple ulcerations* ➡ *and a subtle stricture or spasm of the distal esophagus.* (Right) *This 70-year-old woman with cardiac disease awoke with severe odynophagia the morning after taking her quinidine at bedtime. Barium esophagram demonstrates a long stricture or focal spasm* ➡ *from the thoracic inlet to the aortic arch without definite ulceration.*

KEY FACTS

IMAGING

- Videofluoroscopic esophagram
  - If there is concern for aspiration or fistula, start with nonionic, low osmolar, water-soluble contrast medium [e.g., iohexol (Omnipaque)]
  - Follow with barium if no leak or fistula
- Acute radiation esophagitis (RE)
  - Location: Usually conforms to radiation portal
  - Disordered motility, interruption of primary peristalsis
  - May be seen within days to weeks of radiation therapy (RT)
- Chronic RE
  - Strictures: Concentric, smooth, tapered narrowing
  - Upper or mid esophagus within radiation portal
  - Usually 4-8 months after completion of RT
  - Late-developing deep ulcers; ominous, raising concern for fistula, especially to bronchus
  - Motility disturbance may persist forever

- CT shows radiation port indirectly
  - Scarring of lung in paramediastinal distribution
  - Thick-walled esophagus with narrowed lumen
  - Shows any residual tumor or lymphadenopathy
- PET/CT
  - Caution: Radiation injury to esophagus and mediastinum may be FDG avid

TOP DIFFERENTIAL DIAGNOSES

- Reflux esophagitis
- Caustic esophagitis
- Nasogastric intubation esophagitis
- Tumor recurrence

CLINICAL ISSUES

- **Protocol advice**
  - **CT and fluoroscopic esophagram give complementary information**

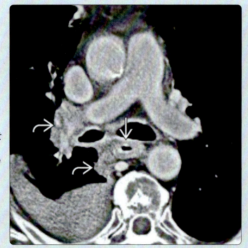
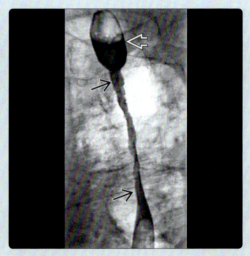

(Left) Axial CECT in an elderly man with lung cancer who developed dysphagia and odynophagia while receiving radiation therapy to his mediastinum shows a right lung tumor and mediastinal lymphadenopathy ➡. The esophageal wall ➡ is thickened and the lumen is narrowed. (Right) Upright spot film from an esophagram in the same patient shows a long stricture ➡ of the mid thoracic esophagus with dilation of the proximal portion ➡, indicating partial obstruction in this classic case of radiation esophagitis.

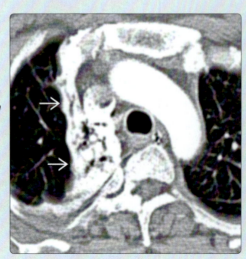
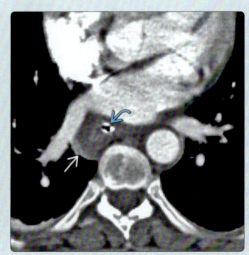

(Left) Axial CECT in a middle-aged man with lung cancer who received radiation and chemotherapy demonstrates extensive fibrosis and volume loss of the right lung ➡ in a paramediastinal distribution, corresponding to the radiation port. (Right) Axial CECT of a patient with dysphagia following radiation therapy for lung cancer shows marked thickening of the esophageal wall ➡ surrounding the nasogastric tube ➡.

Esophageal Webs

TERMINOLOGY

- Thin mucosal fold, narrowing esophageal lumen
  - Lacks muscle layer (unlike distal esophageal B or Schatzki ring)

IMAGING

- **Full column barium esophagram** with rapid-sequence filming, or have patient swallow small marshmallow followed by barium
- Appearance: 1- to 2-mm wide, shelf-like filling defect
  - Usually along anterior wall of cervical esophagus
  - Circumferential, radiolucent ring in some cases
  - May occur at other sites in esophagus
- Mild, moderate, or severe luminal narrowing
- Partial obstruction suggested by
  - Jet phenomenon: Barium spurting through ring
  - Dilation of esophagus or pharynx proximal to web

TOP DIFFERENTIAL DIAGNOSES

- Esophageal strictures
  - Longer length of luminal narrowing of esophagus
- Schatzki ring
  - Lower esophageal or B ring at GE junction

PATHOLOGY

- Esophageal webs may be associated with
  - Plummer-Vinson (Paterson-Kelly) syndrome
  - Eosinophilic esophagitis
  - Epidermolysis, pemphigoid
  - Celiac-sprue disease
  - Chronic GE reflux
  - Graft-vs.-host disease

CLINICAL ISSUES

- Usually asymptomatic
- Dysphagia with impaction of food or pills above web
- Respond to balloon or bougie dilation but often recur

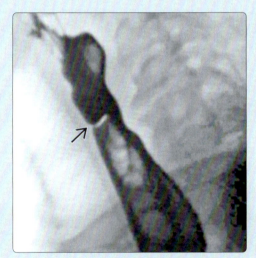

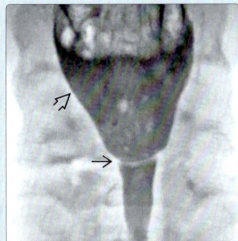

(Left) One of a series of rapid-sequence spot films from a barium esophagram in a 45-year-old woman with dysphagia shows a thin, shelf-like indentation ⇨ from the anterior and lateral walls of the pharyngoesophageal junction. (Right) Frontal esophagram in the same patient shows abnormal distension of the pharynx ⇨ above this web ⇨, confirming that it is causing luminal narrowing and partial obstruction.

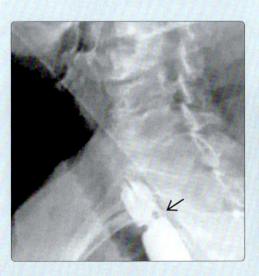

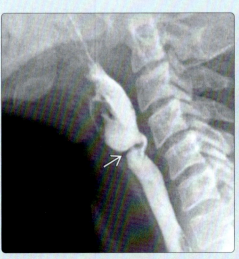

(Left) Barium esophagram in a 50-year-old woman with solid food dysphagia shows a shelf-like narrowing ⇨ of the proximal esophageal lumen. This web is unusually thick and circumferential. (Right) Lateral esophagram in a young patient with epidermolysis bullosa shows a web-like stricture ⇨ near the pharyngoesophageal junction, representing a stricture due to repeated episodes of mucosal ulceration, typical of patients with epidermolysis.

TERMINOLOGY

- Annular, inflammatory, symptomatic narrowing of normal lower esophageal mucosal or B ring

IMAGING

- Most likely results from reflux or eosinophilic esophagitis
- Classification based on ring diameter
  - Ring < 13 mm: Symptomatic
  - Ring 13-20 mm: Occasionally symptomatic
  - Ring > 20 mm: Asymptomatic
- Single contrast barium esophagram
  - Thin (2-4 mm in height), web-like constriction at gastroesophageal junction
  - Margins: Smooth and symmetric
  - Sliding hiatal hernia seen below ring
- Schatzki ring best visualized
  - In prone right anterior oblique position
  - During suspended deep inspiration and Valsalva
  - With lumen distended with barium

TOP DIFFERENTIAL DIAGNOSES

- Reflux esophagitis
- Esophageal webs
- Esophageal carcinoma
- Muscular or contractile or A ring

CLINICAL ISSUES

- **"Cheap steakhouse" syndrome: Due to inadequately chewed piece of meat impacted above ring**
- Recurrent dysphagia; intermittent obstruction by food
  - Treatment: Mechanical disruption by bougienage or pneumatic dilation

DIAGNOSTIC CHECKLIST

- May need deep inspiration, Valsalva, distention to demonstrate Schatzki ring on esophagram
- May give 13-mm barium pill during fluoroscopic esophagram to judge diameter of ring

(Left) Graphic shows a small hiatal hernia ⬎ and an annular ring-like narrowing ➡ at the gastroesophageal junction. (Right) Film from a barium esophagram demonstrates a small hiatal hernia ⬎ and a Schatzki ring ➡ with a luminal diameter of only 5-7 mm. Symptomatic narrowing of the B ring, which constitutes the Schatzki ring, probably results from reflux esophagitis.

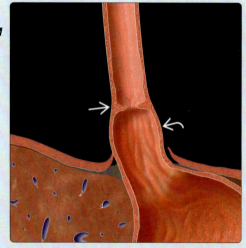
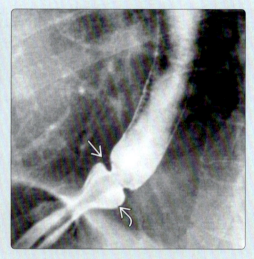

(Left) In this young man with abrupt onset of chest pain after swallowing a piece of meat, a spot film from an esophagram shows a Schatzki ring ➡ with the piece of meat ⬎ impacted above it. (Right) Initial views of the esophagus (not shown) were normal. Repeat films, taken during deep inspiration and Valsalva maneuver, show the Schatzki ring ➡ at the gastroesophageal junction. This lesion can be missed if it is tilted relative to the plane of imaging or if the esophagus is not optimally distended.

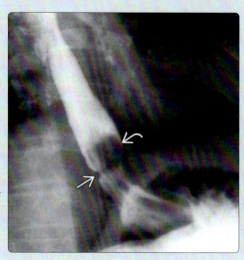
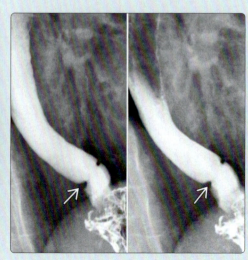

Cricopharyngeal Achalasia

TERMINOLOGY

- Failure of cricopharyngeal muscle (upper esophageal sphincter) relaxation due to hypertrophy or spasm

IMAGING

- Prominent cricopharyngeus muscle at pharyngoesophageal junction with retention of barium in pharynx on lateral view
  - Pharyngoesophageal junction: C5-C6 level
- Videofluoroscopic recording: Frontal, lateral, and oblique
  - Rapid sequence filming is required for demonstration

TOP DIFFERENTIAL DIAGNOSES

- Cervical osteophytes (indentation)
  - Large anterior cervical osteophytes can impinge on pharyngoesophageal junction, simulating cricopharyngeal achalasia
- Esophageal tumor
  - Tumor at pharyngoesophageal junction may constrict lumen concentrically or eccentrically

PATHOLOGY

- Usually just "poor timing" of cricopharyngeal contraction
  - Due to "presbyesophagus" or other cause of dysmotility in most cases
- May occur as isolated abnormality

CLINICAL ISSUES

- Intermittent symptoms: Dysphagia, food "sticking" in throat (at suprasternal level)
- Treat underlying problem
  - e.g., reflux esophagitis with spasm
- Rarely requires cricopharyngeal myotomy or botulinum toxin injection

DIAGNOSTIC CHECKLIST

- Persistent narrowing or just intermittent indentation
- Smoothly outlined, lip-like projection posteriorly at C5-C6 level with jet effect seen via narrowed lumen

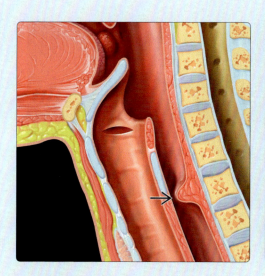

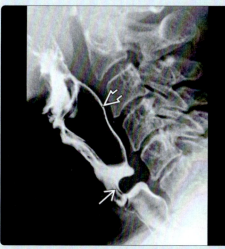

(Left) Graphic shows hypertrophied, contracted cricopharyngeus muscle ⇨ at the pharyngoesophageal junction (usually near the C5-C6 cervical level). (Right) Lateral view from an esophagram shows a typical appearance of cricopharyngeal achalasia with a large filling defect ⇨ along the posterior wall of the pharyngoesophageal junction at the C5-C6 level. Note the distension of the pharynx ⇨ proximal to this process.

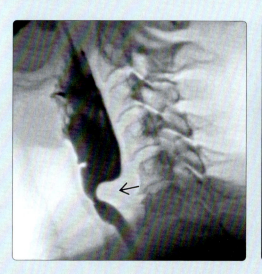

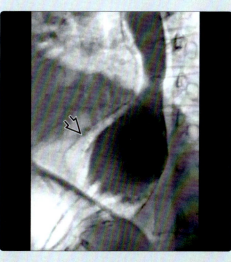

(Left) Lateral film from an esophagram shows a prominent cricopharyngeal "bar" ⇨ at the C5-C6 level in a woman with symptoms of reflux and pills "sticking" in her throat. (Right) Spot film of the lower esophagus in the same woman shows a hiatal hernia ⇨ and marked gastroesophageal reflux. Cricopharyngeal achalasia is most often seen in patients with other esophageal disorders, such as reflux esophagitis or motility disorders.

Achalasia

IMAGING

- Classified based on etiology: Primary or secondary
- Primary (idiopathic)
  - "Bird beak" deformity: Dilated esophagus with smooth, symmetric, tapered narrowing at esophagogastric region
  - Transient flow of fluid into stomach when hydrostatic pressure of fluid column exceeds tonic lower esophageal sphincter (LES) pressure
  - Length of narrowed segment typically < 3.5 cm; widest diameter upstream is often > 4 cm
- Secondary (pseudoachalasia)
  - Intrinsic or extrinsic tumor (especially gastric), peptic stricture, postvagotomy, Chagas disease, others
- Manometric characteristics of achalasia
  - Increased or normal resting LES pressures
  - Incomplete or absent LES relaxation on swallowing
- **Fluoroscopy (esophagram) is complementary to manometry and endoscopy for diagnosis**

- CT or PET/CT when malignancy is present or suspected

TOP DIFFERENTIAL DIAGNOSES

- Esophageal scleroderma
- Esophageal or gastric fundal carcinoma
- Esophagitis with stricture

CLINICAL ISSUES

- Complications
  - Aspiration pneumonitis
  - Superimposed infection (e.g., *Candida* esophagitis)
  - 10x increased risk of carcinoma
- Treatment
  - Medical (Botox injection); endoscopic (balloon dilation)
    - Rarely provide long-term relief of symptoms
  - Heller myotomy (partial-thickness incision of LES)
    - ± partial (Toupet) fundoplication
  - Peroral endoscopic myotomy procedure

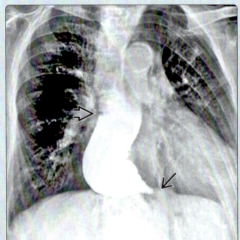
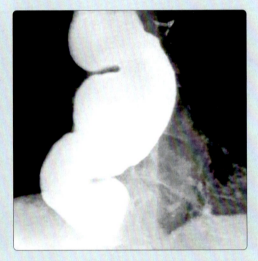

(Left) *Upright spot film from an esophagram shows a dilated esophagus with an abrupt taper ("bird beak") just above the gastroesophageal (GE) junction ➡. Note the absent gastric air bubble and the fluid-barium level ➡ within the esophagus.* (Right) *Spot film from an esophagram shows a grossly dilated, tortuous esophagus with a sigmoid appearance. This is an example of longstanding achalasia.*

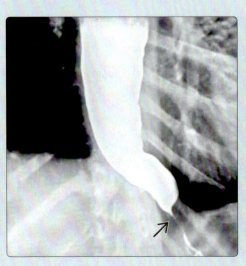
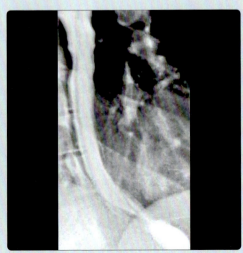

(Left) *Spot film from an esophagram shows a typical appearance of achalasia, pre-Heller myotomy, with "bird beak" deformity of the distal esophagus ➡, marked dilation of the proximal esophageal lumen, and absent peristalsis.* (Right) *Upright film from an esophagram in the same patient following Heller myotomy shows that the esophageal lumen is no longer dilated. The esophagus emptied readily in the upright position, due to gravity, while peristalsis was still absent.*

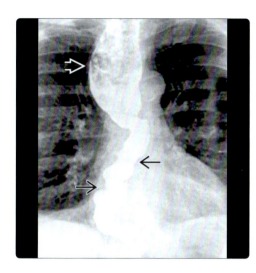 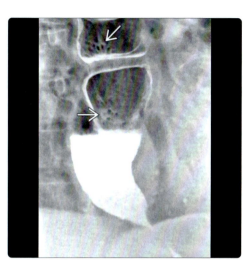

(Left) *Upright spot film from an esophagram shows retained food and fluid ⇨ within the dilated esophagus of a 78-year-old woman with dysphagia. Deep, nonpropulsive tertiary contractions ⇨ are noted. This is an example of vigorous achalasia, in which esophageal contractions are seen but are not effective. Manometry confirmed achalasia.* **(Right)** *Upright spot film from an esophagram shows typical findings of achalasia plus numerous irregular plaques ⇨ due to Candida esophagitis.*

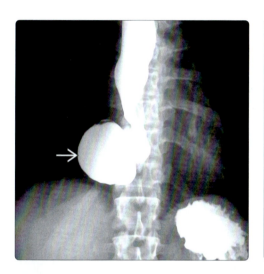 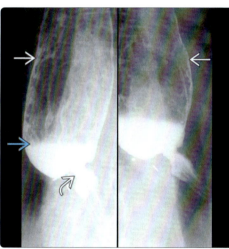

(Left) *Esophagram shows a large pulsion epiphrenic diverticulum ⇨ in a patient with achalasia.* **(Right)** *Two films from an esophagram demonstrate a markedly dilated, atonic esophagus ⇨ with a barium-fluid level ⇨ on these upright films. There is a tight peptic stricture ⇨ at the GE junction. These were the result of longstanding scleroderma, rather than achalasia.*

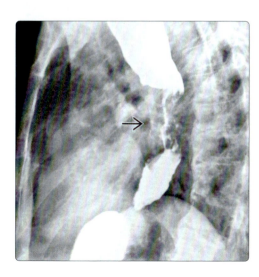 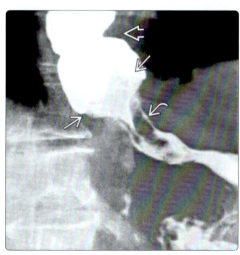

(Left) *Spot film from an esophagram in a patient with longstanding achalasia shows an irregular constricting, "apple core" mass ⇨, which proved to be squamous cell carcinoma.* **(Right)** *Esophagram shows a dilated esophagus with tertiary contractions ⇨ simulating achalasia. The abrupt narrowing of the lumen with overhanging edges ⇨ and presence of nodular thickened folds ⇨ suggests the true diagnosis of gastric carcinoma, causing this pseudoachalasia appearance.*

IMAGING

- Achalasia
  - Idiopathic or neurogenic disorder
  - Incomplete or absent relaxation of lower esophageal sphincter (LES)
  - Absent primary peristalsis; occasional shallow or deep aperistaltic contractions
  - Markedly dilated esophagus, usually > 4 cm
  - Bird beak deformity in esophagogastric region
- Distal (or diffuse) esophageal spasm
  - Absent peristalsis and frequent contractions, often obliterating lumen
    - Esophageal lumen may show corkscrew or rosary bead pattern
  - Often with chest pain during contractions
- Presbyesophagus (nonspecific esophageal motility disorder)

- Not recognized as distinct motility disturbance according to some definitions
- **Extremely common in patients beyond age 60**
- Multiple nonpropulsive (tertiary) contractions and decreased primary peristalsis
- Many patients have symptoms of gastroesophageal reflux disease
  - Reflux may not be demonstrated on barium esophagram
- Scleroderma
  - Decreased or absent resting LES pressure
  - Absence of peristalsis in lower 2/3 of esophagus
  - Patulous gastroesophageal region and reflux → fusiform distal peptic stricture ± hiatal hernia

DIAGNOSTIC CHECKLIST

- **Accurate diagnosis relies on clinical, radiographic, and motility findings**

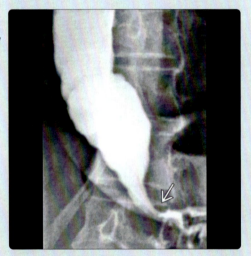
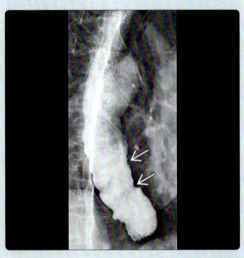

(Left) Upright film from an esophagram in a 28-year-old woman with primary achalasia shows marked dilation of the esophageal lumen, ending in a smoothly tapered bird beak deformity ➡ through the lower esophageal sphincter. (Right) Later film from esophagram in the same patient shows absent primary peristalsis and only weak intermittent tertiary contractions ➡, causing the undulating surface contour. Retained fluid within the esophagus dilutes the barium.

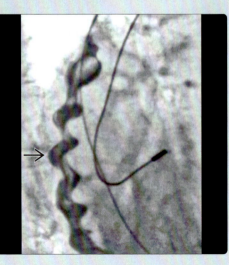
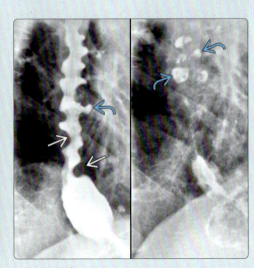

(Left) Spot film from an esophagram in an elderly man with distal esophageal spasm shows intermittent obliterative contractions, imparting a corkscrew appearance ➡ to the esophagus. (Right) Spot films from an esophagram in an elderly woman with distal esophageal spasm show obliterative, deep contractions ➡. Multiple barium-filled pulsion diverticula are evident ➡ especially after the barium bolus has passed. Pulsion diverticula are closely associated with esophageal dysmotility.

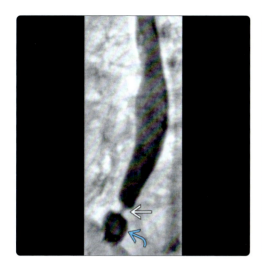

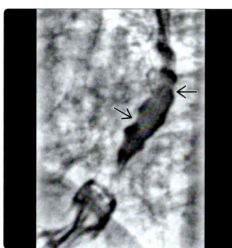

(Left) *Spot film from an esophagram in a middle-aged man with presbyesophagus shows a small hiatal hernia* ⇗ *with the gastroesophageal-esophageal junction marked by a Schatzki ring* ⇒*.* (Right) *Spot film from the esophagram in the same patient shows intermittently evident nonpropulsive tertiary contractions* ⇒*. The Schatzki ring and dysmotility resulted in obstructed passage of a barium pill (not shown).*

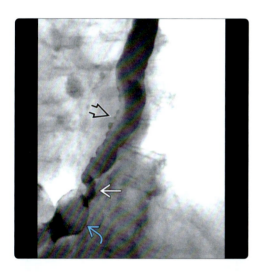

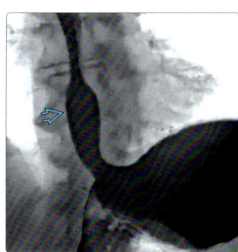

(Left) *Spot film from a barium esophagram in an elderly man with dysphagia and heartburn demonstrates a small hiatal hernia* ⇗ *and a stricture at the gastroesophageal junction* ⇒*. Tertiary contractions are also noted* ⇒*.* (Right) *Esophagram in the same patient shows free gastroesophageal reflux* ⇒ *noted on rolling the patient into a supine position. The esophageal dysmotility in this patient is probably a result of age ("presbyesophagus") as well as the effects of reflux esophagitis (GERD) on motility.*

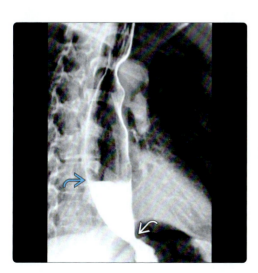

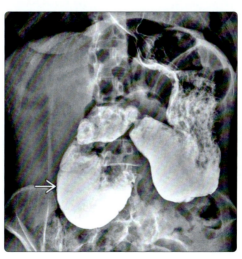

(Left) *Upright spot film from an esophagram in a 38-year-old woman with scleroderma shows a stricture at the gastroesophageal junction* ⇒ *and dilation of the aperistaltic esophagus with an air-fluid level* ⇒ *indicating stasis. These findings mimic those of primary achalasia, leading to the term pseudoachalasia.* (Right) *The same patient also had scleroderma affecting the intestine with a dilated, aperistaltic duodenum* ⇒ *and gastric outlet obstruction noted on this spot film from an upper GI series.*

Zenker Diverticulum

TERMINOLOGY

- Pharyngoesophageal diverticulum or posterior hypopharyngeal diverticulum/outpouching
- Mucosal herniation through area of anatomic weakness of cricopharyngeal muscle (Killian triangle)

IMAGING

- **Contrast (barium) esophagram is best diagnostic study**
- Barium-filled sac posterior to cervical esophagus
  - Opening into pouch at level of cricopharyngeus muscle (cervical vertebral level 5-6)
    - Prominent or thickened cricopharyngeal muscle
  - Luminal narrowing of proximal esophagus due to extrinsic compression by diverticulum
- Almost all patients have associated esophageal dysmotility, often with hiatal hernia and gastroesophageal reflux disease
- Average maximal dimension: 2.5 cm (range: 0.5-8.0 cm)

TOP DIFFERENTIAL DIAGNOSES

- Killian-Jamieson diverticulum
  - Opening below cricopharyngeus muscle; protrudes laterally

CLINICAL ISSUES

- Upper esophageal dysphagia
  - Regurgitation and aspiration of undigested food
- Complications
  - **Risk of perforation during endoscopy or placement of nasogastric or feeding tubes**
  - Aspiration pneumonia (30% of cases)
  - Risk of carcinoma (0.3% of cases)
- Treatment: Surgical diverticulectomy or endoscopic repair

DIAGNOSTIC CHECKLIST

- Following repair of Zenker diverticulum, residual outpouching will still be seen in most cases

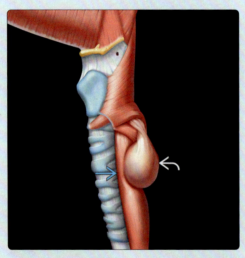
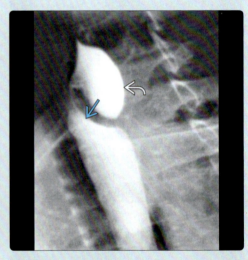

(Left) *Graphic shows a pouch-like herniation ➡ through the Killian dehiscence just above the cricopharyngeal muscle. The distended diverticulum compresses the proximal esophagus ➡.* (Right) *Lateral view of a barium swallow shows a large pouch ➡ arising from the posterior pharyngoesophageal junction, a classic Zenker diverticulum. Note the extrinsic compression ➡ on the proximal esophagus.*

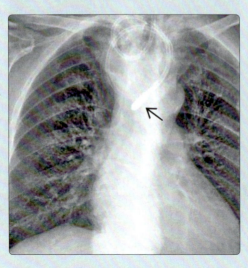
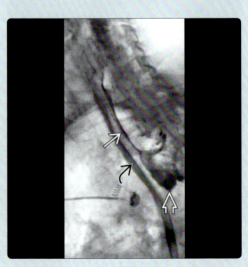

(Left) *Chest film in an elderly woman was obtained following attempted placement of a feeding tube ➡, which is coiled within the mediastinum. A subsequent esophagram confirmed a large Zenker diverticulum.* (Right) *In this elderly man with chest pain following the attempted placement of feeding tube, a film from an esophagram shows a mediastinal collection of gas and contrast medium ➡. The track ➡ runs parallel to the course of the proximal esophagus ➡. A perforated Zenker diverticulum was confirmed.*

KEY FACTS

TERMINOLOGY

- Esophageal saccular protrusion or outpouching; pseudodiverticulum (only mucosal layer)

IMAGING

- Proximal esophagus: Zenker diverticulum
- Mid esophageal pulsion diverticula
  - Barium-filled outpouchings from esophagus
  - Usually smooth, rounded contour and wide neck
  - Diverticula tend to remain filled after most of esophageal barium is emptied due to lack of muscle in wall
  - Single or multiple, of varied sizes
  - Almost all patients have evidence of diffuse esophageal spasm or significant dysmotility
- Distal esophageal (epiphrenic) pulsion diverticula
  - Large, barium-filled sac in epiphrenic area
  - Easily mistaken for hiatal hernia

TOP DIFFERENTIAL DIAGNOSES

- Hiatal hernia (especially type 3 paraesophageal hernia)
  - Look for gastric folds within hernia
- Traction diverticulum
- Esophageal perforation

CLINICAL ISSUES

- Small diverticula: Usually asymptomatic
- Large diverticula: Dysphagia, regurgitation, halitosis
- Complications
  - Perforation, fistula formation, retained foreign body
    - Perforation by feeding tube or endoscope is recognized hazard of pulsion diverticula
  - Squamous cell carcinoma: Rare (~ 1%)
- Treatment: Surgical diverticulectomy (endoscopically)
  - Caution: Patients almost always have some residual diverticulum, which may be mistaken for postoperative leak or recurrence

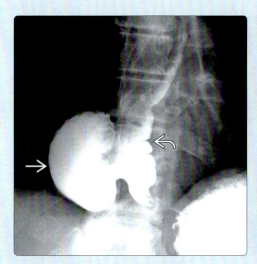
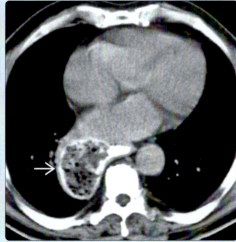

(Left) Spot film from an esophagram in an elderly patient with dysphagia and halitosis shows a large epiphrenic diverticulum ➡ and esophageal dysmotility with tertiary contractions ↗. (Right) Axial NECT in the same patient shows the large epiphrenic diverticulum ➡ containing contrast and retained food. The retained food accounts for the symptom of halitosis.

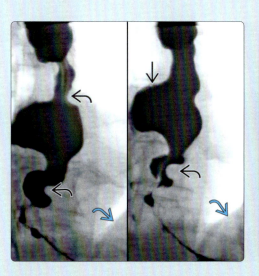
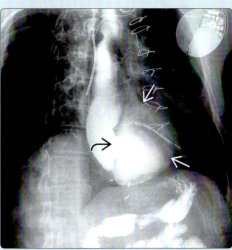

(Left) Two views from an esophagram show deep, nonpropulsive, tertiary contractions ↗ and a pulsion diverticulum ➡. The diaphragm ↗ is noted for reference. Pulsion diverticula are almost always associated with esophageal motility disturbances and become more common with advanced age. (Right) Esophagram shows a large epiphrenic (pulsion) diverticulum ➡ that could be mistaken for a type III paraesophageal hernia. Note the wide mouth ↗ and absence of gastric folds within the diverticulum.

Esophageal Perforation

IMAGING

- Diagnosis depends on high degree of suspicion and recognition of typical clinical features
  - Most are due to esophageal instrumentation or surgery
    - Especially common (4%) after endoscopic mucosal dissections
  - Protocol: Start with **upright chest and abdominal films (radiographs)**
  - Confirmed by **contrast esophagram or CT, which are complementary**
    - **CT with oral and IV contrast material**
- Cervical esophageal perforation (EP)
  - Subcutaneous or interstitial emphysema in neck and mediastinum
- Thoracic EP
  - Consider perforation of Zenker diverticulum
    - Especially following attempted passage of endoscope or feeding tube

- Chest film: Pneumomediastinum, pleural effusion
- EP of intraabdominal segment of distal esophagus
  - Abdominal plain film: Pneumoperitoneum
- EP near GE junction
  - Often due to Boerhaave syndrome (retching, vomiting; increased abdominal pressure)
  - Extravasated contrast from left lateral aspect of distal esophagus into mediastinum, sometimes pleural space, and rarely abdomen (never into abdomen alone)
- CT shows extraesophageal air in almost all cases, fluid and "oral" contrast medium in most cases
- Intramural EP: Extravasated gas and contrast remain within esophageal wall
  - Much better prognosis than for transmural injury
- Esophagography: Technique
  - Nonionic water-soluble contrast media [e.g., iohexol (Omnipaque)] initially, followed with barium if no leak or fistula seen
  - Barium (or CT) may detect small leak not visible initially

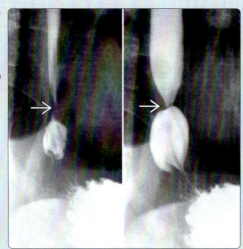
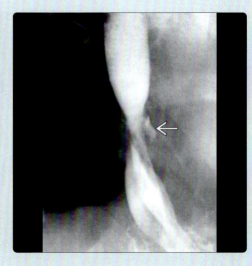

(Left) *Spot films from a barium esophagram reveal a tight stricture ➡️ at the GE junction. Due to concern for Barrett metaplasia or early cancer, an endoscopic biopsy of the lesion was performed following balloon dilation of the stricture.* (Right) *Postbiopsy esophagram in the same patient illustrates a focal intramural contrast collection ➡️ of contrast medium, indicating a localized perforation. These intramural perforations will usually heal spontaneously.*

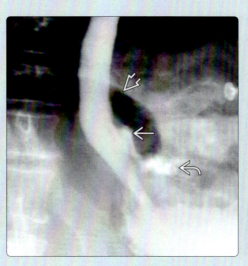
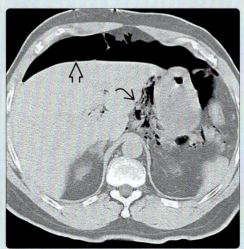

(Left) *Spot film from an esophagram in a man with chest pain following endoscopic removal of an impacted food bolus shows perforation of the distal esophagus ➡️ with extravasation of contrast material ➡️ and gas ➡️ into the upper abdomen and mediastinum.* (Right) *Axial CT in the same patient shows free intraperitoneal gas ➡️ and extraluminal gas ➡️ along the esophagus and proximal stomach. The imaging findings are identical to those seen in Boerhaave syndrome.*

KEY FACTS

IMAGING

- General features: Sudden increase in intraluminal pressure leads to full-thickness esophageal perforation
  - Usually from left side of distal thoracic esophagus
- Chest film
  - Left-side pleural effusion or hydropneumothorax
  - Radiolucent streaks of gas along aorta or in neck
- **Esophagram and CT are both definitive diagnostic tests**
- Esophagography with nonionic, water-soluble contrast agent (e.g., Omnipaque or Isovue), not hyperosmolar agent like Gastrografin (meglumine & sodium diatrizoate)
  - Shows extravasation of ingested or injected (through NG tube) contrast medium
  - From left side of esophagus, just above gastroesophageal junction
  - If initial study with water-soluble contrast medium fails to show leak, examination must be repeated immediately with barium to detect subtle leaks
- CT
  - Extraluminal gas &/or oral contrast medium in lower mediastinum &/or upper abdomen
  - Periesophageal, pleural, pericardial fluid collections

TOP DIFFERENTIAL DIAGNOSES

- Mallory-Weiss syndrome
- Pulsion diverticulum (epiphrenic)
- Iatrogenic (postinstrumentation) injury

CLINICAL ISSUES

- Classic triad: Vomiting, chest pain, subcutaneous emphysema
- Accounts for 15% of total esophageal perforation cases
- Prognosis for large perforation
  - After 24 hours without treatment: Mortality = 70%
  - After immediate surgical drainage: Good
- Treatment: Drains in esophagus, mediastinum, pleural space, &/or abdomen

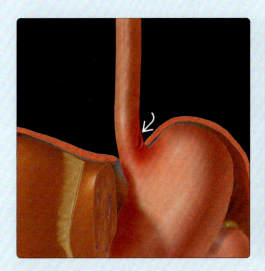

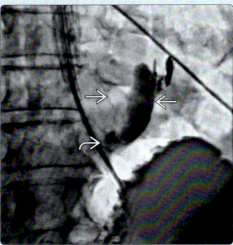

(Left) *Graphic shows a vertically oriented laceration ➦ of the distal esophagus, just above the hiatus and gastroesophageal junction.* (Right) *Film from an esophagram following injection of a water-soluble contrast medium through a nasogastric tube demonstrates a leak of air and contrast medium ➥ from a tear in the left anterior wall of the distal esophagus ➚, a classic appearance for Boerhaave syndrome.*

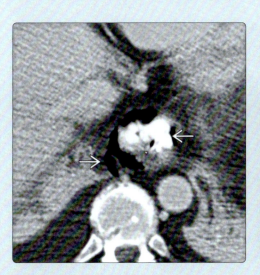

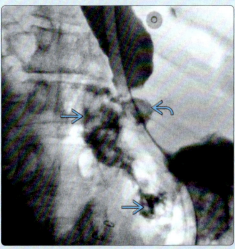

(Left) *Axial CECT in a middle-aged man with severe chest pain after repeated retching shows extraluminal gas and contrast material ➡ surrounding the esophagus in the lower mediastinum and upper abdomen.* (Right) *Film from a fluoroscopic exam in the same patient during injection of water-soluble contrast through a nasogastric tube shows extraluminal contrast in the mediastinum and upper abdomen ➡. The site of the tear is the left anterior wall ➘ of the distal esophagus.*

KEY FACTS

IMAGING

- Many surgical options for surgical excision of esophagus
  - Transthoracic esophagectomy: Usually performed through right intercostal approach (Ivor Lewis procedure)
  - Other options include minimally invasive (laparoscopic; thoracoscopic) procedures
- Stomach is ideal conduit, as it has reliable blood supply and can reach high into thorax or neck for anastomosis
- Perioperative complications
  - Hemorrhage
  - Injury to recurrent laryngeal or vagus nerve (5-10%)
  - Injury to tracheobronchial tree
  - Chylothorax (2-4%)
- Postoperative complications
  - Essentially all patients have some degree of dysphagia, early satiety, and reflux following esophagectomy
  - Anastomotic leak (10-16%)

- Anastomotic stricture (15-25%)
- Diaphragmatic hernia (1-6%)
- Delayed emptying of conduit
  - Causes: Redundant or twisted conduit, mechanical obstruction, functional delay
- Recurrent carcinoma
- Complication rates vary substantially according to experience and skill of surgical team
  - Open surgical procedures: ↑ perioperative morbidity and mortality
  - High (cervical) anastomoses: ↑ incidence of injury to laryngeal or recurrent laryngeal nerve
    - Leaks more easily controlled by drains
- Imaging protocols
  - **Esophagram**: 1st postoperative study is done with water-soluble nonionic contrast agent (e.g., Omnipaque)
  - **CECT**: Complementary to esophagram for strictures, leaks, abscesses, etc.
  - **PET/CT**: Best for detection of recurrent carcinoma

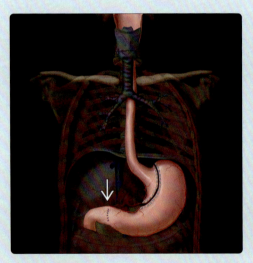
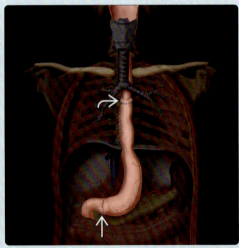

(Left) Graphic illustrates the 1st step in an esophagectomy with gastric interposition. The stomach is divided along its long axis, creating a gastric tube or conduit 5 or 6 cm in diameter, which is pulled up into the chest. This can be done through a right (Ivor Lewis) or left thoracotomy or even through laparoscopic ports. A pyloroplasty ➡ is usually done to facilitate gastric emptying. (Right) Graphic shows the gastric conduit anastomosed to the mid esophagus ➡ and the pyloroplasty ➡.

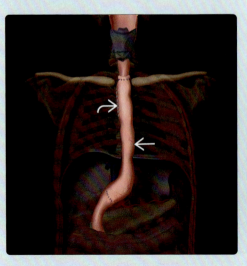
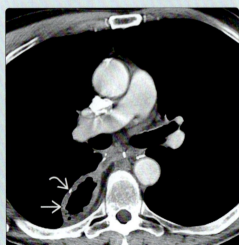

(Left) Graphic shows the gastric conduit ➡ anastomosed to the cervical esophagus. Note the position of the gastric staple line ➡ along the right side of the conduit. (Right) Axial CT shows a mildly dilated, gas-filled gastric conduit ➡ in the paravertebral location. Note the position of the gastric staple line ➡. The conduit is not filled with retained fluid, and there is no evidence of lung injury from reflux.

IMAGING

Surgical Procedures

- Usual indication for surgery
  - Curative or palliative resection of esophageal carcinoma
  - Resection of Barrett esophagus with severe dysplasia
- Many surgical options for surgical excision of portion of esophagus
- Transthoracic esophagectomy
  - Usually performed through right intercostal approach (**Ivor Lewis procedure**)
    - Generally begins with laparotomy for mobilization of stomach, which is then used to create gastric tube/conduit that will replace resected esophagus
    - Pyloroplasty or pyloromyotomy is usually performed to facilitate gastric emptying and to minimize gastroesophageal reflux
    - Esophagus and regional lymph nodes (mediastinum and neck) are resected en bloc
    - Esophagogastric anastomosis is created in thorax, above level of tracheal carina
- Many variations exist
  - e.g., left thoracotomy approach, transhiatal open approach (without thoracotomy), minimally invasive procedures (performed through ports in thorax and abdomen without open incision into either)
  - Experience and preference of surgeon play major role in surgical approach

Complications

- **Perioperative complications**
  - Hemorrhage
  - Injury to recurrent laryngeal or vagus nerve (5-10%)
    - Results in impaired cough and increased risk of aspiration pneumonia
  - Injury to tracheobronchial tree
    - Can result in fistula, aspiration pneumonia
  - Chylothorax (2-4%)
- **Postoperative complications**
  - Essentially all patients have some degree of dysphagia, early satiety, and reflux following esophagectomy
    - Most patients learn to cope with these symptoms, which may decrease over time
    - Mortality
      - 30-day mortality (1-6%)
      - 5-year mortality (70-80%)
  - **Anastomotic leak** (10-16%)
    - Early complication, usually detected within days of surgery
    - Some may respond to conservative management, stent placement, and/or surgical drains left in place
    - May lead to abscess in mediastinum &/or pleural space
  - **Anastomotic stricture** (15-25%)
    - Early or late complication
    - Most due to benign, probably ischemic, stricture
      - Irregular, long stricture raises concern for recurrent malignancy in esophagus or mediastinum
    - Diagnosed by barium esophagram with delayed passage, air-fluid level, dilation of esophagus
    - Usually responds to balloon dilation (may require repeated treatments)
  - **Diaphragmatic hernia** (1-6%)
  - **Delayed emptying of conduit**
    - Very substantial problem leading to significant symptoms in 25-30% of patients
      - Places patient at increased risk of regurgitation and aspiration; impairs nutrition
    - **Redundant conduit** (excess length of gastric tube)
      - Results in horizontal portion of conduit above diaphragm that impairs emptying
      - Looks and behaves like end-stage achalasia
      - Treated by surgical revision (pulling excess conduit back into abdomen)
    - **Mechanical obstruction**
      - At hiatus (too small or tight for gastric conduit): Some degree of narrowing of gastric conduit through diaphragm is expected
    - **Functional delay**
      - Conduit is not very dilated or mechanically obstructed but is slow to empty
      - May be due to vagotomy or injury to vagus nerve
      - Resection of lesser curve of stomach causes loss of gastric pacemaker neurons
  - **Recurrent carcinoma**
    - Majority of patients treated for esophageal carcinoma with esophagectomy will die of recurrent or metastatic disease
      - 5-year mortality exceeds 75% (varies according to aggressiveness of surgeon in operating on patients with early or advanced cancer)

Imaging Recommendations

- Protocol advice
  - Esophagram
    - 1st study is performed with water-soluble contrast medium, preferably nonionic, low-osmolar agent
      - Reduce danger of aspiration pneumonitis from hyperosmolar contrast medium (e.g., Gastrografin)
  - CECT
    - Complementary role to esophagram
    - Protocol: With oral and IV contrast medium
    - Assessment of anastomotic leak, thoracic complications (mediastinitis, pleural effusion, etc.)
  - PET/CT
    - Best test for detection of recurrent carcinoma
      - Usually apparent as FDG-avid sites
    - Uncommonly occurs within esophagus or gastric conduit
    - Pleural or peritoneal seeding are more common
    - Hematogenous metastases to liver, lungs, bones, and other sites

CLINICAL ISSUES

Natural History & Prognosis

- In spite of problems, modern surgical techniques for esophagectomy offer significant improvement in morbidity and mortality compared with prior treatment options

(Left) *Graphic shows a redundant conduit. The horizontal portion of the conduit contributes to the impaired gastric emptying. Note that the point of narrowing is at the diaphragm* ➡️*, not the pylorus, which has been widened by pyloroplasty* ➡️*.* (Right) *Esophagram shows kinking of the redundant conduit* ➡️ *above the diaphragm* ➡️*. The conduit is dilated with an air-fluid level* ➡️*, indicating partial obstruction. The conduit was pulled down into the abdomen at revision laparoscopy with resolution of symptoms.*

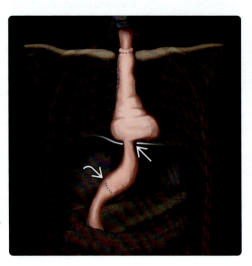
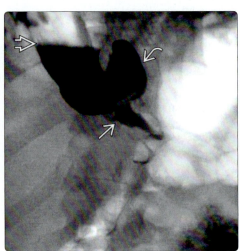

(Left) *Axial CECT in a 65-year-old man post esophagectomy shows the fluid-distended gastric conduit* ➡️ *and indirect evidence of severe aspiration pneumonia and pleural effusion. Note bilateral pleural effusions and lung consolidation* ➡️*.* (Right) *Axial CECT in the same patient shows impaired emptying and fluid distention of the gastric conduit* ➡️ *as well as severe lung disease and pleural effusions.*

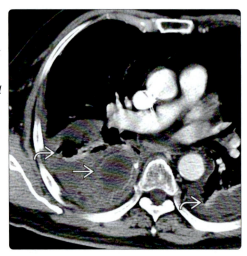
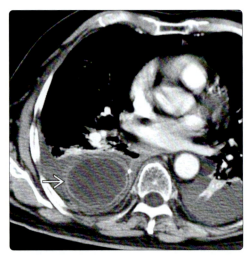

(Left) *Upright film from an esophagram in a patient with obstruction shows a dilated conduit* ➡️ *with air-fluid-barium levels* ➡️*. The stomach is narrowed as it traverses the diaphragm* ➡️*, but the pyloroplasty* ➡️ *is neither the site nor the cause of the delayed emptying.* (Right) *Esophagram film of a redundant conduit with delayed emptying shows marked distention of the gastric conduit* ➡️ *with a horizontal component above the diaphragmatic hiatus. Note the similarity to end-stage achalasia.*

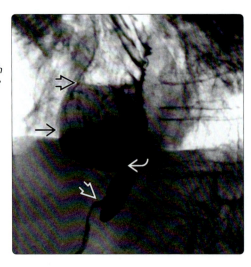
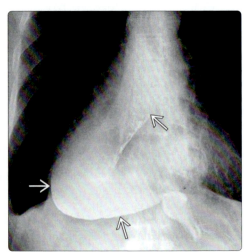

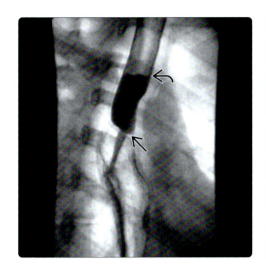

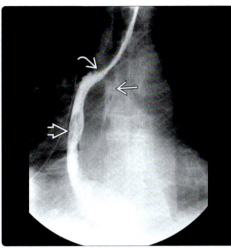

(Left) *Spot film from an esophagram shows a tight stricture ⮌ at the esophagogastric anastomosis with delayed emptying of the esophagus, evident as an air-fluid level ⮕. The stricture would not allow passage of a 13-mm barium pill (not shown).* (Right) *Spot film from an esophagram in a 70-year-old man with fever and chest pain 3 days after partial esophagectomy shows the anastomosis ⮕ between the esophagus and the gastric conduit ⮕. There is an anastomotic leak ⮕ into the mediastinum.*

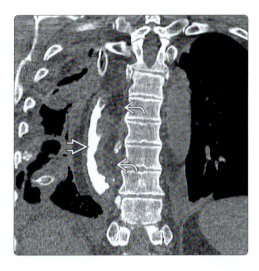

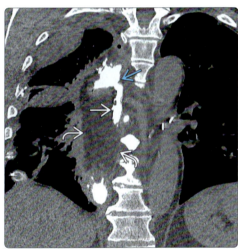

(Left) *Coronal reformatted NECT in a patient with fever following esophagectomy shows oral contrast medium within the gastric conduit ⮕. The conduit is surrounded by complex fluid ⮕.* (Right) *Coronal NECT section in the same patient shows contrast extravasation ⮕ from the esophagogastric anastomosis ⮕ into the mediastinum, accounting for the mediastinal abscess ⮕ (complex fluid collection).*

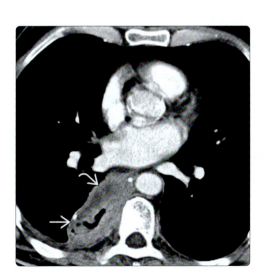

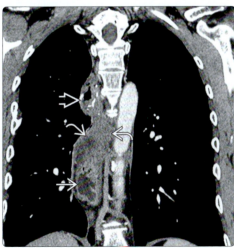

(Left) *Axial CECT 18 months after esophagectomy shows the nondilated gastric conduit ⮕. There is a large soft tissue mass ⮕ abutting the conduit and extending into the mediastinum in this patient with a recurrent tumor.* (Right) *Coronal CECT reformation in the same patient shows the gastric conduit ⮕ and extensive mediastinal mass effect ⮕, representing recurrent esophageal tumor. A portion of the anastomotic staple line ⮕ is seen.*

TERMINOLOGY

- **Nissen fundoplication (FDP)**: Complete (360°) FDP
- **Dor FDP**: Partial anterior hemi-valve
- **Toupet FDP**: Partial (270°) FDP, posterior side
- **Belsey Mark IV** repair: 240° FDP wrap around left lateral aspect
- **Nissen-Collis** procedure creates "neoesophagus"
  - GE junction (at B ring) will be above diaphragm; intact wrap around proximal stomach (neoesophagus) will be below diaphragm

IMAGING

- Preoperative: Identify "short esophagus," hiatal hernia, ulceration, strictures, and dysmotility
- Wrap complications
  - Tight FDP wrap (fixed narrowing and delayed emptying of esophagus)
  - Complete disruption of FDP sutures (recurrent hernia and reflux)

- Partial disruption of FDP sutures (1 or more loose-looking outpouchings of wrap)
  - Intact wrap may slide downward over stomach; hourglass configuration of stomach
  - Intrathoracic migration of wrap upward through hiatus
- Fluid collections in abdomen or mediastinum
  - Herniated abdominal fluid, lymph, hematoma, infection ± leak, abscess
- Fluoroscopic esophagram soon after surgery is mandatory
  - Provides structural information, anatomical abnormalities
  - Wrap complications, leaks, persistence of reflux
- CT for severe abdominal or chest pain, suspected visceral injury, or abscess

DIAGNOSTIC CHECKLIST

- Postoperative fluoroscopic evaluation should be used liberally or even routinely
- CT for suspected leak or bleeding

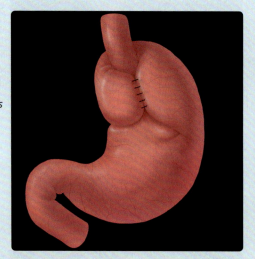
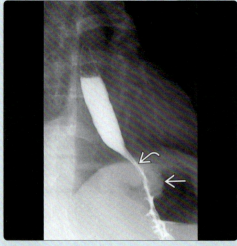

(Left) Graphic shows a Nissen fundoplication (FDP) with the gastric fundus wrapped completely (360°) around the gastroesophageal junction. (Right) Upright spot film from an esophagram performed soon after a Nissen FDP shows an intact wrap ➡ in its expected subdiaphragmatic location as a filling defect within the air-filled fundus. The distal 3 cm of the esophageal lumen is compressed ➡ as it passes through the wrap.

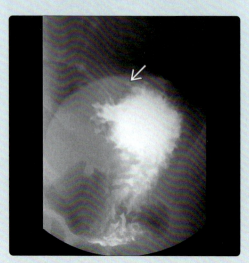
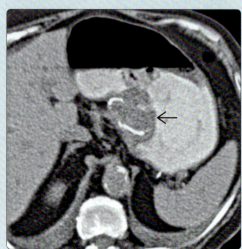

(Left) A supine film from the same study shows the intact wrap ➡ as a filling defect with the barium pool in the fundus. (Right) Axial NECT shows an intact FDP as a soft tissue density mass ➡ within the gastric fundus. The metallic staple line is evident within the wrap. The mass effect of the wrap tends to decrease with time following surgery.

TERMINOLOGY

Abbreviations
- Fundoplication (FDP)

Definitions
- Nissen FDP: Complete (360°) FDP
  o Gastric fundus wrapped 360° posteriorly around intraabdominal esophagus to create antireflux valve
  o Concomitant hiatal hernia (HH) is reduced; diaphragmatic esophageal hiatus sutured
- Dor FDP: Partial (180-200°) anterior to right wrap
  o Anterior hemi-valve
- Toupet FDP: Partial (270°) FDP
  o Posterior hemi-valve created; often from thoracoscopic approach
- Belsey Mark IV repair: Open surgical; 240° FDP wrap around left lateral aspect of distal esophagus
  o Fundus sutured to intraabdominal esophagus; acute esophagogastric junction angle (angle of His)
  o Can also be performed via minimally invasive techniques

IMAGING

Radiographic Findings
- **Fluoroscopy**
- **Preoperative evaluation is critical to identify**
  o Presence, type, and size of HH
  o Irreducible HH or "short esophagus"
    - Stomach is pulled taut into chest; does not return to abdomen on upright positioning
    - May require Collis gastroplasty (effectively lengthening esophagus by creating gastric tube)
    - Wrap goes around "neoesophagus" in abdomen = Nissen-Collis FDP
  o Also evaluate for reflux and esophageal motility
    - FDP is relatively contraindicated in patients with severe dysmotility
- Normal postoperative appearance
  o **Nissen FDP wrap**: Well-defined mass in gastric fundus; smooth contour and surface
    - Distal esophagus tapers smoothly through center of symmetric compression by wrap
    - Tapered segment 2-3 cm long
    - Pseudotumoral defect within gastric fundus = wrap
      □ Defect more pronounced for complete wrap of Nissen than partial wrap of Toupet, Belsey
  o **Toupet and Dor**: Partial FDP
    - Barium may fill portions of wrap
      □ Do not mistake for leak or dehiscence
      □ Distal esophagus should still be "squeezed"
  o **Nissen-Collis** procedure
    - Gastroesophageal (GE) junction (at B ring) will be above diaphragm
    - Intact wrap around proximal stomach (neoesophagus) will be below diaphragm
  o Belsey Mark IV repair
    - Wrap produces smaller defect than Nissen FDP
    - 2 distinct angles form as esophagus passes FDP
- **Wrap complications**
  o Tight FDP wrap
    - Fixed narrowing of distal esophagus with delayed emptying
    - May also see gas distention of stomach (gas bloat syndrome)
  o Complete disruption (dehiscence) of FDP sutures
    - Findings may resemble those of normal patient who has had no surgery
    - Recurrent HH and GE reflux
  o Partial disruption of FDP sutures
    - Partially intact wrap; does not squeeze distal esophagus
  o Slipped Nissen
    - Intact wrap may slide downward over stomach
    - Hourglass configuration of stomach caused by wrap pinching stomach
  o Intrathoracic migration of wrap
    - Intact FDP wrap herniates partially or entirely through esophageal hiatus of diaphragm
- **Nonwrap complications**
  o Leaks, fistula
    - Detected by extravasation of oral contrast medium
    - Uncommon since neither esophageal nor gastric wall is usually cut

CT Findings
- Wrap: Soft tissue density mass surrounding intraabdominal esophagus
  o Extending caudally about 3 cm
- Retraction injury to adjacent organs
  o May result in liver or splenic laceration
  o Right ventricular laceration; cardiac tamponade
  o Bleeding and hematoma in gastric wall or in peritoneal spaces adjacent to stomach and duodenum
- Fluid collections in abdomen or mediastinum
  o Ascites, disrupted lymphatic drainage, hematoma, infection ± leak, abscess
  o Drainage under CT guidance; may obviate reoperation
- Hollow visceral perforation
  o Extraluminal contrast, free air in chest or abdomen
- Superior mesenteric vein and portal vein thrombosis
  o Rare; ~ 2 weeks after laparoscopic FDP

Imaging Recommendations
- Best imaging tool
  o Fluoroscopic esophagram
    - Structural or morphological abnormalities
    - Wrap complications, leaks, persistence of reflux
  o CT for severe abdominal or chest pain, suspected visceral injury, or abscess
- Protocol advice
  o Perform initial postoperative esophagram with water-soluble contrast medium
  o Film initially in standing oblique positions
  o Include supine films to exclude leak or reflux

(Left) *A semirecumbent film from an esophagram shows an intact but "tight" FDP with dilation of the esophagus ⇒ and delayed emptying. The undersurface of the wrap is seen as a filling defect ⇒ within the gastric fundus. The distal esophageal lumen ⇒ is tightly compressed.* (Right) *Spot film from an esophagram shows intrathoracic migration of an intact Toupet FDP. Contrast fills the portions of the fundus ⇒ that constitute the wrap, but the compression of the distal esophagus ⇒ is maintained. The entire wrap lies above the diaphragm ⇒.*

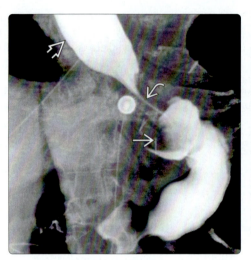
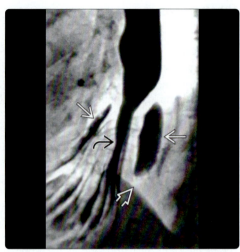

(Left) *Spot film from an esophagram shows extravasation of contrast medium ⇒ and gas ⇒ into the mediastinum, indicating perforation of the esophagus or the wrap.* (Right) *Axial CT in the same case shows large collections of gas and fluid in the mediastinum ⇒ due to perforation of the Nissen FDP.*

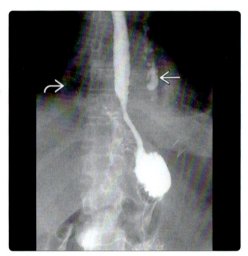
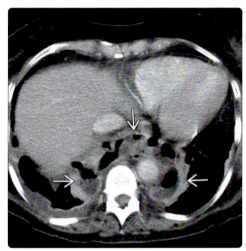

(Left) *This elderly patient recently had repair of a large paraesophageal hernia and FDP. A spot film from an esophagram demonstrates extravasation of contrast medium ⇒ into the mediastinum from the distal esophagus. Very little contrast reaches the stomach.* (Right) *NECT in the same case shows a large mediastinal fluid collection of near-water attenuation ⇒ and residual herniation of the stomach ⇒. The dense collection of extraluminal contrast ⇒ indicates a leak from near the operative site.*

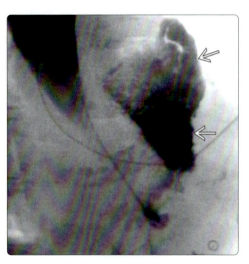
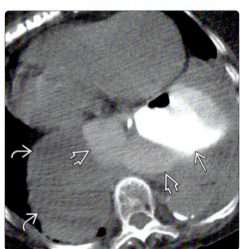

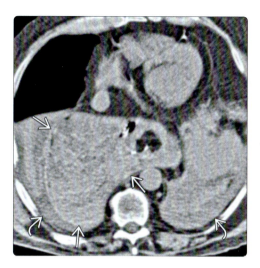
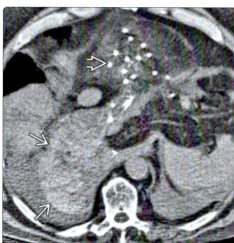

(Left) This elderly man had a falling hematocrit following surgical repair of a large paraesophageal hernia. Axial NECT shows a large mediastinal hematoma ➡ in the space formerly occupied by the herniated stomach. Hemothorax is also evident ➡. (Right) In the same patient, metallic anchors ➡ are present from the mesh repair of the large hernia, and more mediastinal hematoma is seen ➡. This hematoma should not be mistaken for leak of contrast medium.

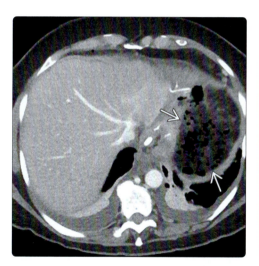
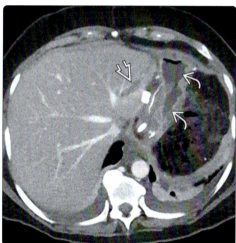

(Left) This 67-year-old man had FDP performed by an inexperienced surgeon. A splenic laceration occurred during surgery leading to splenectomy. A postoperative CT shows gas and fluid in the splenectomy bed ➡. (Right) A more caudal CT section shows a loculated collection of gas and fluid ➡, subsequently confirmed to be due to a leak from the operative site. A small liver laceration ➡ is also seen.

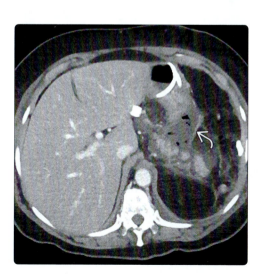
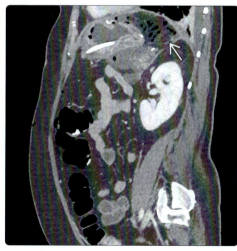

(Left) A more caudal CT section in the same patient shows more of the extravasated gas and fluid ➡ from the FDP site. (Right) Sagittal reformatted CT in the same patient shows the left subphrenic collection of extravasated gas and fluid ➡ near the site of the FDP.

IMAGING

- Types include leiomyoma, gastrointestinal stromal tumor (GIST), granular cell, lipoma, hemangioma, hamartoma
- Fluoroscopic-guided barium studies
  - Discrete mass; solitary (most common) or multiple
  - Round or ovoid filling defects sharply outlined by barium on each side (en face view)
  - Narrowed (tangential view) or stretched and widened (en face view) esophageal lumen
  - Smooth surface lesion, with upper and lower borders of lesion forming right or slightly obtuse angles with adjacent esophageal wall (profile view)
  - Overlying mucosa may ulcerate
- Leiomyoma: ± amorphous or punctate calcifications
- Esophageal GIST
  - May be large mass
  - May ulcerate with gas ± contrast medium entering cavity
- CT: Discrete mass in wall; no signs of invasion or metastases
  - Helps distinguish lipoma (fat density) and other mediastinal masses (e.g., mediastinal cyst)

TOP DIFFERENTIAL DIAGNOSES

- Mediastinal tumor
- Normal mediastinal structures
- Esophageal carcinoma
- Foreign body

CLINICAL ISSUES

- Asymptomatic: No treatment
- Large, symptomatic lesions: Enucleation or esophageal resection with gastric interposition

DIAGNOSTIC CHECKLIST

- Most intramural masses are benign (unlike gastric tumors)
- Leiomyomas are much more common than GIST in esophagus (but not in stomach)
- **Intramural masses may not be evident on endoscopy**

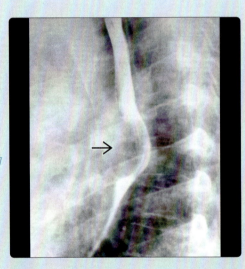
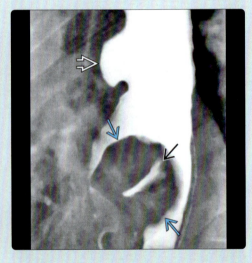

(Left) *Film from a barium esophagram demonstrates a mass ⇨ causing eccentric narrowing of the distal lumen. The mass forms obtuse angles with the wall, and the esophageal folds and mucosa are intact. A leiomyoma was enucleated endoscopically.* (Right) *Single-contrast esophagram shows an en face view of an intramural mass ⇨ in the distal esophagus with central ulceration ⇨ due to leiomyoma. The traction diverticulum ⇨ is an incidental finding.*

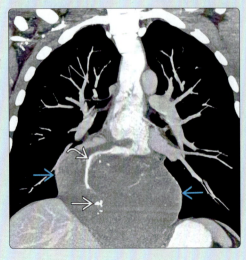
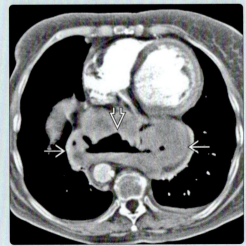

(Left) *Coronal CECT in a 24-year-old man shows a huge, soft tissue-density mass ⇨ that envelops and displaces the distal esophagus ⇨. Small foci of calcification ⇨ are noted. The mass was resected and proved to be a benign leiomyoma arising from the esophageal wall.* (Right) *Axial CECT in a 73-year-old woman shows a huge esophageal mass ⇨ with a large central ulceration ⇨ that contains gas due to communication with the esophageal lumen. The central cavitation is typical of a GIST; the esophagus is an unusual site.*

Fibrovascular Polyp

TERMINOLOGY

- Rare, benign, tumor-like lesion of esophagus
  - Originates within cervical esophageal wall but presents as intraluminal polyp or mass

IMAGING

- Fluoroscopic barium esophagography
  - Smooth, expansile, sausage-shaped, and intraluminal
  - Cervical esophageal mass extending distally to fill esophageal lumen
- CT: Varied density based on content
  - Fat density: Abundance of adipose tissue
  - Heterogeneous: Mixture of fat, soft tissue, focal calcifications

TOP DIFFERENTIAL DIAGNOSES

- Esophageal carcinoma
  - May present as large, polypoid intraluminal mass
  - Margins are irregular and more lobulated

- Esophageal submucosal mesenchymal tumors
  - Leiomyoma and lipoma are most common
  - Rarely as large or long as fibrovascular polyps

PATHOLOGY

- Giant, smooth or lobulated, expansile polyp with discrete pedicle attached to cervical esophagus
- Varying amounts of fibrovascular and adipose tissue covered by normal squamous epithelium

CLINICAL ISSUES

- Uncommonly, regurgitation of mass into pharynx or mouth
  - May cause laryngeal occlusion, asphyxia, and sudden death
- Fibrovascular polyps may bleed
- Malignant degeneration extremely rare
- Treatment
  - Small fibrovascular polyps: Endoscopic resection
  - Gigantic fibrovascular polyps: Surgical resection

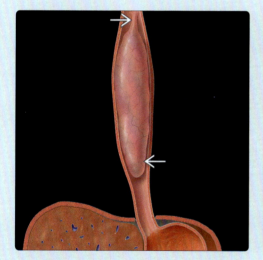

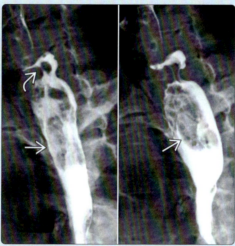

(Left) Graphic shows a long, smooth, sausage-like mass ➡ arising from the proximal esophageal wall, filling most of the esophageal lumen. (Right) Spot films from a barium esophagram demonstrate a large, cylindrical mass ➡ within the esophagus. The mass originates from a pedicle ➡ near the cricopharyngeal level. The mass is so long and bulky that it might be mistaken for an air bubble or debris within the esophagus.

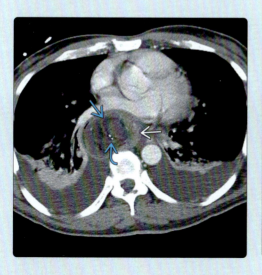

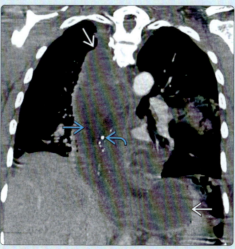

(Left) In this man with chronic dysphagia, axial CT shows massive distention of the esophagus by a tumor ➡ having soft tissue, fat ➡, and calcified components ➡, diagnostic of a fibrovascular polyp. (Right) In the same patient, the coronal reformatted CT shows the mass ➡ that extended from the proximal esophagus into the stomach. Again seen are the calcifications ➡ and fat components ➡ of this fibrovascular polyp.

Esophagus

IMAGING

- **Barium esophagram**
  - May provide 1st evidence of cancer in patient with solid food dysphagia
  - Luminal constriction (stricture) with nodular or ulcerated mucosa
- **CT with IV contrast**
  - Main role in evaluation of known advanced cancer; pre and post therapy
  - May show invasion of tracheobronchial tree, aorta, or other signs of nonresectability
  - Mediastinal and abdominal lymphadenopathy
  - Liver and other metastases
- **PET/CT**
  - Best imaging tool for detecting regional and distal metastases
  - Pre and post therapy
- **Endoscopic ultrasonography**

- Best technique for determining locoregional extent of tumor
- Depth of invasion and mediastinal adenopathy
- **Upper endoscopy**
  - Primary tool for diagnosis

CLINICAL ISSUES

- Squamous cell carcinoma (SCC)
  - 2 major risk factors in USA: Tobacco and alcohol abuse
- Adenocarcinoma
  - Increasing in prevalence relative to SCC, especially in industrialized countries
    - 7x increase over past 20 years
  - Risk factors: Barrett metaplasia; gastroesophageal reflux disease; obesity
- Treatment
  - Surgery, radiation (pre- and postoperative radiation)
  - Esophagectomy with gastric interposition is most common

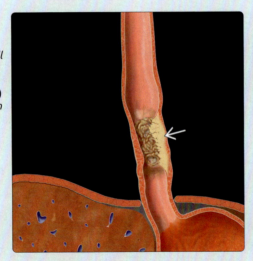
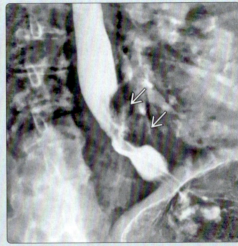

(Left) *Graphic shows a sessile polypoid mass* ➡ *with an irregular surface that infiltrates the esophageal wall and narrows the lumen, a typical appearance of an esophageal carcinoma.* (Right) *Spot film from an esophagram shows a polypoid mass* ➡ *of the distal esophagus with an irregular surface and luminal narrowing. This was a squamous cell carcinoma.*

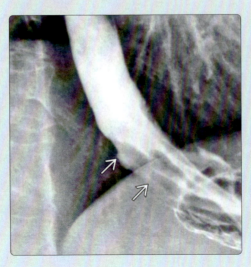
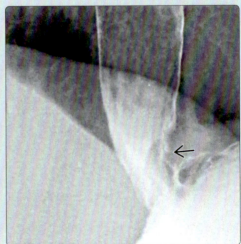

(Left) *The initial 2 films from a barium esophagram (not shown) looked normal. However, a repeat film, with emphasis on suspended deep inspiration and Valsalva maneuver, demonstrates nodular thickened folds* ➡ *in the distal esophagus.* (Right) *Another spot film in the same patient with deep inspiration and Valsalva demonstrates nodular thickened folds* ➡ *and luminal narrowing in the distal esophagus. Biopsy confirmed adenocarcinoma.*

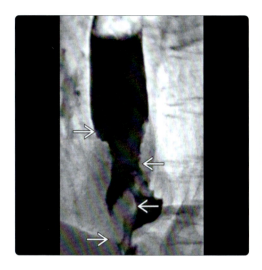
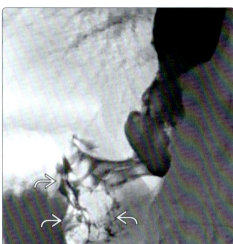

(Left) *Upright spot film from an esophagram shows an "apple core" constricting lesion ➡ of the distal esophagus. There is an abrupt transition, or shoulder, at the proximal end of the tumor as it abuts the normal esophagus. The mucosa through the tumor is destroyed with nodular contours.* (Right) *Esophagram in the same patient shows nodular thickened folds ➡ in the gastric cardia as well, strongly suggesting gastric extension of the tumor. Alternatively, gastric carcinoma may invade the distal esophagus.*

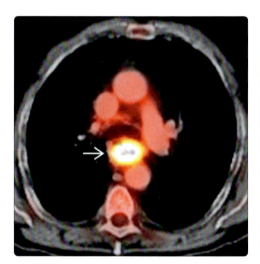
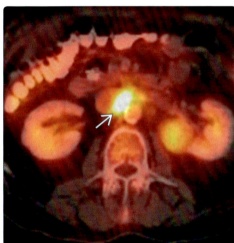

(Left) *A "fused" (combined) axial PET/CT shows intense FDG uptake within a mass ➡ that encircles the midesophagus, a primary esophageal cancer.* (Right) *Axial, more caudal PET/CT section in the same patient shows intense FDG uptake within an aortocaval node ➡, indicating metastases to the upper abdomen. PET/CT is the most effective means of evaluation for the total extent of disease and often affects management decisions.*

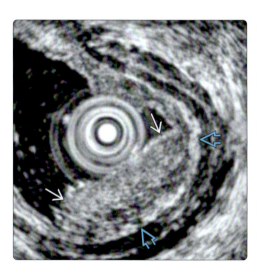
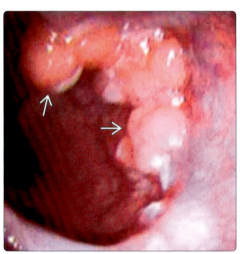

(Left) *Endoscopic ultrasound (EUS) demonstrates an intraluminal mass ➡ that does not penetrate the muscularis propria ➡ (T1a adenocarcinoma). EUS is the best method for determining the depth of tumor invasion.* (Right) *Endoscopic photograph in the same patient shows an irregular polypoid mass ➡ in the distal esophagus. This adenocarcinoma was treated by esophagectomy with gastric interposition in the chest.*

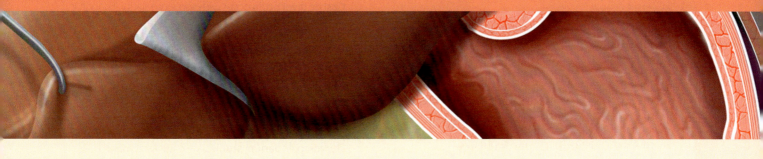

SECTION 5
Stomach and Duodenum

Gastric Anatomy and Terminology

The stomach is the alimentary reservoir for the mixing, grinding, and enzymatic digestion of food. It is divided into the cardia, fundus, body, antrum, and pylorus; each with its own specific function.

The cardia is the portion of the stomach surrounding the esophageal orifice and the site where the lesser and greater curvatures meet. The fundus is the most cephalic part of the stomach and touches the left hemidiaphragm. The body is the main portion of the stomach and the principal site of acid production. The antrum is the prepyloric part of the stomach. The pylorus is the sphincter that controls emptying into the duodenum; it is formed by thickening of the middle layer of smooth muscle and a thin fibrous septum.

Mural Anatomy

The gastric wall consists of 3 layers of smooth muscle; the outermost is the longitudinal muscle layer, the middle is the circular muscle layer, and the inner is the oblique muscle layer. The middle circular muscle layer is the thickest component.

Gastric rugae are the redundant folds of gastric mucosa that are most prominent when the stomach is collapsed. The reservoir and mixing functions of the stomach demand a thick, expansile, muscular vessel, which characterizes gastric morphology.

Gastric mucosa is composed of columnar epithelium. Gastric glands vary in prevalence in different parts of the stomach. These produce mucin (to line and protect the gastric mucosa), pepsinogen (a precursor to pepsin needed for digestion), and hydrochloric acid (which activates digestive enzymes and assists with the breakdown of food).

Other Anatomical Considerations

The stomach has a rich vascular supply with the lesser curve supplied by branches of the left and right gastric arteries that run within the lesser omentum. Numerous collateral pathways arising from branches of the celiac and superior mesenteric arteries make the stomach and duodenum resistant to ischemic injury as well as difficult to control by catheter embolotherapy in the setting of acute upper GI hemorrhage.

The greater curve is supplied by the left and right gastroomental (gastroepiploic) arteries that run within the greater omentum. In planning for partial gastrectomy, surgeons try to ensure an intact arterial supply from at least 1 of its 2 sources, preferably the gastroepiploic vessels.

Venous drainage is into the portal system through the left and right gastric veins and via the splenic and superior mesenteric veins. All of these have **collateral connections** that become important in the event of venous occlusion or portal hypertension, when **gastric varices** may become prominent and hemorrhage.

Lymphatic drainage follows the course of the arteries, then to celiac nodes via efferent lymphatic ducts. Inspection of these nodal groups is important in staging gastric malignancies. The rich lymphatic and venous drainage of the stomach accounts for the high prevalence of metastatic disease at the time of diagnosis of gastric carcinoma.

The vagus nerve carries parasympathetic stimuli to the stomach, stimulating peristalsis and acid secretion. Surgical interruption of the vagus nerve has been used extensively to treat acid-peptic disease, especially in the era before effective medical control. In order to prevent gastric retention, a vagotomy must be accompanied by some form of gastric emptying procedure, such as partial gastrectomy or pyloroplasty.

Gastric diverticula occur with some regularity (though in < 1%) and are likely to be mistaken for more significant abnormalities. These congenital, true diverticula usually arise near the gastric cardia. They often have only a thin connection to the stomach, and it may not be apparent on CT or MR. A completely fluid-filled diverticulum is often mistaken for an adrenal mass, while one containing both gas and fluid might be misdiagnosed as an abscess.

Imaging Issues

Fluoroscopic **barium studies** are complementary to endoscopy and CT for most cases of dyspepsia and abdominal pain, and they are superior to endoscopy in the evaluation of functional abnormalities (e.g., reflux, or gastroparesis).

In many radiology practices, the main role of barium studies is in the pre-/postoperative evaluation of patients undergoing gastric surgical procedures, such as **esophagectomy with gastric pull-through, fundoplication** for gastroesophageal reflux disease, partial gastrectomy for cancer, or some form of **bariatric surgery**. Radiologists and other physicians must become familiar with the range of expected alterations following various surgical procedures as well as the numerous complications that may result. Since clinical signs and symptoms are often lacking or nonspecific in these patients, radiologists are often the 1st to recognize adverse results of surgery.

CT has become the principal means of staging **primary and metastatic tumors involving the stomach**. CT is complementary to upper GI series and endoscopy in diagnosing **gastritis** and **gastric ulcers**, especially with complications, such as perforation. CT has a primary role in diagnosing inflammatory processes that affect the stomach secondarily, such as pancreatitis.

Endoscopy is the most accurate means of diagnosing gastric carcinoma and primary inflammatory conditions, such as gastritis. However, endoscopy may fail to detect submucosal gastric masses, such as **lymphoma** or **GI stromal tumors (GIST)**, in which the overlying mucosa is often normal.

Approach Thick-Walled Stomach

The presence of "**thickened folds**" on an upper GI series is a finding of limited value in isolation because so many intrinsic and extrinsic processes, inflammatory or malignant, may result in this finding.

CT findings help to narrow the differential diagnosis by allowing characterization of the nature of the wall thickening. As with the small bowel and colon, inflammatory processes (such as **gastritis**) result in submucosal edema, which appears as a layer of hypodensity (near water attenuation) between the mucosa and serosa. Soft tissue density within the wall is more likely to be of neoplastic origin.

CT may also allow distinction among the various gastric neoplasms. **Primary carcinoma** usually produces nodular, irregular wall thickening with limited distensibility, often with evidence of metastatic spread to the liver, regional nodes, ± omentum.

Gastric lymphoma often causes massive nodular thickening of folds but uncommonly limits distensibility or causes gastric outlet obstruction. Lymphoma and gastric metastases are often accompanied by extragastric sites of tumor.

A **gastric** GIST usually appears as a submucosal, mostly exophytic gastric mass. While the mucosa is intact over a small GIST, large lesions often have ulcerated mucosa, which, along with central cavitation of the tumor, may be evident as a large perigastric mass containing gas, fluid, and enteric contrast medium.

The "global view" allowed by CT often provides other clues to the etiology of thickened folds, such as evidence of pancreatitis, the presence of a pancreatic neuroendocrine tumors in Zollinger-Ellison syndrome, or cirrhosis and signs of portal hypertension in a patient with gastric varices.

Gastric Distention

Persistent, symptomatic gastric distention may result from gastric outlet obstruction, postoperative complications, gastroparesis, and other causes. CT, nuclear scintigraphy (gastric emptying test), and the upper GI series can play an important role in distinguishing among these etiologies.

Differential Diagnosis

Gastric Mass Lesions
Common
- Gastric carcinoma
- Hyperplastic or adenomatous polyps
- Bezoar (mimic)
- Perigastric mass (mimic): Splenomegaly, renal cell carcinoma, hepatocellular carcinoma, splenosis
- Gastric varices

Less Common
- Gastric metastases and lymphoma
- Mesenchymal tumors (e.g., GIST, lipoma, neural tumor)
- Polyposis syndromes
- Ectopic pancreatic tissue
- Hematoma
- Duplication cyst

Thickened Gastric Folds
Common
- Gastritis
- Gastric ulcer
- Portal hypertension, varices
- Gastric carcinoma
- Pancreatitis, acute; pancreatic pseudocyst

Less Common
- Gastric metastases and lymphoma
- Ménétrier disease
- Zollinger-Ellison syndrome
- Caustic gastroduodenal injury
- Crohn's disease

Rare but Important
- Tuberculosis
- Radiation gastritis
- Amyloidosis
- Eosinophilic gastritis
- Chemotherapy-induced gastritis
- Sarcoidosis

Gastric Distention or Outlet Obstruction
Common
- Gastric or duodenal ulcer
- Gastric carcinoma
- Gastroparesis
- Postoperative state (e.g., fundoplication; vagotomy)
- Gastric volvulus
- Hypertrophic pyloric stenosis
- Gastric ileus

Less Common
- Pancreatitis, acute or chronic
- Metastases and lymphoma
- Duodenal mass or stricture (carcinoma, metastases, annular pancreas)
- Gastric polyps
- Superior mesenteric artery syndrome

Rare but Important
- Infiltrating lesions: Crohn's disease, sarcoidosis, tuberculosis, etc.

Epigastric Pain
Common
- Functional dyspepsia
- Reflux esophagitis
- Duodenal or gastric ulcer
- Gastritis
- Cholecystitis or choledocholithiasis
- Cholangitis (ascending primary sclerosing, recurrent pyogenic)
- Hepatitis
- Pancreatitis, acute or chronic
- Coronary artery disease
- Gastric carcinoma
- Pancreatic tumors
- Sphincter of Oddi dysfunction
- Psychosomatic disorders
- Hiatal or ventral hernia

Less Common
- Crohn's disease
- Other gastric causes: Ménétrier disease, caustic gastroduodenal injury, GIST, gastric metastases, and lymphoma
- Other hepatic causes: Neoplasms, infections, inflammation, ischemia
- Other pancreatic causes: Pancreas divisum
- Other duodenal causes: Carcinoma, metastases, and lymphoma
- Musculoskeletal etiologies

Selected References

1. Foley KG et al: N-staging of oesophageal and junctional carcinoma: is there still a role for EUS in patients staged N0 at PET/CT? Clin Radiol. 69(9):959-64, 2014
2. Yoshikawa T et al: Accuracy of CT staging of locally advanced gastric cancer after neoadjuvant chemotherapy: cohort evaluation within a randomized phase II study. Ann Surg Oncol. 21 Suppl 3:S385-9, 2014
3. Ba-Ssalamah A et al: Texture-based classification of different gastric tumors at contrast-enhanced CT. Eur J Radiol. 82(10):e537-43, 2013
4. Yi JH et al: 18F-FDG uptake and its clinical relevance in primary gastric lymphoma. Hematol Oncol. 28(2):57-61, 2010
5. Noguera JJ et al: Gastric diverticulum mimicking cystic lesion in left adrenal gland. Urology. 73(5):997-8, 2009
6. Shiotani A et al: The preventive factors for aspirin-induced peptic ulcer: aspirin ulcer and corpus atrophy. J Gastroenterol. 44(7):717-25, 2009
7. Chen BB et al: Preoperative diagnosis of gastric tumors by three-dimensional multidetector row ct and double contrast barium meal study: correlation with surgical and histologic results. J Formos Med Assoc. 106(11):943-52, 2007
8. Chen CY et al: Gastric cancer: preoperative local staging with 3D multi-detector row CT–correlation with surgical and histopathologic results. Radiology. 242(2):472-82, 2007

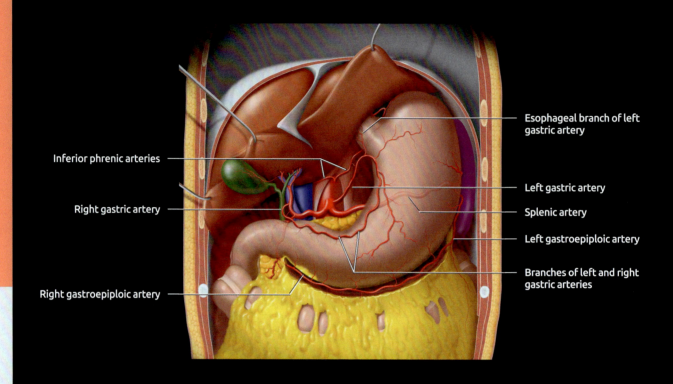

Inferior phrenic arteries

Right gastric artery

Right gastroepiploic artery

Esophageal branch of left gastric artery

Left gastric artery

Splenic artery

Left gastroepiploic artery

Branches of left and right gastric arteries

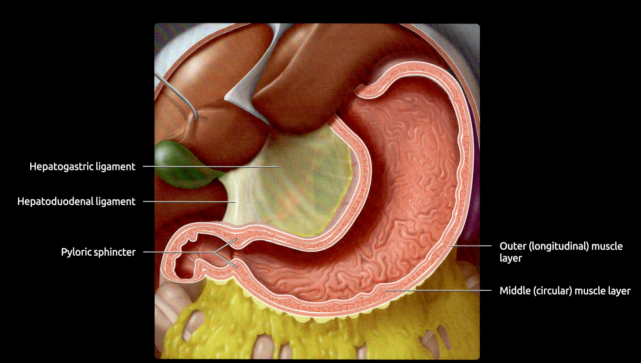

Hepatogastric ligament

Hepatoduodenal ligament

Pyloric sphincter

Outer (longitudinal) muscle layer

Middle (circular) muscle layer

(Top) *In "conventional" arterial anatomy of the stomach and duodenum (present in only 50% of the population), the left gastric artery arises from the celiac trunk and supplies the lesser curvature and anastomoses with the right gastric artery, a branch of the proper hepatic artery. The greater curvature of the stomach is supplied by anastomosing branches of the gastroepiploic arteries with the left arising from the splenic artery.* **(Bottom)** *The lesser omentum extends from the stomach to the porta hepatis and can be divided into the broader, thinner hepatogastric ligament and the thicker hepatoduodenal ligament. Note the layers of gastric muscle with the middle circular layer being the thickest.*

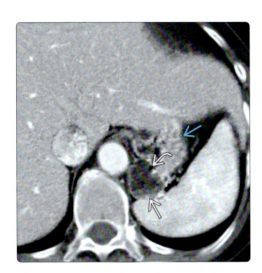

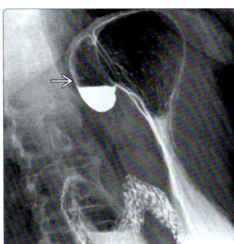

(Left) Axial CECT shows a near water density left upper quadrant mass ➡ that might be mistaken for an adrenal adenoma or other lesion. Its contiguity with the stomach ⇨ and a tiny bubble of gas ➡ suggest the correct etiology of gastric diverticulum. (Right) An upright film from an upper GI series in the same patient shows the juxtacardiac diverticulum ➡ with an air-fluid level.

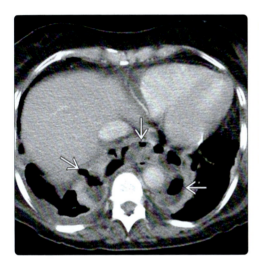

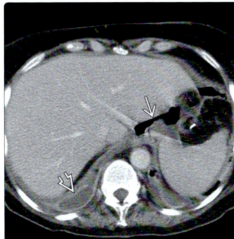

(Left) In this patient who had chest pain following recent Nissen fundoplication and reduction of a large paraesophageal hernia, axial CT shows collections of gas and fluid ➡ within the mediastinum, suggestive, but not diagnostic, of a leak or perforation. (Right) Axial CT in the same patient shows intraabdominal extension of gas ➡. Bilateral pleural effusions ➡ are also noted.

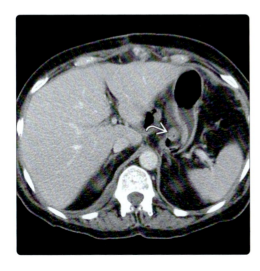

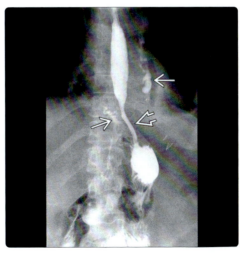

(Left) Another CT section in the same patient shows the intact fundoplication ➡, compressing the distal esophagus and proximal stomach. (Right) Spot film from an esophagram in the same patient shows compression of the distal esophagus ➡ from an intact fundoplication. Leak of contrast material ➡ into the mediastinum and upper abdomen, however, confirms perforation (leak) of the esophagus or the gastric wrap itself.

(Left) *Film from an upper GI series 1 day following gastric banding procedure shows the gastric band ⟹ around the proximal stomach with the correct orientation. A leak of water-soluble contrast medium and gas is evident ⟹.* (Right) *Upright spot film in a patient who had recent Roux-en-Y gastric bypass surgery shows a spherical distention of the gastric pouch ⟹ with an air-fluid level and delayed emptying, signs of a stricture of the anastomosis between the gastric pouch and the Roux limb ⟹.*

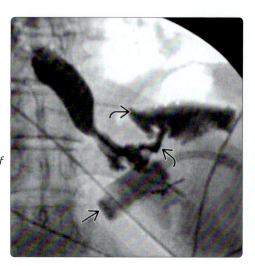
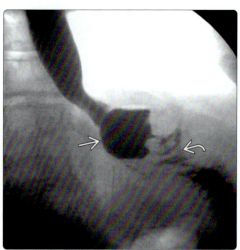

(Left) *Axial CECT in a young man with severe abdominal pain due to NSAID gastritis shows massive thickening and edema of the gastric wall. Note the enhancing mucosa ⟹ as distinct from near water density submucosal edema ⟹.* (Right) *Axial CECT in a patient with gastric carcinoma shows a distended stomach ⟹ (outlet obstruction) with a contracted antrum, thickened wall ⟹, and submucosal soft tissue density. Adjacent lymphadenopathy ⟹ indicates spread beyond the stomach.*

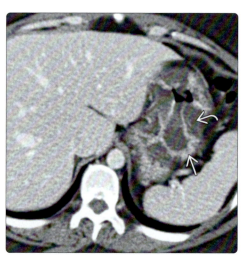
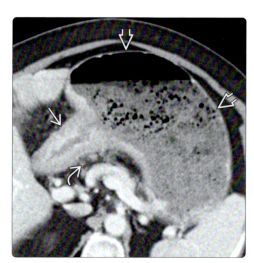

(Left) *In this patient with a palpable left upper quadrant mass, CT shows features of a gastric GI stromal tumor. The stomach ⟹ is indented along its dorsal surface by the mass ⟹, which is necrotic in its center and contains a gas-fluid level ⟹ due to communication with the gastric lumen.* (Right) *Axial CECT in a patient with gastric lymphoma shows massive wall thickening of soft tissue attenuation ⟹ but no outlet obstruction. Note the extensive regional lymphadenopathy and omental tumor deposits ⟹.*

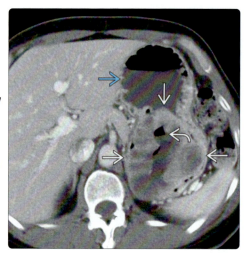
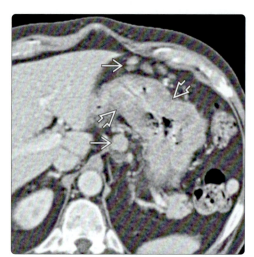

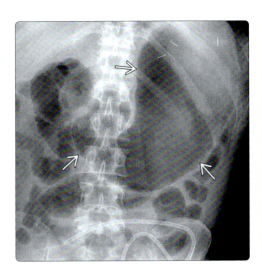

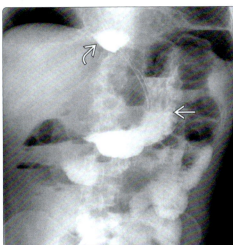

(Left) *In this patient who has had persistent distention and retching for weeks following a fundoplication (antireflux surgery), a supine film demonstrates marked distention of the stomach* ➡. (Right) *In the same patient, an upright film from an upper GI series obtained following placement of a nasogastric tube shows less gastric distention but a persistent gas-fluid-contrast level in the stomach* ➡, *esophagus* ➡, *and small bowel, known complications of fundoplication.*

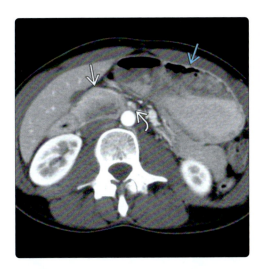

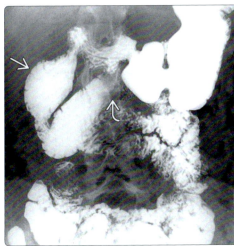

(Left) *In this 25-year-old woman with weight loss, nausea, and vomiting, CT shows marked distention of the stomach* ➡ *and duodenum* ➡ *up to where it crosses the midline, where it is compressed between the aorta and the superior mesenteric vessels* ➡. (Right) *Film from an upper GI series in the same patient shows the straight line demarcation* ➡ *of the midline duodenum with dilation of the upstream duodenal lumen* ➡. *These are classic clinical and imaging features of the superior mesenteric artery syndrome.*

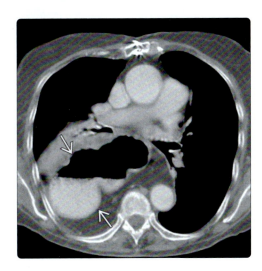

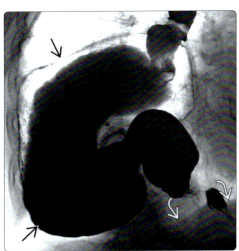

(Left) *In this elderly woman with postprandial abdominal and chest discomfort, CT shows the dilated stomach* ➡ *within a hernia sac in the right thorax and its rotation on its long axis.* (Right) *Film from an upper GI series confirms the presence of the entire stomach* ➡ *within the thorax with an organoaxial volvulus. The diaphragm is marked* ➡ *for orientation.*

KEY FACTS

IMAGING

- Most (> 75%) are congenital, juxtacardiac diverticula
  - Near gastroesophageal junction, on posterior aspect of lesser curvature of stomach
- Usually 1-3 cm, up to 10 cm in diameter
- On upper GI series
  - Barium-filled diverticulum with air-fluid level
- CT findings
  - **Often in left suprarenal location**
    - Mimics adrenal or pancreatic mass
  - Connection to stomach may be subtle
  - Air-filled, fluid-filled, or contrast-filled mass
  - No enhancement of contents

TOP DIFFERENTIAL DIAGNOSES

- Adrenal mass
- Pancreatic tumor
- Abdominal abscess
- Ectopic pancreatic tissue

PATHOLOGY

- Pouch/sac includes all 3 normal layers of gastric lining

CLINICAL ISSUES

- Complications (rare)
  - Bleeding
  - Ulceration
  - Carcinoma
- No treatment needed unless complications occur

DIAGNOSTIC CHECKLIST

- Incidental finding that may be mistaken for adrenal mass on CT or MR
  - **Barium studies or CT in supine and prone position with oral contrast** and gas granules will differentiate diverticulum from mass

(Left) Upright film from an upper GI series shows a typical gastric diverticulum ➡ with an air-contrast level seen within an outpouching near the gastric cardia. (Right) Axial CECT in the same patient shows a near water density mass ➡ projecting posterior to the gastric fundus ➡. The connection to the stomach is much more difficult to see on CT. Distention of the stomach with oral contrast or gas granules may be required to make the diagnosis on a CT scan.

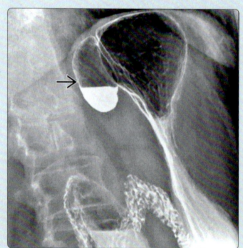
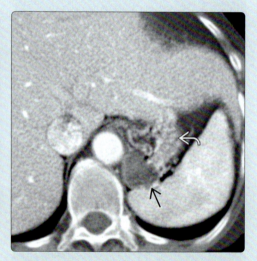

(Left) CECT shows an oval mass ➡ containing water density fluid and gas, seemingly separated from the gastric fundus ➡ by the pancreas ⇨. On more cephalic sections, the "mass" was contiguous with the posterior wall of the fundus. (Right) On a more inferior image, the diverticulum ➡ extends dorsal to the pancreas ⇨ and splenic vein ➜. Without the presence of the air-fluid level it would be difficult to distinguish this from an adrenal mass. An upper GI series confirmed a typical juxtacardiac diverticulum.

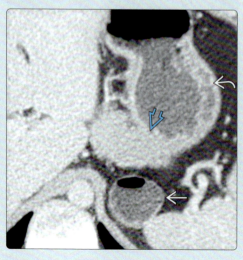
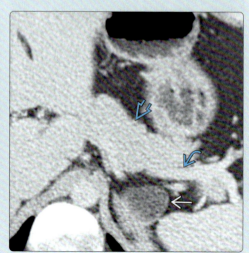

Duodenal Diverticulum

KEY FACTS

IMAGING

- **Easily depicted on barium UGI series and CT**
- Outpouchings from duodenal lumen
  - Location: Medial descending duodenum in periampullary region (70%), 3rd or 4th portion (26%), lateral (4%) descending duodenum
  - Filling defects within diverticulum (food and gas)
  - CT: Fluid-filled diverticulum may simulate cystic mass in pancreatic head
  - CT usually shows air-fluid level within diverticulum
- Intraluminal diverticula
  - Windsock appearance: Barium-filled, globular structure of variable length, originating in 2nd portion of duodenum, fundus extending into 3rd portion; outlined by thin, radiolucent line
  - CT: Contrast medium and gas within diverticulum, surrounded by contrast in duodenal lumen; separated by thin wall of diverticulum

TOP DIFFERENTIAL DIAGNOSES

- Pancreatic pseudocyst
- Pancreatic cystic tumor
- Perforated duodenal ulcer

CLINICAL ISSUES

- May be congenital or acquired
- Very common (~ 25% of population) but uncommonly (< 10% of affected patients) symptomatic
- Periampullary diverticula
  - May predispose to biliary sphincter incompetence, reflux, biliary stones
  - Makes endoscopic sphincterotomy more difficult and dangerous
- Perforation (duodenal diverticulitis)
  - Symptoms and signs are indistinguishable from perforated ulcer or pancreatitis
  - May occur spontaneously or following instrumentation (e.g., endoscopy or passage of feeding tube)

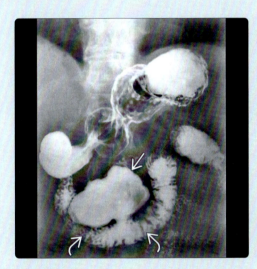
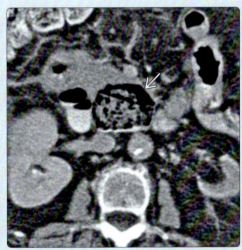

(Left) Film from an upper GI series in an asymptomatic 75-year-old man shows a large, featureless outpouching ➡ arising from the upper margin of the 3rd portion of the duodenum ➡. (Right) Axial CT in the same patient shows the diverticulum ➡ filled with food debris and gas. This could be confused with a gas-containing abscess, but the absence of symptoms or inflammatory changes on CT makes the diagnosis.

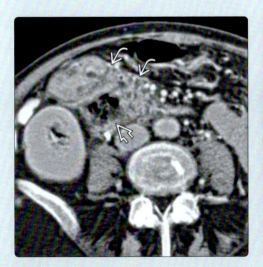
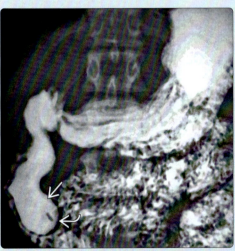

(Left) Axial CT in a 60-year-old woman with acute, severe epigastric pain shows a retroperitoneal collection of gas and fluid ➡. Note the thickened, inflamed wall ➡ of the adjacent 2nd and 3rd portions of the duodenum. A perforated duodenal diverticulum was found at surgery. (Right) Film from an upper GI series shows intraluminal diverticulum ➡ having a windsock appearance within the lumen of the duodenum. Note the thin radiolucent line ➡ at the leading edge.

TERMINOLOGY

- Inflammation of gastric mucosa induced by group of disorders that differ clinically but share similar imaging features
  - Common etiologies include *Helicobacter pylori*, NSAIDs, steroids, alcohol and coffee, stress

IMAGING

- **CT: Thickened gastric wall with submucosal edema**
  - Close to water density
  - CT for global view and concern for extragastric complications (e.g., perforation)
- **Upper GI series best for mucosal detail**
  - Mucosal erosions surrounded by radiolucent halos of edematous, elevated mucosa
  - Scalloped or nodular antral folds
  - Crenulation or irregularity of lesser curvature
  - Location: Gastric antrum on crests of rugal folds
  - Prolapse of antral mucosa through pylorus

- Lack of complete distensibility of stomach (especially antrum)

TOP DIFFERENTIAL DIAGNOSES

- Gastric carcinoma
- Zollinger-Ellison syndrome
- Acute pancreatitis
- Gastric metastases and lymphoma

DIAGNOSTIC CHECKLIST

- CT and upper GI usually just suggest gastritis
- Specific etiology determined by other medical data ± endoscopic biopsy

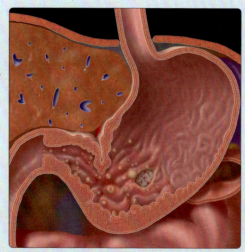
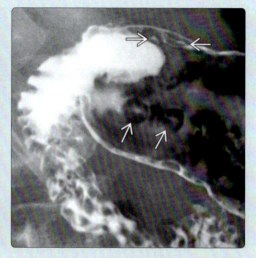

(Left) *Graphic shows an ulcer crater and numerous mucosal erosions, mostly in the antrum along the ridges of hypertrophied folds. The antrum is less than completely distensible.* (Right) *Upper GI series shows rows of varioliform erosions* ➡ *along the tops of hypertrophied gastric antral folds. This is diagnostic of gastritis but not specific as to the etiology.*

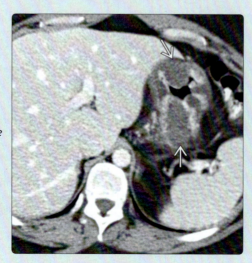
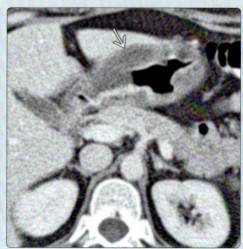

(Left) *CT of an athletic 30-year-old woman with severe abdominal pain and nausea due to NSAID gastritis shows massive thickening of the gastric wall with marked edema of the submucosa* ➡. *The enhancing mucosa imparts a striped appearance to the gastric wall.* (Right) *The body and antrum of the same patient are similarly involved* ➡. *Following cessation of ibuprofen use and beginning antacid therapy, the patient's symptoms resolved, and a repeat CT scan (not shown) was normal.*

TERMINOLOGY

Definitions

- Inflammation of gastric &/or duodenal mucosa induced by group of disorders that differs in etiological, clinical, histological, and radiological findings
- Classification of gastritis
  - Erosive or hemorrhagic gastritis (2 types)
    - Complete or varioliform
    - Incomplete or "flat"
  - Antral gastritis
  - *Helicobacter pylori* gastritis
  - Hypertrophic gastritis (Ménétrier disease)
  - Atrophic gastritis (2 types: A and B)
  - Granulomatous gastritis (Crohn's disease and tuberculosis)
  - Eosinophilic gastritis
  - Emphysematous gastritis
  - Caustic ingestion gastritis
  - Radiation gastritis
  - AIDS-related gastritis: Viral, fungal, protozoal, and parasitic infections

IMAGING

General Features

- Best diagnostic clue
  - Superficial ulcers and thickened folds

Upper GI Findings

- Erosive gastritis, complete or varioliform erosions (most common type)
  - Location: Gastric antrum on crests of rugal folds
  - Multiple punctate or slit-like collections of barium
  - Erosions surrounded by radiolucent halos of edematous, elevated mucosa
  - Scalloped or nodular antral folds
  - Epithelial nodules or polyps (chronic)
- Nonsteroidal antiinflammatory drug (NSAID) induced
  - Linear or serpiginous erosions clustered in body, on or near greater curvature
  - Varioliform or linear erosions in antrum
  - NSAID-related gastropathy: Subtle flattening and deformity of greater curvature of antrum
- Antral gastritis
  - Thickened folds, spasm, or decreased distensibility
  - Scalloped or lobulated folds oriented longitudinally or transverse folds
  - Crenulation or irregularity of lesser curvature
  - Prolapse of antral mucosa through pylorus
- *H. pylori* gastritis
  - Location: Antrum, body, or occasionally fundus; diffuse or localized
  - Thickened, lobulated gastric folds
  - Enlarged areae gastricae (≥ 3 mm in diameter)
- Hypertrophic gastritis (Ménétrier disease)
  - Location: Fundus and body
  - Markedly thickened, lobulated gastric folds
- Atrophic gastritis
  - Narrowed, tubular, nondistensible stomach
  - Smooth, featureless mucosa, ↓ folds
  - Small (1-2 mm in diameter) or absent areae gastricae
- Granulomatous gastritis; Crohn's disease
  - Location: Antrum and body
  - Multiple aphthous ulcers
  - Acute: Indistinguishable from erosive gastritis
  - Advanced disease → large ulcers, thickened folds, nodular or "cobblestone" mucosa
  - Ram's horn sign: Tubular, narrowed, funnel-shaped antrum
- Granulomatous gastritis; tuberculosis
  - Location: Lesser curvature of antrum or pylorus
  - Antral narrowing → obstruction
  - Often involves duodenum as well
- Eosinophilic gastritis and duodenitis
  - Location: Antrum and body, ± duodenum, small bowel, esophagus
  - Mucosal nodularity, thickened folds, antral narrowing and rigidity
- Emphysematous gastritis
  - Gas in wall of stomach; no positional change
  - Note: Use water-soluble contrast for upper GI
- Caustic ingestion (use water-soluble contrast)
  - Acute: Ulceration, thickened folds, gastric atony; mural defects
  - Chronic: Antral narrowing and deformity
    - May progress to linitis plastica or perforation
- Radiation gastritis
  - Acute: Ulceration, thickened folds, gastroparesis or spasm
  - Chronic: Antral narrowing and deformity (scarring)
- AIDS-related gastritis
  - Mucosal nodularity, erosions, ulcers, thickened folds, or antral narrowing

CT Findings

- Decreased wall attenuation (edema or inflammation)
  - Target or halo: Increased mucosal enhancement and decreased density of submucosa (edema)
- Thickened gastric folds or wall
- *H. pylori* gastritis: Circumferential antral wall thickening or focal thickening of posterior gastric wall along greater curvature
- Emphysematous gastritis: Thickened wall and gas within wall
  - May have portal venous gas

Imaging Recommendations

- Best imaging tool
  - Upper GI series for mucosal detail
  - **Contrast-enhanced, multiplanar CT** for global view and concern for extragastric complications (e.g., perforation)
  - **Upper endoscopy is best for evaluation of mucosal disease**

DIFFERENTIAL DIAGNOSIS

Gastric Carcinoma

- Differentiate from gastritis by loss of distensibility and decreased or absent peristalsis in involved portion
  - Nodular, distorted mucosa
  - Submucosa of soft tissue density

Zollinger-Ellison Syndrome

- Thickened gastric folds in fundus and body (edema, inflammation, and hyperplasia)
- ↑ fluid in lumen ± ulcers at unusual locations
- Due to gastrinoma (pancreatic endocrine tumor)

Acute Pancreatitis

- Common cause of gastric wall thickening (posterior wall)

Gastric Metastases and Lymphoma

- CT: Submucosal tumor is soft tissue (not water) density
- Metastases (e.g., malignant melanoma, breast cancer)
  - Tend to restrict distention
- Gastric lymphoma
  - Markedly thickened wall without outlet obstruction

PATHOLOGY

General Features

- Etiology
  - Erosive: NSAIDs, alcohol, steroids, stress, trauma, burns, or infections
  - Atrophic: Fundus and body (autoimmune)
  - Antral: Alcohol, tobacco, coffee, bile, or *H. pylori*
  - Granulomatous: Crohn's disease, sarcoidosis, tuberculosis, syphilis, or candidiasis
  - Emphysematous: *Escherichia coli*, *Staphylococcus aureus*, *Clostridium perfringens*, or *Proteus vulgaris*
  - Caustic ingestion: Strong acids (hydrochloric, sulfuric, etc.) or alkali
  - Radiation > 5,000 rads
  - AIDS related: Cytomegalovirus, cryptosporidiosis, toxoplasmosis, or strongyloidiasis
- Associated abnormalities
  - Atrophic gastritis: 90% of patients have pernicious anemia patients
  - Hypertrophic gastritis: 66% of patients have duodenal ulcers

Gross Pathologic & Surgical Features

- Erosive gastritis: Areas of congested, edematous, or ulcerated mucosa
- Atrophic gastritis: Thin, smooth mucosa, flattened rugae, or tubular stomach
  - Loss of parietal or chief cells

CLINICAL ISSUES

Presentation

- Most common signs/symptoms
  - Asymptomatic in some
  - Epigastric pain, nausea, vomiting, or hematemesis
- Lab data
  - ↑ leukocytes; positive fecal occult blood test
  - Atrophic gastritis: ↓ vitamin B12
  - Positive *H. pylori* (endoscopy, histology, cultures, urea breath, and serologic tests)

Natural History & Prognosis

- Caustic ingestion gastritis: Acute severe phase (1-4 days), ulceration and spasm; chronic phase (3-4 weeks), cicatrization and scarring (linitis plastica)

- Radiation gastritis: Inflammation (1-6 months), scarring and fibrosis (> 6 months)
- Complications
  - Gastric or duodenal ulcer, pernicious anemia, low-grade MALT lymphoma or gastric carcinoma
  - Eosinophilic gastritis: Gastric outlet obstruction
  - Caustic ingestion gastritis: Gastric necrosis
- Prognosis
  - Erosive, antral, *H. pylori*, and atrophic gastritis: Good after treatment
  - Eosinophilic gastritis: Chronic, relapsing disease with intermittent exacerbation and asymptomatic intervals
  - Emphysematous gastritis: 60-80% mortality

Treatment

- Stop offending agents: Alcohol, tobacco, NSAIDs, steroids, and coffee
- *H. pylori* treatment: Metronidazole, bismuth and clarithromycin, amoxicillin or tetracycline
- Hypertrophic gastritis: Antisecretory agents (H2-receptor antagonists or proton-pump inhibitors)
- Atrophic gastritis: Replace vitamin B12
- Eosinophilic gastritis: Steroids
- Emphysematous gastritis: IV fluids, antibiotics, but no nasogastric tube
- Caustic ingestion gastritis: Steroids, antibiotics, parenteral feedings, surgery

DIAGNOSTIC CHECKLIST

Consider

- History and presence of *H. pylori* infection, caustic ingestion, AIDS

Image Interpretation Pearls

- *H. pylori* gastritis: Thickened, lobulated gastric folds with enlarged areae gastricae
- Erosive gastritis: Multiple collections of barium surrounded by radiolucent halos of edematous, elevated mucosa

Reporting Tips

- CT and upper GI usually just suggest gastritis
  - Specific etiology determined by other medical data ± endoscopic biopsy

SELECTED REFERENCES

1. Byrne D et al: Imaging findings in emphysematous gastritis. Ir Med J. 107(2):60-1, 2014
2. Kim HW et al: Atrophic gastritis: a related factor for osteoporosis in elderly women. PLoS One. 9(7):e101852, 2014
3. Makhoul E et al: Emphysematous gastritis. Acta Gastroenterol Belg. 76(4):445-6, 2013
4. Gonen C et al: Magnifying endoscopic features of granulomatous gastritis. Dig Dis Sci. 54(7):1602-3, 2009
5. Yüksel O et al: Erosive gastritis mimicking watermelon stomach. Am J Gastroenterol. 104(6):1606-7, 2009
6. Horton KM et al: Current role of CT in imaging of the stomach. Radiographics. 23(1):75-87, 2003
7. Bender GN et al: Double-contrast barium examination of the upper gastrointestinal tract with nonendoscopic biopsy: findings in 100 patients. Radiology. 202(2):355-9, 1997
8. Sohn J et al: Helicobacter pylori gastritis: radiographic findings. Radiology. 195(3):763-7, 1995

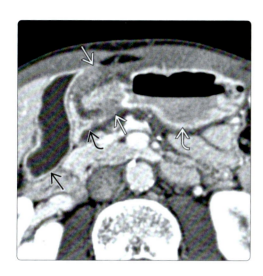

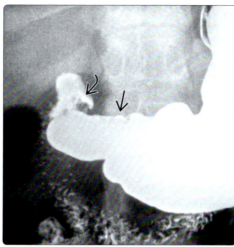

(Left) *Axial CT of antral gastritis in a 54-year-old man shows a thickened and hyperemic gastric wall ➡. The antrum is contracted with a particularly thickened and edematous wall ➡. The gallbladder ➡ is noted. The base of the duodenal bulb ➡ is indented.* (Right) *Upper GI series in the same patient shows a nondistensible antrum with thickened, nodular folds ➡ and herniation of gastric folds into the duodenal bulb ➡. These are classic CT and upper GI features of antral gastritis.*

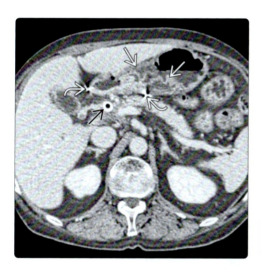

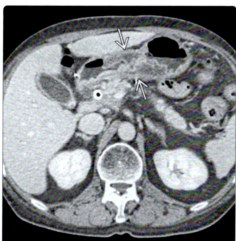

(Left) *Axial CECT of radiation gastritis in a patient with pancreatic cancer shows a stent ➡ in the bile duct and metallic fiducial markers ➡ that were placed at the time of surgical exploration to serve as markers for subsequent radiation therapy. Note the thick-walled stomach ➡ with submucosal edema limited to the radiation port.* (Right) *In the same patient, note the findings of gastritis ➡ limited to the radiation field in front of the pancreatic head and neck tumor.*

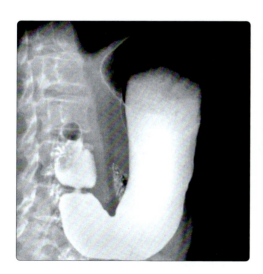

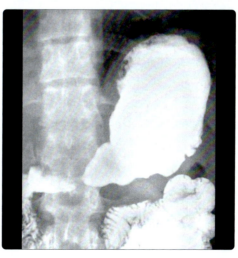

(Left) *An upright spot film from an upper GI series in this patient with atrophic gastritis shows almost complete absence of gastric folds.* (Right) *Upper GI series in a patient with chronic Crohn's gastritis shows a deformed stomach that is reduced in size, with loss of normal gastric folds, and a tubular, funnel-shaped antrum that has been likened to a ram's horn.*

TERMINOLOGY

- Mucosal erosion of duodenum

IMAGING

- 95% of duodenal ulcers are in duodenal bulb, 5% postbulbar
- **Upper GI series**: Sharply marginated barium collection with folds radiating to edge of ulcer crater
  - Deformity of bulb (edema, spasm, and scarring)
  - Pseudodiverticula balloon-out between areas of fibrosis and spasm
  - Postbulbar ulcers: Medial wall of proximal descending duodenum above papilla of Vater
  - **Cloverleaf deformity** of bulb due to pseudodiverticula
- **CT with IV ± oral contrast medium** for diagnosis of perforation
  - Wall thickening, luminal narrowing of duodenum
  - Presence of intra- and extraperitoneal gas in upper abdomen is essentially diagnostic of perforated duodenum
- **Most cases are diagnosed by upper endoscopy**

CLINICAL ISSUES

- 2-3x more frequent than gastric ulcers
- Many cases are asymptomatic
- Burning, gnawing, or aching pain at epigastrium 2-4 hours after meals, relieved by antacids or food
- Pain episodes occurring in clusters of days to weeks followed by longer pain-free intervals

DIAGNOSTIC CHECKLIST

- **Barium upper GI series and CT are complementary to endoscopy in diagnosis of ulcers and complications**
- Eradication of *Helicobacter pylori* is 1st step of treatment
  - Proton-pump inhibitors are also effective
- Effective medical treatment has made surgical treatment much less common

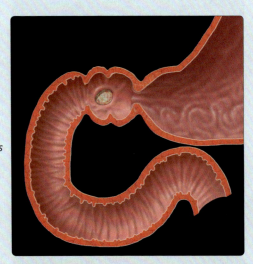
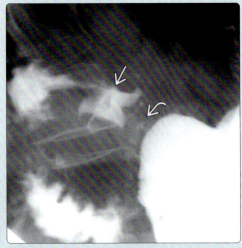

(Left) Graphic illustrates a duodenal ulcer with a deformed bulb due to converging folds and spasm. (Right) Film from an upper GI series shows a cloverleaf deformation of the duodenal bulb with the ulcer ➡ at the center of the cloverleaf. The other lobes of the cloverleaf are the duodenal bulb fornices or recesses. The pylorus ➡ is marked for orientation.

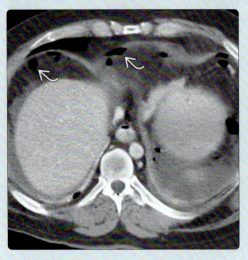
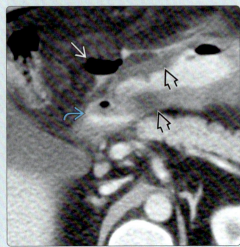

(Left) Axial CECT in a 42-year-old man presenting with acute severe abdominal pain and guarding shows extensive free intraperitoneal gas ➡ from a perforated duodenal ulcer. (Right) Axial CECT in the same patient demonstrates a thickened gastric wall ➡, probably due to gastritis. Ventral to the duodenal bulb ➡ and antrum are small collections of extraluminal gas and oral contrast medium ➡ that confirm an ulcer as the source of perforation.

Gastric Ulcer

IMAGING

- Imaging may suggest diagnosis; **endoscopy is main diagnostic modality**
  - **Multiplanar enhanced CT**: To show complications (± ulcer itself)
  - **Upper GI series can show ulcer**
- Benign gastric ulcer
  - Sharply defined mucosal defect (ulcer); smooth, even, radiating folds to edge of ulcer crater
  - Projects beyond expected contour of stomach (on upper GI and CT imaging)
  - Usually on lesser curve, posterior wall, or antrum
  - CT may show extravasation of gas and oral contrast (lesser sac or greater peritoneal cavity)
- Malignant ulcer
  - Uneven shape; irregular or asymmetric edges; interruption and clubbing of radiating folds
  - Does not project beyond contour of stomach

- CT may show metastasis to nodes, peritoneum, liver
- Sump ulcers: Distal 1/2 of greater curvature (NSAIDs)
- Incisura defect: Smooth or narrow indentation on curvature opposite ulcer (muscle contraction)

TOP DIFFERENTIAL DIAGNOSES

- Gastritis
- Gastric GI stromal tumor
- Gastric metastases and lymphoma
- Artifactual

PATHOLOGY

- 2 major risk factors: *Helicobacter pylori* (60-80%) and NSAIDs (20%)

CLINICAL ISSUES

- Benign (95%), malignant (5%)
- Often multiple: 20-30% prevalence
- Complications: Hemorrhage, perforation, gastric outlet obstruction, and fistula

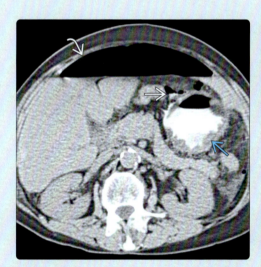
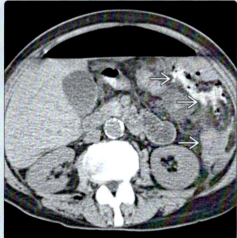

(Left) *NECT of a perforated gastric ulcer shows a thick-walled stomach ⇒ and massive free intraperitoneal gas ⇒. Extraluminal contrast material and gas are present near the anterior surface of the stomach ⇒, representing the perforated ulcer.* (Right) *In the same patient, the extravasated enteric contrast material mixes with ascites to result in high-attenuation ascites ⇒. Note that gastric ulcers may perforate into the lesser sac or the greater peritoneal cavity, as in this case.*

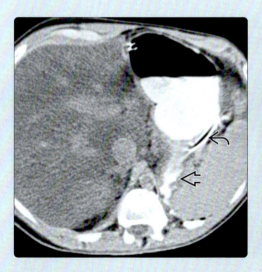
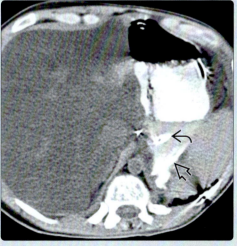

(Left) *NECT of an alcoholic man with pain and hypotension shows diffuse low attenuation of the liver, compatible with steatosis or massive hepatic necrosis. A nasogastric tube ⇒ marks the dependent surface of the stomach. Contrast material spills into the lesser sac ⇒ through a perforated ulcer.* (Right) *CT in the same patient shows the nasogastric tube ⇒ and the lesser sac collection of oral contrast medium ⇒. The ulcer was confirmed and repaired at surgery, but the patient died of acute hepatic failure.*

KEY FACTS

TERMINOLOGY

- Severe peptic ulcer disease associated with marked ↑ in gastric acid due to gastrin-producing pancreatic neuroendocrine tumor (gastrinoma)

IMAGING

- Best diagnostic clue
  - Hypervascular pancreatic or peripancreatic mass with multiple peptic ulcers and thickened gastric folds
- Best imaging tools
  - **Multiphasic, multiplanar CECT or MR** for pancreas and liver (possible metastasis)
  - Endoscopic ultrasonography for additional primary sites; guides biopsy
- Gastrinoma: Pancreas (75%), duodenum (15%), and liver and ovaries (10%)
  - Common site: Gastrinoma triangle
- Ulcers: Stomach and duodenal bulb (75%), postbulbar and jejunum (25%)

TOP DIFFERENTIAL DIAGNOSES

- *Helicobacter pylori* gastritis
- Other gastritides (e.g., Ménétrier disease)

PATHOLOGY

- 20-60% of cases are associated with multiple endocrine neoplasia type 1 (MEN1)

CLINICAL ISSUES

- Most common signs/symptoms
  - Pain, increased acidity, severe reflux, diarrhea, upper gastrointestinal tract ulcers
  - Gastrinomas are often multiple (60%), malignant (60%), and metastatic (30-50%)
- Prognosis
  - Good with surgical resection of primary gastrinoma
  - Poor if gastrinoma, liver metastases, or ulcers recur after surgery

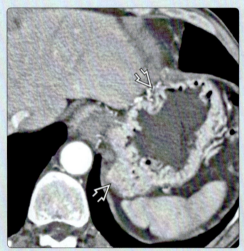
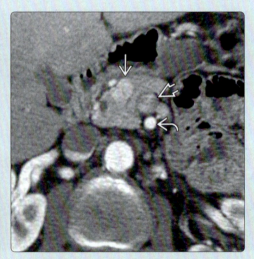

(Left) *Arterial-phase CECT in a 63-year-old man who presented with intractable peptic ulcer disease demonstrates hyperemia and mural thickening ➡ of the stomach.* (Right) *Arterial-phase CECT in the same patient shows a small, hypervascular gastrinoma ➡ in the pancreatic head. It is important to distinguish this from the superior mesenteric artery ➡ and superior mesenteric vein ➡.*

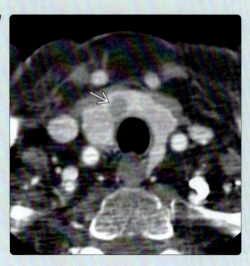
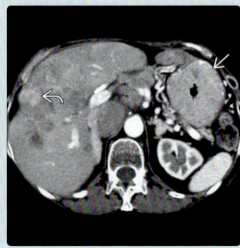

(Left) *Axial CT of a 55-year-old woman with hypercalcemia, diarrhea, and severe abdominal pain as presenting symptoms of MEN1 syndrome shows 1 of several neck masses ➡, representing parathyroid adenomas or hyperplasia.* (Right) *Arterial-phase CECT in the same patient shows marked hypervascularity and thickening of the gastric wall ➡. Multiple liver metastases are present ➡. The serum gastrin levels were strikingly elevated, confirming ZES, though the gastrinoma was not identified on CT.*

Ménétrier Disease

TERMINOLOGY

- Hyperplastic, protein-losing gastropathy

IMAGING

- Rare condition of unknown cause
- Upper GI series: Grossly thickened, lobulated folds in gastric fundus and body with poor barium coating
- **CECT: Massive thickening of mucosa and submucosa;** cerebriform (brain-like) appearance
  - Engorged gastric arteries and veins
  - No extension into perigastric tissues
- **Endoscopic US and upper endoscopy** also show characteristic abnormalities

TOP DIFFERENTIAL DIAGNOSES

- Gastritis
- Zollinger-Ellison syndrome
- Gastric metastases and lymphoma
- Gastric carcinoma

CLINICAL ISSUES

- Histology: Marked foveolar hyperplasia (mucin production)
  - Leads to protein loss and hypoproteinemia
  - Atrophy of acid-producing cells → hypochlorhydria
- Bimodal age distribution
  - Children (usually boys)
  - Associated with CMV and *Helicobacter pylori* infection
- Adults, usually men (mean age: 55 years)
  - Prolonged and progressive illness in most adults
- Complications
  - Gastric carcinoma may have ↑ prevalence (controversial)
  - Increased risk of deep venous thrombosis
  - Risk of atrophic gastritis, gastric ulcer, GI bleeding
- Treatment
  - Medical therapy: Anticholinergic agents, antibiotics, prostaglandins, octreotide
    - Monoclonal antibody (cetuximab) to EGFR
  - May require total gastrectomy

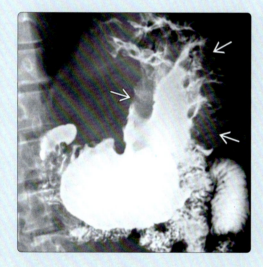
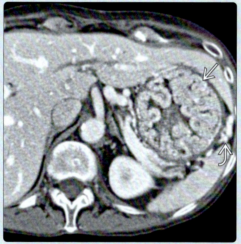

(Left) Film from an upper GI series shows massive fold thickening ➡ throughout the gastric fundus and body with relative sparing of the antrum. Also noted is poor coating of the mucosa by the barium. (Right) CECT in a 68-year-old woman with proven Ménétrier disease shows grossly thickened folds ➡ in the gastric fundus and body along with engorged gastric vessels ➡. The thick, tortuous folds resemble cerebral (brain) convolutions.

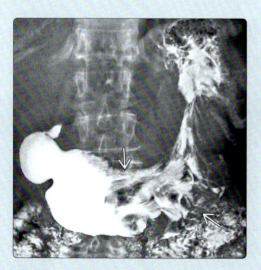
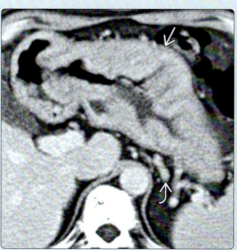

(Left) Film from an upper GI series shows massive fold thickening ➡ of the gastric fundus and body with sparing of the antrum. Note the poor coating of the gastric mucosa with barium to the surface of the stomach, reflecting the excessive mucus discharge of the gastric glands. (Right) In the same patient, CECT shows marked thickening of the gastric mucosa and submucosa ➡, but there is no sign of extension into the perigastric tissues. The gastric arterial and venous branches are engorged ➡, indicating hyperemia of the stomach.

KEY FACTS

TERMINOLOGY

- Objectively delayed gastric emptying in absence of mechanical obstruction

IMAGING

- Best test: Delayed emptying of both solids and liquids on **radionuclide gastric emptying scan**
  - > 10% retention of food at 4 hours is excessive
- Upper GI series or CT
  - Dilated stomach with decreased or absent peristalsis

TOP DIFFERENTIAL DIAGNOSES

- Gastric outlet obstruction
- Postoperative state, stomach

PATHOLOGY

- Idiopathic: No identifiable cause in ~ 50% of cases
- Type 1 diabetes is main identifiable cause
  - Usually longstanding and poorly controlled

- Affects 40% of patients with diabetes
- Narcotic analgesic use is 3rd most common cause
  - Others drugs may also be implicated
- Postsurgical
  - Prior thoracic or gastric surgery may injure vagus nerve
  - Some cases are deliberate
    - e.g., to reduce gastric acid production
  - Others are unintentional (e.g, following fundoplication)
- Neurologic disorders
- Electrolyte disturbances

CLINICAL ISSUES

- Symptoms: Nausea, vomiting, postprandial bloating, early satiety
- Treatment
  - Promotility and antiemetic agents
  - Botulinum toxin injection into gastric pylorus
  - Gastric electrical stimulation device (pacemaker)
  - Surgical pyloroplasty

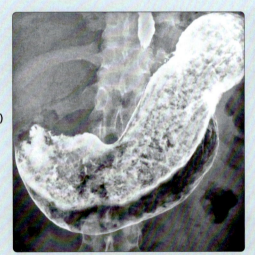
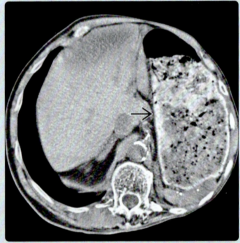

(Left) *Upper GI series of a 34-year-old man with type 1 diabetes and persistent nausea shows stasis of the barium (after a 20-minute delay) and food debris within the stomach, in spite of no oral intake for > 12 hours. No peristalsis was evident.* **(Right)** *NECT in a 61-year-old man with diabetes shows a markedly distended stomach containing contrast material and food ⇨ in spite of the patient having fasted for 12 hours. This indicates delayed gastric emptying and proved to be due to diabetic gastroparesis.*

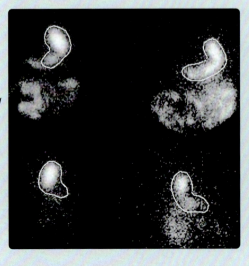
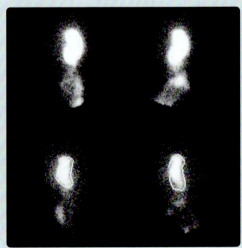

(Left) *Gastric emptying scintigraphy in a patient with diabetic gastroparesis shows mild to moderate gastric emptying delay (30% emptied at 120 minutes, 55% at 240 minutes) on this solid-labeled phase. Similar delay was found for liquids.* **(Right)** *Gastric emptying scan shows severe delay in emptying of ingested solids (32% at 120 minutes). This patient had multiple prior surgeries, including vagotomy and Billroth II partial gastrectomy. Multiple factors most likely contribute to delayed emptying in this patient.*

Gastric Bezoar

TERMINOLOGY

- Intragastric mass composed of accumulated ingested (but not digested) material
  - Phytobezoar: Undigested vegetable matter
    - Persimmons contain tannin, which coagulates on contact with gastric acid
  - Trichobezoars: Accumulated, matted mass of hair
    - Most common in young girls
  - Lactobezoar: Undigested milk concretions (infants)
  - Pharmacobezoar: Bezoar composed of medications

IMAGING

- **CT or fluoroscopy: Intraluminal mass containing mottled gas pattern**
- Mobile intraluminal gastric filling defect
- Mottled appearance is result of air bubbles retained in interstices of mass
- Large bezoars may fill & take shape of stomach
- Small bezoars are rounded or ovoid

- Tend to float on water-air surface surrounded by gastric contents

CLINICAL ISSUES

- Predisposing causes
  - Previous gastric surgery: Vagotomy, pyloroplasty, antrectomy, partial gastrectomy
  - Inadequate chewing, missing teeth, dentures
  - Overindulgence in foods with high fiber content
  - Altered gastric motility: Diabetes, mixed connective tissue disease, hypothyroidism
- Bezoars usually form in stomach
  - May fragment & enter small bowel where they absorb water, increase in size, & become impacted
  - May present with small bowel obstruction
- Drinking several liters of cola ± acetylcysteine may clear all or portions of phytobezoars
- Symptomatic, large phytobezoars or trichobezoars require endoscopic fragmentation or surgical removal

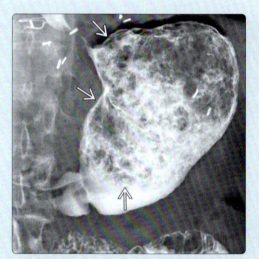
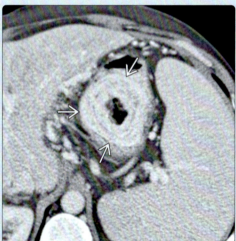

(Left) *Film from an upper GI series in a 60-year-old man with early satiety, many years after vagotomy and Billroth I surgery (antrectomy) shows evidence of the prior surgery and a large heterogeneous "ball" of debris and gas* ➡ *within the stomach mixed with the barium.* (Right) *Axial CECT shows a laminated mass* ➡ *in the stomach due to a phytobezoar.*

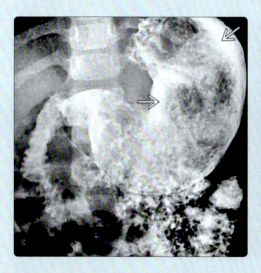
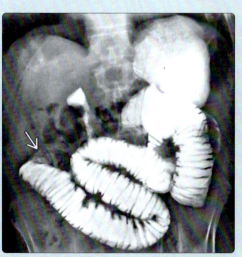

(Left) *Upper GI series in a 3-year-old girl with vomiting shows a fixed filling defect* ➡ *in the stomach with a swirled pattern of gas and solid material found to represent a trichobezoar.* (Right) *Film from a small bowel follow-through shows evidence of a prior Billroth II partial gastrectomy and complete obstruction of antegrade flow of barium in the mid jejunum* ➡. *At surgery, a phytobezoar was removed, which corresponded to the shape and size of the gastric remnant.*

Hiatal Hernia

KEY FACTS

IMAGING

- 2 general types
  - Sliding (axial) hiatal hernia (HH): Gastroesophageal junction (GEJ) and gastric cardia pass through esophageal hiatus
  - Paraesophageal (rolling) hernia: Gastric fundus ± other parts of stomach herniate into chest
- Surgical classification
  - Type I: Sliding HH (only cardia in chest); most common
  - Type II Paraesophageal (PEH): GEJ in normal position under diaphragm, fundus in chest (very rare)
  - Type III PEH: GEJ in chest, along with fundus ± other portions of stomach (2nd most common HH)
  - Type IV PEH: Intrathoracic stomach ± volvulus
- Type I (sliding HH): Signs on upper GI series
  - Lower esophageal mucosal (B) ring & gastric rugae observed ≥ 2 cm above diaphragmatic hiatus
  - Often reducible in erect position
- Paraesophageal hernia (types II to IV)
  - Portion of stomach anterior or lateral to esophagus in chest
  - Frequently nonreducible; almost always with GE reflux
  - Often accompanied by herniation of abdominal fat ± colon & other organs

PATHOLOGY

- Multifactorial etiology; including obesity, deconditioning
- Reflux itself induces irritation that causes spasm of longitudinal muscles of esophagus
  - Shortens esophagus, which pulls stomach up into chest

CLINICAL ISSUES

- Medical treatment and lifestyle modification (treatment same as for GERD)
- Endoscopic techniques, including sphincter augmentation
- ↑ use of laparoscopic fundoplication to treat GERD & to repair all types of HH

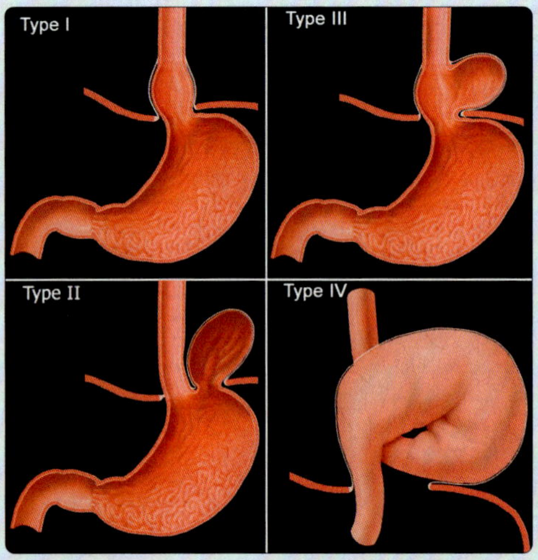

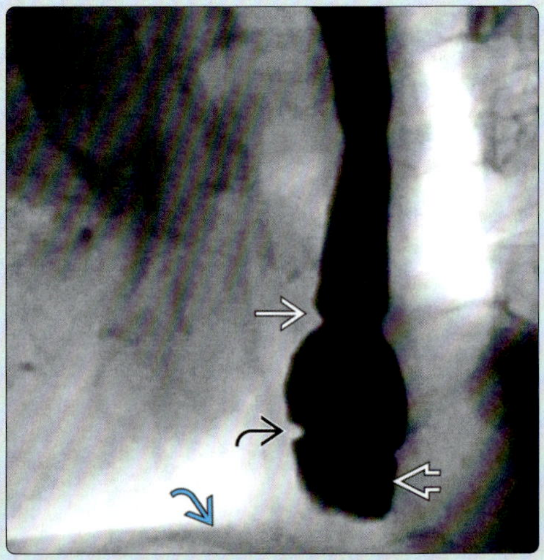

(Left) *Graphic outlines the surgical classification of hiatal hernias (HH). Type I is a sliding HH, and types II-IV are paraesophageal hernias. Type III is the 2nd most common type, but it is uncommon compared to type I (sliding HH).* **(Right)** *Esophagram in a patient with type I sliding HH shows the lower esophageal sphincter, or phrenic ampulla, marked by the A ring → proximally and the B ring ↗ distally. Just below the B ring is the herniated portion of the gastric cardia ⇨, above the diaphragm ↷.*

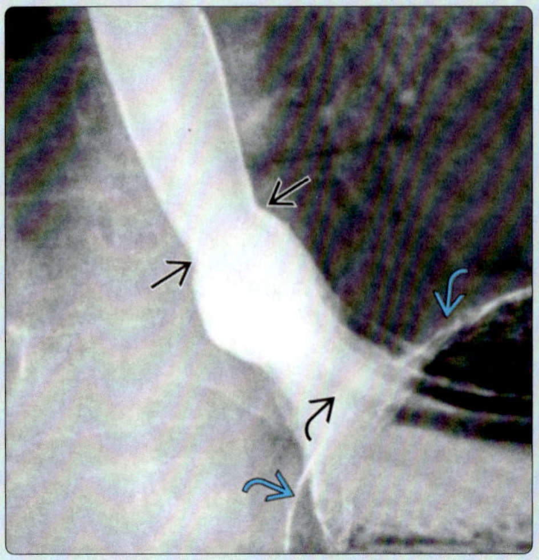

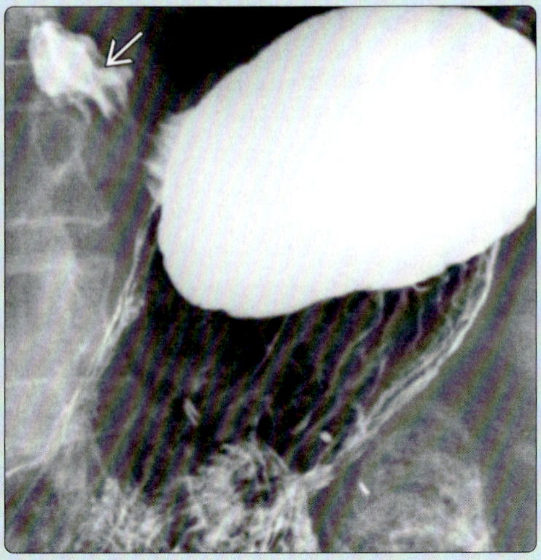

(Left) *Film from a barium esophagram in a patient with type I sliding HH shows the gastroesophageal (GE) junction, marked by the B ring →. Gastric folds ↗ extend up through the hiatus, above the diaphragm ↷.* **(Right)** *Supine film from an esophagram in the same patient reveals reflux →. While reflux is commonly seen in patients with sliding HHs, it is uncertain whether the HH causes the reflux or vice versa.*

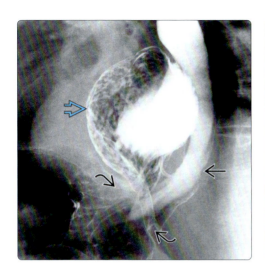

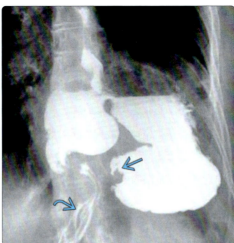

(Left) *The GE junction* ⇨ *in this patient with a type III PEH is in the chest, along with a substantial portion of the stomach* ⇨*. The stomach is pinched as it traverses the diaphragmatic hiatus* ⇨*. Type III PEHs are encountered with increased frequency.* (Right) *Upper GI series in a patient with type IV PEH is shown. The entire stomach is intrathoracic and "upside down," indicating an organoaxial volvulus, although some barium does enter the duodenum* ⇨*. The GE junction is marked* ⇨ *as it enters the cardia & fundus.*

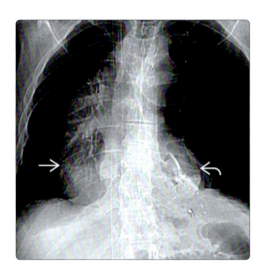

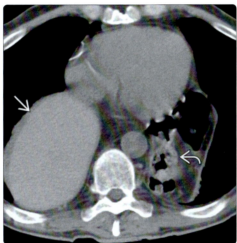

(Left) *Upright chest film in an elderly man with chest pain shows a widened mediastinum with an air-fluid level to the right of the spine* ⇨ *and what appear to be bowel segments* ⇨ *to the left of the thoracic spine.* (Right) *Axial CT in the same patient shows that most of the stomach* ⇨ *lies within the right hemithorax (type iV PEH) and the colon* ⇨ *lies to the left and behind the heart, along with omental fat, all herniating through a wide defect in the esophageal hiatus.*

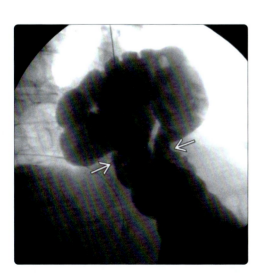

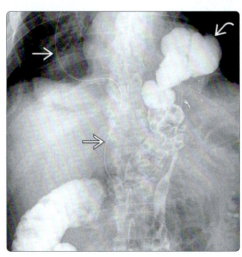

(Left) *A barium enema in the same patient confirms that the splenic flexure of the colon is herniated, and there is a "waist"* ⇨ *or compression of the colon as it traverses the hiatus.* (Right) *Post evacuation film from the barium enema shows barium retained within the herniated colon* ⇨*. Note the position of a nasogastric tube* ⇨ *within the herniated stomach and the duodenum, which is within the abdomen.*

IMAGING

- **Multiplanar, contrast-enhanced CT is 1st-line diagnostic study (after plain film of chest & abdomen); fluoroscopic UGI series is complementary**
  - CT is better at demonstrating associated hernias and gastric ischemia
- Organoaxial volvulus: Rotation of stomach around its long axis
  - Most common type; "upside-down stomach"
  - Occurs in setting of large paraesophageal hernia (PEH)
  - Stomach rotates upward with greater curvature lying above lesser curve
- Mesenteroaxial volvulus: Rotation of stomach about its short axis
  - More common type in children
- Entire stomach may be herniated (type IV PEH) or only part (type III PEH)
  - Either can result in volvulus ± obstruction ± ischemia
  - Gastric wall pneumatosis indicates ischemia

TOP DIFFERENTIAL DIAGNOSES

- Hiatal hernia
  - Types III and IV PEHs increase risk for gastric volvulus
- Postoperative state, stomach
  - Esophagectomy with gastric pull through (conduit may twist and obstruct)
- Epiphrenic pulsion diverticulum

CLINICAL ISSUES

- Endoscopy can decompress stomach and temporarily reduce volvulus in some cases
- Definitive treatment: Open or laparoscopic detorsion and gastropexy

DIAGNOSTIC CHECKLIST

- Presence or absence of obstruction and ischemia are more important than remembering or reporting whether volvulus is organo- or mesenteroaxial

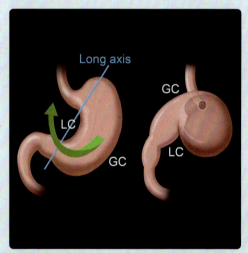
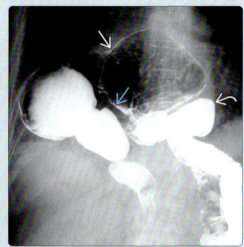

(Left) Graphic illustrates an organoaxial gastric volvulus in which the stomach twists along its long axis, resulting in the greater curvature (GC) lying above the lesser curvature (LC). (Right) Film from an upper GI series in a 73-year-old woman shows a type IV paraesophageal hernia (PEH) with organoaxial volvulus but little or no obstruction. The greater curvature of the stomach ➡ lies above the lesser curvature ➡. The small bowel ➡ is also herniated through a large diaphragmatic defect.

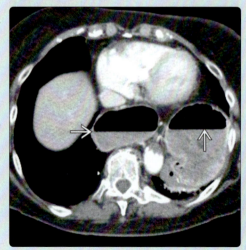
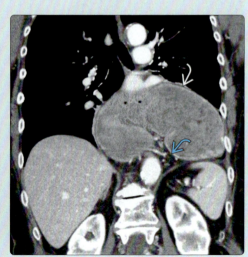

(Left) Axial CECT demonstrates an intrathoracic stomach (type IV PEH) in a 81-year-old woman with mild chest pain and a known brain malignancy. The stomach is dilated with 2 air-fluid levels ➡, indicating obstruction. (Right) Coronal CECT in the same patient demonstrates an upside-down configuration of the stomach, with reversal of the greater ➡ and lesser ➡ curvatures, in keeping with an organoaxial volvulus.

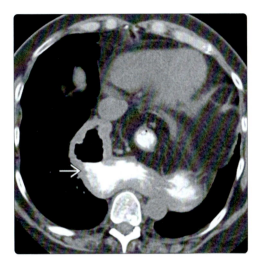
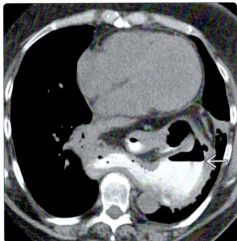

(Left) Axial NECT in a 63-year-old woman with chronic intermittent chest and abdominal pain demonstrates the entirety of the stomach within the thoracic cavity (type IV PEH). Notice the large amount of contrast retained in the stomach ➡ nearly 2 hours after its administration. (Right) Axial NECT in the same patient again demonstrates the intrathoracic stomach ➡ with retained contrast in its lumen.

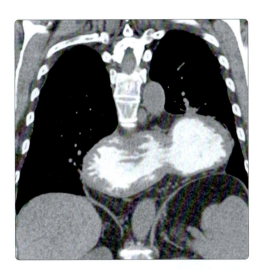
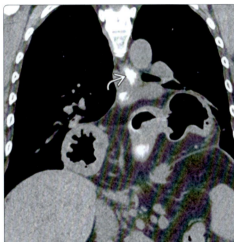

(Left) Coronal NECT in the same patient better demonstrates the twisting of the stomach with the greater and lesser curvatures having reversed. (Right) Coronal NECT in the same patient demonstrates contrast retained within the midthoracic esophagus ➡. The patient was felt to be at least partially obstructed, and underwent operative repair, where the organoaxial volvulus was confirmed.

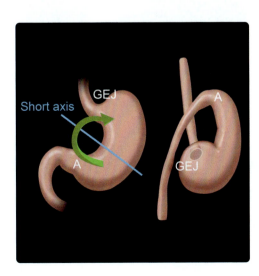
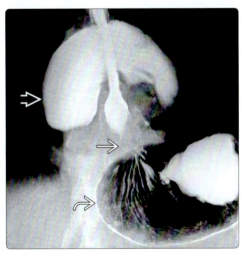

(Left) Graphic illustrates a mesenteroaxial volvulus in which the stomach twists along its short axis, resulting in the antrum (A) lying above the fundus and gastroesophageal junction (GEJ). (Right) Spot film from an upper GI series shows the GEJ ➡ and fundus ➡ in the abdomen. The body and antrum of the stomach ➡ are in the chest and are twisted and compressed as they traverse the diaphragm, constituting a mesenteroaxial volvulus with obstruction.

TERMINOLOGY

- **Billroth 1 (B1) procedure** (antrectomy with gastroduodenostomy)
  - Uncommonly performed today
- **Billroth 2 (B2) procedure** (distal gastrectomy with gastrojejunostomy)
  - Variable length of duodenum and jejunum form proximal or afferent loop
- **Surgery for gastric cancer** (partial or complete gastrectomy)
  - Latter includes esophagojejunal anastomosis

IMAGING

- **Recurrent cancer**: Especially in those with primary gastric cancer
  - Patients who have had B2 surgery for benign ulcer disease are also at ↑ risk (3-6x) of cancer in gastric stump
  - Due to bile gastritis and achlorhydria
- **Dumping syndrome**: 5-50%, varies with type of procedure

- **Bezoar formation**: ↑ after B1 and B2
  - Predisposing factors: Achlorhydria, denervation, edentulous patient, anastomotic stricture
- **Stomal ulceration**: Usually on small bowel side
- **Jejunogastric intussusception**: Rare complication of B2
- **Afferent loop syndrome**: Obstruction of afferent loop at or near anastomosis → dilation of afferent limb
  - Missed by upper GI; shown by CT (dilated afferent limb)
- **Chronic remnant gastritis**: Due to effects of alkaline bile and pancreatic juice on gastric mucosa

DIAGNOSTIC CHECKLIST

- Upper GI series is 1st-line test (along with endoscopy) for detecting mechanical complications of gastric surgery
- CT is optimal test for general surveillance for postoperative complications
- PET/CT is optimal imaging test for surveillance of recurrent gastric carcinoma

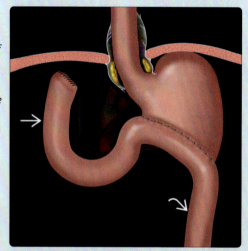
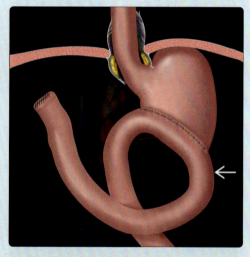

(Left) Graphic depicts an isoperistaltic Billroth 2 gastrojejunostomy. The afferent limb ➡, composed of the duodenum and a variable length of jejunum, carries pancreaticobiliary secretions toward the stomach, while the efferent limb ➡ carries fluid and food downstream. (Right) Graphic depicts an antiperistaltic Billroth 2 procedure in which the afferent loop ➡ enters the anastomosis from a left-to-right direction. This procedure is intended to reduce the prevalence of bile gastritis.

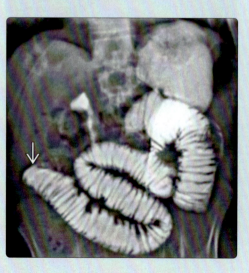
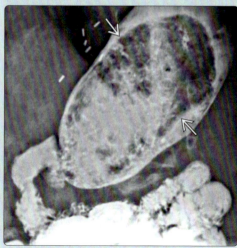

(Left) Film from a small bowel follow-through shows evidence of a prior Billroth 2 procedure and complete obstruction of antegrade flow of barium in the mid jejunum ➡. At surgery, a phytobezoar was removed, which corresponded to the shape and size of the gastric remnant. (Right) Film from an upper GI series shows evidence of a prior Billroth 1 procedure along with persistent filling defects ➡ within the stomach that conform to the shape of the stomach, a bezoar.

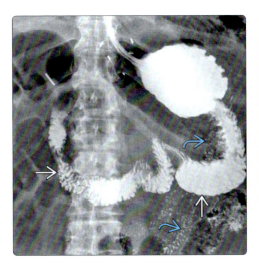

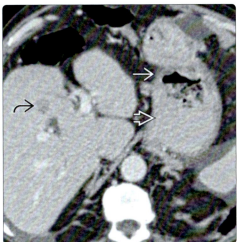

(Left) This 30-minute delayed film from a small bowel follow-through in an elderly man who had a Billroth 2 procedure for benign ulcer disease 15 years prior shows preferential filling of the afferent limb ➡ and delayed and decreased filling of the efferent limb ➡. (Right) Axial CECT in the same patient shows luminal distention and wall thickening of the gastric remnant ➡ near the gastroenteric anastomosis ➡ due to gastric carcinoma. Liver metastases are evident ➡.

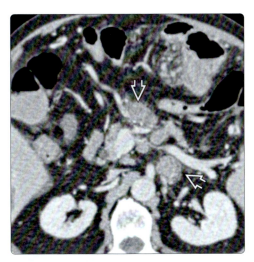

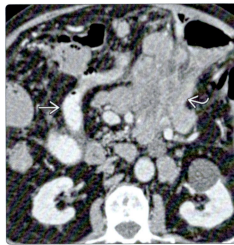

(Left) Axial CECT in the same patient shows extensive mesenteric and retroperitoneal lymphadenopathy ➡ from lymphatic metastases. (Right) Axial CECT in the same patient shows a large mesenteric tumor encasing the efferent limb ➡. The contrast-filled lumen of the afferent limb is seen ➡. Gastric cancer occurs with increased frequency following this type of ulcer surgery, usually 15 or more years later.

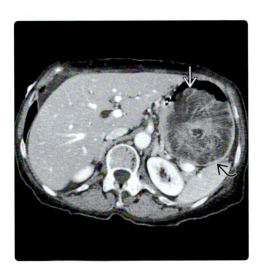

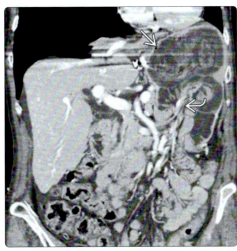

(Left) CT demonstrates a loop of thick-walled and ischemic jejunum ➡ within the distended gastric remnant ➡, a jejunogastric intussusception as a complication of partial gastrectomy with Billroth 2 anastomosis. (Right) Coronal CECT reformation in the same patient shows the retrograde intussusception ➡ with invagination of bowel, mesenteric fat, and vessels ➡ into the gastric remnant (intussuscipiens). This is a rare complication but may result in bowel obstruction and ischemia.

IMAGING

- **Endoscopy is primary diagnostic tool**
  - **Multiplanar enhanced CT and barium upper GI series are complementary**
- Polyps classified based on pathology
  - Hyperplastic, adenomatous, and hamartomatous
- Fundic gland polyps: Now most common type
  - Sometimes considered variant of hyperplastic polyps
- Hyperplastic polyps
  - Typical: Small (< 1 cm), multiple, sessile
  - Virtually no malignant potential
  - Location: Fundus and body
- Adenomatous polyps
  - Usually solitary, > 1 cm
  - Less common (< 20% of benign polyps)
  - Increased risk of malignant change
- Hamartomatous polyps
  - Peutz-Jeghers syndrome (multiple small gastric polyps)

TOP DIFFERENTIAL DIAGNOSES

- Retained food and pills
- Gastric carcinoma (polypoid type)
- Gastric metastases and lymphoma
- Gastric gastrointestinal stromal tumor
- Ectopic pancreatic tissue

CLINICAL ISSUES

- Prevalence of gastric polyps in patients who have upper endoscopy = 6% (2009 study)
- Fundic (77%), hyperplastic (18%), malignant (4%), adenomas (< 1%)
- Much higher percentage of fundic polyps than in earlier studies
  - Caused by increased use of proton pump inhibitor medications
- Syndromic polyps have high association with cancer risk in stomach and other organs
  - e.g., familial polyposis, Peutz-Jeghers syndrome

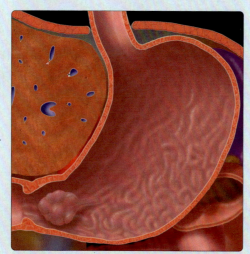

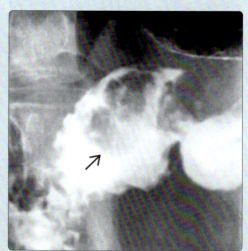

(Left) Graphic shows a pedunculated polyp in the gastric antrum, prone to prolapse through the pylorus with peristalsis. Any type of large polyp may prolapse in this fashion, including large hyperplastic, adenomatous, and even polypoid masses arising from the submucosa, such as lipomas. (Right) Upper GI series shows a polypoid mass ➡ in the duodenal bulb that is a prolapsed gastric antral polyp (adenoma).

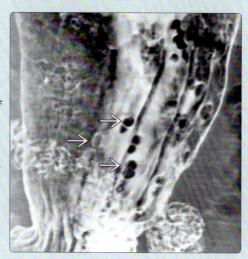

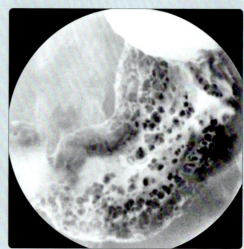

(Left) Film from an upper GI series in a 57-year-old man shows multiple small, sessile polyps ➡ in the gastric body. The appearance and age of the patient are typical for hyperplastic polyps. (Right) Film from an upper GI series of adenomatous polyps in a patient with familial polyposis shows innumerable small polyps throughout the stomach. These are somewhat larger, more numerous, and more irregular in shape than most hyperplastic polyps.

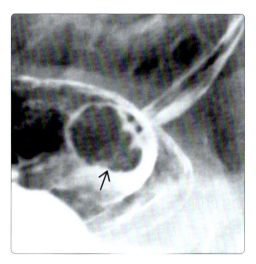

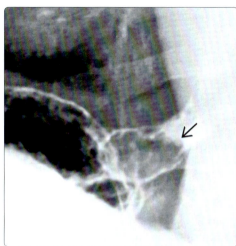

(Left) *Film from an upper GI series in an elderly man with dysphagia shows a well-defined polyp* ➡ *at the gastroesophageal junction.* (Right) *Another spot film from the upper GI in the same patient shows the polyp* ➡ *prolapsing into the distal esophagus. Endoscopy and resection revealed an adenomatous gastric polyp.*

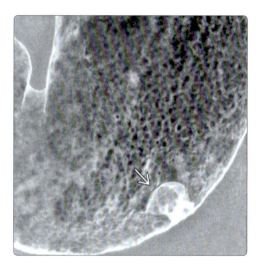

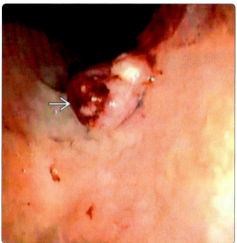

(Left) *Film from an upper GI series shows a well-defined polyp* ➡ *in the gastric body.* (Right) *Endoscopic photograph in the same patient shows an ulcerated mass* ➡ *that was a benign adenoma. A band was placed around the base of the polyp, and it was resected at endoscopy.*

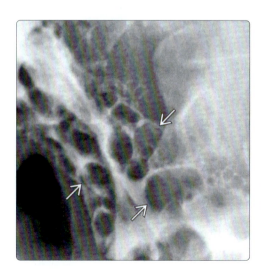

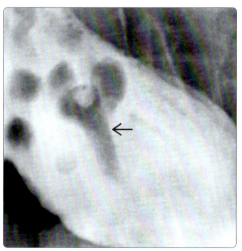

(Left) *Film from an upper GI series in an elderly man with dyspepsia shows a cluster of polypoid lesions* ➡ *arising from the gastric cardia and body. These have a smooth surface and most appear sessile.* (Right) *Upper GI series in the same patient shows that some of the polyps appear to have a stalk* ➡*. Endoscopy revealed multiple polyps with a villous adenoma histology.*

TERMINOLOGY

- Intramural mass comprised of 1 or more tissue elements of gastric wall
  - Gastrointestinal stromal tumor (GIST) is most common
  - Others include lipoma, carcinoid, leiomyoblastoma, lymphangioma, neural tumors

IMAGING

- **Upper endoscopy** may not detect intramural mass that lacks intraluminal or mucosal extension
- **Contrast-enhanced, multiplanar CT is 1st-line test**
  - Shows intraluminal, intramural, and extragastric extent of mass
  - Shows density (attenuation) of mass (e.g., soft tissue, water, fat)
- **Lipoma**: Most common in antrum
  - May prolapse through pylorus into duodenum
  - Well-circumscribed areas of uniform fat density = definitive diagnosis

- **GIST**: Often large with central necrosis and ulceration of overlying mucosa on CT
  - Most GIST > 2 cm have necrosis ± cavitation
  - Gas or ingested contrast medium may enter necrotic center of GIST
- **Carcinoid (neuroendocrine) tumors**: May be multiple as result of excess gastrin secretion (Zollinger-Ellison syndrome or atrophic gastritis)
- **Others: e.g., neural tumors, hemangiomas, or lymphangiomas**
  - These have no distinctive features on imaging studies

TOP DIFFERENTIAL DIAGNOSES

- Gastric carcinoma, metastases, and lymphoma
- Ectopic pancreatic tissue
- Pancreatic pseudocyst
- Splenosis
- Hematoma/seroma

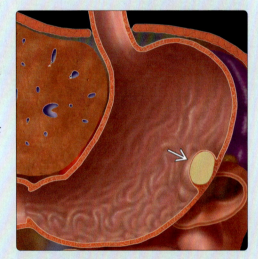
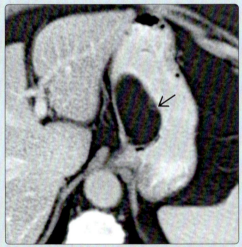

(Left) Graphic shows a "generic" intramural gastric mass ➡ with intact mucosa and slightly obtuse or right angles at the interface with the gastric wall. (Right) Axial CECT shows a discrete fat-density mass ➡ within the gastric wall with intact, stretched mucosa, diagnostic of a lipoma.

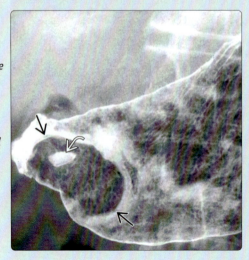
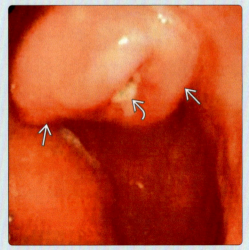

(Left) Upper GI series shows a gastric antral mass ➡ with a central ulceration ➡, typical of a gastric gastrointestinal stromal tumor (GIST). Note the otherwise intact mucosa over the mass, even with preservation of the areae gastricae. (Right) Endoscopic photograph in the same patient shows the submucosal benign gastric GIST ➡ with central ulceration ➡.

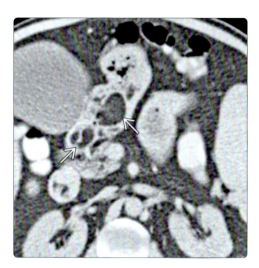
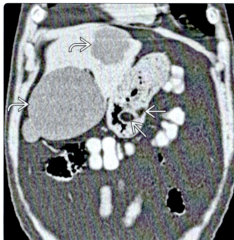

(Left) Axial CECT in a patient with multiple gastric lipomas demonstrates several fat-containing masses ➡ within the wall of the stomach. Some are pulled by peristalsis into the lumen as polyps on a stalk. (Right) In the same patient, 2 of the lipomas ➡ can also be identified. Hepatic lesions ➡ are simple cysts. It is uncommon to detect multiple lipomas within the stomach, but these lesions are invariably benign and require no treatment or further evaluation unless they bleed or prolapse into the duodenum with obstructive symptoms.

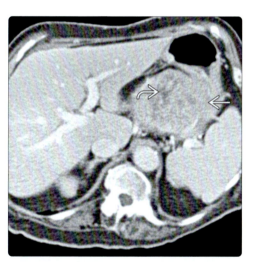
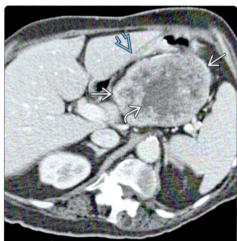

(Left) Axial CECT in this patient with a benign GIST shows a large, exophytic mass ➡ arising from the lesser curve of the stomach. It is relatively vascular with central areas of necrosis ➡. (Right) In the same patient, the GIST ➡ has prominent and characteristic central necrosis ➡. The stomach ➡ is displaced ventrally.

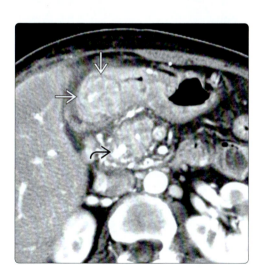
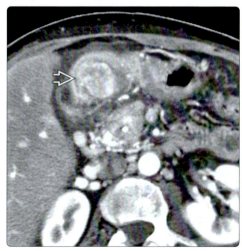

(Left) Axial CECT in a middle-aged woman with chronic pancreatitis shows calcifications ➡ within the head of the pancreas. An unexpected finding was a vascular mass ➡ within the posterior wall of the stomach. (Right) Axial CECT in the same patient shows that the vascular intramural mass has intact gastric mucosa ➡ "draped" over it. This was resected and proven to be a neurolemmoma of the gastric wall.

Gastric Carcinoma

IMAGING

- Best imaging tools to complement endoscopy
  - **Double-contrast upper GI series, CECT, EUS**
- Best diagnostic clue
  - Polypoid or circumferential gastric mass with no peristalsis through lesion
- CT findings
  - Polypoid mass ± ulceration
  - Wall-thickening with infiltration of perigastric fat
  - Scirrhous carcinoma: Thickened wall, nondistensible lumen (**linitis plastica**)
  - Hematogenous metastases (liver, peritoneum, lungs, bones)
  - **Krukenberg tumor**: Metastases to ovaries via peritoneal seeding
- **Pseudoachalasia**: Gastric fundus carcinoma may invade & obstruct distal esophagus

TOP DIFFERENTIAL DIAGNOSES

- Gastric metastases and lymphoma
- Gastric stromal tumor (GIST)

PATHOLOGY

- Risk factors
  - *Helicobacter pylori* (3-6x ↑ risk), pernicious anemia
  - Diet heavy in nitrites or nitrates; salted, smoked food

CLINICAL ISSUES

- Most common signs/symptoms
  - Anorexia, weight loss, anemia
- Diagnosis by endoscopic biopsy and histology

DIAGNOSTIC CHECKLIST

- Protocol advice
  - Distend stomach with water prior to CT
  - IV contrast enhancement + multiplanar reformations are essential

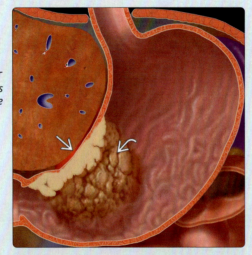
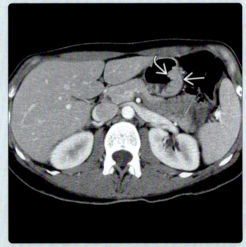

(Left) *Graphic shows a large intraluminal mass with a broad base and irregular surface ⟳. The gastric wall ⟳ is thickened by tumor infiltration.* (Right) *Axial CECT in a 41-year-old woman shows mural thickening of soft tissue density ⟳, representing an infiltrative gastric carcinoma. Note the irregular surface ⟳ of the mass.*

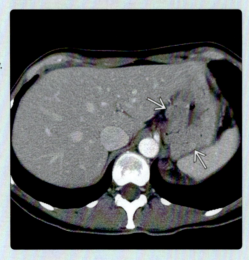
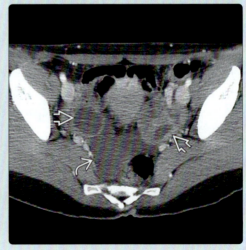

(Left) *More cephalad section in the same patient shows circumferential thickening of the gastric wall ⟳ that severely limits its distensibility.* (Right) *In the same case, CT through the pelvis shows a collection of ascites ⟳ and bilateral adnexal masses ⟳. The right adnexal mass is mostly cystic with a contrast-enhancing rim of soft tissue, while the left mass is more solid than cystic. At surgery, gastric carcinoma and bilateral ovarian metastases (Krukenberg tumors) were confirmed.*

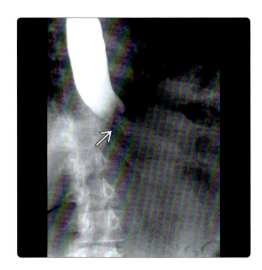

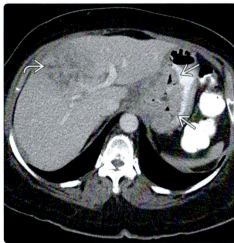

(Left) *Spot film from an esophagram in an 80-year-old woman with dysphagia shows moderate dilation and delayed emptying of the esophagus in the upright position. The lumen is abruptly and irregularly narrowed at the GE junction* ➡. *(Right) Axial CECT section in the same patient shows a gastric cancer* ➡ *that obstructed the esophagus, in addition to a hepatic metastasis* ➡.

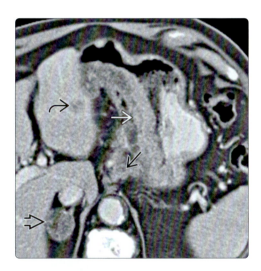

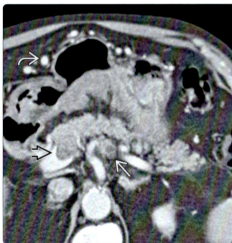

(Left) *Axial CECT in a 77-year-old man shows a large mass* ➡ *infiltrating and thickening the lesser curve from the gastric cardia to the pylorus. Liver* ⊡ *and adrenal* ➡ *metastases are evident, along with regional lymphadenopathy* ➡. *(Right) Axial CECT in the same patient reveals involvement of the splenic vein* ➡, *which has resulted in splenic vein narrowing and perigastric collaterals* ➡. *Celiac nodal metastases* ➡ *are also noted.*

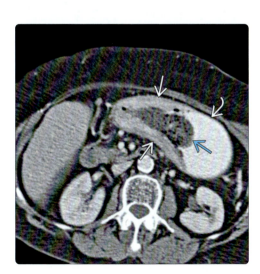

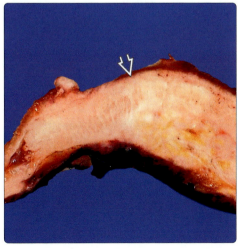

(Left) *Axial CECT in an elderly woman with early satiety & weight loss shows soft tissue density infiltration of the wall of the distal stomach* ➡, *with gastric outlet obstruction suggested by the presence of retained food* ➡ *within the stomach. Note the normal thin gastric wall* ➡ *for comparison. (Right) Gross pathology photograph of the resected specimen shows the scirrhous, fibrotic appearance of the gastric wall* ➡ *where it is infiltrated by the tumor. Tumors of this type limit peristalsis and distention (linitis plastica appearance).*

Stomach and Duodenum

IMAGING

- **Best imaging tools: Multiplanar CT or PET/CT**
  - Most comprehensive display of primary tumor and metastatic foci
- **Hematogenous spread** of metastases to stomach
  - Malignant melanoma: Bull's-eye or "target" lesions, nodular intramural cavitated lesions
  - Breast cancer: Linitis plastica or "leather bottle"
    - Markedly thickened gastric wall with enhancement, folds preserved
    - Mimics primary scirrhous carcinoma of stomach
- **Direct invasion or lymphatic spread** to stomach
  - Distal esophageal carcinoma: Polypoid, lobulated mass in gastric fundus
  - Transverse colon cancer → gastrocolic ligament → greater curvature
    - Thickened wall or mass in greater curvature ± gastrocolic fistulous tract

- **Omental and peritoneal metastases**
  - Ovary, uterus, breast, pancreas, GI tract
  - Lacy reticular pattern to bulky masses (omental cake) displace and indent gastric wall
- **Gastric lymphoma**
  - Markedly thickened gastric wall, regional or widespread adenopathy
  - Rarely causes linitis plastica or gastric outlet obstruction

DIAGNOSTIC CHECKLIST

- Check for history or evidence of primary cancer or *Helicobacter pylori* gastritis
- Image interpretation pearls
  - Imaging important to suggest and stage malignancy, but biopsy is required
  - Imaging findings easily mimic primary gastric carcinoma in some cases

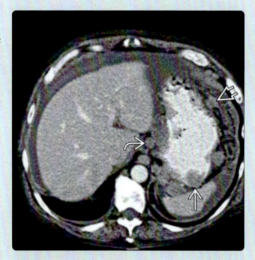 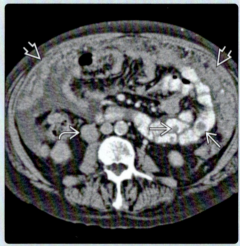

(Left) *Axial CECT in a 69-year-old man shows widespread metastases from the patient's known metastatic melanoma, including the gastric wall ➡, lymph nodes ➡, and omentum ➡.* (Right) *Axial CECT in the same patient again illustrates classic widespread metastases from melanoma, here involving the small bowel ➡, lymph nodes ➡, and omentum ➡, with both nodular and diffuse metastases seen.*

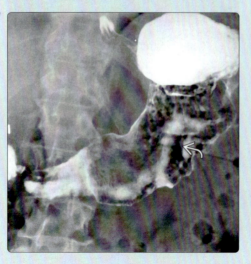 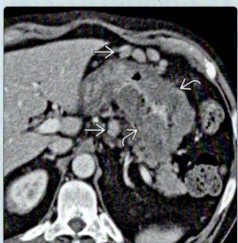

(Left) *Upper GI in a 70-year-old man with weight loss and dyspepsia reveals distortion and blunting of the gastric folds ➡. In spite of what appears to be diffuse involvement of the stomach, there is no outlet obstruction, and the stomach is distensible.* (Right) *Axial CECT in the same patient shows massive thickening of the gastric wall of soft tissue attenuation ➡. Note the extensive regional lymphadenopathy and omental tumor deposits ➡. These findings are typical of primary gastric lymphoma.*

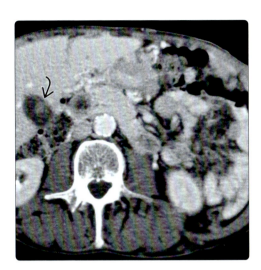

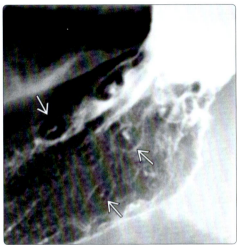

(Left) Axial CECT in a 57-year-old man with a known history of malignant melanoma, now presenting with weight loss and dyspepsia, shows metastases to the liver and gallbladder ➡. The stomach is not well distended or easily assessed. (Right) Upper GI in the same patient illustrates classic bull's-eye lesions ➡ consisting of small, intramural masses with a central ulceration.

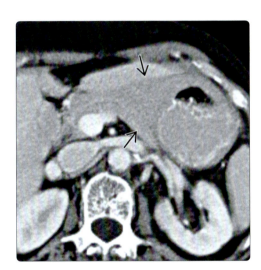

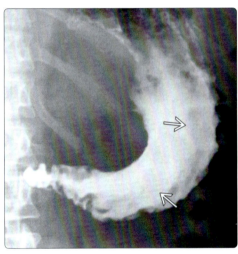

(Left) Axial CECT in a 75-year-old man who presented with weight loss and dyspepsia demonstrates a soft tissue density mass ➡ that diffusely infiltrates the gastric wall. There is no outlet obstruction. (Right) Upper GI in the same patient reveals marked thickening and blunting of the gastric folds ➡ but nearly normal distensibility and no obstruction, findings typical of lymphoma.

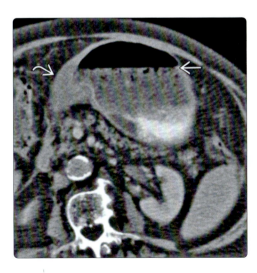

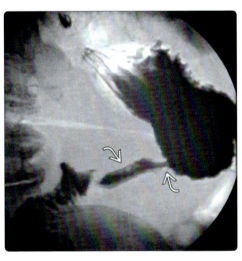

(Left) Axial CECT in an 84-year-old woman with a known history of breast cancer and a recent onset of early satiety and nausea reveals gastric distension ➡ and retention of food. The antrum is nondistensible and is infiltrated with a soft tissue density mass ➡. (Right) Upper GI in the same patient confirms a scirrhous lesion of the gastric antrum ➡ causing delayed gastric emptying. These imaging findings are indistinguishable from primary gastric carcinoma but were due to breast metastases to the stomach.

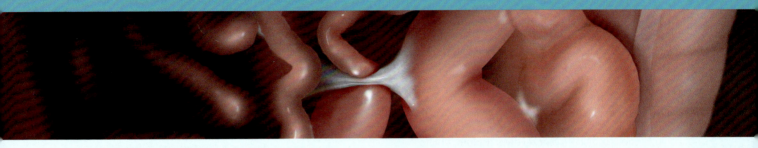

SECTION 6
Small Intestine

Embryology and Congenital Malformations

The small intestine and the right side of the colon constitute the embryologic midgut, which herniates into the umbilical cord during the process of marked elongation in fetal development. Following a 270° counterclockwise rotation, the midgut returns to the peritoneal cavity. Errors during this complex series of events are common, resulting in varying degrees of **malrotation** ± volvulus. This may result in bowel obstruction and ischemia and may present in infancy or be delayed into adult life.

In the fetus, the omphalomesenteric or vitelline duct connects the distal small bowel (SB) with the yolk sac. By birth, the vitelline duct has usually atrophied and disappeared; failure of involution results in a **Meckel diverticulum**, a blind outpouching from the distal ileum.

Gross Anatomy

The jejunum begins at the duodenojejunal flexure, which is often acutely angulated, as it is suspended by the suspensory ligament of the duodenum (ligament of Treitz), an extension of the right crus of the diaphragm. The jejunum constitutes ~ 40% of the SB and is ~ 2-3 meters long.

The jejunum normally lies primarily in the left upper quadrant and is distinguished by having a thicker, more vascular wall than the ileum. Its circular folds (valvulae conniventes and folds of Kerckring) are taller and more closely spaced (4-7 per inch).

The ileum constitutes the distal 60% of the small intestine, though there is no clear line of delineation, and usually lies in the right side of the abdomen and pelvis. Relative to the jejunum, the wall of the ileum is thinner and less vascular but has more prominent lymphoid follicles in the submucosal layer.

The small intestine is supplied entirely by the superior mesenteric artery (SMA) and vein (SMV). Occlusion of the SMA by thrombus or embolus results in **SB ischemia**, but arterial occlusion may be difficult to diagnose on clinical or imaging evaluation until frank infarction with bowel wall pneumatosis develops. SMV occlusion results in more impressive edema of the bowel wall and mesentery. Various vasculitides affect long segments of the bowel and are manifested by impressive bowel wall edema and luminal dilation.

Lymphatic drainage begins at the level of the villi (tiny projections of the mucous membrane) with the lacteals, specialized lymphatic vessels that absorb fat from the gut lumen. The lacteals empty milky, lipid-rich chyle into the regional lymphatic plexus in the mesentery and then progressively into the lymph nodes, intestinal lymphatic trunks, cisternal chyli, and thoracic duct. The thoracic duct transports dietary lipids directly into the bloodstream as it empties into the left subclavian vein. Intestinal lymphangiectasia results from a congenital abnormality of lymphatic development or from lymphatic obstruction in the SB wall or mesentery. The resulting interference with lipid absorption from the gut can result in malnutrition, chylous ascites, and other complications.

Mural Small Bowel Anatomy

There are 5 layers of the SB wall. The innermost is the mucosa, the absorptive surface of the bowel. The jejunal mucosa is extensively plicated (folded), and these transverse ("circular") folds lie perpendicular to the long axis of the bowel. The other layers are the submucosa, circular muscle, longitudinal muscle, and serosa. The serosa is the peritoneal lining of the bowel. The mucosal surface of the jejunum is increased by prominent villi, which are finger-like projections of mucosa. The submucosa has a network of capillaries, lymphatics, and a nerve plexus (of Meissner) within loose areolar tissue.

The ileum has the same 5 layers, but its wall is thinner and less vascular, with less prominent transverse folds and villi. This fold pattern of the jejunum and ileum can be altered by various disease processes or even reversed, as seen in some patients with celiac-sprue.

Imaging Issues

Plain films of the abdomen remain of value for initial detection or exclusion of SB obstruction, free intraperitoneal air, and calculi, though CT offers greater sensitivity and specificity in these and other investigations of abdominal and SB disorders.

The role of the **barium SB follow through** and enteroclysis studies has diminished markedly with advances of CT and MR, capsule endoscopy, and standard endoscopy. The advent of CT and MR enterography in particular has greatly improved our ability to diagnose specific SB disease processes along with their distribution, degree of severity, complications, etc. **CT and MR enterography** have become 1st-line modalities in evaluation of patients with known or suspected inflammatory bowel disease, GI bleeding, bowel ischemia, and SB neoplasms. Enterography entails distention of the SB lumen with a neutral contrast agent, bolus administration of IV contrast medium, and multiplanar viewing, especially in the coronal plane. **Newer CT techniques**, such as iterative reconstruction, allow imaging with **markedly reduced radiation dose**, an important consideration especially for repeat examinations of young patients with chronic illness, such as Crohn's disease. MR offers the additional advantage of "real-time" sequences that may be useful to assess SB peristalsis.

Approach to the Abnormal Small Bowel

Almost all acute bowel injuries result in thickening of the submucosal layer (thickened folds). The etiology of the injury may be suggested by the **attenuation of the submucosal layer** on CT evaluation, making this an essential element in the interpretation of CT for SB disorders.

Submucosal gas (**pneumatosis**) often indicates bowel infarction, but there are many other "benign" (nonischemic and less threatening) causes, including various medications and prior interventions, such as surgery or endoscopy. Analysis of other CT findings, such as the presence or absence of ascites and ileus, along with correlation with clinical features, such as severe abdominal pain and lactic acidosis, are critical for accurate diagnosis.

At the other extreme of attenuation, intramural hemorrhage may be detected as higher than soft tissue density within the bowel wall and may result from trauma or coagulopathy.

Soft tissue density within the submucosa is the least specific finding and may be caused by a variety of inflammatory and neoplastic processes.

Most acute inflammatory, infectious, or ischemic injuries to the bowel result in submucosal edema, seen as near water attenuation. This observation is important in excluding neoplastic processes as considerations.

Submucosal fat density may be a normal finding, particularly in obese patients. Other causes include chronic, quiescent inflammatory bowel disease (Crohn's especially), cytoreductive therapy for patients with hematologic malignancies, and celiac disease.

In addition to identifying the character of the submucosal wall thickening, it is useful to **identify the site and length of SB disease**. Some processes are very focal (e.g., tumor), while others affect short segments (bowel wall hematoma), or long segments (vasculitis, radiation enteritis, some forms of ischemia). Others affect the SB diffusely (shock bowel, SMA or SMV thrombosis). While a specific diagnosis may not be made by imaging alone, the combination of imaging, laboratory, and clinical data will often indicate the disease process.

Intussusception is an indication or sign, rather than a disease per se. Intussusceptions in adults that were symptomatic and persistent enough to be diagnosed by barium studies have been regarded as likely due to a lead mass. However, intussusceptions that are nonobstructing and involve only short segments of SB are commonly observed on CT scanning and are uncommonly due to neoplastic lesions. In most cases, the underlying bowel is normal, although intrinsic diseases, such as celiac disease, or extrinsic processes, such as adhesions, are associated with transient intussusception.

SB obstruction is a common condition, usually the result of adhesions (scar tissue from prior abdominal surgery) that constrict the bowel lumen. Adhesive SB obstruction is suggested by abrupt transition from dilated to collapsed bowel along with angulation of the lumen &/or SB folds. Most often, it is a diagnosis of exclusion, made by imaging evidence of an absence of internal or external hernia, mass lesion, intussusception, etc.

SB neoplasms are relatively uncommon or at least are less likely to come to medical attention. As in the colon, primary SB carcinoma is seen as a short segment of abrupt luminal narrowing, causing bowel obstruction. Metastases to the SB may have a similar appearance but are more frequently intramural, multiple, and less likely to obstruct.

Carcinoid (neuroendocrine tumor) is one of the more common SB tumors, but it is usually diagnosed by virtue of its clinical (carcinoid syndrome) or imaging signs of metastatic disease, including mesenteric and hepatic masses.

As with other portions of the GI tract, imaging studies are employed with increasing frequency to evaluate various postoperative alterations of bowel anatomy. It is important to become familiar with the spectrum of enterostomies, enterectomies, anastomoses, and even transplantations in order to be able to recognize complications of these procedures and to differentiate these from expected postsurgical changes.

Differential Diagnosis

Segmental or Diffuse Small Bowel Wall Thickening
Common
- Crohn's disease
- Celiac-sprue
- Infectious enteritis
- Ischemic enteritis
- Intramural hemorrhage
- Shock bowel (hypotensive complex)
- Portal hypertension
- Hypoalbuminemia

Less Common
- Radiation enteritis
- Opportunistic intestinal infections
- Vasculitis
- Metastases and lymphoma, intestinal
- Carcinoid tumor
- Angioedema, intestinal
- Lymphangiectasia, intestinal
- Graft-vs.-host disease

Pneumatosis of Small Intestine or Colon
Common
- Ischemic enteritis or colitis
- Postoperative or postendoscopy
- Medication-induced pneumatosis
- Pseudopneumatosis (mimic, in right colon)
- Barotrauma; chronic obstructive pulmonary disease; asthma
- Cystic fibrosis
- SB obstruction
- Collagen vascular disease
- Necrotizing enterocolitis

Less Common
- Pneumatosis cystoides intestinalis
- SB transplantation
- Inflammatory bowel disease
- Toxic megacolon
- Graft-vs.-host disease
- Caustic gastroduodenal injury
- Gas in wall of an ileal conduit

Small Bowel Obstruction
Common
- Adhesions
- External or internal hernias
- Peritoneal metastases
- Crohn's disease
- Congenital stenosis; atresia; malrotation
- Cystic fibrosis

Less Common
- Iatrogenic; SB intubation
- Intussusception
- Primary SB malignancy
- Intestinal trauma
- Vasculitis
- Gallstone ileus
- Radiation enteritis
- Ischemic enteritis

Rare but Important
- Intestinal parasitic disease
- Meckel diverticulum

(Left) *CT of a man with abdominal distention months after stem cell transplantation shows extensive pneumatosis ➡ but no ascites or ileus. These findings, along with no clinical evidence for bowel ischemia, correctly suggested benign, medication-induced pneumatosis.* **(Right)** *Axial CECT shows diffuse small bowel (SB) wall thickening with near water density submucosal edema and intense mucosal enhancement ➡ in a patient with "shock bowel" following abdominal trauma. This is a form of reversible bowel ischemia.*

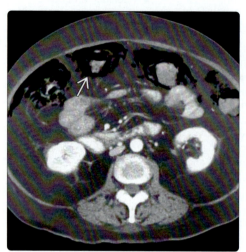
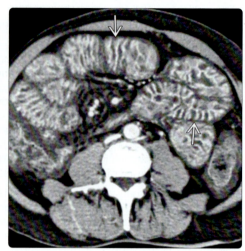

(Left) *CT of a young woman with acute onset of abdominal pain shows wedge-shaped and striated zones of decreased attenuation ➡ within the kidneys.* **(Right)** *CT in the same patient shows long segmental SB wall thickening with submucosal edema ➡. This, along with the renal inflammatory or ischemic changes in a young patient, suggested the diagnosis of vasculitis as the underlying disease process, subsequently confirmed by renal biopsy.*

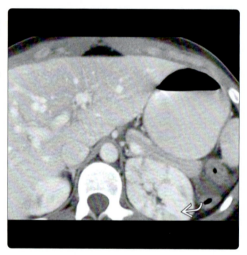
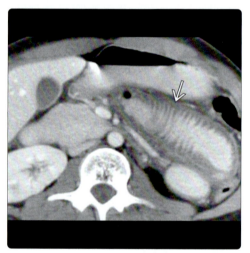

(Left) *CT in a 58-year-old man with malignant melanoma and presenting with acute abdominal pain shows a classic SB intussusception with the intussusceptum and its mesenteric fat and vessels ➡ inside the intussuscipiens ➡.* **(Right)** *CT in the same patient shows the lead point of the intussusception ➡, a metastasis in the wall of the intussusceptum.*

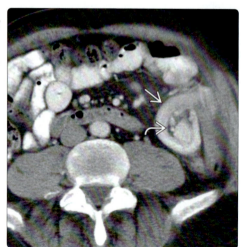
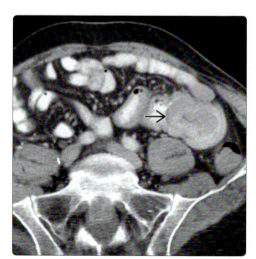

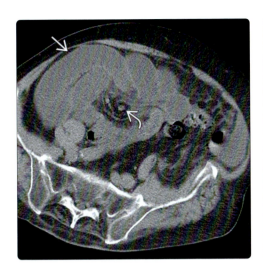
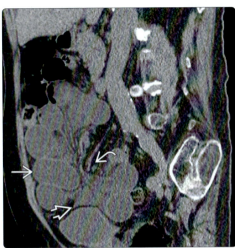

(Left) *NECT in an elderly woman with abdominal pain and vomiting shows a cluster of dilated, fluid-distended SB segments ➡ with twisting and distortion of the mesenteric vessels ⬀. (Right) CT reconstruction shows the dilated SB ➡, arrayed as balloons on strings representing the engorged mesenteric vessels ⬀, classic findings of a closed loop SB obstruction (SBO). Interloop ascites ⬀, mesenteric edema, and poor definition of the SB walls suggest ischemia. Closed loop SBO with infarcted bowel was confirmed at surgery.*

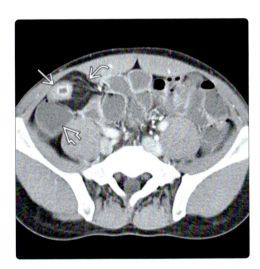
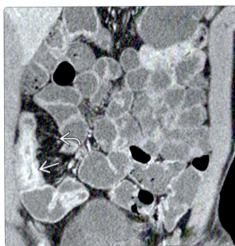

(Left) *CT enterography in a young man with abdominal pain and diarrhea shows good distention of the SB and colon ➡ with water density contrast medium. The SB is normal except for the terminal ileum ➡, which shows luminal narrowing, wall thickening, and mucosal hyperenhancement. Mesenteric vascular engorgement is present ⬀. (Right) Coronal CT in the same patient shows the active inflammation of the terminal ileum ➡ and local fibrofatty proliferation ⬀, typical features of Crohn's disease.*

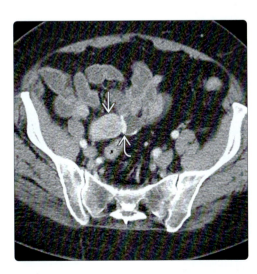
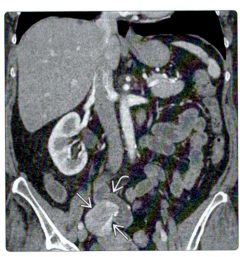

(Left) *CECT enterography in an elderly woman with acute GI bleeding shows a brightly enhancing mass ➡ arising from the ileum. Within the affected segment of bowel, there are high-density foci of extravasated contrast material ⬀ indicating active bleeding from the mass. (Right) Coronal CT in the same patient shows the hypervascular mass ➡ having an endoluminal and exophytic component, arising from an ileal segment ⬀, typical of a GI stromal tumor, confirmed at surgery.*

KEY FACTS

TERMINOLOGY

- Rotational abnormality of gut due to arrest of gut rotation and fixation during fetal development

IMAGING

- Many variations and classifications
- Complete nonrotation
  - Jejunum lies to right of spine
  - Ileum lies to left of spine or in pelvis
- Best imaging studies
  - Upper GI series with small bowel follow-through
  - Normal barium enema does not exclude small bowel malrotation nor volvulus
  - Classic malrotation
    - Cecum lies in midline or to left of midline
    - Fixed in position by adhesive bands from undersurface of liver (Ladd bands)
    - Ladd bands cross duodenum and may cause obstruction

- Oral contrast medium ends abruptly or in corkscrew pattern within duodenum
- CT: Superior mesenteric vein ventral to or to left of superior mesenteric artery
  - Volvulus of midgut indicated by whirlpool or swirl sign of twisted mesenteric vessels and bowel
  - CT shows congenital anomalies and complications (e.g., bowel ischemia)

TOP DIFFERENTIAL DIAGNOSES

- Paraduodenal hernia

CLINICAL ISSUES

- Up to 40% diagnosed by 1 week of age
  - 50% by 1 month
  - 75% by 1 year
  - 25% after 1 year
- Some cases of volvulus or obstruction occur in older children or adults

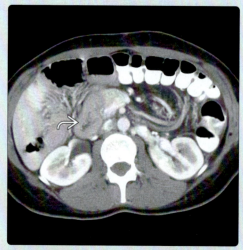 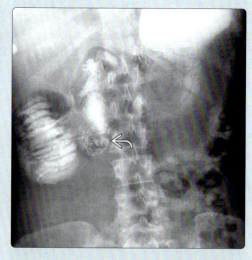

(Left) Axial CECT in a 27-year-old man with pain and vomiting shows all of the small bowel, even the duodenum ➡, lying to the right of midline. The cecum is midline, and the remaining colon lies to the left of midline. (Right) Upper GI series in the same patient shows partial obstruction at the level of the distal duodenum. The duodenum never crosses the midline but has a peculiar Z or corkscrew configuration ➡. Malrotation and duodenal obstruction by bands were confirmed at surgery.

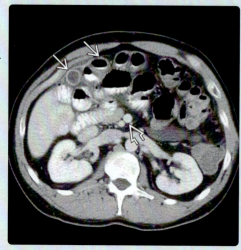 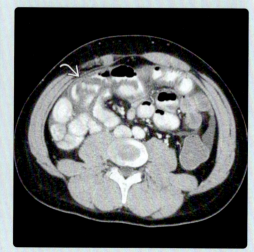

(Left) Axial CECT in a 47-year-old woman presenting with pain shows reversal of the position of the superior mesenteric artery and superior mesenteric vein ➡ with all of the small bowel lying on the right side of the abdomen. Jejunal wall thickening and focal ascites ➡ are noted along with luminal distention. (Right) Axial CECT in the same patient shows additional jejunal segments with mural thickening ➡. The malrotation was confirmed at surgery along with ischemic jejunum that was trapped between adhesions.

Duplication Cyst

TERMINOLOGY

- Named according to GI site from which they arise

IMAGING

- Barium fluoroscopic exams and multiplanar, contrast-enhanced CT are complementary studies
- Most common sites are ileum (33%), esophagus (20%), large bowel (13%), jejunum (10%), stomach (7%), and duodenum (5%)
  o 82% are spherical cysts: No communication with lumen
  o 18% are tubular: Often communicate with lumen of adjacent gut
  o Submucosal or extrinsic mass, indenting or displacing lumen of GI tract

TOP DIFFERENTIAL DIAGNOSES

- Depends on location of cyst and imaging modality
  o Stomach or duodenum: Pancreatic pseudocyst or cystic tumor
  o Ileum: Meckel diverticulum
  o Various sites: Cystic degeneration of solid mass

PATHOLOGY

- Usually lined by GI tract epithelium with smooth muscle in wall
  o Ectopic mucosa within cysts includes gastric, squamous, transitional, and ciliated mucosa
- Associated: Vertebral anomalies, esophageal atresia, other GI tract duplications

CLINICAL ISSUES

- Most are discovered in infancy or early childhood
  o Most common symptoms are related to luminal obstruction (tracheal compression, painful abdominal cramps, dysphagia, constipation)
  o Large cysts in neonates are easily palpable
- Symptoms: Usually low grade and chronic in adults (bleeding, pain, obstruction)

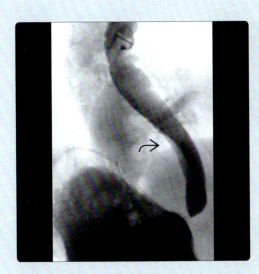
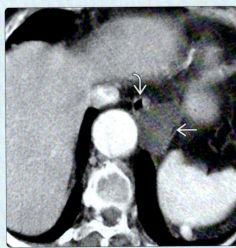

(Left) Spot film from esophagram in an elderly man with an esophageal duplication cyst shows deviation of the distal 1/3 of the esophagus ➡, suggesting an extrinsic mass. (Right) Axial CECT in the same patient shows a water-density mass ➡ indenting the wall of the distal esophagus ➡. Most duplication cysts have a similar spherical or tubular morphology with near water-density, nonenhancing contents.

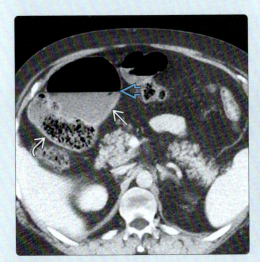
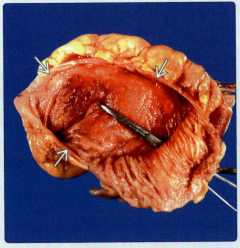

(Left) Axial CECT in a 48-year-old man with chronic painful abdominal cramps shows a large mass ➡ in communication with the bowel, accounting for the air-fluid levels ➡ within it. The mass results in partial small bowel obstruction, accounting for the small bowel feces sign ➡ and dilation of upstream loops. (Right) Gross pathology photograph of the same patient shows the opened cyst ➡ with a probe passing from the lumen of the ileum into the cyst, demonstrating its communication.

TERMINOLOGY

- Ileal outpouching due to persistence of omphalomesenteric or vitelline duct
  - 50% contain ectopic gastric mucosa
  - 90% present with GI bleeding in children

IMAGING

- Rule of 2s
  - Seen in ~ 2% of population
  - Located within 2 feet of ileocecal valve
  - Length of 2 inches (on average)
  - Symptomatic usually before age 2
  - 2 main complications in adults: Diverticulitis (20%) and intestinal obstruction (40%)
- Scintigraphic "Meckel scan": Tc-99m pertechnetate
  - More valuable for diagnosis in children; indirectly detects aberrant gastric mucosa
  - Children often present with pain and GI bleeding

- For diagnosis in adults: Multiplanar, contrast-enhanced CT
  - Adult presentation: Meckel diverticulitis or bowel perforation
  - Meckel diverticulitis
    - Mural thickening and hyperenhancement of MD
    - Diverticulum may perforate
      - Extraluminal gas and lymphadenopathy
      - Mesenteric fat infiltration and fluid
  - ± partial or complete small bowel obstruction
    - Inflammation of adjacent small bowel may cause spasm
    - Inverted diverticulum may form lead mass to intussusception
  - Blind-ending pouch containing fluid, air, &/or particulate matter (including calculi)

TOP DIFFERENTIAL DIAGNOSES

- Appendicitis and other causes of acute RLQ pain in adults

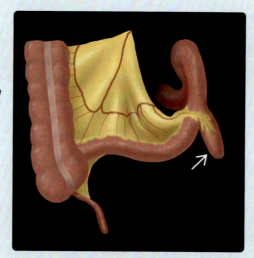
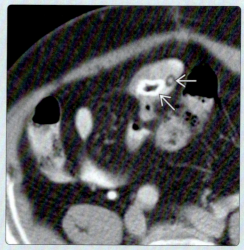

(Left) Graphic shows a blind-ended outpouching ➔ from the antimesenteric border of the distal ileum, typical of a Meckel diverticulum. (Right) Axial CECT shows enteroliths ➔ within a blind-ended sac in the right lower quadrant that proved to be a Meckel diverticulum at surgery.

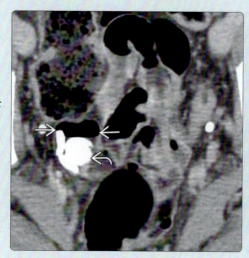
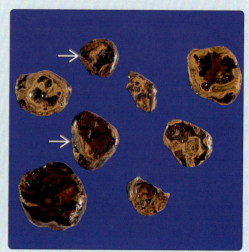

(Left) Axial CECT in a 27-year-old man with right lower quadrant pain shows calcified enteroliths ➔ lying within a blind-ending sac ➔ in the RLQ. (Right) Surgery confirmed a Meckel diverticulum with mild chronic inflammation of the wall and multiple calcified enteroliths ➔ within it.

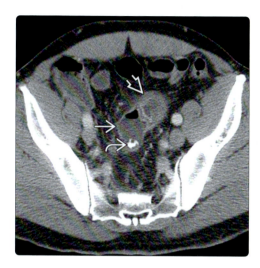
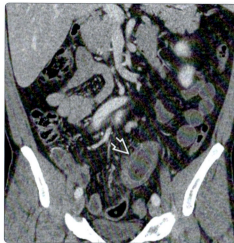

(Left) *Axial CT shows a dilated small bowel with wall thickening* ➡ *of a distal small bowel segment. An adjacent blind-ending sac* ➡ *represents the Meckel diverticulum that contains calcified enteroliths* ➡ *in its dependent portion. Meckel diverticulitis was confirmed at surgery.* (Right) *Coronal reformatted CT in the same patient shows the inflamed and obstructed small bowel segment* ➡ *that was adherent to the Meckel diverticulum.*

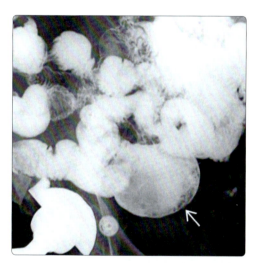
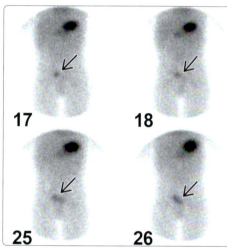

(Left) *Film from a barium small bowel follow-through shows a blind-ending pouch* ➡ *arising from the distal ileum. Barium mixes with enteric debris within the diverticulum, which shows no evidence of obstruction or perforation. Like most Meckel diverticula, especially in adults, this one was probably an asymptomatic incidental finding.* (Right) *Tc-99m pertechnetate scan from a child with GI bleeding and pain shows accumulation of isotope* ➡ *in the RLQ due to ectopic gastric mucosa within a Meckel diverticulum.*

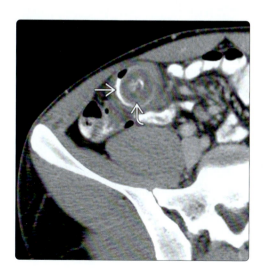
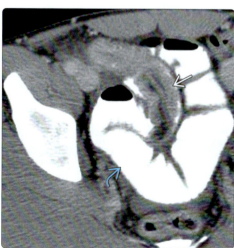

(Left) *Axial CECT in a 17-year-old girl with painful abdominal cramps and RLQ tenderness shows a distal ileal intussusception. The intussuscepted segment* ➡ *is outlined by contrast within the lumen of the intussuscipiens* ➡. (Right) *Axial CECT in the same patient shows a long-segment intussusception* ➡ *with dilation of the small bowel upstream* ➡, *due to obstruction. An inverted Meckel diverticulum was found as the lead mass at surgery.*

Small Intestine

IMAGING

- **Small bowel follow-through**
  - Relatively inexpensive and well tolerated
  - Patient drinks large volume of barium; fluoroscopic spot films and other radiographs follow course of barium throughout small bowel to colon
- **Enteroclysis**
  - Most sensitive, more expensive, less comfortable, identifies smaller diverticula
- **CT enterography**
  - May be more difficult to distinguish diverticula from bowel segments
  - Multiplanar reformations can help recognition
  - Extraluminal gas, fluid, inflammatory infiltration = diverticulitis (usually with perforation)
  - Portal venous gas may result from septic mesenteric or portal vein thrombophlebitis (rather than ischemia)

TOP DIFFERENTIAL DIAGNOSES

- Crohn's disease
- Intestinal scleroderma
- Meckel diverticulum

CLINICAL ISSUES

- Most common signs/symptoms: Usually asymptomatic unless perforated
- Diverticulitis: Usually result of perforation of diverticulum
- Malabsorption or anemia
  - Stasis within large or numerous diverticula with bacterial overgrowth
  - Bacteria consume vitamins (including B12) and nutrients
- Bleeding
  - Thin-walled vessels in wall of diverticulum may bleed
- Small bowel obstruction
  - Large diverticula may cause adhesions, intussusception, or volvulus

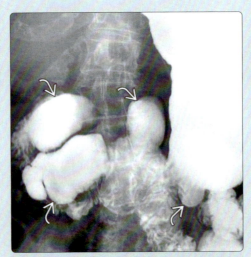
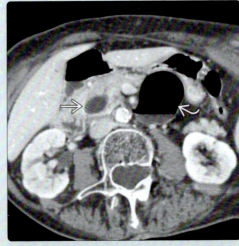

(Left) Small bowel follow-through shows multiple large duodenal and small bowel diverticula ➡ in a patient with no relevant symptoms. (Right) Axial CECT in the same patient shows 1 of the large diverticula as a thin-walled cystic structure with a gas-fluid level ➡. One of the duodenal diverticula ➡ is fluid-filled and might be mistaken for a cystic lesion in the head of the pancreas.

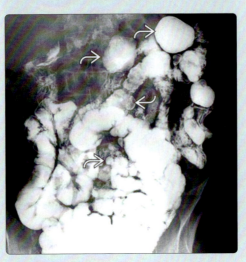
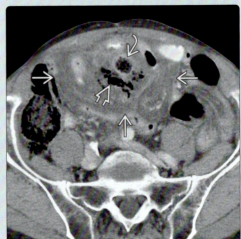

(Left) Small bowel follow-through performed at a time when the patient was asymptomatic shows several small bowel diverticula ➡. (Right) Axial CECT at a time of acute symptoms in the same patient shows extraluminal gas and fluid ➡ with a large inflammatory process ➡ centered in the small bowel mesentery. A diverticulum filled with gas and particulate debris is seen ➡. A perforated diverticulum and mesenteric abscess were confirmed at surgery.

Gallstone Ileus

TERMINOLOGY

- Mechanical bowel obstruction due to impacted gallstone(s)

IMAGING

- **Best imaging study: Multiplanar contrast-enhanced CT**
  - Rigler triad of small bowel obstruction, gas in biliary tree, and ectopic gallstone
  - Described on plain film interpretation; better seen on CT
- CT findings
  - Gallstone surrounded by gas in bowel loop
    - Cholesterol stones are near water density, often with calcified rim
  - Collapsed gallbladder (GB), pneumobilia (gas within GB ± bile duct lumen)
  - Dilated bowel with transition to collapsed bowel at impacted gallstone
- Location: Stone obstructs at points of luminal narrowing; duodenum, ligament of Treitz, ileocecal valve, sigmoid colon

PATHOLOGY

- Occurs with chronic cholecystitis
- Diagnosis is frequently delayed or missed
- May occur as a complication of ERCP

CLINICAL ISSUES

- Most common signs/symptoms: Fever, distension, obstipation
  - Intermittent acute colicky abdominal pain (20-30%)
  - Nausea, vomiting; abdominal distention
- Gallstone erodes into inflamed GB wall, passes into GI tract (usually duodenum) → bowel obstruction

DIAGNOSTIC CHECKLIST

- Consider in elderly woman with recurrent right upper quadrant pain, recently more severe, with prolonged vomiting

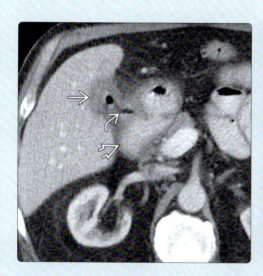
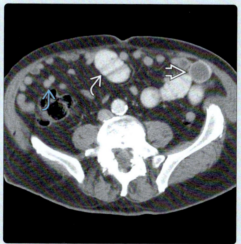

(Left) Axial CECT in a 65-year-old woman presenting with crampy abdominal pain demonstrates a thick-walled gallbladder ➡ with air within its lumen and a gas-filled fistula ➡ to the duodenum ➡. (Right) Axial CECT in the same patient identifies the obstructing gallstone ➡, which is impacted in the distal jejunum. The cholesterol stone is low density with a calcified rim. The proximal small bowel ➡ is dilated, while the distal small bowel ➡ and colon are collapsed.

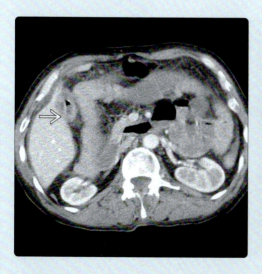
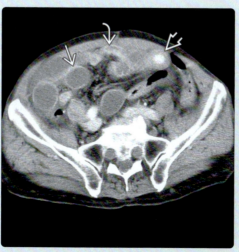

(Left) Axial CECT in a patient presenting with bloating and abdominal pain demonstrates gas within a thick-walled gallbladder ➡, a typical finding in gallstone ileus, also known as gallstone obstruction. (Right) Axial CECT in the same patient demonstrates dilation of the proximal small bowel ➡ and decompressed, nondilated distal small bowel ➡. The high-density obstructing gallstone ➡ is seen, as a laminated calcification, at the site of transition from the dilated to the decompressed bowel.

KEY FACTS

TERMINOLOGY

- Proportional gaseous dilatation of large and small bowel (SB) due to lack of intestinal peristalsis, not mechanical obstruction

IMAGING

- CT or abdominal plain films (supine, upright, decubitus)
- Proportional dilatation of SB and colon with no transition point
  - SB > 3 cm on plain films, 2.5 cm on CT
  - Air-fluid levels on upright and decubitus films

TOP DIFFERENTIAL DIAGNOSES

- SB or colonic obstruction
- Intestinal pseudoobstruction
- Ogilvie syndrome
- Aerophagia

CLINICAL ISSUES

- Postoperative ileus is most common cause of delayed discharge from hospital
  - Usually resolves spontaneously in 3-7 days
- Most common signs/symptoms
  - Tympanic abdomen on percussion, lack of flatus
  - Gaseous distension, abdominal pain, nausea, and vomiting
  - Absence of bowel sounds on auscultation
- Treatment
  - Treat underlying etiology (e.g., hypokalemia, sepsis)
  - IV fluids, nasogastric suction

DIAGNOSTIC CHECKLIST

- Pitfalls: Ileus plus ascites, and recent bowel surgery, mimic small bowel obstruction (SBO) on plain films
  - CT can be used to resolve issue if necessary

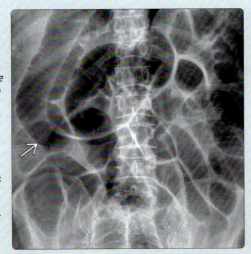
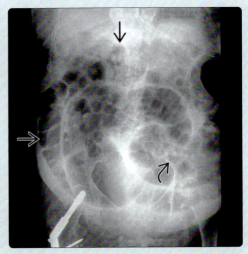

(Left) Supine abdominal radiograph in an 88-year-old man with abdominal distension and hypokalemia from diuretic use shows proportional dilation ➡ of the large and small bowel with no clear transition point. The ileus resolved with electrolyte replacement. (Right) Supine radiograph in a 90-year-old woman with abdominal distension and pain following a hip "pinning" shows gaseous dilation of the colon ➡ and the small bowel ➡ in a uniform pattern with no point of transition.

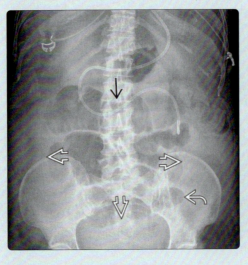
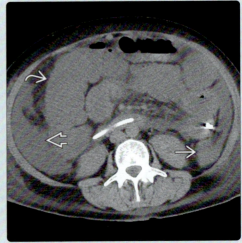

(Left) This 52-year-old woman has cirrhosis with increasing abdominal distention and nausea. A supine abdominal film, requested to evaluate possible SBO, shows a dilated transverse colon ➡ and small bowel ➡, but no gas in other colon segments. Ascites ➡ fills the pelvis and paracolic gutters. (Right) CT in the same patient shows ascites ➡ and fluid-distended bowel ➡. Gas fills only a portion of the nondependent bowel, while the dependent SB & colon ➡ are fluid-filled & less dilated. This may be misinterpreted as SB obstruction.

TERMINOLOGY

Definitions

- Proportional gaseous dilatation of large and small bowel (SB) due to lack of intestinal peristalsis, not mechanical obstruction

IMAGING

General Features

- Best diagnostic clue
  - Proportional dilatation of large and small intestine on plain films with no transition point

Imaging Recommendations

- Best imaging tool
  - Plain abdominal radiography, including supine and upright or decubitus views
  - Multiplanar CT is more accurate with fewer imaging pitfalls
- Protocol advice
  - Oral contrast may not be tolerated and is rarely necessary for CT

Radiographic Findings

- Radiography
  - Symmetric dilatation of large and small bowel
    - SB diameter > 3 cm (larger than on CT measurements due to magnification on plain radiography)
  - Air-fluid levels on upright and decubitus films
  - **Pitfall: Ileus plus ascites mimic small bowel obstruction (SBO)**
    - Gas collects mostly in mesenteric bowel (SB, transverse, and sigmoid colon)
    - Retroperitoneal colon segments remain mostly gas-free, invisible on supine films
    - CT can easily resolve this, showing generalized dilation of SB and colon without transition point
  - **Recent bowel surgery; plain film findings mimic SBO**
    - SB will be dilated to point of bowel incision
    - This can be form of ileus and usually resolves spontaneously

Fluoroscopic Findings

- Upper GI
  - Delayed transit of contrast through SB
  - No mechanical obstruction or transition to collapsed SB
- Contrast enema
  - No colonic obstruction
  - Contrast flows to ileocecal valve without difficulty

CT Findings

- Dilated large and SB
  - SB diameter > 2.5 cm

DIFFERENTIAL DIAGNOSIS

Small Bowel or Colonic Obstruction

- Bowel dilated upstream from transition point, obstructing lesion
- SB feces sign found just proximal to point of obstruction

Intestinal Pseudoobstruction

- Etiologies include
  - Visceral myopathy or neuropathy
  - Degenerative neurologic disorders (Parkinson disease)
  - Scleroderma

Ogilvie Syndrome

- Acute colonic pseudoobstruction (common in postoperative and septic patients)
- Often involves right colon and cecum > transverse colon

Aerophagia

- Air-swallowing, common in hospitalized patients
- Especially those with enteric feeding tubes
- Excess gas within nondilated stomach, SB, colon

PATHOLOGY

General Features

- Etiology
  - Abdominal surgery, general anesthesia
  - Opioid (narcotic) drug use
  - Electrolyte disturbance (especially hypokalemia), hypothyroidism
  - Stress-induced sympathetic reflexes, cytokine-mediated inflammatory factors
  - Sepsis (especially peritonitis), mesenteric ischemia, ureteral colic
  - Retroperitoneal hemorrhage, acute myocardial infarction, spinal cord injury

CLINICAL ISSUES

Presentation

- Most common signs/symptoms
  - Gaseous distension, abdominal pain, nausea, and vomiting
- Other signs/symptoms
  - Constipation, bloating, lack of bowel sounds on auscultation
  - Tympanic abdomen on percussion, lack of flatus

Demographics

- Epidemiology
  - **Postoperative ileus is most common cause of delayed discharge from hospital**

Natural History & Prognosis

- Postoperative ileus most often resolves spontaneously in 3-7 days; persistent or ↑ bowel dilation should prompt intervention

Treatment

- Treat underlying etiology (e.g., hypokalemia, sepsis)
- IV fluids, nasogastric suction

SELECTED REFERENCES

1. Blumenfeld YJ et al: Risk factors for prolonged postpartum length of stay following cesarean delivery. Am J Perinatol. ePub, 2015
2. Gan TJ et al: Impact of postsurgical opioid use and ileus on economic outcomes in gastrointestinal surgeries. Curr Med Res Opin. 1-28, 2015
3. Moss G: The etiology and prevention of feeding intolerance paralytic ileus - revisiting an old concept. Ann Surg Innov Res. 3:3, 2009

Small Bowel Obstruction

TERMINOLOGY

- Obstruction or blockage of ≥ 1 small bowel (SB) segments by intrinsic or extrinsic narrowing of SB lumen

IMAGING

- SB > 3 cm diameter on radiographs, 2.5 cm on CT
  - Air-fluid levels on upright or decubitus radiograph
- **Small bowel feces** sign: Gas bubbles mixed with particulate matter in dilated loops just proximal to site of obstruction
- **Closed loop obstruction**
  - SB segments are usually markedly distended (> 4 cm) by fluid, little gas
  - Relatively little dilatation of bowel proximal to closed loop obstruction
  - **Whirl sign** due to tightly twisted mesenteric vessels
  - "**Balloons-on-strings**": Dilated SB tethered by stretched mesenteric vessels
- **Strangulating SBO**: Impaired blood supply to SB
  - Absent, decreased, or delayed bowel wall enhancement

  - Bowel wall thickening (edema or hemorrhage)
  - Mesenteric and interloop edema ± ascites
  - Vessels: Congested, thrombosed, or obscured
  - Obscured margins among affected SB segments

TOP DIFFERENTIAL DIAGNOSES

- Adynamic or paralytic ileus
- Colonic obstruction
- Cystic fibrosis

CLINICAL ISSUES

- Most common causes: Adhesions (~ 60%), hernias (15%), tumors (~ 15%; metastases > primary tumor)
- Up to 80% of adhesive SBOs resolve spontaneously
- Mortality is ~100% for untreated strangulated SBOs

DIAGNOSTIC CHECKLIST

- CT diagnosis of closed loop or strangulated (ischemic) SBO is crucial for directing prompt surgical intervention
- **Know the CT signs for closed loop or ischemic SBO**

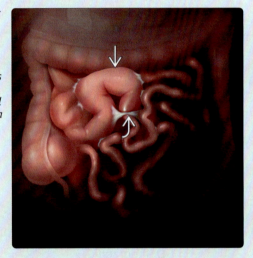
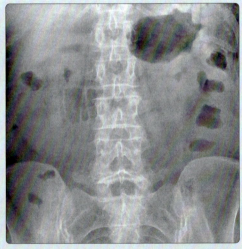

(Left) *Anteroposterior graphic depiction of a small bowel obstruction (SBO) due to an adhesive band is shown. Note the dilation of the proximal small bowel (SB)* ➡ *as well as the adhesive band* ➡. *(Right) In this patient with abdominal pain, distention, and nausea, a supine film of the abdomen shows no obvious dilation of SB.*

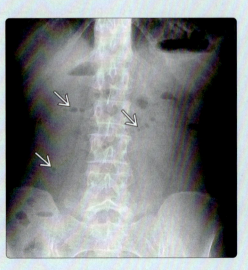
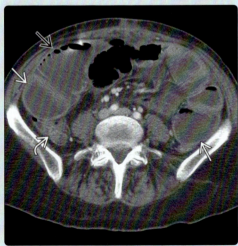

(Left) *An upright film in the same patient shows a string-of-pearls sign* ➡, *indicating gas within fluid-distended, obstructed segments of SB. (Right) Axial CT section in the same patient shows collapsed distal SB* ➡, *but massive dilation of proximal SB segments* ➡ *with only small bubbles of intraluminal air* ➡, *accounting for the string-of-pearls sign. An adhesive SBO was confirmed at surgery.*

Small Bowel Obstruction

TERMINOLOGY

Abbreviations

- Small bowel obstruction (SBO)

IMAGING

General Features

- Best diagnostic clue
  - Identification of transition zone between dilated and collapsed bowel is critical to define presence, site, and cause of obstruction (all better determined on CT than on plain films)
- Size
  - Small bowel loops > 3 cm diameter on radiographs, 2.5 cm on CT (due to magnification effect on plain films)

Radiographic Findings

- Radiography
  - Supine abdomen with upright or decubitus views
    - Dilated SB loops with air-fluid levels on upright or decubitus radiograph
  - Can miss SBO (fluid-distended bowel not evident on plain films)
  - String-of-pearls sign: Small air bubbles within fluid-distended bowel seen on supine view

Fluoroscopic Findings

- Enteroclysis or SB series
  - Passage of contrast into colon excludes complete SBO
  - Transition may define location, degree, cause of obstruction
    - e.g., angulated segment with distortion of folds suggests adhesive SBO

CT Findings

- Dilated SB loops > 2.5 cm diameter ± air-fluid levels
- **Small bowel feces sign**: Gas bubbles mixed with particulate matter in dilated loops just proximal to site of obstruction
- **Extrinsic lesions**
  - Adhesions
    - Short, abrupt transition, angulation of course of SB, minimal mural thickening
    - Adhesions themselves are not identified on CT
    - Adhesive SBO is diagnosis of exclusion; no hernia, mass, intussusception
  - Hernia
    - External hernias (inguinal, femoral, spigelian, obturator, etc.)
      - □ Most common type of hernia to cause SBO
    - Internal hernia: Cluster of dilated SB segments; crowding, twisting, displacement of mesenteric vessels, ± mesenteric edema
    - Dilated segment of SB leading into hernia; collapsed segment leaving hernia
    - Strangulated hernia: Thickened bowel wall ± intramural hemorrhage
  - Peritoneal carcinomatosis: Omental and peritoneal masses, dilated bowel loops, multiple transition zones
    - Metastases may cause luminal obstruction or functional obstruction due to serosal coating (impairs peristalsis)

- Other inflammatory causes (appendicitis, diverticulitis, etc.)
- **Intrinsic lesions**
  - Malignant tumor (adenocarcinoma, GIST, carcinoid, etc.)
    - Thickened enhancing wall and luminal narrowing at transition zone
  - Crohn's disease
    - Mucosal hyperenhancement, submucosal edema over long segment of distal SB
  - Intussusception
    - Bowel-within-bowel
    - Layers of bowel wall interspersed with mesenteric fat and vessels
  - Other infectious, ischemic, or inflammatory
    - e.g., radiation or ischemic stricture, tuberculous enterocolitis
- **Intraluminal lesions**: Gallstones, foreign bodies, bezoars, *Ascaris*
  - Classic triad: Ectopic calcified stone and gas in gallbladder/biliary tree and SBO = gallstone ileus
  - Bezoar: Intraluminal mass with air in interstices at point of transition
- **Closed loop obstruction**: Obstruction at 2 points, involves mesentery
  - Usually due to internal hernia or adhesions
  - Affected SB segments are usually markedly distended (> 4 cm) by fluid, little gas
  - Relatively little dilatation of bowel proximal to closed loop obstruction
  - Mesenteric vessels converging toward site of torsion
  - Beak sign: Fusiform tapering at point of torsion/obstruction
  - Volvulus: C-shaped, U-shaped, or "coffee bean" SB configuration
    - **Whirl sign** due to tightly twisted mesenteric vessels
    - **"Balloons-on-strings"**: Appearance of dilated SB tethered by stretched mesenteric vessels
- **Strangulating SBO**: Blood flow to affected SB is blocked
  - Absent, decreased, or delayed bowel wall enhancement in affected SB
  - Bowel wall thickening (edema or hemorrhage)
    - High density of SB wall on NECT = hemorrhage = ischemia
  - Mesenteric and interloop edema ± ascites
  - Combination of factors obscures margins among affected SB segments
  - Mesenteric vessels: Congested, thrombosed, or obscured by adjacent edema

Imaging Recommendations

- Best imaging tool
  - Multiplanar CECT: Sensitivity 95%, specificity 96% in high-grade SBO
    - CT evaluation is mandatory in patients with history of inflammatory bowel disease or cancer, or:
      - □ Suspected bowel ischemia
      - □ Suspected abdominal sepsis
- Protocol advice
  - **Administration of positive oral contrast medium is rarely useful** and may impede CT detection of complications of SBO, such as ischemia

(Left) This patient had a prior surgical history and now presents with nausea and vomiting. Axial CT shows the dilated proximal SB ➡ and decompressed bowel ➡ distal to the transition site. **(Right)** A coronal-reformatted CT in the same patient shows the transition ➡ from dilated to collapsed SB. No mass, hernia, or other specific cause was identified, leading to the inference that this was an adhesive SBO, subsequently confirmed at surgery.

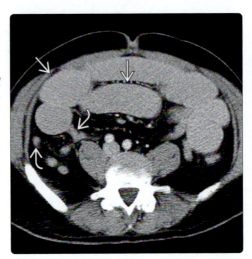
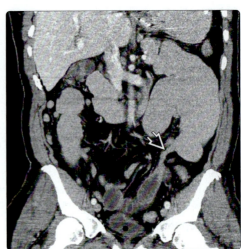

(Left) This elderly woman has abdominal pain, distention, and vomiting. Axial CT shows markedly dilated proximal SB segments ➡, while distal SB and colon are decompressed ➡. **(Right)** A more caudal CT section in the same patient shows dilated SB ➡ entering a right femoral hernia, the site and cause of the obstruction.

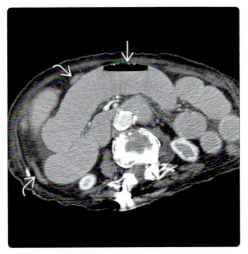
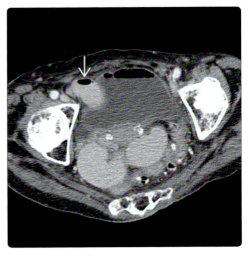

(Left) A more caudal CT section in the same patient shows a "knuckle" of SB ➡ trapped within the femoral hernia, establishing this as the transition point and etiology of the SBO. **(Right)** A coronal-reformatted CT section in the same patient shows the transition point, as the dilated SB ➡ enters the right femoral hernia ➡. Hernias are the 2nd most common etiology for SBO, though much less common than adhesive SBO.

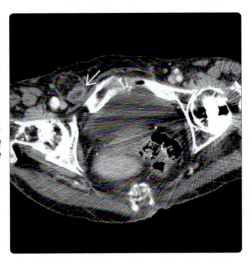
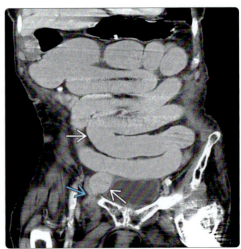

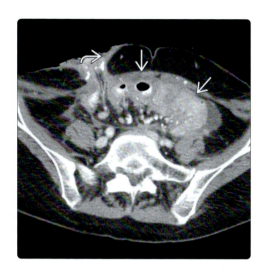

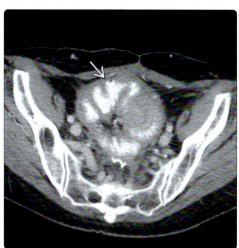

(Left) *This woman has metastatic ovarian carcinoma and has had prior bowel resection and ileostomy for SBO. CT shows the ileostomy ➡ and SB segments that are matted together ➡ without definable mesenteric fat between SB segments.* (Right) *Another CT section in the same patient shows SB loops that are encased and angulated ➡ due to serosal implants of recurrent ovarian carcinoma. Almost 1/2 of all women with ovarian carcinoma will develop symptoms of SBO.*

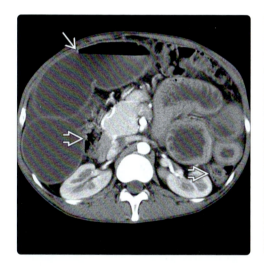

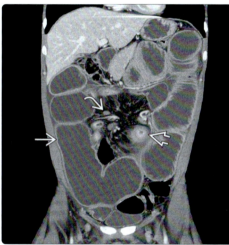

(Left) *This young man has longstanding Crohn's disease with progressive abdominal distention and pain. Axial CT shows massive dilation of some SB segments, some of which have air-fluid levels ➡. The colon ➡ is decompressed.* (Right) *Coronal CT section in the same patient shows the dilated, more proximal SB ➡ with the transition point being more distal SB, featuring mucosal hyperenhancement, submucosal edema, and luminal narrowing ➡. Mesenteric lymphadenopathy ➡ is another typical feature of Crohn's disease.*

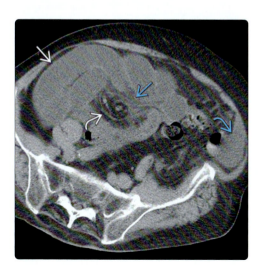

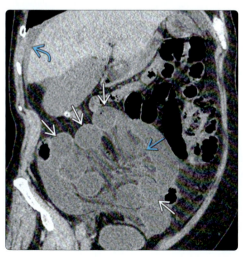

(Left) *In this elderly man with abdominal pain & distention, CT shows dilated, fluid-filled SB ➡ and a whirl sign ➡, twisting of the SB mesenteric vessels. Mesenteric edema ➡ and ascites ➡ are also noted, all indicative of closed loop SBO with bowel ischemia.* (Right) *Coronal CT in the same patient shows a "balloons-on-strings" appearance of the fluid-distended SB segments ➡ tethered by their stretched mesenteric vessels. Mesenteric edema ➡ and ascites ➡ are noted. A closed loop SBO with ischemic SB was confirmed at surgery.*

Mesenteric Adenitis and Enteritis

TERMINOLOGY

- Benign inflammation of lymph nodes in ileocolic mesentery, often with terminal ileitis

IMAGING

- **Multiplanar, contrast-enhanced CT is optimal imaging test**
  - **Sonography (US) is preferred 1st-line imaging in children & young women**
- Cluster of mildly enlarged ileocolic mesenteric lymph nodes (≥ 5 mm)
  - Mesenteric adenopathy is often much more evident on coronal-reformatted CT
- Ileal ± cecal wall thickening, sometimes with regional ileus
  - Mucosal hyperenhancement, submucosal edema
- **Normal-appearing appendix (essential for confident diagnosis)**

TOP DIFFERENTIAL DIAGNOSES

- Appendicitis
- Crohn's disease
  - Early Crohn's disease may be impossible to distinguish
  - Time course & likelihood of recurrence are different
- Cecal or appendiceal carcinoma
  - Affects older adults, not children

PATHOLOGY

- Reactive lymph node enlargement secondary to enteric pathogens
- Viral (most common)
- Bacterial (especially *Yersinia* & *Campylobacter* species)

CLINICAL ISSUES

- **Common cause of RLQ pain in children & young adults (~ 10%)**
- Pain, fever, nausea, vomiting; leukocytosis
- Self-limited, usually resolves without treatment

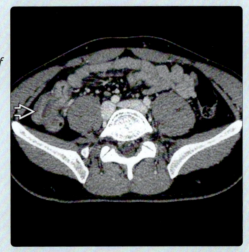
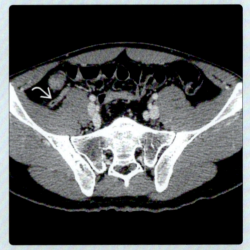

(Left) *Axial CECT in a 25-year-old woman presenting with fever and RLQ tenderness shows wall thickening and mucosal hyperenhancement of the terminal ileum and cecum ⟹. (Right) Another CECT section in the same patient shows a normal appendix ⟹, excluding appendicitis as the diagnosis.*

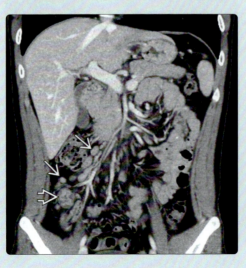
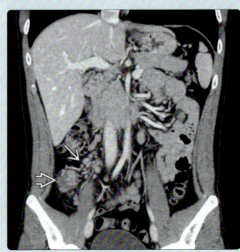

(Left) *Coronal reformatted CECT in the same patient shows a cluster of mildly enlarged, ileocolic mesenteric nodes ⟹ along with the thick-walled, inflamed terminal ileum ⟹. (Right) Another coronal CECT section shows enlarged nodes and engorged vessels in the ileocolic mesentery ⟹ along with the thick-walled terminal ileum ⟹. These are classic imaging and CT features of mesenteric adenitis and enteritis, and the patient made an uneventful recovery without specific therapy.*

Intestinal Lymphangiectasia

TERMINOLOGY

- Primary intestinal lymphangiectasia (Waldmann disease)
  - Rare congenital disorder characterized by hypoproteinemia, peripheral edema, and lymphocytopenia resulting from loss of lymphatic fluid into intestine
  - Important cause of protein-losing enteropathy
- Secondary: Much more common
  - Causes include mesenteric or retroperitoneal node dissection (obliterates lymphatics)
  - Right heart failure; fibrosing mesenteritis; retroperitoneal fibrosis are also implicated

IMAGING

- **Contrast-enhanced, multiplanar CT is 1st-line imaging test**
- Diffuse small bowel (SB) wall thickening with submucosal edema
- Infiltration of small bowel mesentery

- ± mesenteric and retroperitoneal lymphadenopathy
- ± short segment, nonobstructing SB intussusceptions
- For secondary form of lymphangiectasia
  - May see signs of surgery, cardiac failure, retroperitoneal fibrosis or tumor, tuberculosis, etc.

TOP DIFFERENTIAL DIAGNOSES

- Whipple disease, lymphoma, intestinal opportunistic infections

PATHOLOGY

- Both primary & secondary forms result in decreased absorption of chylomicrons and fat-soluble vitamins, excessive leakage of lymph into bowel lumen, and excessive loss of protein
- Laboratory findings: Low serum albumen, gamma globulins, cholesterol, fat-soluble vitamins
- Diagnosis is made by intestinal biopsy

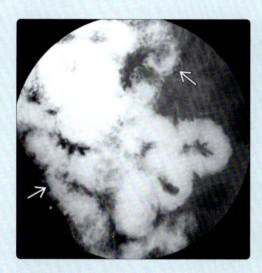

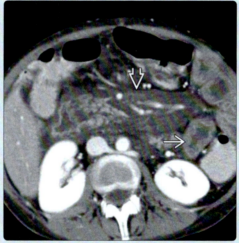

(Left) This young man had lower extremity edema, hypoproteinemia, and diarrhea. A film from a small bowel (SB) follow-through shows diffuse, nodular, thickened folds ➡ throughout the entire SB, proven to be due to lymphangiectasia. (Right) This 36-year-old woman presented with chronic diarrhea and lower extremity edema. CT shows fluid-distended SB with submucosal edema ➡. More striking is the marked edema within the mesentery ➡.

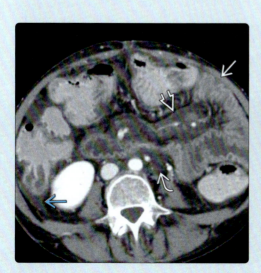

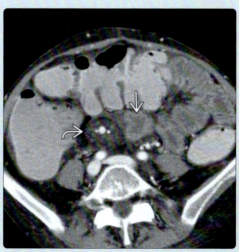

(Left) CT in the same patient shows more of the SB wall thickening ➡ and mesenteric edema ➡ as well as ascites ➡ and enlarged, low density lymph nodes ➡. (Right) CT in the same patient shows more of the fluid-distended SB ➡ and colon and additional hypodense nodes or infiltration at the root of the SB mesentery ➡. Intestinal lymphangiectasia was the final diagnosis.

TERMINOLOGY

- Symptomatic gastrointestinal infection of immunocompromised host by organisms that usually cause no or minor illness in immunocompetent individuals

IMAGING

- **Contrast-enhanced, multiplanar CT**
- **Cytomegalovirus**
  - Favors distal small bowel (SB) and colon
  - Mucosal hyper- or hypoenhancement; submucosal edema
  - Infiltration of mesenteric fat
  - Lymphadenopathy is very uncommon
- **Mycobacterial**
  - *Mycobacterium avium-intracellulare*: Thickened SB folds with relatively little submucosal edema
  - *Mycobacterium tuberculosis*: Favors ileocecal distribution
  - Mesenteric lymphadenopathy, often with low density (caseation)

- Exudative ascites (may mimic peritoneal carcinomatosis)
- **Protozoan** (*Cryptosporidium*, Microsporidia, and *Giardia*)
  - Duodenum and jejunum, sparing distal SB and colon
  - Fold thickening without much submucosal edema
  - Excess fluid (luminal distention) of proximal SB
  - No ascites; uncommon lymphadenopathy
- **Bacterial** (*Clostridium difficile* colitis, *Campylobacter*, and others)
  - Segmental or, more commonly, pancolitis
  - Striking mucosal hyperenhancement and submucosal edema
  - Ascites (present in 40% of cases)
  - May progress to toxic megacolon or perforation

DIAGNOSTIC CHECKLIST

- Specific diagnosis can be suggested by CT (with IV, not oral, contrast medium)
- Diagnosis depends on microbiological confirmation by analysis of bowel content, serologic markers, or even biopsy

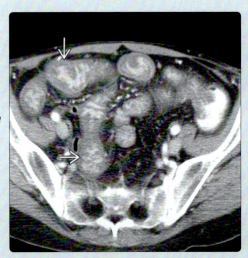
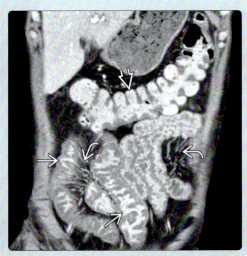

(Left) *This young woman has cystic fibrosis and lung transplantation with new onset diarrhea. Axial CECT shows mucosal hyperenhancement and submucosal edema ➡ affecting most of the small bowel.* (Right) *Coronal CECT in the same patient shows the widespread enteritis ➡ with engorged mesenteric vessels ⬏. The colon ⬌ is spared. Endoscopy and biopsy confirmed cytomegalovirus (CMV) enteritis.*

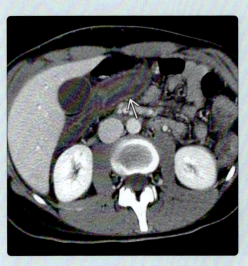
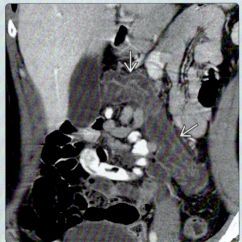

(Left) *This 35-year-old man with AIDS developed profuse diarrhea and abdominal pain. Axial CECT shows pancolitis with marked submucosal edema ➡ but no hyperenhancement of the mucosa.* (Right) *Coronal CECT in the same patient shows more evidence of pancolitis ➡, proven to be due to CMV, which may induce ischemic injury to both the small bowel and colon in immunocompromised patients.*

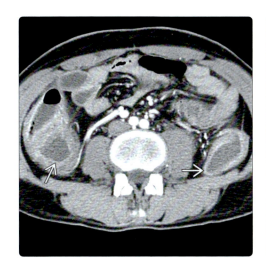

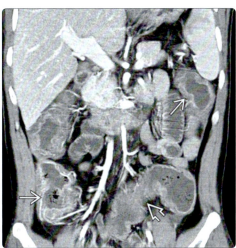

(Left) *Axial CECT in a 34-year-old HIV-positive man presenting with diarrhea shows the typical appearance of CMV colitis. Note the diffuse thickening of the colon wall and mucosal hyperenhancement* ➡ *with fluid-distended lumen (diarrhea).* (Right) *Coronal CECT in the same patient illustrates the global nature of this colitis with involvement of the ascending and descending colon* ➡ *as well as sigmoid* ➡*. CMV colitis infects an immunocompromised host with a virus that causes vasculitis.*

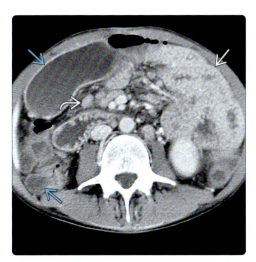

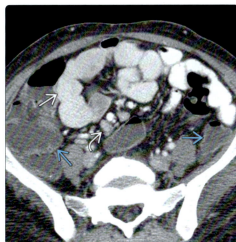

(Left) *Axial CECT in a young man with HIV and intractable diarrhea shows the typical appearance of Mycobacterium avium-intracellulare (MAI) enteritis. Note marked mucosal enhancement* ➡ *and mesenteric adenopathy* ➡ *with fluid-distended bowel* ➡*.* (Right) *This young woman is HIV-positive with new-onset diarrhea. Axial CECT shows fluid distention of both small* ➡ *and large bowel* ➡ *along with mesenteric lymphadenopathy* ➡*. Cryptosporidium was the causative organism and typically causes diarrhea.*

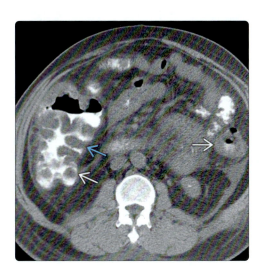

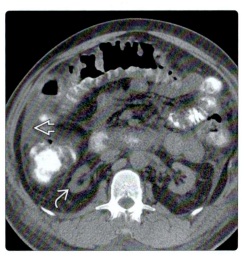

(Left) *This man has a functioning renal allograft and developed acute bloody diarrhea due to Clostridium difficile. Axial NECT shows massive submucosal edema* ➡ *of the entire colon (pancolitis) with some segments having an accordion appearance* ➡*.* (Right) *Axial NECT in the same patient shows ascites* ➡ *and mesenteric edema. Note the atrophic native kidneys* ➡*. In spite of prompt diagnosis and treatment, the colitis progressed to perforation and emergency colectomy.*

KEY FACTS

TERMINOLOGY

- Celiac disease: Chronic intolerance of gluten that induces intestinal injury in genetically predisposed individuals
- Nontropical sprue or celiac-sprue disease, gluten-sensitive enteropathy

IMAGING

- **CT or MR enterography is best imaging tool**
- SB wall may be thick or thinned
  - Mucosal hyperenhancement accompanies active ulceration
  - Reversal of jejunoileal fold patterns (atrophied jejunal, thickened ileal)
  - Submucosal edema, fat, or gas
  - Small bowel intussusceptions; intermittent, nonobstructing
  - Eccentric soft tissue density mass in bowel wall (tumor)
  - Mesenteric adenopathy (may be cavitated)
- Excess fluid within SB lumen

- **Conformation** of flaccid SB segments (indent each other)
  - Distends lumen and dilutes contrast medium
- Colonic luminal dilation
  - Excess gas, fluid, fat within lumen
- Eccentric soft tissue density mass in bowel wall
  - Strongly suggests lymphoma or carcinoma

CLINICAL ISSUES

- Common: Affects 1 in 200 in USA, but < 10% are currently diagnosed
  - Most common cause of SB disease and malabsorption in some countries
- Steatorrhea, abdominal distension, flatulence
  - Diarrhea, weight loss, glossitis, anemia
- Refractory disease
  - Enteritis that does not respond to at least 6 months of gluten-free diet
  - GI malignancies are main cause of death in celiac disease

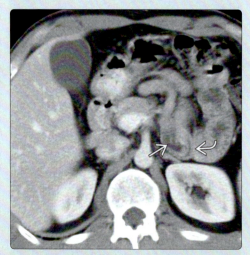
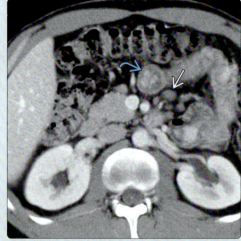

(Left) Axial CECT in a 37-year-old man with painful abdominal cramps shows 1 of several sites of intussusception ⊐, typically short segment and nonobstructing. Note the presence of mesenteric fat ⊐ accompanying the intussuceptum. (Right) Axial CECT in the same patient demonstrates that the jejunal fold pattern seems blunted ⊐. Also noted is mesenteric lymphadenopathy ⊐.

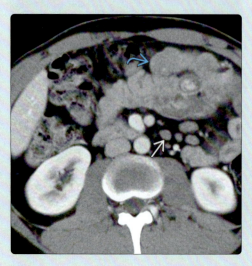
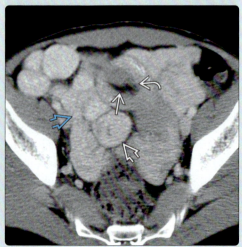

(Left) Axial CECT in the same patient shows more mesenteric lymphadenopathy ⊐ along with the abnormally blunted jejunal fold pattern ⊐. (Right) Axial CECT in the same patient shows another intussusception ⊐ with its accompanying mesenteric fat ⊐. There is a suggestion of abnormal fold prominence in the ileum ⊐. The flaccid, dilated pelvic SB loops ⊐ press on each other without intervening space, known as the conformation sign.

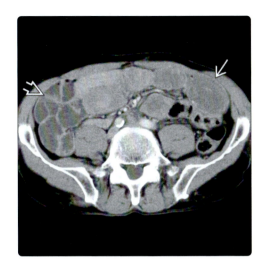
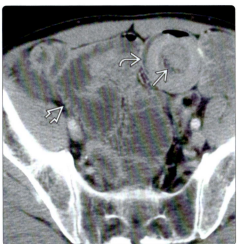

(Left) *Axial CT in a 69-year-old woman with chronic diarrhea & pain shows fluid distention of SB ➡ with conformation of the flaccid segments ⮞. The fold pattern of the jejunum is blunted.* (Right) *Axial CT in same patient shows a short segment, nonobstructing intussusception ➡ with a target appearance and intraluminal mesenteric fat ➡. The fold pattern of the ileum ⮞ is more prominent than that of the jejunum, a reversal of the normal situation. Biopsy & response to a gluten-free diet confirmed celiac disease.*

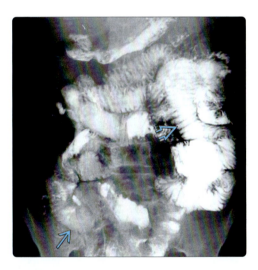
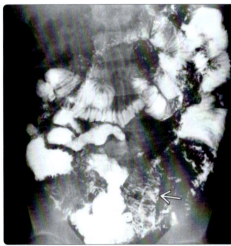

(Left) *Films from a barium small bowel follow-through (SBFT) in a 30-year-old woman with steatorrhea show a typical malabsorption pattern, consisting of dilution of the barium ➡ and dilation of the lumen ⮞. The folds within the jejunum appear blunted. There is poor coating of the mucosa by the barium.* (Right) *SBFT in the same patient illustrates intermittent intussusception with a coiled spring appearance in the mid jejunum ➡. Celiac disease is the most common specific cause of malabsorption.*

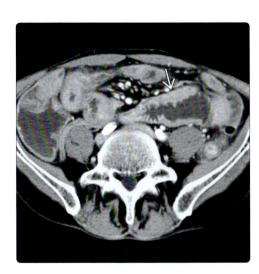
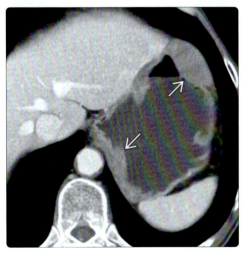

(Left) *Axial CECT in a patient with sprue shows fluid-distended bowel. One segment of jejunum has focal, soft tissue density thickening ➡ of the wall, which was found to be due to lymphoma.* (Right) *Axial CECT in the same patient shows multifocal, soft tissue density gastric wall thickening ➡, which was also due to lymphoma. Patients with refractory sprue are at increased risk for both lymphoma and carcinoma of the bowel.*

TERMINOLOGY

- Disease of unknown etiology characterized by transmural inflammation of GI tract

IMAGING

- CT and MR enterography have supplanted most barium studies for diagnosis in adults and children
  - Faster to perform, less operator dependent, more sensitive and specific
  - Allow assessment of extraintestinal disease (e.g., cholangitis; arthritis)
- Multiplanar CT or MR enterography
  - Distend bowel with water ± neutral contrast agent (e.g., VoLumen)
  - Bolus IV contrast medium at 3-4 mL/second
  - Multiplanar reconstructions
- Noncicatrizing, acute phase
  - Target or double halo sign
  - Hyperenhancing inner ring (mucosa)
  - Low-density middle ring (submucosal edema)
  - Engorged vasa recta: Comb sign
  - Proliferation of mesenteric fat and lymphadenopathy
- Chronic or cicatrizing phase
  - Strictures ± dilated small bowel (SB) upstream
  - Abscesses, fistulas, sinus tracts
- Pelvic MR for perianal and rectal Crohn's disease
- Barium enema, enteroclysis can depict strictures and fistulas
- Colonoscopy is best to assess colonic involvement, guide biopsy of colon and terminal ileum (TI)
- Capsule endoscopy may complement imaging studies
  - Not of proven value following negative CT or MR enterography

TOP DIFFERENTIAL DIAGNOSES

- Ulcerative colitis ("backwash" ileitis)
- Mesenteric enteritis and adenitis
- Infectious ileitis or colitis

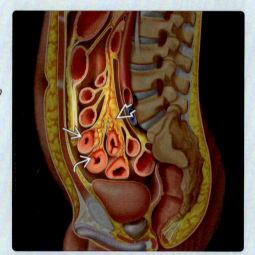

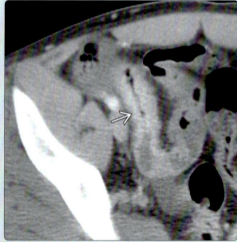

(Left) Graphic in the sagittal plane illustrates typical features of Crohn's disease, including segmental small bowel (SB) wall thickening, mucosal hyperemia ➡, transmural inflammation with deep ulcers ➡, mesenteric vessel engorgement, and fibrofatty proliferation ➡. (Right) This 19-year-old man has an acute flare of his Crohn's disease. CT shows mucosal hyperenhancement, wall thickening, and luminal narrowing of the terminal ileum ➡.

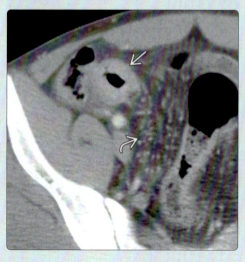

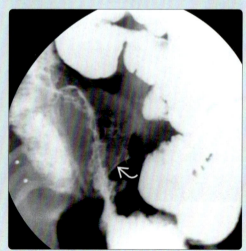

(Left) CT in the same patient shows the inflamed terminal ileum ➡ as well as local mesenteric fibrofatty proliferation and engorged vasa recta ➡. (Right) Spot film from a SB follow-through (SBFT) in the same patient shows diseased terminal ileum and colon with longitudinal and transverse ulcerations of the ileal mucosa (cobblestone pattern) and luminal narrowing. At least 2 sinus tracts ➡ are opacified. Traditional barium studies may be valuable for evaluation of strictures, fistulas, and sinus tracts.

Crohn's Disease

TERMINOLOGY

Definitions

- Disease of unknown etiology characterized by transmural inflammation of GI tract

IMAGING

General Features

- Best diagnostic clue
  - Segmental, discontinuous inflammation of small bowel (SB) ± colon with mucosal hyperenhancement, submucosal edema, engorged vasa recta
    - Usually accompanied by clusters of prominent mesenteric nodes
- Location
  - Anywhere along GI tract, from mouth to anus
    - Most common: Terminal ileum (TI) and proximal colon
  - Distribution
    - 80% of patients have SB involvement
    - 50% have ileocolitis
    - 20% have disease limited to colon
      - □ Crohn's ("granulomatous") colitis
      - □ Only 10% have rectal involvement
- Morphology
  - Transmural inflammation
    - Predisposes to strictures, fistulas, sinus tracts, abscesses
  - Skip lesions (segmental or discontinuous)

Fluoroscopic Findings

- Barium studies: Early changes
  - Target or bull's-eye appearance of aphthoid ulcerations: Punctate, shallow central barium collections surrounded by halo of edema
  - "Cobblestoning": Combination of longitudinal and transverse ulcers
  - Deep fissuring ulcers
- Barium studies: Late changes
  - Skip lesions: Segmental disease with normal intervening segments
  - Sacculations seen on antimesenteric border
  - Postinflammatory pseudopolyps, haustral loss, intramural abscess
  - String sign: Luminal narrowing and ileal stricture
  - Sinus tracts, fissures, fistulas are hallmarks of disease
  - Anorectal lesions: Ulcers, fissures, abscesses, hemorrhoids, stenosis

CT Findings

- **CT enterography**
  - Axial and multiplanar reformations throughout abdomen and pelvis
  - Distend SB with oral water ± neutral contrast agent (VoLumen)
  - Bolus administration of IV contrast to demonstrate signs of active inflammation
- **Noncicatrizing, acute phase**
  - Stratified wall thickening of discontinuous SB segments
    - Target or double halo sign
    - Hyperenhancing inner ring (mucosa)

- Low-density middle ring (submucosal edema)
- Soft tissue-density outer ring (muscularis propria and serosa)
  - Comb sign: Engorged vasa recta
    - Supply actively inflamed SB segments
  - Proliferation of mesenteric fat and lymphadenopathy
    - Nodes rarely > 1 cm in diameter
- **Chronic or cicatrizing phase**
  - Luminal narrowing ± dilated SB upstream
  - Mural stratification lost: Indistinct mucosa, submucosa, muscularis propria
    - Alternatively, submucosal fat may proliferate, preserve stratification
  - Abscesses, fistulas, sinus tracts
    - **Fistulas** connect 2 epithelialized surfaces (e.g., bowel to bowel, bladder, vagina, or skin)
    - **Sinus tracts** are blind ending (e.g., bowel to abscess)
  - Mesenteric changes: Abscess, fibrofatty proliferation, mildly enlarged nodes
  - Perianal disease: Fistulas and sinus tracts

MR Findings

- **MR enterography**
- Breath holding, fat suppression, and gadolinium enhancement show extent and severity of inflammation
  - Mucosal hyperenhancement, submucosal edema, engorged vasa recta in acute inflammation
- Allows real-time imaging to assess peristalsis in segments of suspected disease
- Sensitive in detecting and characterizing **fistulas, sinuses, abscesses in perianal Crohn's disease**
- Diffusion-weighted imaging can reveal active inflammation even without IV contrast administration

Ultrasonographic Findings

- Grayscale ultrasound
  - Transrectal sonography
    - Mural thickening, abscesses, fistulas

Other Modality Findings

- Colonoscopy is best modality to assess colon
  - Often allows inspection and biopsy of TI
- Capsule endoscopy is commonly used to complement imaging studies
  - Not of proven value following "negative" CT or MR
  - Contraindicated in patients with enteric strictures

Imaging Recommendations

- Best imaging tool
  - **Multiplanar CT or MR enterography**
    - Distend bowel with water ± neutral contrast agent (e.g., VoLumen)
    - Bolus IV contrast medium at 3-4 mL/second
    - For CT, use low-dose protocols (e.g., iterative reconstruction) to reduce radiation risk
  - Barium enema, enteroclysis, SB follow-through
    - Can be useful for depiction of strictures and fistulas
  - MR for perianal and rectal Crohn's disease

SELECTED REFERENCES

1.   Allen BC et al: MR enterography for assessment and management of small bowel Crohn disease. Radiol Clin North Am. 52(4):799-810, 2014

(Left) *In this 37-year-old man, CT shows 2 segments of inflamed SB ➡ that were separated by normal segments of bowel, the classic "skip lesions" of Crohn's disease. Note the engorged vasa recta (comb sign) ⇗ supplying the more distal segment of inflamed bowel. (Right) CT in the same patient shows additional segments of inflamed bowel ➡ with mucosal enhancement, wall thickening, and luminal narrowing.*

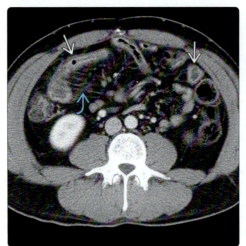
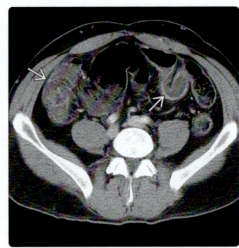

(Left) *Coronal reformatted CECT in the same patient shows separate segments of inflamed bowel ➡ along with mesenteric lymphadenopathy ➡ and prominent vessels. (Right) Coronal CECT in the same patient shows inflamed bowel ➡ and mesenteric lymphadenopathy ➡. The diagnosis of Crohn's disease was confirmed on colonoscopy with biopsy of the terminal ileum.*

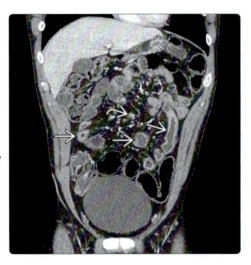
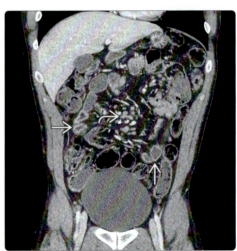

(Left) *Axial CECT in a 48-year-old woman presenting with recent weight loss and diarrhea shows segmental SB wall thickening characterized by excessive submucosal fat deposition ➡, indicative of chronic inflammation. Nonepithelialized fistulas ➡ extend from 1 bowel segment to the others. (Right) Coronal CECT in the same patient again demonstrates the extension of the nonepithelialized fistulas ➡ between the bowel segments that appear to be tethered together.*

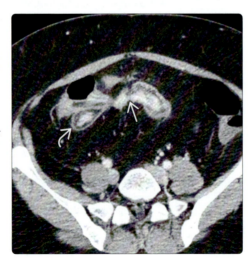
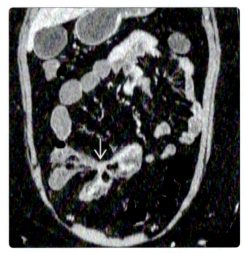

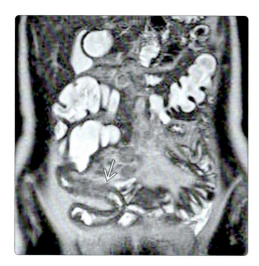

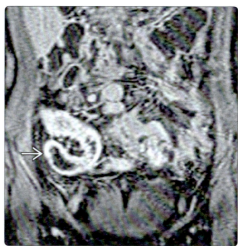

(Left) *This patient had prior ileocecal resection for Crohn's disease and has recurrent symptoms. Coronal T2WI MR (part of the MR enterography protocol) shows mural thickening of a SB segment ➡ representing the neoterminal ileum where recurrent disease often occurs.* (Right) *Coronal T1WI C+ FS MR in the same patient shows vivid mucosal enhancement of the affected segment ➡. The adjacent SB and colon do not enhance with the same intensity.*

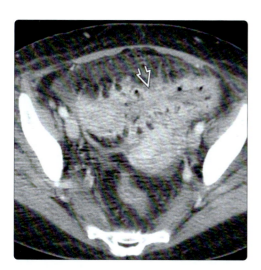

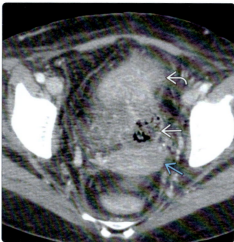

(Left) *This 52-year-old woman has chronic Crohn's colitis with recent recurrent urinary tract infections. CT shows markedly inflamed sigmoid colon ➡ and mesentery.* (Right) *CT in the same patient shows an extraluminal collection of gas and fluid ➡ interposed between the colon, uterus ➡, and top of the bladder ➡.*

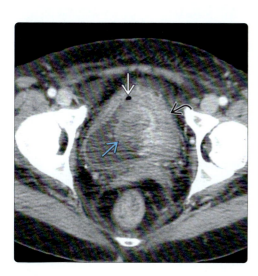

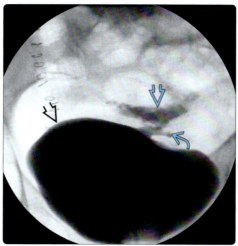

(Left) *CECT in the same patient shows a markedly thickened wall of bladder ➡ along with gas ➡ and debris ➡ within the bladder.* (Right) *Retrograde injection of contrast material into the bladder ➡ opacifies the sigmoid colon ➡ through a fistulous tract ➡. Fistulas are a key feature of the transmural inflammation caused by Crohn's disease.*

Intestinal (Angioneurotic) Angioedema

TERMINOLOGY

- Noninflammatory transient edema of intestinal wall due to increased vascular permeability and extravasation of intravascular fluid

IMAGING

- **Contrast-enhanced, multiplanar CT is diagnostic test of choice**
- Ascites (100% of cases): Small to moderate volume
- Bowel wall thickening: Submucosal edema, mucosal and mesenteric hyperemia
  - Involves long segment of jejunum &/or ileum
- Luminal dilation (> 2.5 cm) without obstruction
- Imaging findings are entirely reversible, seen only during acute phase

TOP DIFFERENTIAL DIAGNOSES

- Vasculitis
- Ischemic enteritis
- Intestinal trauma

PATHOLOGY

- **Hereditary** angioedema: Autosomal dominant
  - C1-INH (C1 esterase) deficiency (C1-inhibitor)
  - Personal and family history of recurrent attacks
- **Acquired C1-INH deficiency**: Associated with hepatitis, lymphoproliferative, neoplastic, and autoimmune disorders
- **Allergic** angioedema
  - Angioedema secondary to medication (**ACE inhibitors**, aspirin, iodinated contrast)

CLINICAL ISSUES

- Abdominal pain, vomiting, laryngeal and cutaneous edema
- Many patients are not diagnosed and undergo laparotomy
- 40 million patients take ACE-inhibitor medication to control hypertension (e.g., lisinopril, enalapril)
  - ~ 0.5% of these will develop intestinal angioedema (200,000 patients)

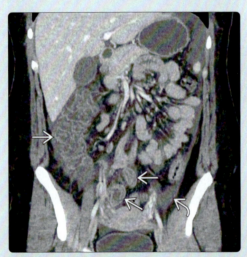
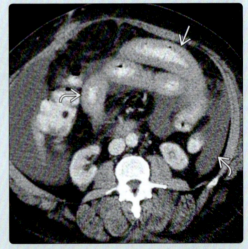

(Left) This 21-year-old woman with hereditary angioedema had multiple episodes of laryngeal edema and abdominal pain. Coronal CECT, taken during one acute episode, shows striking submucosal edema ➡ within the walls of the right colon and distal small bowel, along with ascites ➡. (Right) In this case of acquired angioedema due to hepatitis, axial CECT shows long segmental jejunal thickening ➡ and ascites ➡. Laboratory tests confirmed C1 esterase deficiency and complement activation.

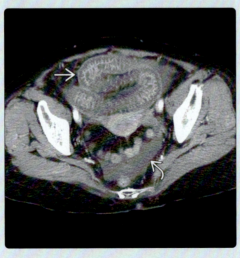
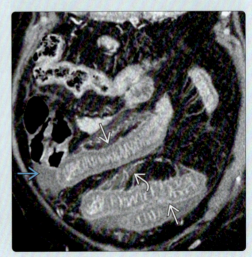

(Left) This elderly woman has hypertensive heart disease and presents with acute abdominal pain. Axial CECT shows a long segment of small bowel wall thickening and submucosal edema ➡ with associated ascites ➡. (Right) Coronal CECT from the same patient shows the long segment bowel wall edema ➡, mesenteric edema ➡, and ascites ➡. Intestinal angioedema was attributed to the patient's ACE-inhibitor medication, which was withheld; symptoms resolved within 36 hours.

Small Bowel NSAID Stricture

TERMINOLOGY

- Focal stricture(s) in small bowel (SB) due to NSAID use

IMAGING

- Barium SB follow-through or enteroclysis
  - Single or multiple short-segment annular strictures ± partial SB obstruction
  - Strictures may resemble normal plicae circulares on enteroclysis
- CT findings
  - Strictures: Short segmental narrowing of lumen with dilation of bowel upstream
  - Mucosal inflammation: Mucosal hyperenhancement and submucosal edema

TOP DIFFERENTIAL DIAGNOSES

- Crohn's disease: Longer segments of transmural involvement

- Celiac-sprue disease: Jejunoileal fold pattern reversal; intussusceptions
- Ischemic enteritis: Bowel wall thickening; strictures can be late result
- SB carcinoma: "Apple core" constricting, obstructing lesion
- Radiation enteritis: Longer strictures; pelvic SB segments
- Small intestine vasculitis: Long segments of submucosal edema

PATHOLOGY

- All NSAID (including aspirin) formulations can cause enterocolitis
  - Slow-release formulations affect distal SB and colon

CLINICAL ISSUES

- Often asymptomatic; may have symptoms of bowel obstruction
- May require surgery or endoscopic balloon dilation or needle-knife electroincision for bowel obstruction

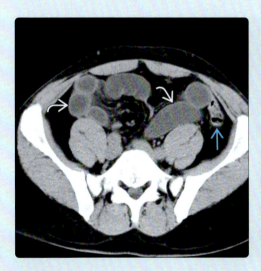 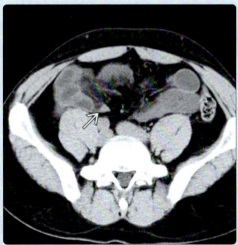

(Left) Axial NECT in a 40-year-old man shows a dilated proximal and mid small bowel ⇗ and collapsed colon ➡. These findings indicate mechanical small bowel obstruction but not its specific etiology. (Right) Axial NECT in the same patient shows an abrupt transition from dilated to collapsed small bowel in the ileum ➡. There was no history of prior abdominal surgery, making adhesive bowel obstruction a less likely etiology.

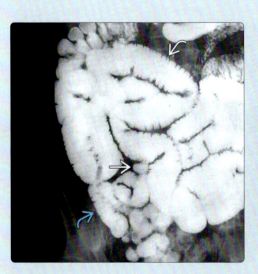 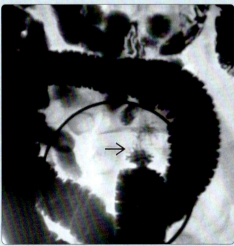

(Left) Small bowel follow-through in the same patient shows dilation of the proximal small bowel ⇗ and a short stricture in the ileum ➡ with collapsed bowel ⇗ distal to this point. (Right) Spot film from the small bowel study in the same patient shows a short stricture ⇗ in the ileum. At surgery, the stricture was confirmed, resected, and determined to be due to injury from chronic use of NSAIDs.

Pneumatosis of the Intestine

TERMINOLOGY

- Pneumatosis is descriptive sign, not disease or diagnosis
  - Cystic or linear collections of gas in subserosal or submucosal layers of GI tract wall
- Pneumatosis intestinalis: Most common form of intramural gas, found in small bowel more often than colon
- Pneumatosis coli: Rounded collections of gas in distal colonic wall, usually asymptomatic finding

IMAGING

- **Contrast-enhanced multiplanar CT**
  - **Bolus IV contrast; water as oral contrast medium**
- Pneumatosis of ischemic etiology
  - Dilated bowel lumen (ileus), thickened wall, abnormal wall enhancement
    - Ascites, may be of blood density (> 35 HU)
    - ± pneumoperitoneum or pneumoretroperitoneum
    - ± mesenteric or portal venous gas
- **Portal venous gas is not always due to bowel infarction**

TOP DIFFERENTIAL DIAGNOSES

- Etiologies
  - Bowel infarction
  - Medication induced
  - Postoperative or post endoscopy
  - Autoimmune disease
  - Pulmonary disease (gas dissecting from thorax to abdomen)

CLINICAL ISSUES

- Most common signs/symptoms
  - Nonischemic causes: Patients are often asymptomatic
  - Bowel ischemia: Nausea, abdominal pain, distension, melena, fever, vomiting, cough (depending on etiology)
  - Labs: Increased lactate, WBC, amylase, serum glucose
- Treatment and prognosis depend on etiology
- **Direct communication between radiologist and clinical team is essential**

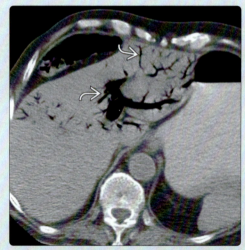 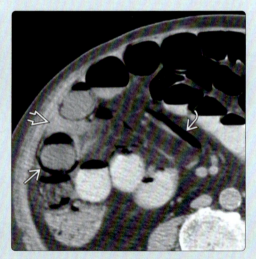

(Left) Axial CECT in an acutely ill elderly man demonstrates extensive gas within the intrahepatic portal veins ➜. (Right) Axial CECT in the same patient reveals ascites ⊇, extensive small bowel dilation (ileus), and pneumatosis ➜ as well as gas within mesenteric veins ⇗. This combination of findings is essentially diagnostic of transmural bowel infarction.

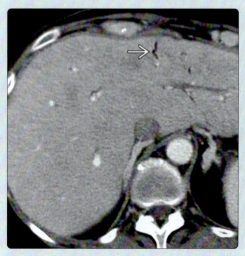 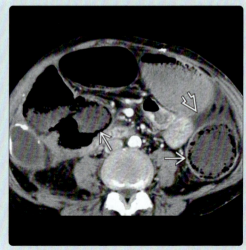

(Left) Axial CECT in a 75-year-old man who presented with abdominal pain and prior bowel ischemia demonstrates relatively subtle gas within the peripheral intrahepatic branches of the portal vein ➜. (Right) Axial CECT in the same patient reveals extensive pneumatosis ➜ within dilated segments of the bowel. Ascites is also noted ⊇ near the damaged bowel. The patient went to surgery for resection of the infarcted bowel.

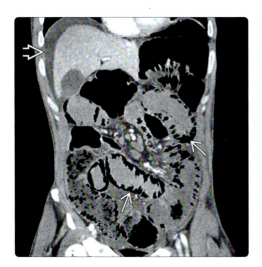

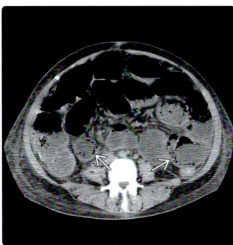

(Left) Coronal CECT reformation in the same patient shows extensive small bowel pneumatosis ➡. Also note the dilation of the bowel lumen and the presence of ascites ➡, findings that help confirm that this pneumatosis is likely due to bowel ischemia. **(Right)** Axial NECT in a 44-year-old woman with cirrhosis and hypotension demonstrates pneumatosis within the bowel walls ➡ and luminal distention with fluid (ileus) due to bowel infarction.

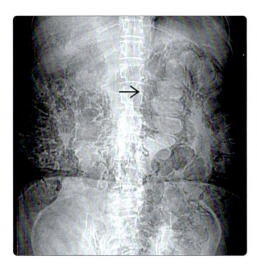

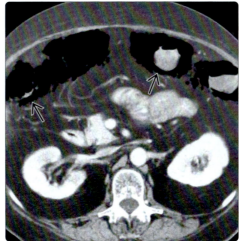

(Left) This 54-year-old woman had a recent stem cell transplant and had abdominal distention. A supine film shows extensive pneumatosis ➡ within the colonic and small bowel walls. **(Right)** CECT in the same patient shows gas within the bowel wall ➡ but no ascites or ileus. The patient remained relatively asymptomatic, confirming this as "benign" (nonischemic) pneumatosis, likely due to medications.

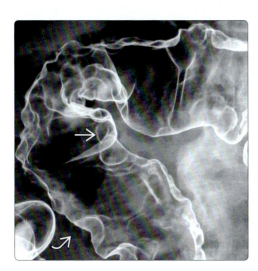

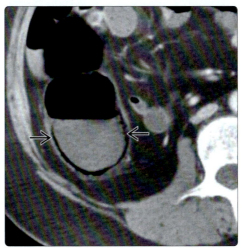

(Left) Air-contrast barium enema shows polypoid gas "cysts" ➡ within the colonic wall. The submucosal gas ➡ (pneumatosis) is due to benign pneumatosis coli. **(Right)** CECT shows gas along the dependent wall of the cecum and ascending colon ➡ that might be misinterpreted as pneumatosis. This finding is limited to where the colonic contents abut the inside wall of the colon and does not extend around the circumference of the colon. Gas trapped against the inner wall of the cecum is a common and innocuous finding.

KEY FACTS

TERMINOLOGY

- Small bowel (SB) ischemia resulting from mesenteric arterial or venous narrowing or occlusion, leading to inadequate supply of nutrients and oxygen

IMAGING

- Imaging findings vary, based on etiology and acuity of ischemic injury
- **Acute arterial thrombosis or embolus**
  - Little SB wall thickening, mesenteric edema, or ascites
  - **Lack of bowel mucosal enhancement due to compromised arterial flow**
  - CT signs of embolic ischemic injury to other organs
- **Chronic arterial occlusive disease**
  - Narrowing or occlusion of SMA with collateral vessels
- **Mesenteric venous thrombosis**
  - Fluid-distended SB with thick walls
  - Infiltrated mesentery and ascites
  - Occurs in prothrombotic (hypercoagulable) disorders

- **Pneumatosis intestinalis and portal venous gas**
  - Not sensitive nor specific for bowel ischemia
  - Branching gas extending to periphery of liver
- **Nonocclusive bowel ischemia**
  - Common etiologies: Closed-loop SB obstruction; cocaine or methamphetamine use; hypotensive episode; vasculitis
- **Multiplanar, multiphasic CECT is best imaging tool**
  - Can generate CT angiogram; makes arterial or venous occlusion more apparent and quantifiable
  - Shows etiology of nonocclusive ischemia (e.g., closed-loop SB obstruction)
- **Catheter angiography**
  - Diagnostic confirmation and treatment of arterial occlusive disease

DIAGNOSTIC CHECKLIST

- **Diagnosis of bowel ischemia demands correlation of clinical, laboratory, and imaging findings**

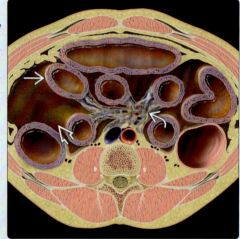
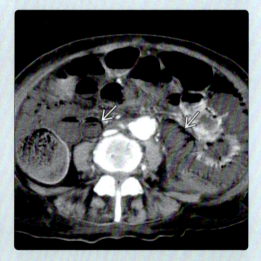

(Left) Graphic shows a dilated small bowel (SB) ➡ with thickened wall, ascites ➡, and edematous mesentery ➡, all findings seen with occlusion of the superior mesenteric vein. (Right) Axial CECT in an elderly woman with abdominal pain demonstrates dilated SB with pneumatosis ➡. Portal venous gas was also present on other sections (not shown). No enhancement of SB mucosa is seen, indicating arterial occlusion as the etiology. Infarcted bowel was confirmed at surgery, and the patient died.

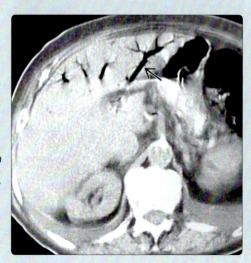
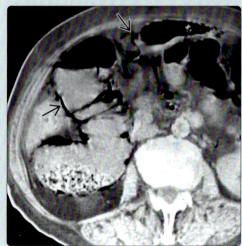

(Left) In this elderly man complaining of severe abdominal pain, axial CT section, viewed at "lung windows," shows portal vein gas ➡ as a branching air density extending to the periphery of the liver. (Right) In the same patient, CT shows pneumatosis and gas in the wall of the colon ➡ and SB. These findings, in concert with the symptoms and laboratory evidence of lactic acidosis, are diagnostic of bowel ischemia.

TERMINOLOGY

Synonyms

- Acute mesenteric ischemia

Definitions

- Small bowel (SB) ischemia resulting from mesenteric arterial or venous narrowing or occlusion, leading to inadequate supply of nutrients and oxygen

IMAGING

General Features

- Best diagnostic clue
  - Pneumatosis (SB wall gas) ± portal vein gas
    - This is late sign; neither sensitive nor specific for bowel infarction
  - Imaging findings vary, based on etiology and acuity of ischemic injury

Radiographic Findings

- Radiography
  - Dilated bowel with air-fluid levels; ileus pattern
  - Thickening of valvulae conniventes
  - Linear distribution of gas (pneumatosis intestinalis)

CT Findings

- CECT
  - **Acute arterial thrombosis or embolus**
    - Superior mesenteric artery (SMA) or branches may be occluded by thrombus, arterial dissection, or other causes (e.g., tumor invasion)
    - Emboli are usually near origin SMA, distal to middle colic artery
    - Bowel wall is usually not thickened in acute mesenteric arterial occlusion
      - Acute arterial bowel ischemia usually has little mesenteric infiltration or ascites
    - **Lack of bowel mucosal enhancement due to compromised arterial flow**
    - CT signs of embolic ischemic injury to other organs (e.g., spleen and kidneys)
    - CT or clinical signs of embolic source (e.g., enlarged left atrium; prosthetic cardiac valves or assist devices)
  - **Chronic arterial occlusive disease**
    - Narrowing or occlusion of SMA and celiac axis
    - Collateral vessels to celiac and inferior mesenteric arteries
  - **Mesenteric venous thrombosis**
    - Fluid-distended bowel loops (very sensitive but nonspecific sign)
    - Long segmental SB wall thickening, usually hypodense (edema)
      - ↑ attenuation of bowel wall due to submucosal hemorrhage or hyperemia (reperfusion)
    - Mesenteric fat infiltrated by edema
    - Ascites, often loculated between bowel segments
    - Often occurs in prothrombotic (hypercoagulable) disorders
    - **Pneumatosis intestinalis** (venous > arterial thrombus)
      - Band-like or bubble-like appearance in bowel wall

        - Linear, curvilinear, or cystic gas-filled spaces
        - Not sensitive nor specific for bowel ischemia
    - **Portal vein gas**
      - Appearance: Branching intrahepatic gas extending to periphery of liver
      - When evident on plain films of abdomen: Usually indicates bowel infarction with 75% mortality
      - CT much more sensitive in detecting portal venous gas: Not necessarily due to bowel ischemia; only 25% mortality
  - **Nonocclusive bowel ischemia**
    - Common etiologies: Closed-loop SB obstruction; cocaine or methamphetamine use; severe hypotensive episode; vasculitis
      - Closed-loop SB obstruction: Cluster of fluid-distended SB with twisted mesenteric vessels ("balloons on strings"); infiltrated mesentery; ascites
      - Vasculitis: Long segmental SB wall thickening; ischemic injury to other organs (e.g., kidneys); ascites
      - Hypotension: More common cause of ischemic colitis

Angiographic Findings

- Acute arterial ischemia: Clot/stenosis of SMA or branches
- Acute venous ischemia: Superior mesenteric vein (SMV) occlusion with collaterals
- Nonocclusive ischemia: Slow flow in SMA
- Chronic ischemia: Narrowing/occlusion of celiac artery &/or SMA
  - ↑ collateral arteries from celiac to SMA, or SMA to inferior mesenteric artery

Imaging Recommendations

- Best imaging tool
  - **Multiplanar, multiphasic CECT is best imaging tool**
    - Shows etiology of nonocclusive ischemia (e.g., closed-loop SB obstruction)
    - Can generate CT angiogram; makes arterial or venous occlusion more apparent and quantifiable
    - Lung window setting for detection pneumatosis intestinalis
    - Water is used as "oral contrast medium" (dense enteric contrast precludes evaluation of SB mucosal enhancement)
  - **Catheter angiography**
    - Diagnostic confirmation and treatment of arterial occlusive disease

DIAGNOSTIC CHECKLIST

Consider

- **Diagnosis of bowel ischemia demands correlation of clinical, laboratory, and imaging findings**

Image Interpretation Pearls

- Imaging findings vary due to many factors (e.g., acute vs. chronic; arterial vs. venous)
- Mesenteric venous occlusion causes more impressive wall thickening, mesenteric infiltration, and ascites than arterial occlusion

(Left) Axial CECT shows a severely atherosclerotic aorta. SB is dilated with extensive gas in the bowel wall ➡ and mesenteric veins ⮞. (Right) Axial CECT shows an aortic dissection with the intimal flap ⮞ extending into the superior mesenteric artery, resulting in bowel ischemia.

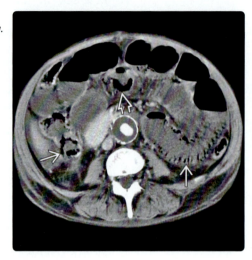
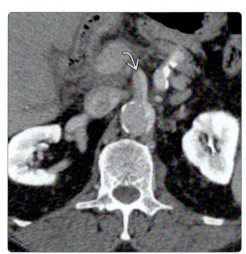

(Left) Supine film of the abdomen in this elderly man with severe abdominal pain shows a generalized ileus and branching gas density within the liver, representing portal vein gas ⮞. (Right) Axial nonenhanced CT in the same patient shows gas in the wall of colon ⮞ and SB ➡, attributed to ischemic injury from hypoperfusion.

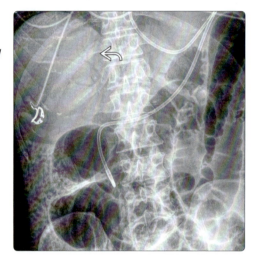
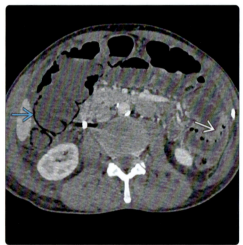

(Left) Axial CECT in a 24-year-old man with pain shows thrombus ⮞ within the lumen of the superior mesenteric vein. SB is markedly dilated and fluid filled ➡. The wall is thickened, and ascites ⮞ is present, findings worrisome for transmural ischemic injury. Mesenteric venous thrombosis often results from a prothrombotic condition. (Right) In the same patient, axial CT shows mesenteric edema, engorged veins ⮞, and ascites ⮞. Bowel infarction and a hypercoagulable disorder were confirmed.

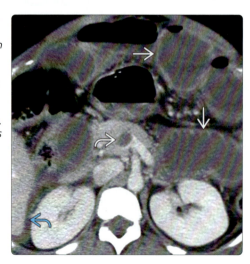
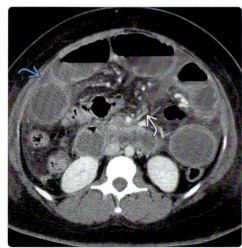

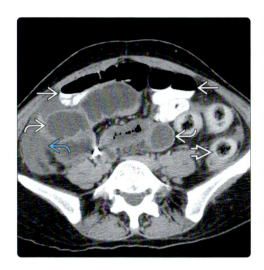

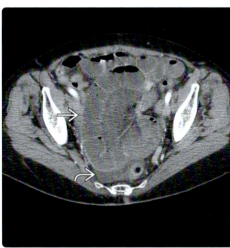

(Left) *Axial CT shows focal ascites ⟶ and mesenteric infiltration near a segment of SB with mural thickening and fluid dilation ⟶, very concerning for closed-loop obstruction with ischemia. The proximal SB ⟶ and colon ⟶ are of normal caliber.* (Right) *Lower CT section in the same patient shows the ischemic bowel ⟶ and ascites ⟶. A closed-loop SB obstruction with infarcted bowel was confirmed at surgery.*

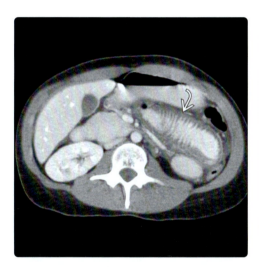

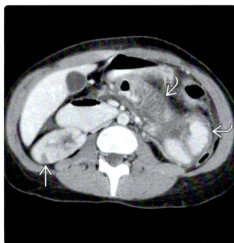

(Left) *Axial CECT in a 21-year-old woman with severe abdominal pain illustrates long-segment bowel wall thickening and submucosal edema ⟶ compatible with enteric ischemia.* (Right) *Axial CECT in the same patient again reveals the long segment bowel wall thickening and submucosal edema ⟶ as well as wedge-shaped defects in the kidneys ⟶ that represent acute ischemic injury. In a young patient, these findings are essentially diagnostic of vasculitis.*

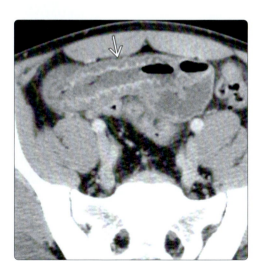

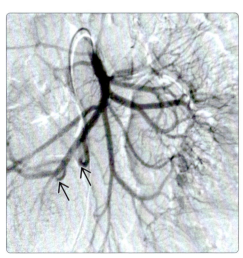

(Left) *In this young man with acute, severe abdominal pain and a history of IV drug abuse, CT shows long segmental bowel wall thickening ⟶.* (Right) *In the same patient, a digitally subtracted catheter angiogram shows occlusion of several ileocolic arteries ⟶, attributed to IV use of amphetamines and cocaine.*

TERMINOLOGY

- Invagination or telescoping of proximal segment of bowel (**intussusceptum**) into lumen of distal segment (**intussuscipiens**)

IMAGING

- Location: Ileoileal > ileocolic > colocolic
- **For intussusception in children**: US and clinical evaluation are diagnostic
  - Much more common; attributed to lymphoid hyperplasia
  - US: Target, doughnut, or bull's-eye sign
  - Air enema is usually successful in confirming and reducing intussusception
- **In adults**: Most short-segment, nonobstructing intussusceptions are of little clinical concern
  - May be due to adhesions, celiac disease, or other nonneoplastic disorders
  - Longer segment or obstruction suggests presence of lead mass

- **Contrast-enhanced, multiplanar CT is 1st-line test**
- Bowel-within-bowel appearance: Alternating layers of mesenteric fat and soft tissue-density bowel walls
- Enhancing mesenteric vessels accompany intussusceptum

PATHOLOGY

- Mass-related lead point
  - Benign: Polyp, leiomyoma, lipoma
  - Malignant: Primary (more common in colon), metastases and lymphoma (more common in small bowel)
- Physical cause but no neoplasm
  - Postoperative causes are most common (e.g., adhesions, anastomoses)

CLINICAL ISSUES

- **Obstruction and ischemia are more common in long-segment intussusception with lead mass**

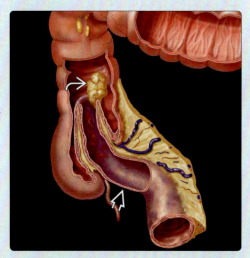
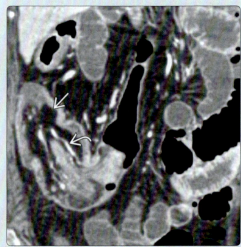

(Left) Graphic shows an ileocolic intussusception with a tumor in the bowel wall ➜ as the lead mass. Note the vascular compromise and ischemia of the intussusceptum ➟. (Right) Coronal CECT shows invaginated mesenteric fat ➜ and vessels ➚ from an ileocolonic intussusception. The lead mass proved to be carcinoma.

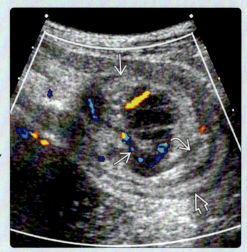
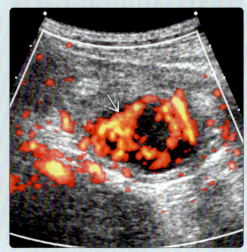

(Left) Transverse color Doppler ultrasound of small bowel intussusception shows vascular flow within an intraluminal mass ➜ and 2 echogenic submucosal rings representing intussusceptum ➟ and intussuscipiens ➜. (Right) Transverse power Doppler ultrasound in the same patient reveals marked hyperemia ➜ within the mass, which proved to be a metastatic melanoma.

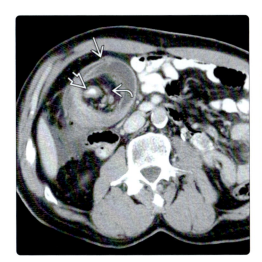
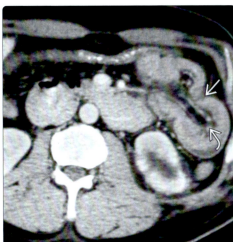

(Left) Axial CECT in a patient with ileocolic intussusception shows an outer ring intussuscipiens ⇉ of the colon wall, while the intussusceptum is a small intestinal segment ⇉. Mesenteric fat and vessels ⇉ accompany the intussuscepted small bowel segment. (Right) Axial CECT shows a reniform (kidney-shaped) small bowel ⇉ due to jejunal intussusception. Note the intussuscepted mesenteric fat and vessels ⇉.

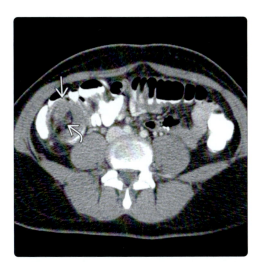
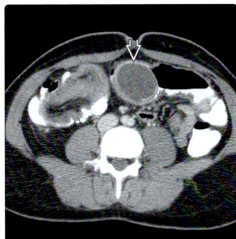

(Left) Axial CECT shows an intussusceptum ⇉ with its mesenteric fat ⇉ within the contrast-opacified lumen of the ascending colon, the intussuscipiens in this case. (Right) Axial CT in the same patient shows that the lead mass of the intussusception is a low-density, spherical mass ⇉ with a calcified rim, a characteristic appearance of an appendiceal mucocele. Long-segment, obstructing intussusceptions, such as this, often have a lead mass when seen in adults.

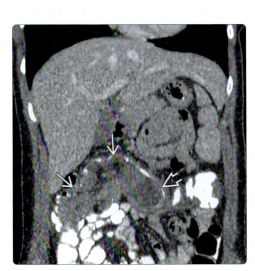
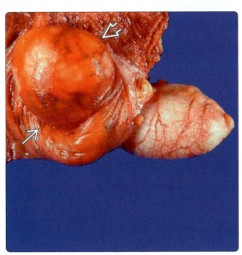

(Left) Coronal CECT in the same patient shows the long-segment intussusception ⇉ and the mucocele ⇉ as the lead mass. (Right) Resected specimen in the same patient, consisting of the terminal ileum and ascending colon, shows the mucocele of the appendix ⇉ and the intussusception ⇉.

TERMINOLOGY

- Damage of small bowel or colonic mucosa and wall due to therapeutic or excessive irradiation

IMAGING

- **Multiplanar, contrast-enhanced CT or MR**
  - Barium enema useful for colorectal involvement
- Bowel wall thickening
  - Acute: Submucosal edema (near water density on CT; high intensity on T2WI MR)
    - Edema suggests submucosal edema, not tumor invasion
  - Chronic: Closer to soft tissue density
- Stenoses → bowel obstruction with dilation of bowel loops "upstream"
  - Single or multiple strictures of varying length
- ± sinuses or fistulas (from bowel to skin, vagina, bladder, other bowel)

- Fluid in tract appears as high signal on MR, contrasted by soft tissue and fat
- Adhesions → angulation between adjacent loops, fixation of loops
- Mesenteric or perirectal infiltration (acute) or fibrosis (chronic)

TOP DIFFERENTIAL DIAGNOSES

- Crohn's disease
- Metastases and lymphoma
- Ischemic and infectious enteritis/colitis

CLINICAL ISSUES

- Usually follows radiotherapy for primary pelvic tumors
  - Acute radiation enteritis or colitis often resolves spontaneously within weeks
  - Moderate to severe chronic radiation enteritis/colitis develops in 5-15%
- Diagnosis is suggested by clinical and imaging features, confirmed by endoscopy and biopsy, if necessary

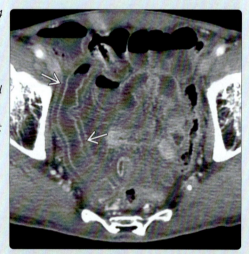
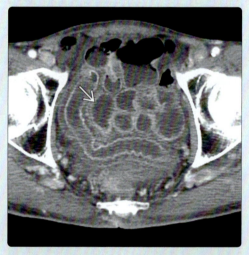

(Left) This 63-year-old man is 4 weeks status post radiation therapy for rectal cancer, and now with pelvic pain and diarrhea. CT shows submucosal edema ➡ within a rigid-appearing loop of distal ileum, compatible with acute radiation enteritis. (Right) Axial CECT in the same patient reveals numerous fluid-filled loops ➡ of proximal bowel, suggesting functional obstruction due to the radiation. The patient was treated with steroids and symptoms resolved over a 2-week period.

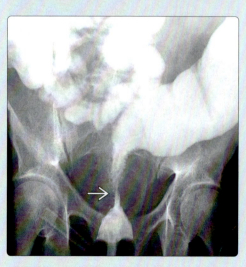
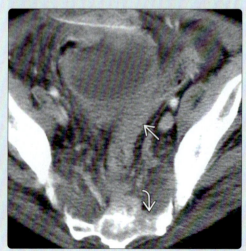

(Left) This 63-year-old man with a history of radiation therapy for sacral metastases now presents with constipation. Spot film from a contrast enema reveals a persistent and high-grade stricture of the rectum ➡, typical for radiation proctitis. (Right) Axial CECT in the same patient confirms the narrowed lumen and thickened wall of the rectosigmoid colon ➡. Also evident is the lytic process in the sacrum ➡, representing the metastatic focus that was the target of the radiation therapy.

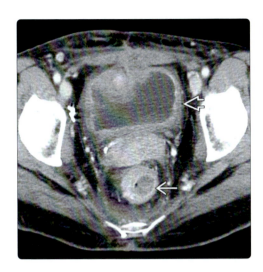
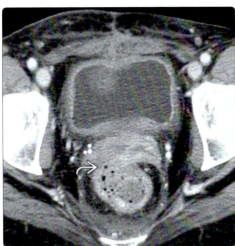

(Left) *This 66-year-old woman had ovarian cancer status post debulking procedure and radiation therapy, and now presents with stool per vagina. CT shows rectal wall thickening and mucosal hyperenhancement ➡. There is similar thickening of the bladder wall and hyperenhancement of the bladder mucosa, consistent with radiation cystitis ➡.* (Right) *CT in the same patient shows obliteration of the fat plane ➡ between the vagina and the rectum and fluid within the vagina, due to colovaginal fistula.*

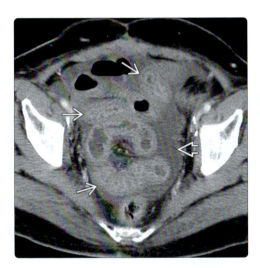
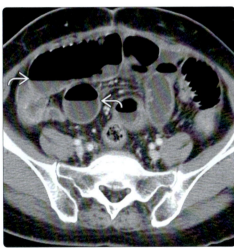

(Left) *This 54-year-old woman had surgery and radiation therapy 2 months prior for endometrial carcinoma. CT shows ascites ➡, submucosal edema, and luminal narrowing ➡ of multiple small bowel segments in the pelvis.* (Right) *In the same patient, CT shows the bowel segments upstream from the pelvic segments are dilated with air-fluid levels ➡, indicating bowel obstruction. The clinical and imaging features are typical of subacute radiation enteritis.*

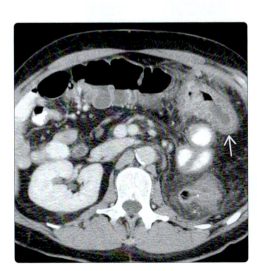
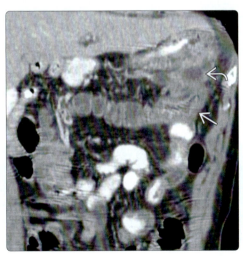

(Left) *This 54-year-old man had pancreatic cancer metastatic to the stomach with subsequent radiation therapy. CT shows mucosal hyperenhancement ➡ and submucosal edema of the distal transverse colon, adjacent to the gastric metastasis (not shown).* (Right) *Coronal CECT in the same patient shows the segmental radiation colitis ➡ as well as the metastasis ➡ in the stomach. Ischemic or infectious colitis could have a similar appearance, but colonoscopic biopsy confirmed radiation colitis.*

Small Intestine Transplantation

TERMINOLOGY

- Isolated small bowel transplant (SB Tx) is primarily for "short gut syndrome"
- Multivisceral Tx (SB, liver, ± pancreas, ± part of stomach)
  - Usually for liver failure due to chronic total parenteral nutrition (TPN)

IMAGING

- Vascular complications: Thrombosis, stricture, pseudoaneurysm (arteries or veins)
  - Less common than for other Tx procedures
- Mesenteritis: Present to some degree in all SB Tx recipients
- Opportunistic infections: May affect any organ, including allograft
- Pneumatosis: Usually not due to ischemia
- Ascites: Usually loculated, nonspecific finding
  - Chylous ascites: Presence of fat-fluid levels
- Post-Tx lymphoproliferative disorder
  - More common in SB (up to 30%) and multivisceral Tx than most other solid organ Tx recipients
  - More common within SB allografts than in host organs
- Rejection and graft-vs.-host disease
  - Both common, cannot be distinguished on imaging
- Dilation of SB lumen
  - May result from dysmotility, adhesion, ischemia, or rejection
- Imaging protocols: Multiplanar CT, ± CT angiography, displays most important anatomical and pathophysiological information pertinent to SB Tx
- Upper GI series to evaluate motility and status of proximal bowel anastomosis

CLINICAL ISSUES

- SB Tx: 1-year patient survival (90%); graft survival (~ 75%)
  - Multivisceral Tx: 1-year patient survival (80%)
  - 5-year patient survival: 60%
- Worse than for solid organ Tx recipients

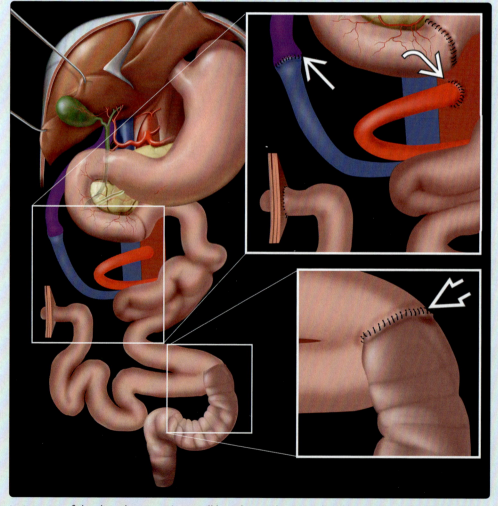

Graphic demonstrates some of the altered anatomy in a small bowel transplantation (SB Tx) procedure. The SB allograft is usually anastomosed proximally to the distal duodenum or proximal jejunum of the recipient, and distally to the sigmoid ➡, with a temporary "chimney" ileostomy in the right lower quadrant. This ostomy allows convenient access to the allograft in the perioperative period for endoscopic visualization and biopsy procedures and may be permanent. The donor superior mesenteric vein (SMV) is anastomosed to the host SMV or portal vein ➡. The donor superior mesenteric artery is anastomosed to the host aorta ➡.

TERMINOLOGY

Abbreviations
- Small bowel transplantation (SB Tx)

Indications for Small Bowel Transplantation
- Primarily for short gut syndrome but also other causes of intestinal failure
  - SB length or function insufficient to provide adequate nutrition
    - Result of various etiologies
      - Superior mesenteric arterial (SMA) or venous (SMV) thrombosis with bowel ischemia, Crohn's disease, midgut volvulus, familial polyposis/Gardner (especially with mesenteric desmoids)
    - Much less commonly due to intestinal pseudoobstruction or other functional deficiency of SB
  - Patients can be maintained on total parenteral nutrition (TPN) indefinitely, except for complications
    - Lack of central venous access to administer TPN, TPN catheter-related sepsis, and TPN-induced cholestatic liver disease
- Indications for multivisceral Tx (liver, ± pancreas, ± part of stomach)
  - Advanced liver disease due to TPN or unrelated cause (e.g., chronic hepatitis)
  - Advanced pancreatic disease
  - Extensive mesenteric thrombosis (with multivisceral ischemia)
  - Severe mesenteric neuropathy
- Special considerations for SB Tx
  - Donor intestine contains large number of immunocompetent lymphocytes in bowel wall (i.e., Peyer patches) and mesenteric nodes
    - ↑ prevalence of graft-vs.-host and graft rejection
  - Donor intestine contains large number of bacteria and other potential pathogens
    - ↑ prevalence of postoperative infections
  - Early diagnosis by imaging of graft-related complications helps to ↓ morbidity and mortality

IMAGING

General Features
- Anatomy of SB and multivisceral Tx
  - Stomach (if included, usually in multivisceral Txs)
    - Donor greater curvature is preserved with gastroepiploic arteries, and donor stomach is anastomosed to proximal recipient stomach
    - Usually includes donor duodenum and pancreas
  - Intestine
    - Most common proximal anastomosis (if not multivisceral Tx): Side-to-side donor jejunum to host duodenum or proximal jejunum
    - Leftward displacement of gastric antrum and duodenum can result from surgical mobilization
    - Most common distal anastomosis: Donor ileum to host sigmoid colon
      - "Chimney" ileostomy at end of donor ileum (temporary or permanent)

- Percutaneous gastrostomy and jejunostomy tubes are placed initially
  - Liver (if included, as part of multivisceral Tx)
  - Pancreas (if included)
    - With intact duodenum, SB, liver as part of multivisceral Tx (usually)
  - Vasculature
    - Arterial
      - Isolated SB Tx: Donor SMA anastomosed to host aorta
      - Multivisceral Tx: 10-cm portion of donor aorta is taken, with celiac trunk and SMA intact, then grafted end to side to host aorta
    - Venous
      - Isolated SB Tx: Donor SMV is anastomosed to host SMV or portal vein
      - Multivisceral Tx: Donor and recipient inferior vena cavas may be anastomosed end to end
      - Portal venous system from donor remains intact; transplanted en bloc

Radiographic Findings
- Upper GI series with oral contrast medium
  - Examine allograft, anastomoses, tone, and motility
  - Pathology: Adhesions, volvulus, stenosis, leak
    - Usually straightforward diagnosis
    - Introduce water-soluble contrast material via stomach (drinking or percutaneous endoscopic gastrostomy tube)
      - Via right lower quadrant ileostomy site
      - Via jejunostomy tube (present in all patients soon after SB Tx)
      - Via rectum
  - Measure transit time with radiopaque markers or oral barium contrast medium
    - Range: 0.2-17.8 hours
    - Most patients display delayed gastric emptying associated with decreased gastric peristalsis
      - 76% of patients have delayed gastric emptying in first 2 months but only 16% at 6 months
      - May be from use of narcotics during perioperative period
- Complications
  - Usually detected on CT; less often on MR
    - Catheter angiography usually performed only after CT, MR, or US has shown evidence of vascular complication
  - Vascular complications
    - Thrombosis
      - Lumen of affected artery or vein fails to opacify with vascular contrast medium
    - Anastomotic strictures
      - Relatively less common in SB Tx due to larger vessels involved
    - Pseudoaneurysm
      - Ballooning out of lumen of vessels, usually artery and usually at site of anastomosis
      - May be due to surgical error or infection
      - Requires surgical revision or intervention (e.g., stent graft)
  - Mesenteritis

- Almost all SB Tx recipients develop some degree of infiltration and thickening of allograft mesentery
  □ Usually persists for up to 1 month
- Usually associated with bowel wall thickening
- May be asymptomatic and of no concern in perioperative period
- Probably represents combination of lymphedema (transected lymphatics) and mild rejection
- Severe mesenteric ± bowel wall thickening usually due to rejection
○ Rejection and graft-vs.-host disease
  - Both are common, cannot be distinguished on imaging
  - Nonspecific findings of allograft wall thickening
  - Diagnosis: Mucosal biopsy of stomach, duodenum, or SB
    □ SB biopsy usually via ileostomy
○ Opportunistic infections
  - May affect any organ (e.g., pneumonia)
  - May affect allograft itself (e.g., CMV enteritis)
  - Cannot be diagnosed on imaging or differentiated from other causes of SB wall edema
○ Dilation of SB lumen
  - In 2/3 of patients in 1st month post SB Tx
  - Nonspecific ileus (denervation of SB, general response to major surgery)
  - May result from dysmotility, adhesion, ischemia, or rejection
  - Endoscopy through ileostomy helps evaluation
○ Pneumatosis
  - May represent ischemia
  - **Most cases are "benign" due to medications, ± influence of bowel dilation, endoscopy, etc.**
  - Endoscopy used to differentiate
○ Ascites
  - Present in most patients, at least temporarily
    □ Usually regresses without treatment
  - Usually somewhat loculated between bowel loops
  - Difficult to distinguish from infected ascites
    □ May require image-guided aspiration of fluid for diagnosis and treatment
  - Chylous ascites
    □ Suggested by presence of fat-fluid levels
    □ Due to interrupted bowel lymphatics
○ Abscess
  - Increased incidence in SB and multivisceral Tx compared to solid organ Tx
  - May appear as loculated ascites with thick, enhancing wall, ± gas bubbles
  - May result from or cause bowel anastomotic leak or fistula
    □ Fistula may extend to skin or, as sinus tract, to retroperitoneum or body wall
○ Mesenteric adenopathy
  - Present to some degree in most SB Tx recipients (clusters of mildly enlarged nodes)
  - Reflects inflammation, infection, or rejection (limited ability to distinguish by imaging)

- Marked or generalized lymphadenopathy suggests additional disease, especially post-Tx lymphoproliferative disorder (PTLD)
○ Motility disturbance
  - Denervated bowel often shows some degree of decreased motility
  - Usually accompanied by generalized dilation of bowel lumen
  - More severe cases may be suggested by "gasless" SB on plain radiographs (fluid distended on CT)
  - Bowel motility can be observed directly by real-time US
    □ Especially useful in children due to lack of ionizing radiation
○ PTLD
  - More common in SB (up to 30%) and multivisceral Tx than most other solid organ Tx recipients
  - More common within allografts themselves than in host organs
    □ Poorly defined hypodense hepatic masses, ± portal adenopathy
    □ Eccentric SB Tx wall thickening, ± intussusception, obstruction, cavitation ("aneurysmal dilation" of lumen)
    □ Soft tissue density masses anywhere in body
  - Only 25% present as markedly enlarged lymph nodes, usually retroperitoneal or generalized, not limited to mesenteric nodes

Imaging Recommendations

- Best imaging tool
  ○ Multiplanar CT, ± CT angiography, displays most important anatomical and pathophysiological information pertinent to SB Tx
  ○ Upper GI series to evaluate motility and status of proximal bowel anastomosis

CLINICAL ISSUES

Natural History & Prognosis

- SB Tx: 1-year patient survival (90%); graft survival (~ 75%)
- Multivisceral Tx: 1-year patient survival (80%)
  ○ 5-year patient survival: 60%
- Worse than for solid organ Tx recipients

DIAGNOSTIC CHECKLIST

Consider

- Imaging is valuable adjunct
  ○ Reasonable accuracy for morphologic abnormalities (e.g., vascular, bowel obstruction, abscess, tumor)
- Diagnosis of allograft rejection, infection, or ischemia is usually dependent on endoscopy and biopsy

SELECTED REFERENCES

1. Ruiz P: Updates on acute and chronic rejection in small bowel and multivisceral allografts. Curr Opin Organ Transplant. 19(3):293-302, 2014
2. van Dijk G et al: Liver, pancreas and small bowel transplantation: current ethical issues. Best Pract Res Clin Gastroenterol. 28(2):281-92, 2014
3. Selvaggi G et al: Intestinal and multivisceral transplantation: future perspectives. Front Biosci. 12:4742-54, 2007

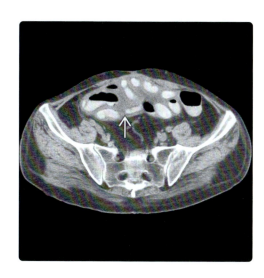 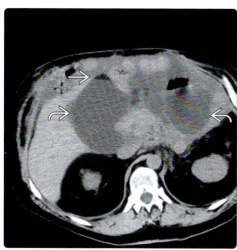

(Left) *Axial nonenhanced (NE) CT shows extensive infiltration of the SB allograft mesentery* ➡ *along with mural thickening of the bowel wall. Both are common and nonspecific findings in recipients of SB Tx.* (Right) *Axial NECT shows fat-fluid levels* ➡ *that indicate the chylous nature of the loculated ascites* ➡ *interposed between loops of the SB allograft. Leakage from SB lymphatics usually resolves over time as the lymphatic connections reform but may require percutaneous drainage.*

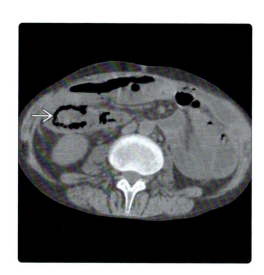 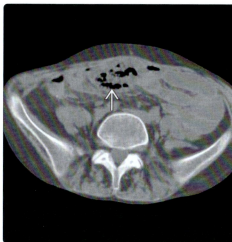

(Left) *NECT shows that the SB allograft is dilated with a thickened wall and pneumatosis* ➡, *raising concern for infarction of the bowel.* (Right) *NECT in the same patient shows pneumatosis* ➡ *in an adjacent part of the SB allograft. At endoscopy (through the ileostomy), the mucosa appeared normal. Pneumatosis within the wall of a SB allograft is not rare and may result from infarction, antirejection medications, bowel obstruction, or other "benign" causes.*

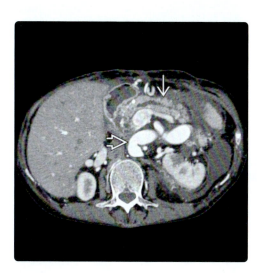 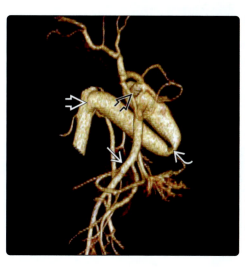

(Left) *Axial CECT in a patient with multivisceral Tx shows the pancreatic* ➡ *and liver allografts. The aortic anastomosis* ➡ *appears to be widely patent.* (Right) *Volume-rendered CT arteriogram in the same patient shows aortic anastomosis* ➡. *The aortic allograft is kinked or acutely bent back upon itself* ➡, *which may compromise flow to the allografts. Note the donor SMA* ➡ *supplying the SB allograft, while the donor celiac axis* ➡ *supplies the pancreatic and hepatic allografts.*

Hamartomatous Polyposis Syndromes

TERMINOLOGY

- Spectrum of hereditary and nonhereditary polyposis syndromes characterized by gastrointestinal (GI) tract polyps and other associated lesions

IMAGING

- **CT enterography is best imaging tool** (multiplanar, contrast enhanced)
- Best diagnostic clue
  - Cluster of small filling defects in small bowel (SB) with intussusception
- Peutz-Jeghers syndrome (PJS)
  - Polyps in jejunum and ileum > duodenum > colon > stomach

TOP DIFFERENTIAL DIAGNOSES

- Familial adenomatous polyposis and related syndromes
- Brunner gland hyperplasia (hamartomas)
- Lymphoid follicles (hyperplasia)

- Metastases and lymphoma (GI tract)

PATHOLOGY

- Sessile/pedunculated; carpet-like, clustered, or scattered polyps

CLINICAL ISSUES

- Most common signs/symptoms
  - PJS: Pain, mucocutaneous pigmentation, melena
- PJS complications
  - Intussusception, SB obstruction, malignant neoplasms
    - Bowel > breast > pancreas > reproductive tract
    - Prognosis: 40% risk of cancer by age 40
- **Intestinal polyposis syndromes encompass wide spectrum of diseases with considerable overlap**
  - Gene mutations and phenotypes
  - Polyp histology; disease severity; extraintestinal manifestations
  - Blurs distinction between polyposis syndromes

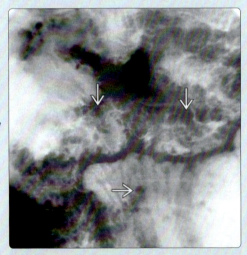
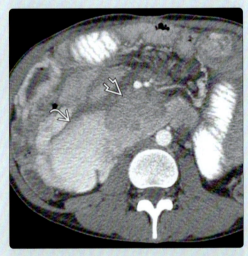

(Left) *This 28-year-old man has known Peutz-Jeghers syndrome (PJS). Film from a small bowel follow-through shows some of the hundreds of small polyps ➡, presumably hamartomas, throughout his bowel.* **(Right)** *Axial CT section in the same patient shows a large mass ⇒ causing partial obstruction of the duodenum ➚, which is markedly dilated. The mass proved to be a metastasis from a testicular nonseminomatous germ cell tumor.*

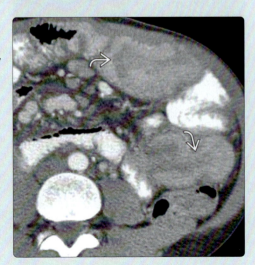
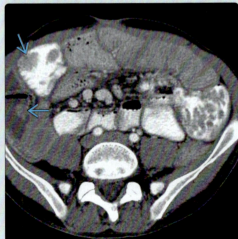

(Left) *Another CECT section from the same patient shows 2 segmental, nonobstructing intussusceptions ⇗, probably due to the hamartomatous polyps.* **(Right)** *Another CECT section in the same patient shows some of the innumerable small bowel polyps ➡. As illustrated by this case, some patients with PJS may develop malignant tumors, not just of the bowel, but also of the breast, pancreas, or reproductive tract.*

TERMINOLOGY

Abbreviations
- Peutz-Jeghers syndrome (PJS)
- Multiple hamartoma (Cowden) syndrome (MHS)
- Juvenile polyposis (JP)
- Cronkhite-Canada syndrome (CCS)

Definitions
- Spectrum of hereditary and nonhereditary polyposis syndromes characterized by gastrointestinal (GI) tract polyps and other associated lesions

IMAGING

General Features
- Best diagnostic clue
  - PJS: Cluster of small filling defects in small bowel (SB) with intussusception
- Location
  - PJS: Jejunum and ileum > duodenum > colon > stomach
  - MHS + JP: Most polyps in rectosigmoid colon
  - CCS: Stomach (100%), colon (100%), SB (50%)

Radiographic Findings
- Fluoroscopic-guided double-contrast studies
  - Multiple, variably sized radiolucent filling defects
- Polyps in PJS occur from stomach to rectum; mouth and esophagus spared
  - SB involved in 95%
    - Usually multiple, broad-based polyps
    - Clustered appearance more than carpeting bowel

Imaging Recommendations
- Best imaging tool
  - Double-contrast barium studies (multiple views)
  - CT enterography

DIFFERENTIAL DIAGNOSIS

Familial Adenomatous Polyposis and Related Syndromes
- Hundreds or thousands of polyps carpeting colonic mucosa
- Tubular or tubulovillous; colorectal cancer risk 100%

Brunner Gland Hyperplasia (Hamartoma)
- Duodenal bulb and descending duodenum
- Hyperplasia: Multiple nodules (Swiss cheese pattern)

Metastases and Lymphoma (Gastrointestinal Tract)
- Rarely as numerous as in polyposis syndromes

PATHOLOGY

General Features
- Etiology
  - Hereditary autosomal dominant (AD): PJS, MHS, only 25% of JP cases
  - Nonhereditary: CCS, 75% of JP cases
- Genetics
  - Spontaneous mutation of gene on chromosome 19 (PJS) and 10 (MHS)
  - *PTEN* is tumor suppressor gene

- Loss or mutation associated with variety of rare syndromes known collectively as PTEN hamartoma tumor syndromes
  - Includes Cowden (MHS) and Bannayan-Riley-Ruvalcaba syndromes

Staging, Grading, & Classification
- Classification: Hamartomatous polyposis syndromes
  - PJS: AD
    - Hamartomatous GI tract polyps, mucocutaneous pigmentation of lips, oral mucosa, palms, and soles
  - MHS (Cowden): AD genodermatosis
    - Mucocutaneous: Facial papules, oral papillomas, keratosis
    - Breast: Fibrocystic (50%), ductal-type cancer (30%)
    - Thyroid (65%): Adenomas, goiter, follicular cancer
    - Pancreatic ductal and intraductal papillary mucinous tumors
  - JP: 2 types
    - Isolated juvenile polyps of childhood (nonhereditary)
    - JP of colon or entire GI tract (AD)
  - Cronkite-Canada: Inflammatory polyps with ectodermal defects

Gross Pathologic & Surgical Features
- Sessile/pedunculated; carpet-like, clustered, or scattered polyps

CLINICAL ISSUES

Presentation
- Most common signs/symptoms
  - PJS: Pain, mucocutaneous pigmentation, melena

Demographics
- Age
  - PJS: 10-30 years
  - MHS: 30-40 years
  - CCS: > 60 years
- Epidemiology
  - PJS = 1:10,000

Natural History & Prognosis
- PJS complications: Intussusception, SB obstruction, malignant neoplasms
  - Bowel > breast > pancreas > reproductive tract
- Prognosis: 40% risk of cancer by age 40
- **Intestinal polyposis syndromes encompass wide spectrum of diseases** with considerable overlap
  - Gene mutations and phenotypes
  - Polyp histology; disease severity; extraintestinal manifestations
  - Blurs distinction between polyposis syndromes

Treatment
- Follow-up and surveillance; surgery for malignant neoplasms

SELECTED REFERENCES

1. Kobayashi Y et al: A tumor of the uterine cervix with a complex histology in a Peutz-Jeghers syndrome patient with genomic deletion of the STK11 exon 1 region. Future Oncol. 10(2):171-7, 2014

Small Bowel Carcinoma

TERMINOLOGY

- Primary adenocarcinoma of small intestine (excluding duodenum)

IMAGING

- **CT enterography is best imaging tool**
  - Multiplanar, contrast-enhanced CT with water distention of bowel
- Most commonly in jejunum, within 30 cm of ligament of Treitz
  - Duodenum is more common location but is often considered as separate entity
- Infiltrating tumor: "Apple core" or annular lesion
  - Short, well-demarcated, circumferential narrowing
  - Irregular lumen, overhanging edges, ± ulceration
  - Narrow, rigid stricture with prestenotic dilatation
- Polypoid sessile tumor: Small, plaque-like growth
- Often presents with intussusception
- ± enlarged mesenteric nodes; perivascular invasion

- ± metastases: Liver, peritoneal surfaces, ovaries

TOP DIFFERENTIAL DIAGNOSES

- Intestinal metastases and lymphoma
  - Non-Hodgkin lymphoma: Bulky mass with lymphadenopathy; rarely causes small bowel obstruction
  - Metastases: Multiple, from melanoma, lung, breast, etc.
- Intestinal GI stromal tumor
  - Usually larger, more exophytic and vascular mass
- Carcinoid tumor [most common primary small bowel (SB) malignancy]
  - Hypervascular submucosal mass with mesenteric invasion; most commonly in ileum
- Crohn's disease: longer segment od wall thickening, mucosal enhancement

CLINICAL ISSUES

- Celiac and Crohn's disease, polyposis syndromes ↑ risk
- Malignant tumors of SB are ~ 3% of all GI tumors

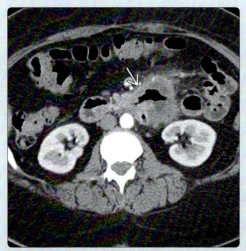
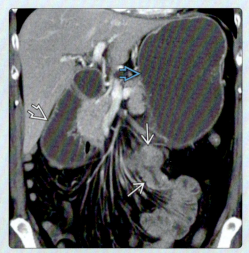

(Left) Axial CECT in a 47-year-old woman demonstrates mass-like wall thickening ➡ of the proximal jejunum. (Right) Coronal CECT in the same patient demonstrates the focal wall thickening in the jejunum ➡. Note the fluid-filled distension of the duodenum ➡ and stomach ➡, secondary to bowel obstruction by the mass. This was found to be a jejunal adenocarcinoma at surgical resection.

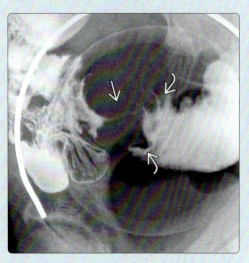
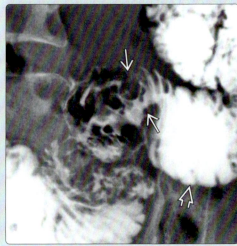

(Left) Spot film from a small bowel follow-through (SBFT) shows an "apple core" stricture of the terminal ileum ➡ with luminal narrowing, mucosal destruction, and overhanging margins ➡. These are classic features of a primary SB carcinoma. (Right) Spot film from a SBFT shows a jejunal mass ➡ with nodular thickened folds, mucosal destruction, and luminal narrowing, characteristic findings of a primary SB carcinoma. The bowel upstream from this tumor is dilated ➡.

KEY FACTS

TERMINOLOGY

- Intestinal metastases from extraintestinal primary cancer
- Primary small bowel (SB) lymphoma
  - Limited to bowel ± mesenteric nodes
- Secondary lymphoma
  - Involvement of spleen, liver, or thoracic nodes

IMAGING

- **Intestinal metastases**
- Malignant melanoma is most common primary site
  - Enhancing masses within SB mesentery and bowel wall
  - Bull's-eye or target lesions; intussusception
- Lung and breast carcinoma metastases
  - Are scirrhous tumors; likely to cause SBO
- Intraperitoneal metastatic spread (e.g., from ovarian and GI primary tumors)
  - Serosal metastases cause clustered adhesion and fixation of SB loops with functional SB obstruction
- **Intestinal lymphoma**

- Circumferential type: Sausage-shaped mass(es)
  - Rarely obstructs; may cause aneurysmal dilation
- Polypoid form: Bull's-eye or target lesions
- Mesenteric form: SB masses and nodes

TOP DIFFERENTIAL DIAGNOSES

- Primary small bowel carcinoma
  - Solitary mass causing luminal obstruction
- Mesenchymal SB tumors (e.g., leiomyoma, lipoma, etc.)
- Infectious and inflammatory etiologies
  - Mucosal hyperenhancement and submucosal edema

CLINICAL ISSUES

- **Metastases**: Most common with melanoma > lung, breast, others
  - May arise many years after primary tumor removal
- **Lymphoma** accounts for 1/2 of all malignant SB tumors
  - More common in patients with celiac disease or immune suppression (e.g., transplant recipients, AIDS)

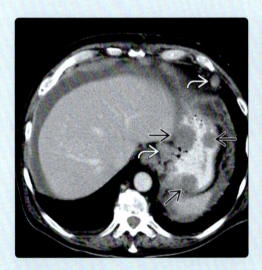
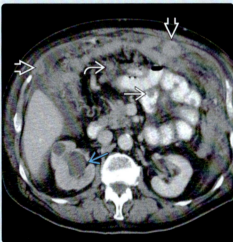

(Left) Axial CECT in a man with metastatic melanoma demonstrates classic widespread metastases from melanoma, including the gastric wall ➡ and lymph nodes ➡. The gastric wall metastases may ulcerate, leading to the classic target or bull's-eye appearance. (Right) CT in the same patient shows widespread metastases, including the small bowel ➡, lymph nodes ➡, & omentum ➡, with both nodular and diffuse metastases seen. The right ureter was obstructed due to a ureteral metastasis, causing hydronephrosis ➡.

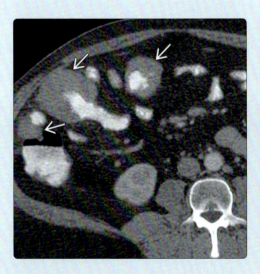
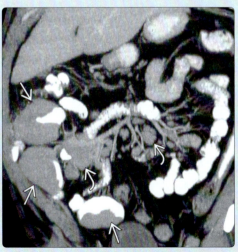

(Left) Axial CECT in a 46-year-old man who presented with a known history of non-Hodgkin lymphoma demonstrates extensive, multifocal, bowel wall thickening ➡. (Right) Coronal CECT reconstruction in the same patient illustrates extensive mesenteric lymphadenopathy ➡ and encasement of the mesenteric vessels but no bowel or vascular obstruction. Multifocal masses of lymphoma ➡ are also seen.

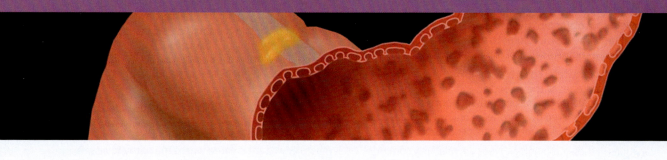

SECTION 7
Colon

Embryology and Congenital Malformations

The ascending and transverse colon, along with the small intestine, are part of the embryologic midgut, which undergoes marked elongation beginning in the 6th week of fetal development. To accommodate this increased length, the midgut herniates into the base of the umbilical cord. During the 10th week, it returns to the abdomen while undergoing a complex series of rotations and fixations.

All portions of the fetal colon are suspended on mesenteries, but the mesenteries of the ascending and descending colon usually fuse to the retroperitoneal fascia, normally leaving these portions covered by peritoneum only on their anterior surface and are thus regarded as retroperitoneal organs.

Variations in these embryologic steps are relatively common and may have clinical consequences. Failure of rotation results in the cecum and ascending colon lying on the left side of the abdomen. Accompanying malrotations of the other portions of the midgut may result in neonatal or adult **midgut volvulus** or adhesive band small bowel obstruction. A left-sided cecum carries with it a left-sided appendix, and appendicitis may present with confusing left lower quadrant pain in these individuals.

The cecum and portions of the ascending colon often maintain a mesentery of variable length into adulthood. This makes the cecum more mobile and prone to twist on its mesentery, especially with gaseous distention of its lumen, and may result in **cecal volvulus**. The sigmoid mesocolon is also often long with a narrow base of attachment to the posterior abdominal wall, predisposing it to twist. **Sigmoid volvulus** often obstructs the lumen, compresses blood vessels, and may lead to ischemia and perforation.

Gross Anatomy

The cecum is the 1st part of the colon and is ~ 7 cm long. It receives the terminal ileum through the ileocecal valve whose "lips" usually contain abundant fat, allowing them to be identified as a useful landmark on CT scans. The appendix is a blind diverticulum, 6-15 cm in length, that has its own mesentery (the mesoappendix). The appendix always arises from the tip of the cecum but may lie in many locations with over 60% of patients having a retrocecal appendix.

The ascending colon extends from the 1st semilunar fold, at the ileocecal valve, to the transverse colon. Its vascular supply is from the right colic branches of the superior mesenteric artery and vein (SMA and SMV, respectively). The transverse colon includes the "radiologic" hepatic and splenic flexures and is supplied by middle colic branches of the SMA and SMV. The descending colon is supplied by the inferior mesenteric artery and vein (IMA and IMV, respectively) and is retroperitoneal. Despite frequent anastomoses between branches of the SMA and IMA, including the marginal artery (of Drummond) and arc of Riolan, the splenic flexure through the descending colon is a common site of **hypoperfusion and ischemia** and may be the result of a congenital deficiency of vascular anastomoses ("watershed area").

The sigmoid colon is quite variable in its length, redundancy, and location. The rectum is the final 15-20 cm of colon. The rectosigmoid junction is usually at the lumbosacral junction and lies in the extraperitoneal pelvis. The rectum has both a mesenteric (superior rectal branches of IMA and IMV) and systemic (middle and inferior rectal branches in the internal iliac vessels) vascular supply. Because of its dual blood supply,

rectal carcinoma may metastasize to systemic sites (lungs, bones, etc.) as well as to the liver (via its IMV drainage), while colon carcinoma almost always metastasizes to the liver 1st.

Mural (Wall) Anatomy

The longitudinal layer of muscle in the colon is not as continuous as it is in the small intestine. Instead, it is separated into taeniae, which are 3 thickened, flat bands of smooth muscle. The rectum has a continuous layer of longitudinal muscle, rather than the taeniae.

The haustra are sacculations of colon wall caused by contraction of the taenia coli and are separated by the semilunar folds. The rectum has valves, which are analogous to the semilunar folds of the colon. Areas of weakness in the muscular wall are created where the nutrient vessels penetrate. Mucosa and submucosa can herniate through these areas of weakness, resulting in diverticulosis.

The colonic submucosa contains numerous, discrete lymphoid follicles that may be apparent as subtle 3- to 4-mm nodules on a double-contrast barium enema, especially in the right colon. The mucosa, unlike the small intestine, is smooth and not covered with villous projections.

Epiploic (omental) appendages (or appendices) are subserosal pockets of fat extending off the colonic surface. These may twist and infarct, causing epiploic appendagitis with symptoms that mimic those of diverticulitis or appendicitis.

Imaging Issues

The double-contrast barium enema, while an excellent study for the diagnosis of colonic diseases, has seen a precipitous decline in use since the advent of colonoscopy, which allows both direct visualization and the ability to biopsy suspicious lesions.

CT is the exam of choice for evaluating local invasion and nodal involvement of neoplasms, colonic inflammatory conditions, the mesenteric vasculature, and pericolonic soft tissues. IV contrast medium is very useful to diagnose various ischemic and infectious/inflammatory conditions. Administration of "positive" rectal contrast medium may be useful, especially to diagnose colonic fistulas.

CT colonography, in experienced hands, has proven to be an excellent screening modality but is time-intensive and requires added expertise in both the performance and interpretation of the study.

Approach to Abnormal Colon

When evaluating a colonic abnormality, the 1st question to address is whether the lesion is diffuse, segmental, or focal. Wall thickening should be characterized as submucosal edema (infectious, inflammatory, or ischemic, never neoplastic) or soft tissue density (less specific, includes possible neoplasm and diverticulitis). Gas density represents pneumatosis but could represent infarction or several nonischemic causes, including the benign, idiopathic pneumatosis coli.

Mucosal lesions form acute borders with the wall and may be pedunculated. Small, solitary mucosal lesions are likely polyps, while a polyposis syndrome should be considered if multiple polyps are present. Large or irregular lesions should raise a suspicion for colon cancer.

Submucosal lesions are found within the bowel wall and form less acute borders ("right angles") with smooth overlying mucosa, although larger lesions can ulcerate. These are much less common than mucosal lesions with lymphoma being the most common example. A pattern of multiple submucosal filling defects ("thumbprinting") is seen with edema, which may result from an inflammatory, infectious, or ischemic process.

Extrinsic lesions displace bowel, and the mass effect creates obtuse borders on contrast studies.

Colonic strictures are common, and, like focal lesions, analyzing the appearance will help in formulating a differential. Malignant strictures (e.g., colon cancer) are generally short segment with abrupt narrowing and overhanging edges ("apple core" lesion). A benign stricture (e.g., postinflammatory or ischemic) is generally longer with smooth, tapered ends.

The length and location of colonic involvement is also integral to making the appropriate diagnosis. The most common lesions include the following.

- **Colon cancer**: Short segment (typically < 10 cm), soft tissue density, may occur anywhere; associated nodal, peritoneal, and hepatic metastases
- **Diverticulitis**: Segmental involvement (typically > 10 cm), most commonly in sigmoid, spares rectum; chronic sequelae include myochosis, a combination of hypertrophy of circular muscle layer, shortening of taeniae, and narrowing of lumen
- **Ulcerative colitis**: Long segment or pancolitis, begins at rectum with contiguous involvement proximally
- **Crohn's (granulomatous) colitis**: Variable length segmental involvement with skip areas, terminal ileum usually involved, may see perirectal involvement
- **Ischemia**: Segmental (90%), usually splenic flexure or sigmoid colon, spares rectum
- **Infectious colitis**: Long segment or pancolitis, involves rectum
- **Neutropenic colitis (typhlitis)**: Moderate length, involving cecum and ascending colon

Differential Diagnosis

Colonic Ileus or Dilation
Common
- Ileus
- Colon carcinoma
- Rectal carcinoma
- Sigmoid volvulus
- Cecal volvulus
- Diverticulitis
- Ogilvie syndrome
- Fecal impaction

Less Common
- Ischemic colitis
- Toxic megacolon
- Endocrine disorders
- Distended urinary bladder
- Neuromuscular disorders

Colonic Fistula
Common
- Diverticulitis
- Colonic carcinoma
- Cervical carcinoma
- Endometrial carcinoma
- Ovarian cancer

- Cystitis
- Bladder instrumentation (mimic)
- Postoperative state, bowel

Less Common
- Crohn's disease
- Bladder carcinoma
- Abscess, abdominal
- Infectious colitis
- Foreign body
- Trauma, colorectal

Colonic Submucosal Wall Thickening
Common
- Diverticulitis
- Infectious colitis
- Ischemic colitis
- Portal hypertension
- Ulcerative colitis
- Crohn's disease
- Obesity (mimic)

Less Common
- Colon carcinoma
- Typhlitis (neutropenic colitis)
- Chemical proctocolitis
- Colonic metastases and lymphoma
- Intramural hemorrhage
- Pneumatosis of intestine
- Hemolytic uremic syndrome
- Intestinal angioedema

Acute Right Lower Quadrant Pain
Common
- Appendicitis
- Crohn's disease
- Pelvic inflammatory disease
- Pyelonephritis
- Urolithiasis (renal calculi)
- Mesenteric adenitis

Less Common
- Diverticulitis
- Infectious colitis
- Epiploic appendagitis
- Omental infarct
- Cholecystitis
- Gynecologic and obstetric causes: Uterine fibroids, hemorrhagic ovarian cysts, ovarian torsion, endometriosis, ruptured ectopic pregnancy
- Ischemic enteritis
- Colon carcinoma
- Appendiceal carcinoma
- Pancreatitis, acute

Rare but Important
- Intussusception
- Meckel diverticulitis
- Typhlitis (neutropenic colitis)
- Mucocele of appendix

Selected References

1. Olpin JD et al: Beyond the bowel: extraintestinal manifestations of inflammatory bowel disease. Radiographics. 160121, 2017
2. Childers BC et al: CT evaluation of acute enteritis and colitis: is it infectious, inflammatory, or ischemic?: resident and fellow education feature. Radiographics. 35(7):1940-1, 2015

(Left) *Surface-rendered endoluminal view from a CT colonography study shows a pedunculated polyp* ➡. *This 6-mm lesion was subsequently removed via conventional colonoscopy and found to be a benign adenomatous polyp.* (Right) *Axial image from the same CT colonography study shows the pedunculated polyp* ➡ *outlined by the insufflated carbon dioxide.*

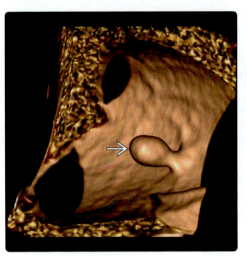
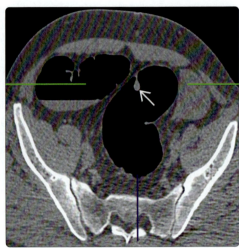

(Left) *Axial CT in a 19-year-old man with acute and chronic right lower quadrant pain and a palpable, tender mass shows mural thickening of the cecum* ➡ *with infiltration of the mesentery and enlarged regional nodes* ➡. (Right) *Axial CT in the same patient shows similar mural thickening of the terminal ileum* ➡. *These are typical features of Crohn's disease, confirmed in this case, but infectious enteritis may have a similar appearance.*

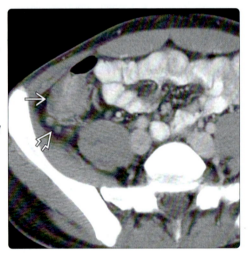
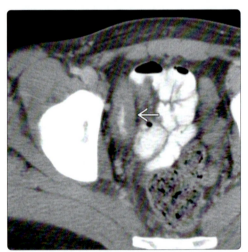

(Left) *Axial CT in an elderly man with acute right lower quadrant pain and a palpable mass shows a dilated appendix* ➡ *and a circumferential soft tissue density mass* ➡ *in the cecum with extensive invasion into adjacent tissues.* (Right) *Axial CT in the same patient shows an omental soft tissue mass* ➡, *essentially diagnostic of metastatic malignancy. At surgery, this and the cecal carcinoma were confirmed and resected.*

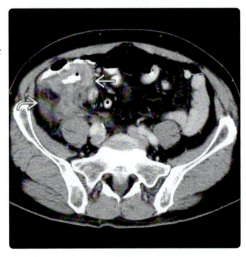
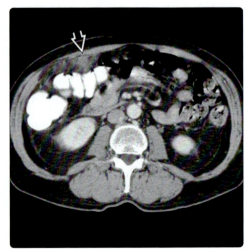

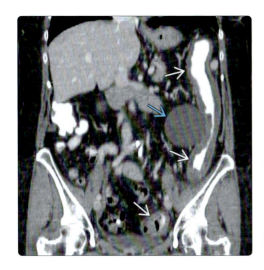
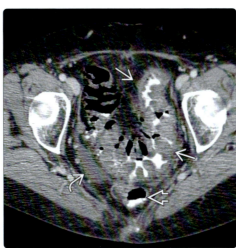

(Left) *Coronal CT in a 69-year-old woman with aortic valve disease, hypertension, acute pain, and hematochezia shows low-density wall thickening of the entire descending and sigmoid colon ➡. Incidentally noted is a renal cyst ⇨.* (Right) *Axial CT in the same patient shows "thumbprinting" ➡ of the sigmoid colon and ascites ⬊. The rectum ➡ was normal. These are classic clinical and CT features of ischemic (hypoperfusion) colitis.*

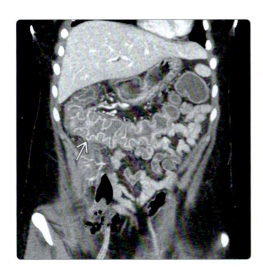
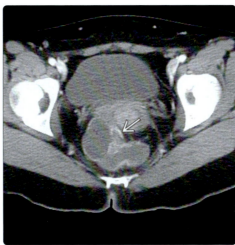

(Left) *An 18-year-old girl (and some friends) had acute onset of profuse, bloody diarrhea after eating hamburgers. Coronal CT shows massive submucosal edema ➡ affecting the entire colon, including the rectum. These are classic clinical and imaging features of infectious colitis. Enteropathic Escherichia coli (0157: H7 subtype) was the etiology.* (Right) *Axial CT in the same patient shows fluid distention of a thick-walled rectum ➡. The rectum is rarely involved in ischemic colitis.*

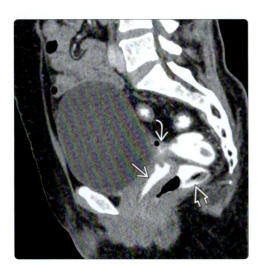
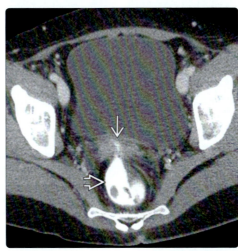

(Left) *This 50-year-old woman had foul-smelling vaginal discharge. Sagittal CT following rectal administration of contrast medium shows contrast filling the rectum ➡, the vagina ➡, and a colovaginal fistulous tract ➡. The cause was diverticulitis, infecting a hysterectomy scar.* (Right) *Axial CT in the same patient shows adherence of the rectosigmoid colon ➡ to the vaginal cuff with contrast filling the vaginal lumen ➡.*

TERMINOLOGY

- Colonic inflammation due to bacterial, viral, fungal, or parasitic infections

IMAGING

- **Best imaging tool: CECT with multiplanar reformations**
  - Mucosal hyperenhancement, marked submucosal edema, ascites
  - Multiple air-fluid levels, inflamed pericolonic fat
- *Clostridium difficile, Campylobacter, Escherichia coli*, CMV
  - Accordion sign: Alternating bands of enhancing mucosa and submucosal edema with compressed lumen
- May progress to hemorrhagic necrosis and perforation; toxic megacolon

TOP DIFFERENTIAL DIAGNOSES

- Ulcerative colitis (UC)
  - Wall thickening is generally less prominent with UC
- Crohn's disease

- Ischemic colitis
  - Usually located in watershed areas, rarely pancolitis
  - Rectum is rarely affected by ischemic colitis

CLINICAL ISSUES

- *C. difficile* colitis occurs mostly in institutionalized patients or those on antibiotic, chemotherapy, or immunosuppressive medication
- Acute infectious diarrhea is most often foodborne or waterborne disease
- Most common bacterial causes of infectious colitis in USA
  - *C. difficile, Salmonella, Campylobacter*, and *E. coli*
- Symptoms: Watery or bloody diarrhea, fever
  - Painful abdominal cramps and tenderness
  - Usually acute onset, except TB (chronic)
- Diagnosis: Stool cultures, blood cultures, endoscopic biopsy, serology studies
- Often self-limited or responsive to antimicrobial therapy in previously healthy patients

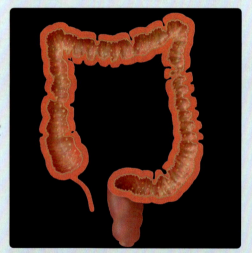
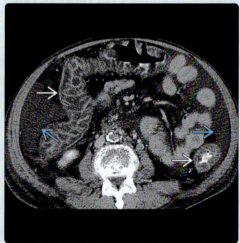

(Left) Graphic illustration demonstrates pancolitis with marked mural thickening and multiple elevated yellow-white plaques, or pseudomembranes, typical for Clostridium difficile colitis. (Right) Axial CECT in a 62-year-old man who presented with diarrhea and dehydration demonstrates a classic case of pseudomembranous (Clostridium difficile) colitis. Note the severe bowel wall thickening throughout the entire colon ➡, and ascites ➡. C. difficile colitis typically presents as a pancolitis, as in this example.

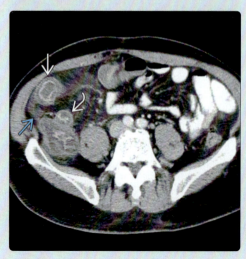
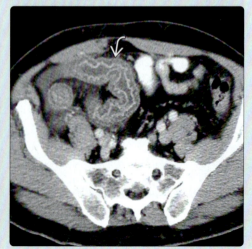

(Left) CECT of a young man presenting with acute abdominal pain and diarrhea shows marked mural thickening and submucosal edema affecting both the ascending colon ➡ and distal ileum ➡. A small amount of ascites ➡ is also seen. (Right) Another CT section in the same patient shows more of the inflammation of the distal small bowel ➡. The etiology was C. difficile infection, an unusual cause of small bowel inflammation.

TERMINOLOGY

Definitions

- Colonic inflammation due to bacterial, viral, fungal, or parasitic infections
- Pseudomembranous colitis: Descriptive term usually applied to *Clostridium difficile* colitis

IMAGING

General Features

- Best diagnostic clue
  - Usually pancolitis, including rectum
- Location
  - Dependent on etiology
    - *C. difficile*: Segmental or pancolitis
      □ Entire colon usually involved; distal small bowel (SB) uncommonly
    - Campylobacteriosis: Pancolitis ± SB
    - *Escherichia coli* (O157:H7): Pancolitis
    - Cytomegalovirus (CMV): Distal ileum and right colon or pancolitis
    - *Yersinia* enterocolitis: Predominantly right colon, occasionally left; invariably in terminal ileum
      □ Right lower quadrant clusters of enlarged nodes
    - Typhoid fever (salmonellosis): Cecum or right colon, invariably in ileum
    - Shigellosis: Predominantly in left colon
    - TB: Right and proximal transverse colon, involves ileum
    - Actinomycosis: Rectosigmoid colon (intrauterine devices), ileocecal region (appendectomy)
    - Gonorrhea, chlamydia, herpes, syphilis: Rectosigmoid colon
    - Histoplasmosis: Ileocecal region
    - Mucormycosis: Right colon
    - Anisakiasis: Occasionally in right colon, rarely in transverse colon
    - Amebiasis: Right colon ± terminal ileum
    - Schistosomiasis: Left or sigmoid colon

Fluoroscopic Findings

- Contrast enema
  - Used less frequently than before; now supplanted by CT, US, and endoscopy
  - Narrowed lumen, haustral thickening (edema/spasm)
  - Colonic wall, ulceration → mucosal irregularity, superficial or deep "collar button" ulcers
  - Discrete punctate, aphthous, or large, oval ulcers; may simulate Crohn's disease
  - TB
    - Oval/circumferential transverse ulcers; loss of demarcation between distorted terminal ileum and ascending colon
    - Fleischner sign: Right angle intersection between ileum and cecum, marked ileocecal valve hypertrophy
    - "Apple core" colonic stricture, indistinguishable from carcinoma

CT Findings

- **Multiplanar, contrast-enhanced CT is imaging test of choice**
- *C. difficile, Campylobacter, E. coli*, CMV
  - Mucosal hyperenhancement, marked submucosal edema, ascites
  - Accordion sign: Alternating bands of enhancing mucosa and submucosal edema with compressed lumen
  - Multiple air-fluid levels, infiltrated pericolonic fat
  - Deep ulcers and marked wall thickening
    - May progress to hemorrhagic necrosis and perforation
    - **Toxic megacolon**
- TB: Marked low-density enlargement of mesenteric lymph nodes
  - Enterocolitis is often due to ingestion of *Mycobacterium bovis*
  - Lungs may not be involved
- Histoplasmosis: Mesenteric adenopathy, hepatosplenomegaly ± calcifications
- Schistosomiasis: Changes in mesenteric or hemorrhoidal vein
  - ± calcification of bowel wall or liver
  - Bladder wall thickening and calcification
- Salmonellosis: May show SB thickening and effacement
- Actinomycosis: Large inflammatory masses
- Mucormycosis: Sinus, lung, and central nervous system changes

Imaging Recommendations

- Best imaging tool
  - CECT with multiplanar reformation

Ultrasonographic Findings

- Wall thickening with increased symmetric thickening and submucosal echogenicity
- Increased mural flow on color Doppler

DIFFERENTIAL DIAGNOSIS

Ulcerative Colitis

- Wall thickening is generally less prominent with ulcerative colitis vs. infectious colitis
- Barium enema
  - Pancolitis with decreased haustration and multiple ulcerations
  - Mucosal "islands" or inflammatory pseudopolyps
  - Diffuse and symmetric thickening of colon wall
  - Chronic phase → "lead pipe" colon

Crohn's Disease

- Concurrent SB (distal ileum) disease
- Transmural skip lesions, sinuses, fistulas
- Mesenteric lymphadenopathy (uncommon in most infectious colitides)

Ischemic Colitis

- Usually located in watershed areas, rarely pancolitis
- **Rectum is rarely affected by ischemic colitis**
- CT: May show pneumatosis, portomesenteric venous gas, ± thrombus within splanchnic vessels

DIAGNOSTIC CHECKLIST

Consider

- Diagnosis by clinical presentation, imaging, lab tests

(Left) *A previously healthy young woman developed diarrhea and tenesmus. CT shows evidence of pancolitis with marked submucosal edema ➡ causing an accordion appearance of the colonic wall.* (Right) *CT in the same patient shows involvement of the rectosigmoid colon ➡ but not the small bowel ⬈. Campylobacter colitis was the final diagnosis.*

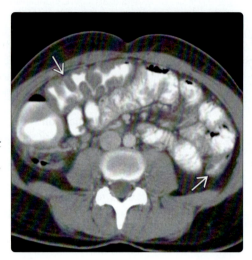
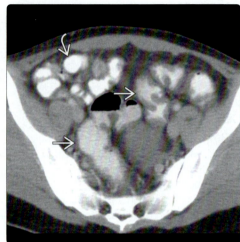

(Left) *A young man with AIDS developed diarrhea and hematochezia. A supine radiograph shows massive thickening of the colonic folds with a thumbprint appearance ⬌.* (Right) *CT in the same patient shows anasarca ⬈, ascites ⬈, and dilation of the small bowel lumen. The wall of the entire colon ⬌ is massively thickened. On endoscopy (not shown), the colonic mucosa was ischemic, and biopsy showed cytomegalovirus (CMV) infiltrating the colonic wall and inducing hemorrhagic necrosis.*

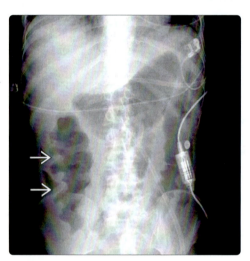
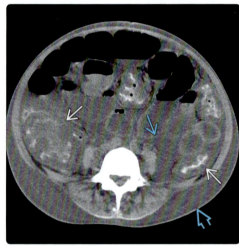

(Left) *A young man developed right lower quadrant (RLQ) pain, fever, and diarrhea. CT shows mural thickening of the ascending colon ⬌ and RLQ lymphadenopathy ⬈.* (Right) *Another CT section in the same patient shows wall thickening of the terminal ileum ⬌ and additional enlarged nodes ⬈. This is a typical example of Yersinia enterocolitis with mesenteric adenitis. Most forms of infectious colitis spare the distal small bowel.*

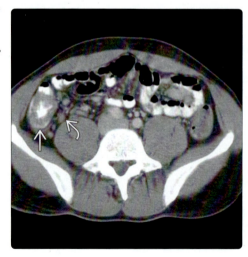
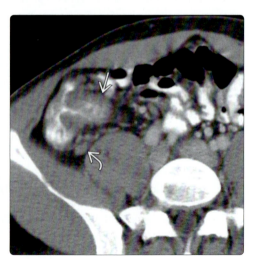

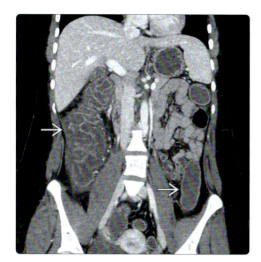
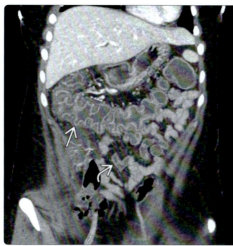

(Left) A teenage girl developed acute bloody diarrhea due to Escherichia coli colitis from contaminated hamburger. Coronal CT shows pancolitis with marked submucosal edema and fluid distention of the entire colon ➡. (Right) Another coronal CT section in the same patient shows more of the mucosal hyperenhancement and submucosal edema ➡ throughout the colon. The small bowel ➘ was spared.

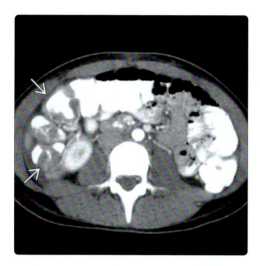
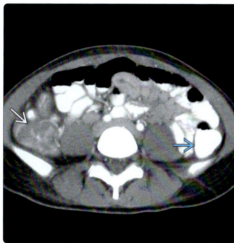

(Left) CECT of a 50-year-old woman with confirmed Salmonella colitis shows marked colonic fold thickening ➡ primarily affecting the ascending colon. Note that the presence of dense contrast material within the colon impairs evaluation for mucosal inflammation. (Right) CECT in the same patient shows marked submucosal edema in the cecum ➡. The left side of the colon ⇨ seems uninvolved. Preferential involvement of the right colon is characteristic of Salmonella (typhus), which is endemic in some populations.

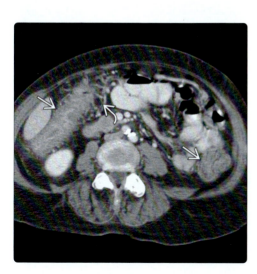
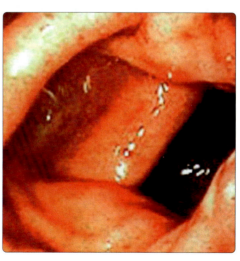

(Left) An elderly woman developed acute diarrhea and tenesmus. CECT shows pancolitis with thickening of the wall ➡ and adjacent mesenteric hyperemia ➘. The rectum and small bowel were spared. Campylobacter colitis was confirmed. (Right) Endoscopic image of the ascending colon in the same patient shows marked fold thickening due to Campylobacter colitis.

Stercoral Colitis and Fecal Impaction

TERMINOLOGY

- Hardened and impacted mass of feces that cannot be passed and obstructs colonic lumen
- Stercoral ulceration
  - Pressure necrosis of bowel lumen by fecal mass

IMAGING

- **CECT (multiplanar, contrast-enhanced)** to evaluate for perirectal and intraperitoneal complications
  - Fecaloma: Entirely intraluminal mass
  - Calcification or high-density matter in or around fecal mass
  - Laminated, radiopaque mass of feces
  - Focal thickening of bowel wall and pericolonic fat stranding (suggests stercoral colitis)
  - Pneumatosis, free air (confirms perforation)

TOP DIFFERENTIAL DIAGNOSES

- Diverticulitis
  - Thickens wall of colon, narrows lumen
  - Usually not accompanied by impacted feces
  - Pericolonic inflammation is dominant finding
- Villous adenoma, colon
  - Bulky but soft intraluminal and mural mass

PATHOLOGY

- Stercoral colitis: Focal inflammatory colitis due to ↑ pressure on bowel wall by fecal mass
- Stercoral ulcer: Pressure necrosis of bowel mucosa on antimesenteric aspect of bowel

CLINICAL ISSUES

- Can be life-threatening and is underdiagnosed
  - Perforation: Associated with 35% mortality
- Usually seen in elderly, debilitated patients
  - Or patients on anticholinergic or narcotic medications
- Requires urgent catharsis, enema, manual disimpaction
- Emergency surgery for perforation

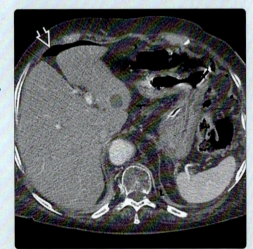
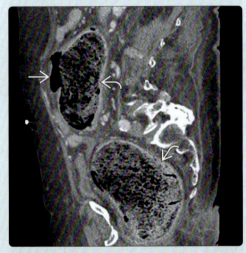

(Left) CT in an 85-year-old woman with chronic constipation and acute abdominal pain shows free intraperitoneal gas and fluid ⇉. (Right) Sagittal reformatted CT section in the same patient shows massive fecal distention of the rectosigmoid colon ⇗ with disruption ⇉ of the anterior wall of the sigmoid colon.

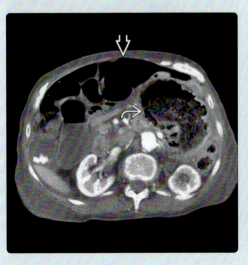
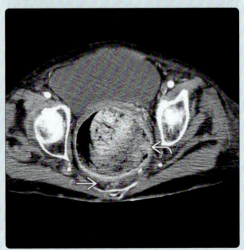

(Left) Axial CECT in an 80-year-old woman presenting with chronic constipation and acute abdominal pain shows free intraperitoneal gas ⇉ and massive distention of the left colon with gas and impacted feces ⇗. (Right) Axial CECT in the same patient shows the rectum massively distended with high density feces ⇉. Infiltration of the perirectal fat ⇉ suggests stercoral ulceration, confirmed at surgery. The rectal perforation by stercoral colitis was fatal in this case.

Rectal Prolapse and Intussusception

TERMINOLOGY

- Partial prolapse
  - Rectal mucosa protrudes no more than 1 inch below anus (shown on defecography)
- External (complete) prolapse (procidentia)
  - All layers of rectum protrude through anus
  - Diagnosis made on physical exam or defecography
- Rectosigmoid (internal) intussusception
  - Proximal rectal ± sigmoid mucosa telescopes into distal rectum; rarely through anus
    - Often "pinches off" base of anterior rectocele
    - Contributes to sensation of incomplete evacuation
  - Diagnosed on defecography or MR
- Rectal ulcer syndrome
  - Traumatic or ischemic ulceration of rectal mucosa associated with disordered evacuation
  - Diagnosed on barium enema or sigmoidoscopy
  - 95% of affected patients have internal intussusception

IMAGING

- Complex disorders of muscles, fascia, and supporting structures of pelvic floor
  - Involves posterior pelvic compartment
- **MR for complete and direct visualization of pelvic organs** and supporting structures of all 3 compartments
- **Barium evacuation proctography** for rectal disorders

PATHOLOGY

- Pelvic floor disorders often overlap
  - e.g., urinary and fecal incontinence; prolapse of bladder and rectum

CLINICAL ISSUES

- > 90% of adult cases are women
  - Some degree of pelvic floor weakening is present in > 50% of women over age 50

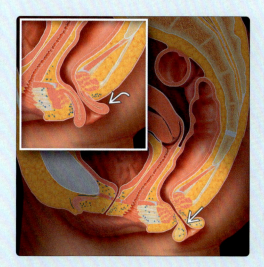
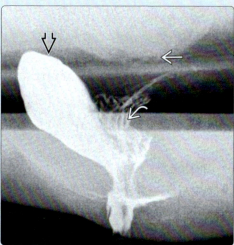

(Left) Graphic shows partial prolapse of rectal mucosa ➡ ~ 1 inch below the anus. Insert shows external (complete) rectal prolapse (procidentia) ➡ with herniation of all layers of the rectal wall. (Right) Film from defecography shows downward intussusception ➡ of the rectal mucosa, pinching of the neck of a large anterior rectocele ➡. Note the low position of the rectum and anus relative to the ischial tuberosities ➡.

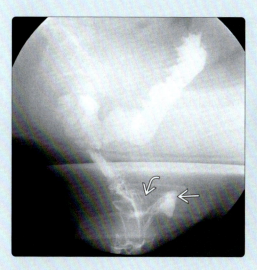
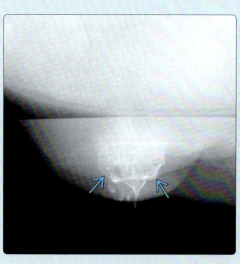

(Left) Lateral spot film from a defecography study shows downward intussusception ➡ of rectal mucosa into the lower rectum, pinching off an anterior rectocele ➡. (Right) In the same case a few seconds later, the rectum has herniated completely through the anus and is seen as a barium-coated mass ➡ outside the anus. This is called external (complete) prolapse or procidentia.

Colon

TERMINOLOGY

- Life-threatening, necrotizing enterocolitis occurring primarily in severely neutropenic patients

IMAGING

- **Best imaging tool: CECT with multiplanar reformations**
  - Massive mural thickening of cecal ± ascending colon wall
    - Other segments of colon and small bowel can be affected
  - Mucosal hyperenhancement and submucosal edema (marked)
  - Infiltration of pericolonic fat
- Less common, more severe findings
  - Pneumatosis, extraluminal gas and fluid (perforation)

TOP DIFFERENTIAL DIAGNOSES

- Pseudomembranous colitis
- Cecal diverticulitis
- Crohn's colitis

- Graft-vs.-host disease

PATHOLOGY

- Severely neutropenic patients
- Majority of cases are those with leukemia &/or hematopoietic stem cell transplant recipients
- Pathogenesis: Probably due to combination of factors
  - Mucosal injury by cytotoxic drugs
  - Profound immunosuppression
  - Invasion of bowel wall by microorganisms (polymicrobial)
  - Progressive necrosis of bowel wall

CLINICAL ISSUES

- Fever, RLQ tenderness in immunosuppressed patient
- Watery diarrhea ± hematochezia

DIAGNOSTIC CHECKLIST

- Consider history of chemotherapy for leukemia or bone marrow transplantation

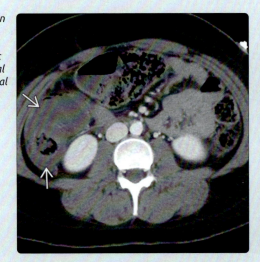
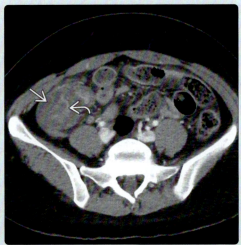

(Left) This 25-year-old woman was receiving chemotherapy for synovial sarcoma and became severely neutropenic with complaints of abdominal pain, fever, and diarrhea. Axial CECT shows marked submucosal edema of the cecum and ascending colon ➡. (Right) Another CECT section in the same patient shows mucosal hyperenhancement ➡ and submucosal edema ➡.

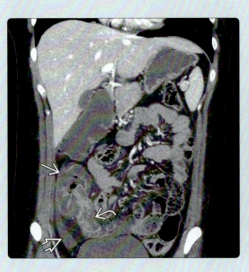
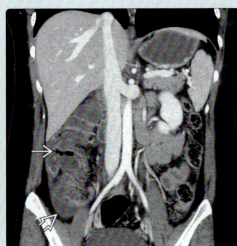

(Left) Coronal reformatted CECT in the same patient shows inflammation of the ascending colon ➡ and terminal ileum ➡ along with pericolonic ascites ➡. (Right) Another coronal CECT section in the same patient shows pneumatosis ➡ within the colonic wall, which, along with ascites ➡, suggests perforation, subsequently proven at surgery. Necrotizing, neutropenic colitis was the diagnosis.

TERMINOLOGY

Synonyms

- Neutropenic enterocolitis, ileocecal syndrome

Definitions

- Life-threatening, necrotizing enterocolitis occurring primarily in severely neutropenic patients

IMAGING

General Features

- Best diagnostic clue
  - Massive mural thickening of cecal ± ascending colon wall
- Location
  - Cecum, ascending colon ± distal ileum
    - Other segments of colon and small bowel can be affected

Radiographic Findings

- Radiography
  - "Thumbprinting" in wall of ascending colon, ± pneumatosis

CT Findings

- CECT
  - Involvement of cecum, ascending colon ± distal ileum
  - Mucosal hyperenhancement
  - Submucosal edema (marked)
  - Infiltration of pericolonic fat
  - Less common, more severe findings
    - Pneumatosis in affected segments of bowel
    - Extraluminal gas or focal fluid (perforation)

Ultrasonographic Findings

- Grayscale ultrasound
  - Hypoechoic or hyperechoic thickened bowel wall
  - Anechoic free fluid, ± mixed echoic abscess

Imaging Recommendations

- Best imaging tool
  - CECT with multiplanar reformations

DIFFERENTIAL DIAGNOSIS

Infectious Colitis

- Due to *Clostridium difficile* or other organisms, usually pancolitis
- Patients are usually not so severely neutropenic

Cecal Diverticulitis

- Bowel wall thickening, fat stranding, free fluid/air, cecal outpouching
- Mucosal hyperenhancement usually absent

Crohn's Colitis

- Usually affects small bowel ± other colonic segments in addition

PATHOLOGY

General Features

- Etiology

  - Severely neutropenic patients (absolute neutrophil count < 500 cells/µL)
    - Majority of cases are those with leukemia &/or hematopoietic stem cell transplant recipients
      - Especially those with acute myeloid leukemia
    - Myelodysplastic syndromes (lymphoma, aplastic anemia, myeloma)
    - Acquired immunodeficiency syndrome (AIDS)
    - Aggressive chemotherapy for solid malignancies
  - Pathophysiology
    - Mucosal injury by cytotoxic drugs
    - Profound immunosuppression
    - Invasion of bowel wall by microorganisms (bacterial and fungal)
    - Progressive necrosis of bowel wall
    - Probably due to combination of factors

Gross Pathologic & Surgical Features

- Hemorrhagic, thick, boggy cecum and ascending colon

Microscopic Features

- Inflammatory, ischemic, necrotic, ulcerative changes
- Polymicrobial infection of bowel wall is often seen

CLINICAL ISSUES

Presentation

- Most common signs/symptoms
  - Fever, RLQ tenderness in immunosuppressed patient
  - Watery diarrhea, ± hematochezia
  - Abdominal distention, nausea, vomiting
  - Peritoneal signs and shock suggest perforation

Demographics

- Age
  - Children > adults
- Gender
  - M = F

Natural History & Prognosis

- Complications: Abscess, necrosis, perforation, sepsis
- Prognosis: Early stage (good), late stage (poor)
  - Mortality has decreased to < 10% in recent series due to earlier diagnosis and better medical and surgical intervention

Treatment

- Medical: High doses of antibiotics and IV fluids
- Complicated case: Granulocyte transfusions; surgical resection for perforation

DIAGNOSTIC CHECKLIST

Consider

- History of chemotherapy for leukemia or bone marrow transplantation

SELECTED REFERENCES

1. del Campo L et al: Abdominal complications following hematopoietic stem cell transplantation. Radiographics. 34(2):396-412, 2014
2. Talebian Yazdi A et al: Neutropenic colitis. JBR-BTR. 94(3):138-9, 2011

TERMINOLOGY

- Chronic, idiopathic, diffuse, inflammatory disease primarily involving colorectal mucosa

IMAGING

- **CECT with multiplanar reformations is best imaging tool**
  - Air-contrast BE is excellent modality for diagnosis of ulcerative colitis (UC) but is rarely requested/performed
- Distal or pancolitis with mucosal hyperenhancement & only moderate submucosal edema
  - Moderate wall thickening (< 10 mm) & luminal narrowing in acute phase
- Target or halo sign
  - Enhancing inner ring of bowel wall (mucosa)
  - Nonenhancing middle ring of bowel wall (submucosa)
  - Enhancing outer ring of bowel wall (muscularis propria & serosa)
- Sites of involvement: Rectum only (30%), rectum & distal colon colon (40%), pancolitis (30%)

- Terminal ileitis seen in minority of patients with right-sided colitis, thought due to "backwash" ileitis
- Foreshortened & ahaustral colon in chronic phase
  - Submucosal fat density; pericolonic fibrofatty proliferation; narrowed lumen are seen
- **Toxic megacolon**
  - Colon is dilated with loss of fold & mucosal pattern
  - Ascites & ileus are common ± pneumatosis, pneumoperitoneum

TOP DIFFERENTIAL DIAGNOSES

- Crohn's: More segmental distribution, wall thickening, small bowel involvement, & mesenteric adenopathy
  - In ~ 10% of cases of inflammatory bowel disease, cannot distinguish Crohn's from UC
- Infectious colitis: More mucosal hyperenhancement & submucosal edema than in UC
- Ischemic colitis: **Rectum is almost always spared in ischemic colitis**

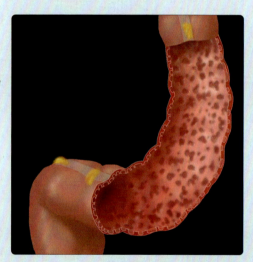
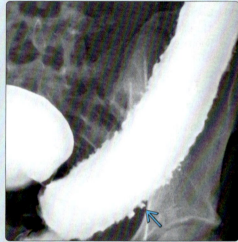

(Left) *Graphic demonstrates innumerable "collar button" ulcers and a loss of haustra throughout the descending and sigmoid colon.* (Right) *Single-contrast barium enema shows innumerable "collar button" ulcers ⟶ and loss of haustra throughout the descending colon.*

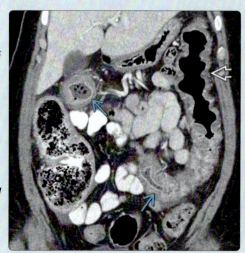
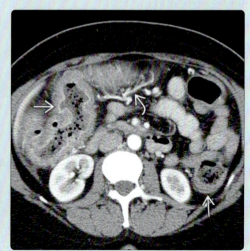

(Left) *This 51-year-old woman presented with an acute flare of chronic ulcerative colitis. Coronal CECT shows pancolitis with mucosal hyperenhancement and submucosal edema ⟶ with blunted transverse folds ⟶.* (Right) *Axial CT in the same patient shows the mucosal hyperenhancement and submucosal edema ⟶ involving all of the colon (and rectum on other sections). Note the prominent vessels ⟶ supplying the inflamed colon.*

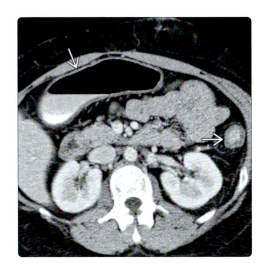

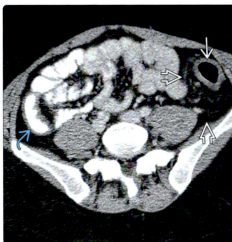

(Left) *Axial CECT in a woman with ulcerative colitis and primary sclerosing cholangitis shows diffuse colon fibrosis and loss of transverse folds ➡ (lead pipe appearance). Primary sclerosing cholangitis is strongly associated with ulcerative colitis.* (Right) *Axial CECT in the same patient shows mural thickening of the distal terminal ileum ⬀, known as backwash ileitis. Note the proliferated fat ➡ around the descending colon ➡, a sign of chronic inflammation.*

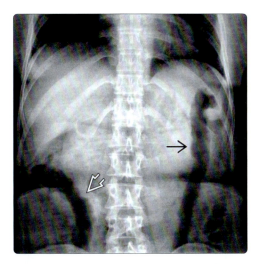

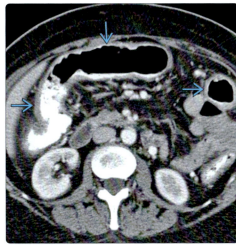

(Left) *Supine film in a 55-year-old woman with longstanding ulcerative colitis and abdominal pain shows the relatively straight and ahaustral colon ➡ with superimposed "thumbprinting" ⮞.* (Right) *Axial CT in the same patient shows mild diffuse colonic wall thickening ➡ without significant hyperenhancement of the mucosa, nor submucosal edema, typical findings of longstanding ulcerative colitis with fibrosis. Colonoscopy proved this patient to have active inflammation only of the sigmoid colon (not shown).*

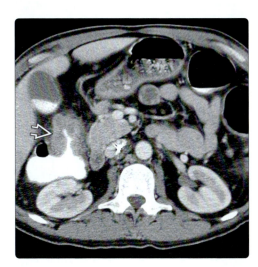

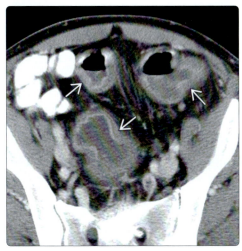

(Left) *Axial CT in a 49-year-old man with weight loss and anemia with chronic intermittent mucous diarrhea shows a circumferential soft tissue density mass ⮞ that narrows the lumen of the ascending colon. The mass proved to be a primary carcinoma.* (Right) *Axial CT in the same patient shows signs of pancolitis with mucosal hyperenhancement and submucosal edema ➡. Longstanding ulcerative colitis predisposes to colon cancer.*

Toxic Megacolon

TERMINOLOGY

- Acute transmural fulminant colitis with colonic dilation and systemic toxicity

IMAGING

- **Plain film: Marked colonic dilatation with abnormal or absent fold pattern**
- **Contrast-enhanced, multiplanar CT is best imaging tool**
- Dilated colon with air-fluid levels and abnormal or absent mucosal and transverse fold patterns
  - ○ > 8 cm (as measured on supine radiograph); > 5 cm on CT
  - ○ Transverse colonic folds may be thickened (edema or hemorrhage) or lost (sloughed mucosa and submucosa)
- Colon distended with gas, fluid ± blood
- ± intramural and intraperitoneal gas ± blood

TOP DIFFERENTIAL DIAGNOSES

- Colonic obstruction or Ileus

- ○ Preservation of mucosal and transverse fold pattern excludes toxic megacolon

PATHOLOGY

- *Clostridium difficile* and other infectious colitis
  - ○ Now most common etiology
  - ○ Ulcerative colitis was more common in past
  - ○ Ischemic colitis can rarely cause toxic megacolon

CLINICAL ISSUES

- Patients appear toxic, very ill
- Fever, pain, abdominal distension, bloody diarrhea
- Complications: Perforation, peritonitis, death
- Lab data: Increased WBC and ESR; positive fecal occult blood test
- Treatment: Colectomy and treatment of complications
- Prognosis: Good following colectomy without perforation
  - ○ Poor if colonic perforation and sepsis precede colectomy

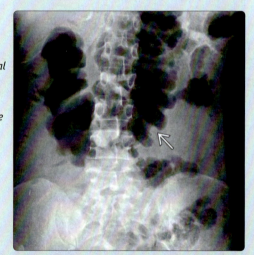
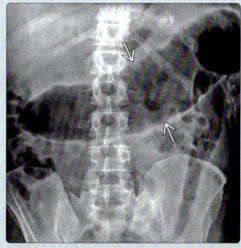

(Left) *Supine radiograph in a 58-year-old woman, who presented with severe abdominal pain and bloody diarrhea, illustrates the typical appearance of toxic megacolon on plain film. The transverse colon is dilated with marked thickening of the transverse folds* ➡. **(Right)** *This 35-year-old man with a history of ulcerative colitis presents with acute severe abdominal pain and distention. This supine radiograph shows a dilated, ahaustral transverse colon with a "shaggy" surface contour* ➡.

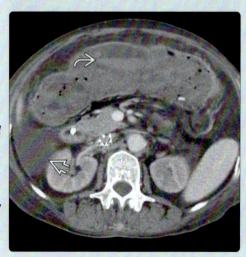
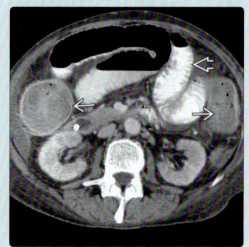

(Left) *This woman developed Clostridium difficile colitis while hospitalized for other reasons. CT shows ascites* ➡, *marked dilation of the transverse colon with loss of its folds, and intraluminal high-density material* ➡ *representing hemorrhage and sloughed mucosa.* **(Right)** *Axial CECT in the same patient shows a generalized ileus with dilated small bowel* ➡. *The colon* ➡ *is massively distended with blood and debris, and its wall is relatively thin. Soon after this scan, the colon perforated and a total colectomy was required.*

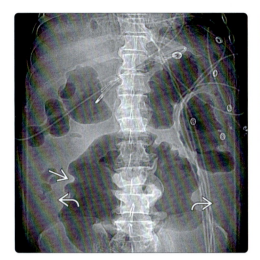

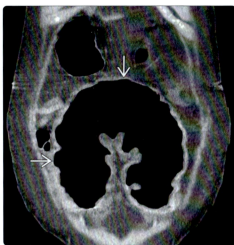

(Left) *This 61-year-old man was hospitalized for unrelated reasons and developed acute pain, diarrhea, hypotension, and tachycardia. This supine film shows bulging flanks ➡ due to ascites. The colon is diffusely dilated with a loss of the normal transverse fold pattern. The folds that are seen are grossly thickened and have a thumbprint appearance ➡.* (Right) *Coronal reformatted CT section in the same patient shows the markedly distended sigmoid colon ➡ with a complete loss of its normal transverse fold pattern.*

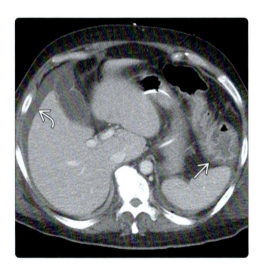

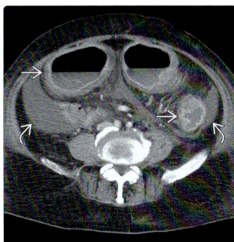

(Left) *Axial CECT in the same patient confirms a large amount of ascites ➡. Colon has a thickened wall with mucosal hyperenhancement ➡.* (Right) *Another CT section in the same patient shows the colon is distended with gas and fluid to a diameter of 7 cm. The mucosa is hyperenhancing, and the wall is thickened by submucosal edema ➡. No normal transverse folds are evident. Ascites fills paracolic gutters ➡, accounting for the bulging flanks seen on plain films. Soon after this study, the patient had a total colectomy.*

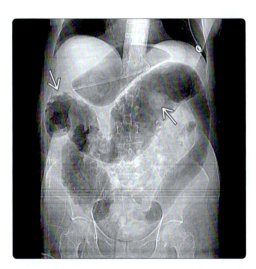

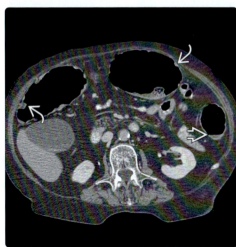

(Left) *This 68-year-old woman has longstanding Crohn's colitis with acute exacerbation. Supine film shows marked dilation of transverse colon with a featureless ahaustral appearance. Irregularity of the luminal surface ➡ suggests mucosal sloughing or pseudopolyps.* (Right) *Axial CT in the same patient shows gas and fluid ➡ distention and thinning of colonic wall as well as mucosal pseudopolyps ➡. Patient was refractory to medical management, and a total colectomy was performed.*

Ischemic Colitis

TERMINOLOGY

- Compromise of mesenteric blood supply leading to colonic injury

IMAGING

- Best imaging tool: **contrast-enhanced CT** with multiplanar reformations **without enteric contrast medium**
  - Allows better assessment of mucosal enhancement
- **Findings vary by acuity, etiology, and severity**
- **Acute arterial thromboembolic**
  - Emboli to superior mesenteric artery (SMA) from cardiac sources most commonly
    - Cardiac assist devices; prosthetic valves, etc.
  - Affects right colon ± small bowel
  - CT findings often subtle (ileus, lack of mucosal enhancement, no wall thickening acutely)
  - Occlusion or filling defect in lumen of SMA
  - Pneumatosis, mesenteric venous gas; more definitive but less common findings

- **Mesenteric venous thrombosis**
  - Thrombosis or filling defect in superior mesenteric vein
  - Marked submucosal edema of affected colon (right > left) ± small bowel
  - Marked infiltration of mesentery ± ascites
  - More common in hypercoagulable patients
- **Hypoperfusion ischemia**
  - Elderly, cardiac patients; recent hypotensive episode
  - Affects "watershed" areas of colon (splenic flexure and descending colon > sigmoid)
  - Long segmental colonic wall thickening on CT
  - **Rectum is rarely affected by ischemic colitis**
    - Due to dual blood supply
  - **Probably most common cause of colonic ischemia**

TOP DIFFERENTIAL DIAGNOSES

- Infectious and ulcerative colitis: Often involve rectum

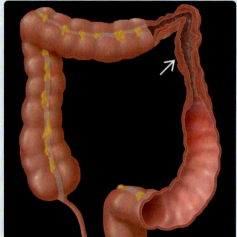
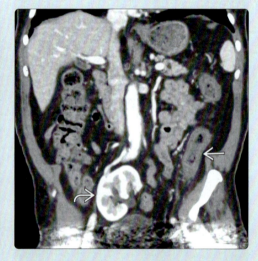

(Left) Graphic shows luminal narrowing and wall thickening ➡ near the splenic flexure, a "watershed" area between the vascular distribution of the superior mesenteric artery (SMA) and inferior mesenteric artery (IMA). (Right) This 89-year-old man had pain and bloody diarrhea several hours after a hip arthroplasty procedure. Coronal reformatted CECT shows wall thickening and mucosal and mesenteric hyperemia affecting the descending colon ➡. Incidental renal allograft noted ➡.

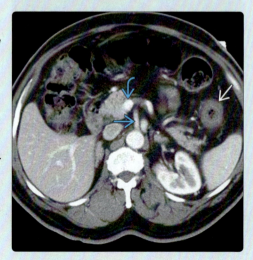
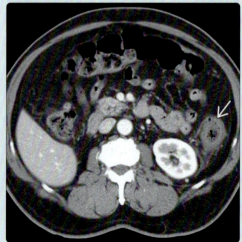

(Left) Axial CECT in the same patient shows submucosal edema and luminal narrowing of the descending colon ➡. The SMA ➡ and superior mesenteric vein (SMV) ➡ are patent. (Right) Another CT section in this patient shows wall thickening and pericolonic stranding of the descending colon ➡, while the remaining colon is normal. The rectum (not shown) was normal. These are classic clinical and CT features of ischemic colitis due to a hypotensive episode in an elderly patient.

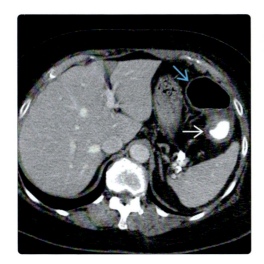
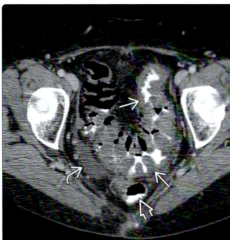

(Left) *This 69-year-old woman has aortic stenosis and was receiving medication for hypertension. She had sudden onset of abdominal pain and hematochezia. CT shows wall thickening in the proximal descending colon ➡, while the more proximal colon ⇨ is gas distended with a normal wall.* (Right) *Axial CECT section in this patient shows massive wall thickening ("thumbprinting") of the sigmoid colon ➡. The rectum ⇨ is spared. Ascites ⇨ is noted. These are classic clinical and CT features of ischemic colitis.*

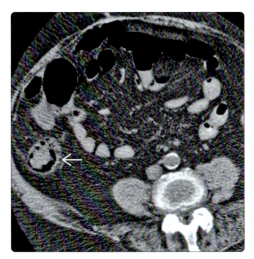
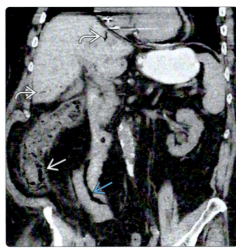

(Left) *This elderly patient has severe atherosclerosis and presents with abdominal pain and hypotension. NECT shows gas within the wall of the ascending colon ➡, which is otherwise relatively normal in appearance.* (Right) *Coronal NECT in the same patient shows gas within the wall of the distal small bowel ⇨ as well as the ascending colon ➡. Portal venous gas ➡ is also present. These are typical features of thromboembolic occlusion of the SMA.*

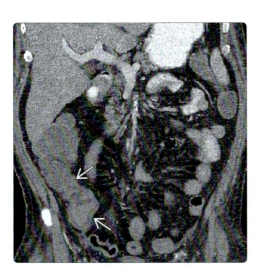
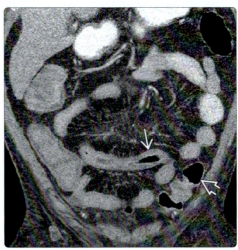

(Left) *This man had abdominal pain and hematochezia following resuscitation for cardiac arrest during dialysis. CT shows mural thickening with submucosal edema throughout the ascending ➡ and transverse colon (not shown).* (Right) *Coronal CT in the same patient shows mural thickening and edema of the small bowel ➡, while the distal colonic wall ⇨ is normal. This distribution of ischemic injury likely resulted from a combination of atherosclerotic narrowing of the SMA and the hypotensive episode.*

TERMINOLOGY

- Acute appendiceal inflammation due to luminal obstruction and superimposed infection

IMAGING

- **US is 1st-line imaging tool in children and young women**
  - **Multiplanar, contrast-enhanced CT has highest sensitivity and specificity (> 90%)**
- US: Distended, thick-walled, noncompressible appendix (≥ 7 mm)
  - Sonographic McBurney sign with focal pain over appendix
  - Shadowing, echogenic appendicolith
  - Increased flow within wall of appendix, indicating inflammation
  - Increased echogenicity of inflamed periappendiceal fat
- CT: Abnormal mural enhancement of distended appendix
  - Inflamed mucosa may show hyperenhancement
  - Necrotic wall may show no enhancement
  - Periappendiceal fat stranding
  - Appendicolith may be present (15-40%)
  - ± periappendiceal abscess or phlegmon
- **MR is good alternative to CT in pregnant patients and children when US is nondiagnostic**

TOP DIFFERENTIAL DIAGNOSES

- Mesenteric adenitis and enteritis
- Ileocolitis
- Crohn's disease
- Gynecologic causes
- Cecal diverticulitis
- Appendiceal tumor
- Cecal carcinoma

CLINICAL ISSUES

- Clinical diagnosis is frequently incorrect in children, young women, and elderly adults

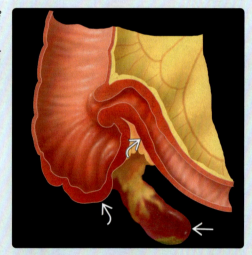

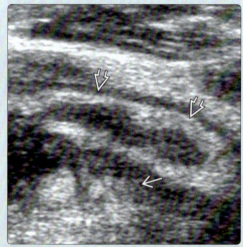

(Left) Graphic illustrates some of the characteristic features of acute appendicitis, including the distended, thick-walled, inflamed appendix ➡ and inflammatory thickening of the adjacent walls of the cecum and terminal ileum ➡. (Right) Longitudinal ultrasound demonstrates a distended, thick-walled appendix ➡, 10 mm in diameter with adjacent hyperechoic periappendiceal inflammation of fat ➡, indicative of an inflammatory process and diagnostic for appendicitis.

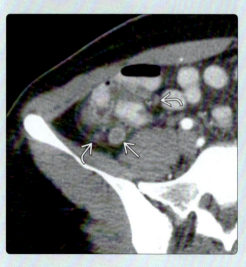

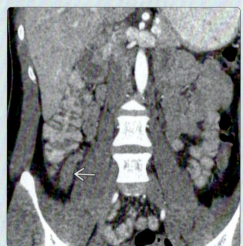

(Left) This young woman had acute right lower quadrant pain with an equivocal US exam. Axial CT shows inflammation of the fat planes and nodes ➡ around a thick-walled appendix ➡. (Right) Coronal reformatted CT in the same patient helps to identify the inflamed appendix ➡ and its retrocecal location, a common variant that may make it difficult to visualize the appendix on ultrasound.

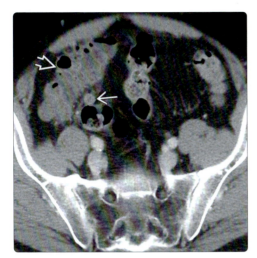 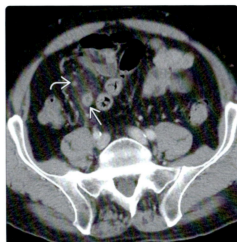

(Left) *This 61-year-old man had atypical signs and symptoms of right abdominal pain. Axial CT shows the inflamed appendix ➡ in an unusually medial position relative to the hepatic flexure of the colon ⇗.* (Right) *Another axial CT section in the same patient shows typical signs of appendicitis, including the thickened, enhancing wall ➡ and inflammation of the local fat and nodes ⇗.*

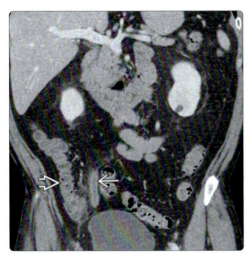 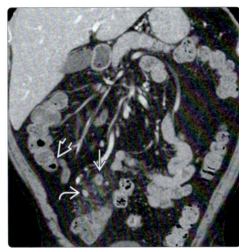

(Left) *Coronal reformatted CT in the same patient helps to identify the inflamed appendix ➡ lying medial to the ascending colon ⇗.* (Right) *Coronal CT in the same patient shows the appendix arising from the tip of the cecum ⇗. The inflamed portion of the appendix ➡ along with the inflamed fat and nodes ⇗ are at some distance from the cecal tip, accounting for the atypical site of maximum tenderness on exam.*

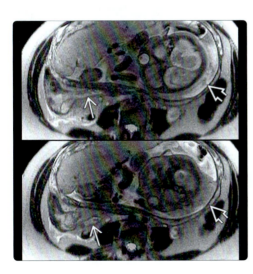 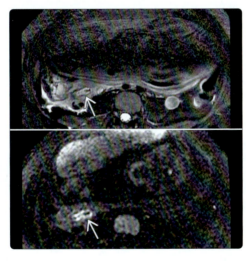

(Left) *This woman presented in her 2nd trimester of pregnancy with acute abdominal pain and fever. Following a nondiagnostic US exam, she had an MR study. On these T2 images, the gravid uterus and fetus ⇗ are evident along with a dilated, thick-walled appendix ➡ arising from the cecal tip.* (Right) *In the same patient, a STIR image (top) and a DWI (bottom) show the edematous, thickened wall of the appendix ➡ that also shows restricted diffusion. Acute appendicitis was confirmed at surgery.*

Colonic Diverticulosis and Diverticulitis

TERMINOLOGY

- Outpouching of colonic mucosa and submucosa, most commonly in sigmoid colon

IMAGING

- Best imaging tools: CT and barium enema
  - CT shows diverticula as outpouchings from colonic wall, filled with gas or feces
  - **Circular muscle hypertrophy (myochosis coli)** causes irregularly spaced indentations and narrowing of lumen of colon; causes symptoms of partial colonic obstruction

TOP DIFFERENTIAL DIAGNOSES

- "Giant sigmoid diverticulum"
  - Represents chronic, walled-off abscess that communicates with colonic lumen
- Diverticulitis
  - Due to perforation of 1 or more diverticula

PATHOLOGY

- Etiology
  - Sedentary lifestyle, high-fat, low-fiber diet predispose to diabetes, obesity, and diverticulosis among other ailments

CLINICAL ISSUES

- Affects > 50% of population > 60 years of age in USA
- Most common colonic disease in Western world
  - Diverticulosis is increasing in prevalence parallel to obesity epidemic
  - Diverticulosis in patients 20-40 years old is no longer rare
- Most common signs/symptoms
  - Most often asymptomatic
  - Alternating constipation and diarrhea (due to circular muscle hypertrophy)
  - Most common cause of rectal bleeding in patients > 40 years of age
  - Diverticulitis or abscess

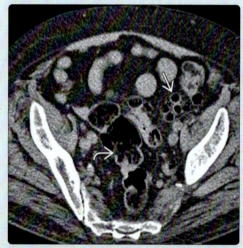
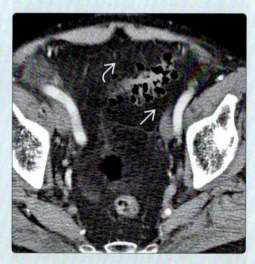

(Left) Axial NECT in a 74-year-old man with a 10-year history of obstipation presenting with lower abdominal pain shows a large amount of stool in the sigmoid colon ➡ and a cluster of gas-filled diverticula ➡ in the descending colon. (Right) Axial CECT in the same patient illustrates the normal fat planes of the sigmoid mesocolon ➡ and the small bowel mesentery ➡ without evidence of mural thickening or pericolonic stranding to suggest diverticulitis.

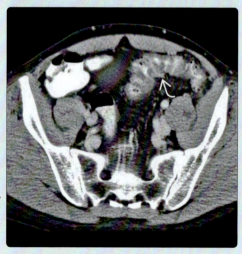
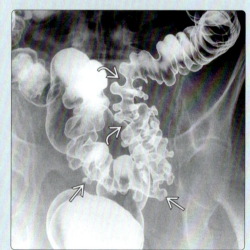

(Left) Axial CECT in a patient presenting with constipation and intermittent painful lower abdominal cramps shows thickening of the sigmoid colon wall ➡ due to myochosis, a combination of hypertrophy of the circular muscle layer, shortening of the taeniae, and lumen narrowing. (Right) Spot film from an air-contrast barium enema shows distortion of the colonic lumen. Luminal outpouchings ➡ are diverticula, while the irregularly spaced infoldings of the wall ➡ represent myochosis (circular muscle hypertrophy).

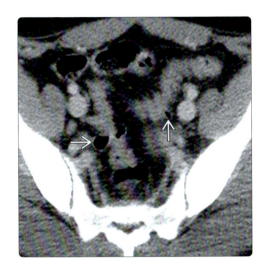
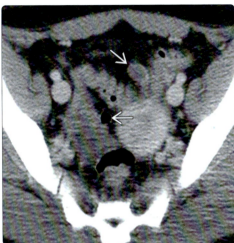

(Left) *This 21-year-old woman was obese and diabetic with complaints of alternating constipation and diarrhea. Numerous diverticula* ➡ *are evident, projecting from the surface of the sigmoid colon.* (Right) *Another CT section in this case shows additional diverticula* ➡. *Along with the epidemic of obesity, diverticulosis is now seen even among young adults, such as this young woman. Both obesity and diverticulosis are related to a diet high in fat and low in fiber, and both are more common among inactive individuals.*

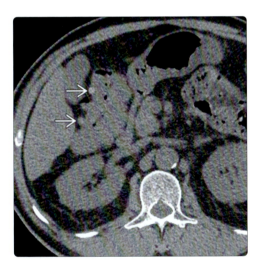
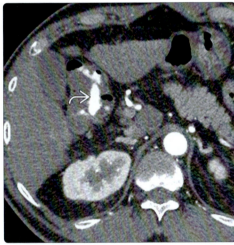

(Left) *This 75-year-old man had rectal bleeding (hematochezia). Axial NECT section shows right colonic diverticula* ➡. (Right) *Arterial-phase CECT in the same patient shows active extravasation of blood* ➡ *into the lumen of the ascending colon, essentially diagnostic of an acute and severe hemorrhage from diverticulosis.*

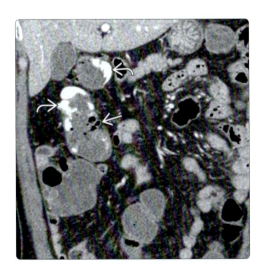
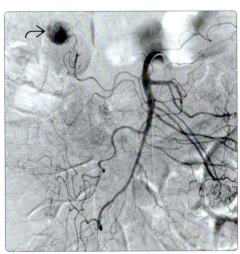

(Left) *Coronal reformatted CECT from the same patient shows the accumulation of opacified blood* ➡ *within the lumen of the colon. Also note the right side diverticula* ➡. (Right) *In the same patient, a film from the superior mesenteric angiogram confirms active bleeding* ➡ *into the lumen of the colon from a branch of the right colic artery. Diverticulosis is a relatively common cause for rectal hemorrhage.*

TERMINOLOGY

- Acute inflammation or infarction of epiploic appendages (EA, fat-filled serosal outpouchings on colonic surface)

IMAGING

- **Multiplanar, contrast-enhanced CT is optimal test**
- Best diagnostic clue: Small, oval pericolonic fatty nodule with hyperdense ring and surrounding inflammation
- More common in left lower quadrant
  - Rectosigmoid (57%), ileocecal (26%), ascending colon (9%)
- CT findings
  - Pericolonic, oval, fat-containing mass with thin hyperattenuating ring
  - ± central "dot" of increased attenuation within inflamed appendage (thrombosed vein)
  - Infarcted EA: Likely accounts for smooth, calcified "stones" occasionally found in dependent peritoneal recesses

TOP DIFFERENTIAL DIAGNOSES

- Omental infarction
  - Appears as larger (3- to 5-cm) ball of "dirty" fat adjacent adjacent to ascending colon
- Diverticulitis
  - Bowel wall and fascial thickening, luminal narrowing; pericolonic fat stranding ± free fluid and air
- Infectious colitis
  - Long segmental or pancolitis
- Ulcerative colitis
- Acute appendicitis

CLINICAL ISSUES

- Clinically, closely mimics diverticulitis and other acute inflammatory conditions
  - **Diagnosis is definitive by CT; obviates surgery**
  - Management by oral analgesics for ~ 3-12 days
- Occurs in all age groups

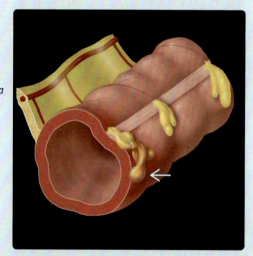

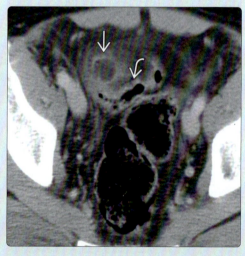

(Left) Graphic illustrates 2 normal epiploic appendages and 1 that is twisted and infarcted ➡. (Right) CT in a young man with epiploic appendagitis and presenting with acute pelvic pain shows a small, oval mass ➡ adjacent to the sigmoid colon. It has a fat-density core and a contrast-enhanced rim with inflammation of the adjacent mesenteric fat. The adjacent colon ➡ appears normal.

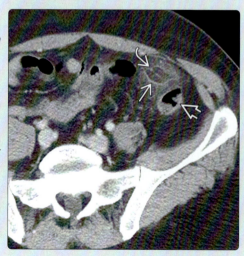

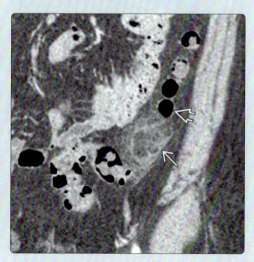

(Left) In this 36-year-old man with acute LLQ pain, CT shows a small, oval, fat-density lesion ➡ adjacent to the surface of the descending colon ➡. The lesion has a thin, enhanced capsule, and there is a thin linear density in its center ➡ that probably represents the thrombosed vein at the center of an infarcted epiploic appendage. (Right) Coronal CT in the same patient shows the small, oval, encapsulated, infarcted epiploic appendage ➡. The surrounding fat is inflamed, but the descending colon ➡ itself appears normal.

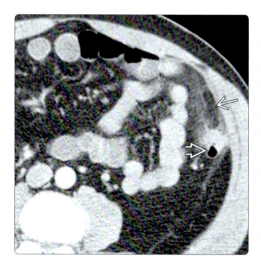 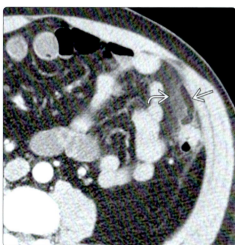

(Left) *Axial CECT in a 63-year-old man presenting with LLQ pain and fever demonstrates an elongated fatty appendage ➡ adjacent to the descending colon ➡. (Right) Axial CECT in the same patient illustrates pericolonic fat stranding ➡ adjacent to the inflamed epiploic appendage ➡.*

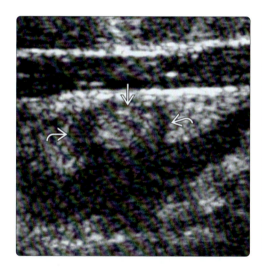 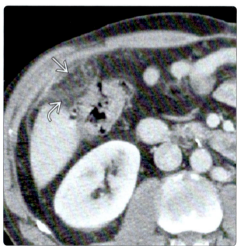

(Left) *Transverse US of the RLQ in a 19-year-old man presenting with RLQ pain demonstrates an echogenic appendage ➡ surrounded by a hypoechoic rim ➡. The lesion was tender and noncompressible. (Right) Axial CECT in the same patient illustrates an oval fatty appendage ➡ adjacent to the ascending colon with surrounding fat stranding ➡, characteristic findings for epiploic appendagitis. Omental infarction may have a similar presentation but usually appears as a larger ball of dirty fat.*

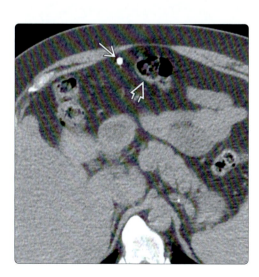 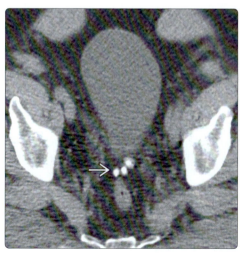

(Left) *In this somewhat obese patient, CT shows a small calcified lesion ➡ near the transverse colon ➡ that represents a calcified, infarcted epiploic appendage. (Right) In the same patient, similar calcified, small loose bodies are identified in a dependent peritoneal recess ➡ and presumably represent infarcted appendages that have detached from the colon. Similar findings can result from "dropped" gallstones, but this patient had an intact gallbladder.*

Sigmoid Volvulus

TERMINOLOGY

- Torsion or twisting of sigmoid colon around its mesenteric axis, resulting in progressive dilation & possible perforation

IMAGING

- **Plain radiographs are diagnostic in 75% of cases**
  - Dilated sigmoid colon with inverted U configuration & absent haustra
  - Vertical or oblique dense white line: Apposed inner walls of sigmoid colon pointing toward pelvis
  - Gas in dilated proximal small intestine & colon; absence of gas in rectum
  - Northern exposure sign: Dilated, twisted sigmoid colon projects above transverse colon on supine radiograph
- **Axial & coronal reformatted CT is most definitive test**
  - Coronal reformatted CT is especially useful in diagnosis
  - "Beaking": Progressive tapering of afferent & efferent limbs leading into twist

- Whirl sign: Tightly twisted mesentery & bowel near base of volvulus
- Contrast enema: Can demonstrate twisted, occluded sigmoid colon (usually not necessary nor therapeutic)

PATHOLOGY

- Major predisposing factors
  - Diet: Fiber increase → increased bulk of stool, elongation & dilatation of colon
  - Chronic constipation & obtundation from medications

CLINICAL ISSUES

- Most common signs/symptoms
  - Acute or insidious onset of pain + distention
- Treatment: Sigmoidoscopic decompression of obstruction ± stabilization via rectal tube insertion
  - Usually followed by surgical resection of sigmoid colon

DIAGNOSTIC CHECKLIST

- Rule out other causes of distal colonic obstruction

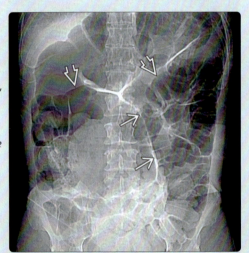
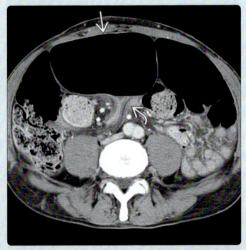

(Left) Supine film of the abdomen shows marked dilation of the sigmoid colon. The sigmoid is folded back upon itself, and the apposed walls ➡ of the redundant sigmoid colon form the "seam" of the football (or coffee bean) shape. The sigmoid extends into the upper abdomen above the transverse colon ⇒. (Right) Axial CECT in the same patient shows the dilated sigmoid lumen ➡ with abrupt narrowing at its base ⇗.

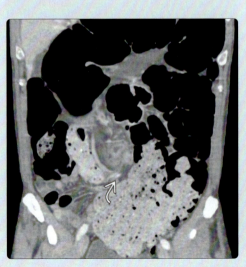
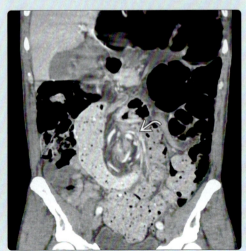

(Left) Coronal reformatted CT in the same patient shows twisting and displacement of the base of the sigmoid colon and its mesentery ➡. The dilated colonic segments upstream from the volvulus may be easier to distinguish on coronal sections. (Right) Another CT section in this case shows the whirl sign ➡ of a twisted colon and vessels at the base of the sigmoid mesentery.

Cecal Volvulus

TERMINOLOGY

- **Cecal volvulus**: Rotational twist of right colon on its axis, resulting in progressive distention and potential ischemia
- **Cecal bascule**
  - **Cecum is distended and lumen narrowed by medial folding and displacement, without twist**

IMAGING

- **Contrast-enhanced, multiplanar CT is best imaging tool**
- Radiography: Dilated, air-filled cecum, with tip in LUQ or abdominal midline
  - Single, long air-fluid level within cecum (upright or decubitus film)
  - Moderately distended gas or fluid-filled small bowel, little gas in distal colon
  - Markedly dilated cecum that appears upside down and backward with ileocecal valve directed laterally
- Additional CT signs
  - Whirl sign: Tightly twisted colonic wall and ileocolic mesenteric vessels

TOP DIFFERENTIAL DIAGNOSES

- Sigmoid volvulus
- Colonic ileus (Ogilvie syndrome)
  - Lacks twist of colon & its vessels
- Distal colon obstruction

CLINICAL ISSUES

- Accounts for 1/3 of colonic volvulus cases
- Complications: Ischemia, necrosis, perforation
- Treatment: Colonoscopy is **not** recommended to reduce volvulus
- Surgery: For immediate decompression & cecopexy

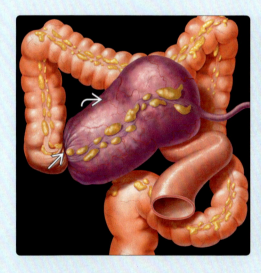

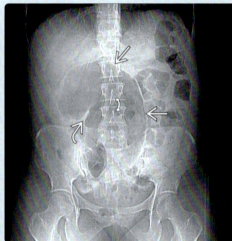

(Left) *Graphic shows a twist (volvulus)* ➙ *of the ascending colon, obstructing the lumen and blood supply. The cecum* ➙ *on the mesentery is dilated, ischemic, and displaced toward the left upper quadrant (LUQ).* (Right) *Supine radiograph shows a gas-distended segment of bowel (cecum)* ➙ *within the mid abdomen. The base of the cecum is directed toward the upper quadrant, and the ileocecal valve* ➙ *is directed laterally. Small bowel is gas-distended, whereas the left colon is relatively collapsed.*

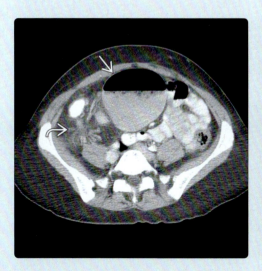

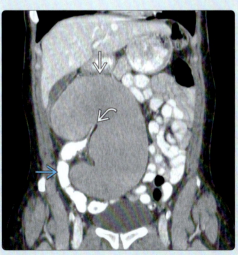

(Left) *Axial CT in the same patient shows a markedly distended cecum* ➙ *with an air-fluid level, and a twisted ("whirled") ileocolic mesentery & vessels* ➙ *within the right lower quadrant.* (Right) *Coronal reformatted CT in the same case shows the markedly distended midline cecum* ➙. *The cecum is upside down and backward, with the ileocecal valve* ➙ *pointed laterally. The SB* ➙ *is opacified with oral contrast medium. Coronal-reformatted CT is usually the most definitive study to show the characteristic features of cecal volvulus.*

Colonic Ileus and Ogilvie Syndrome

TERMINOLOGY

- Ogilvie syndrome, colonic pseudoobstruction, adynamic ileus, functional obstruction
  - Acute: Reversible, occurring with severe medical illness and major surgeries
  - Chronic: Constipation, no etiology for ileus, and repeated obstructive symptoms

IMAGING

- Proximal colon (cecum) dilates more than rest of colon
- Plain radiographs and CT for initial diagnosis
  - Follow closely to resolution
- Colonic ileus: Transitional zone often at splenic flexure
  - **Descending colon is often less distended than more proximal colon**
- **Contrast enema (water soluble)**
  - Very accurate for distinguishing obstruction from ileus
  - Danger of contrast extravasation if perforation has occurred

- **CT**: Differentiates mechanical obstruction from pseudoobstruction
  - No risk of peritoneal contrast extravasation
  - Can identify obstructing lesions, primary colonic pathology, (e.g., cancer, colitis, volvulus) or extracolonic pathology that might cause colonic dilation (e.g., peritoneal carcinomatosis; pancreatitis)

CLINICAL ISSUES

- May progress to ischemia and perforation
  - High morbidity and mortality
- Treatment: Pharmacologic or interventional decompression

DIAGNOSTIC CHECKLIST

- **Cecal diameter > 12 cm (on plain supine radiographs) is considered at risk for perforation**
- Colon diameter will always measure less on CT
  - Diameter > 8 cm on CT is significant dilation

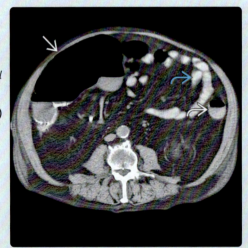
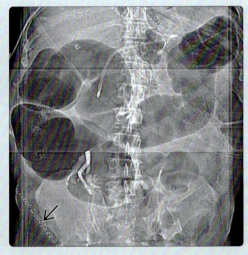

(Left) Axial NECT shows disproportionate dilation of the cecum and ascending colon ➡ in comparison with the normal-appearing descending colon ➡ and small bowel ➡. There was no evidence of a colonic obstruction or volvulus. (Right) Supine radiograph in a patient with postoperative colonic ileus shows distention of the entire colon but minimal gas within the small bowel. Skin clips ➡ are evident in the right lower quadrant from a recent renal transplant procedure.

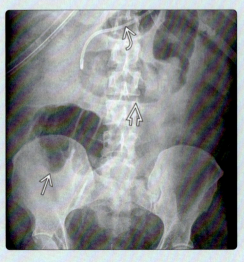
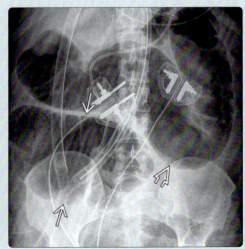

(Left) Supine radiograph of a young women, who recently had open heart surgery and now has a distended abdomen, shows dilation of a mobile cecum ➡ to 10 cm and slightly less dilation of the transverse colon ➡. A feeding tube ➡ marks the stomach. (Right) Repeat film in the same patient the following morning shows progressive dilation of the cecum (to 14 cm) ➡ and transverse colon ➡. Following a call to the referring physicians, the colon was decompressed using IV neostigmine and colonic intubation and suction.

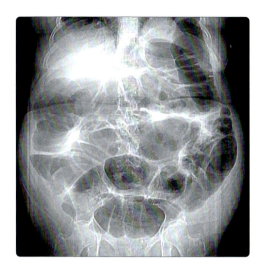 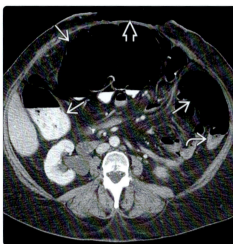

(Left) *Supine radiograph of a 63-year-old woman who recently had repair of a ventral hernia shows diffuse dilation of an elongated colon without definite dilation of the small bowel.* (Right) *CT in same patient shows an open wound ➡ from hernia repair. The colon ➡ is diffusely dilated, while small intestine is normal in caliber. The colonic distention persisted all the way to the rectum, although the descending colon ➡ is less dilated, a common finding in ileus that should not be confused with an obstructing lesion.*

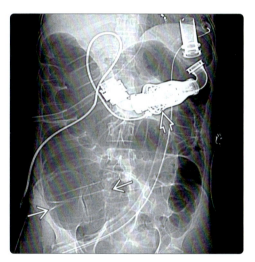 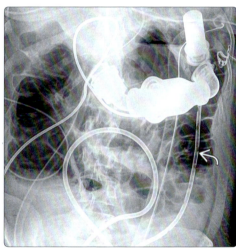

(Left) *This 42-year-old woman has cardiomyopathy treated with a left ventricular assist device ➡. Complaints of abdominal pain and distention led to this supine film showing massive distention of the colon. The cecum ➡ was 11 cm and the transverse colon 8 cm in diameter. On CT, however, the cecum measured 8 cm, and the transverse colon measured 6 cm in diameter.* (Right) *In the same patient, endoscopic placement of a colonic tube ➡ allowed decompression and relief of symptoms.*

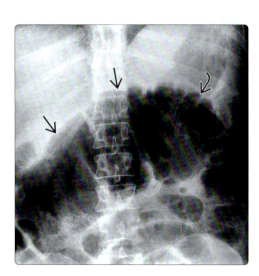 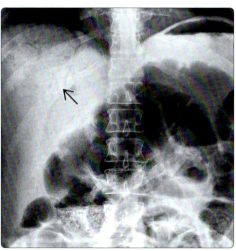

(Left) *Anteroposterior supine radiograph shows a dilated, gas-filled segment of colon ➡ in the upper abdomen with its cecal tip ➡ pointing to the left upper quadrant.* (Right) *Upright radiograph in the same patient shows gas ➡ within the liver in a peripheral branching pattern, consistent with portal venous gas. At surgery, the cecum was twisted on its mesentery (cecal volvulus) with ischemic necrosis of its wall.*

Enteric Fistulas and Sinus Tracts

TERMINOLOGY

- **Enteric fistula**: Abnormal connection between bowel and another epithelial-lined surface (e.g., bladder, vagina, skin)
- **Enteric sinus tract**: Blind-ending tract originating from bowel

IMAGING

- **Fluoroscopy**
  - **Fistulogram**: Best modality for enterocutaneous fistulas
  - **Small bowel follow-through**: Complementary to CT or MR enterography for Crohn's disease
  - **Contrast enema**: Often definitive for colonic fistulas (to bladder, vagina, etc.)
- **CT: Primary or complementary role**
  - Definitive or suggestive signs are present with most enteric & colonic fistulas

- e.g., fistulous tract filled with ectopic gas or contrast medium; tethered bowel adherent to abdominal wall, other bowel or viscera
- **MR is best modality for perianal fistulas**
  - Perianal fistula in active setting usually T2 hyperintense, T1 hypointense and enhancing on T1 C+ MR
  - Parks classification of perianal fistulas
    - **Intersphincteric fistula**: Fistula traverses internal anal sphincter and extends downwards to skin surface
    - **Transsphincteric fistula**: Fistula traverses both internal and external anal sphincters
    - **Extrasphincteric fistula**: Fistula extends from supralevator space into ischioanal fossa without involving sphincter complex
    - **Suprasphincteric fistula**: Fistula crosses internal sphincter, rises into supralevator space, and then crosses into ischioanal fossa

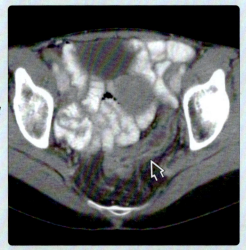
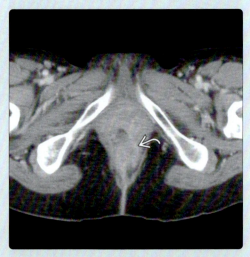

(Left) *Axial CECT shows sigmoid colonic mucosal hyperenhancement, submucosal edema ⇒, and pericolonic infiltration in a 54-year-old woman with a long history of Crohn's disease who developed foul-smelling vaginal discharge.* (Right) *Axial CECT section in the same patient through the low rectum shows severe inflammation and the enhancing walls of a fistulous tract ⇒ extending toward the vagina.*

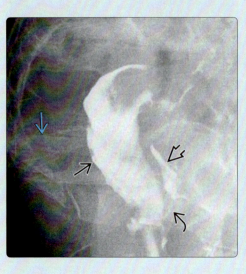
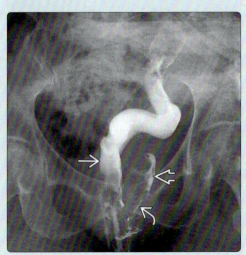

(Left) *Spot film from a water soluble contrast enema in the same case shows opacification of the rectosigmoid colon ➡ and the vagina ⇒ through a fistulous tract ⇒ starting low in the rectum. Contrast spilling out of the anus and vagina stains the overlying sheets ⇒.* (Right) *After removing the soiled sheets, a repeat film from the contrast enema in the same patient shows contrast medium within the rectum ⇒, vagina ⇒, and fistula ⇒.*

IMAGING

Fluoroscopic Findings

- Upper GI
  - May be helpful to demonstrate enteroenteric fistulas, but can be difficult to detect
    - Unlike fistulograms, provide global view of GI tract which may help surgical planning
- Contrast enema
  - Water soluble contrast enema may demonstrate colovesical and colovaginal fistulas
  - Better than upper GI for demonstrating fistulas that involve colon due to increased intraluminal pressures
- Fistulagram
  - Injection of contrast via catheter placed into cutaneous fistula opening
    - Defines presence & location of communication to gut
    - Greater sensitivity for enterocutaneous fistulas compared to small bowel follow-through
    - Provides only limited information about disease upstream or downstream from fistula

CT Findings

- **Gut-to-gut fistula (e.g., enteroenteric, enterocolic, colocolic)**
  - Can be difficult to reliably identify on cross-sectional imaging, although discrete tract filled with enteric contrast or gas may sometimes be visualized
- **Enterocutaneous fistula**
  - May be difficult to demonstrate with certainty on CT
    - Administration of positive oral contrast may be helpful
  - Involved bowel loops are often thickened & tethered to anterior abdominal wall close to ectopic gas in abdominal wall
- **Colovesical fistula**
  - Should be suspected in presence of gas, debris, or rectal contrast material within bladder even if direct track is not visible
  - Bladder wall may appear focally thickened at site of contact between inflamed colon and bladder
- **Colovaginal fistula**
  - Look for gas, debris, or contrast within vagina
- **Diverticulitis with fistula**
  - Wall thickening, luminal narrowing and pericolonic inflammation (± ectopic gas) in site with multiple diverticula (usually sigmoid colon)
  - Can result in fistulas between colon and bladder, vagina, or other bowel loops
- **Crohn's disease with fistula**
  - Strong tendency to form fistulous tracts (e.g., to other small bowel loops, colon, skin, bladder, vagina) or sinus tracts into mesenteric fat
  - Perianal fistulas and abscesses are common
  - Even if direct fistulous tracts are not visible, presence of ectopic gas in mesentery with surrounding thickened, tethered loops of inflamed small bowel should raise concern for "complex fistulizing Crohn's disease" (e.g., multiple complex interloop fistulas and sinus tracts)
  - CT and MR enterography show disease extent best

MR Findings

- MR is imaging modality of choice for evaluation of perianal fistulas
  - MR can determine relationship of fistulous tract with anal sphincters, identify exact site of opening of fistulous tract into anal canal, and differentiate fistulas which arise from distal rectum from those that arise from anal canal
  - Very accurate, with sensitivity of 97% and specificity of 100%

PATHOLOGY

General Features

- Etiology
  - **Spontaneous** (nonsurgical) causes
    - Diverticulitis: Most common cause of fistulization in industrialized countries
    - Crohn's disease: Accounts for 20-30% of all enterocutaneous fistulas
  - **Surgical** causes
    - Probably represents most common cause; usually result from bowel injury during surgery, including inadvertent enterotomy, anastomotic leak, or erosion of foreign body into bowel
      - Associated risk factors: Malnutrition, infection, immunosuppression, radiation therapy, or emergent surgical procedure
    - Abdominoperineal or low anterior resection (LAR) for rectal cancer is especially prone to anastomotic leak and development of fistulas
      - Commonly associated with fistulas to vagina (5-10% of women after LAR)
    - Hysterectomy associated with increased risk of fistula when performed for endometrial or cervical carcinoma
      - Radiation therapy or coexisting diverticulitis increases risk of colovaginal or rectovaginal fistula
  - **Perianal fistulas**
    - 90% are idiopathic and arise due to impaired drainage of anal glands leading to infection and subsequent development of perianal abscess or fistula
      - Inadequately treated abscesses often result in development of fistula, explaining high incidence of both abscess and fistula in same patient (~ 90% with perianal abscess go on to develop fistula)

DIAGNOSTIC CHECKLIST

Image Interpretation Pearls

- Active perianal fistulas demonstrate high signal on T2WI and enhancement on T1 C+ MR, whereas old, healed fistulas are nonenhancing with low signal on T1 and T2WI

SELECTED REFERENCES

1. Amiot A et al: Long-term outcome of enterocutaneous fistula in patients with Crohn's disease treated with anti-TNF therapy: a cohort study from the GETAID. Am J Gastroenterol. 109(9):1443-9, 2014

2. de Miguel Criado J et al: MR imaging evaluation of perianal fistulas: spectrum of imaging features. Radiographics. 32(1):175-94, 2012

(Left) Axial CECT of a morbidly obese young woman with pain and a foul-smelling discharge from a cutaneous site shows a walled-off abscess ⊒ adjacent to the sigmoid colon. There is a tract of gas and fluid ⊒ leading to the anterior abdominal wall defect. (Right) Fistulagram (injection of a catheter ⊒ inserted into the abdominal wall defect), in the same patient, opacifies an abdominal abscess cavity ⊒ and the sigmoid colon lumen ⊒. Diverticulitis was the etiology of this spontaneous colocutaneous fistula.

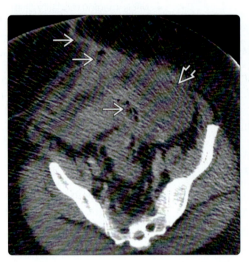
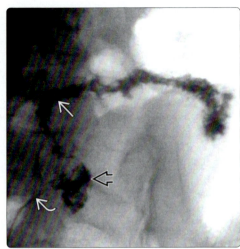

(Left) Axial CECT in the same patient shows rectally administered contrast medium within the vagina ⊒, confirming a colovaginal fistula. (Right) Sagittally reformatted CECT section in the same patient shows the fistula ⊒ from the distal colon (or rectum) ⊒ to the vagina (or cervix) ⊒. Diverticulitis and hysterectomy are both associated with colovaginal fistula.

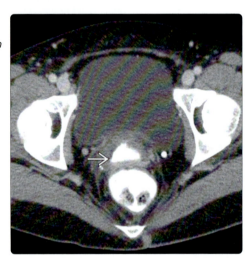
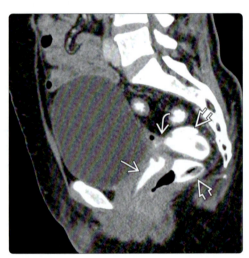

(Left) Axial CECT shows extensive diverticulosis ⊒ in an elderly woman who presented with urinary sepsis and high fever. The colonic lumen is opacified by rectal contrast medium. (Right) Axial NECT in the same patient shows a thick-walled urinary bladder ⊒ that is filled with gas, particulate (fecal) debris, and rectally administered contrast medium ⊒, confirming a colovesical fistula. Diverticulitis was confirmed as the etiology.

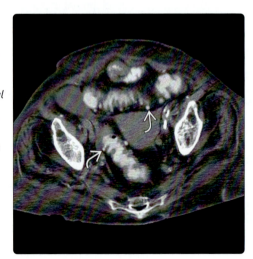
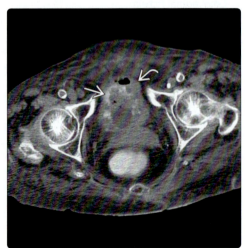

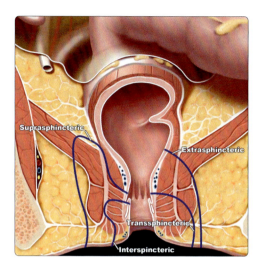

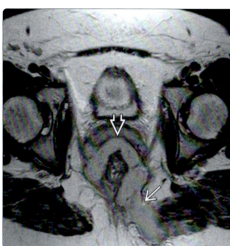

(Left) Graphic illustration of the perianal region demonstrates the 4 different types of perianal fistulas in the Parks classification and their relationship to the internal/external anal sphincters and the levator musculature. (Right) Axial T2 MR demonstrates a large transsphincteric perianal fistula ➡ crossing the external sphincter and extending into the posterior soft tissues on the left. Notice that the fistula is contiguous with a large T2 hyperintense "horseshoe" type abscess ➡ in the intersphincteric space.

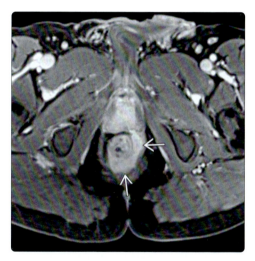

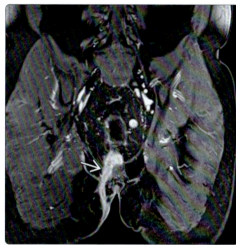

(Left) Axial T1 C+ FS MR in a patient with Crohn's disease demonstrates avid enhancement and thickening of the rectum, compatible with Crohn's colitis. Note the fistulous track ➡ arising from the rectum above the levator muscle complex. (Right) Coronal T1 C+ FS MR in the same patient nicely demonstrates the extrasphincteric fistula ➡ in this patient arising in the supralevator space and directly crossing the levator muscle complex into the ischioanal fossa without involving the anal sphincters.

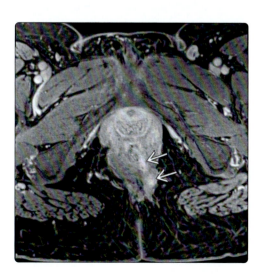

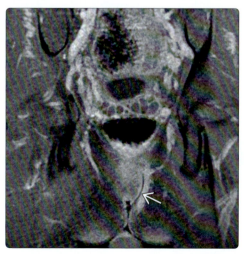

(Left) Axial T1 C+ FS MR demonstrates enhancement along the track of a transsphincteric perianal fistula ➡ arising from the anal canal at the 5 o'clock position. Enhancement along fistulous tracts suggests that the fistula is active, rather than chronic and healed. (Right) Coronal T1 C+ FS MR demonstrates a transsphincteric fistula with an internal low-signal seton catheter ➡. Seton catheters, often utilized to keep fistulous tracts open and facilitate drainage, appear low signal on all pulse sequences.

TERMINOLOGY

- Blunt or penetrating injury to rectum or colon

IMAGING

- Transverse and descending colon are most common sites for blunt traumatic injury
  - Rectum is most common site for penetrating injury
- Best diagnostic clue
  - Colonic wall thickening with adjacent mesenteric hemorrhage or ectopic gas
- **Best imaging tool: CECT with multiplanar reformations**
  - Rectal and intravenous contrast for penetrating injuries
- CT signs
  - Discontinuity or thickening of colonic wall
  - Extracolonic gas (intra- or retroperitoneal), pericolonic fluid or feces
  - Extravasated blood is nearly isodense to opacified blood vessels

- Extravasated endoluminal contrast medium = perforation of colon

TOP DIFFERENTIAL DIAGNOSES

- Pneumoperitoneum from other causes
- Nontraumatic bowel wall thickening

PATHOLOGY

- Associated abnormalities
  - Injuries of small intestine, mesentery, solid viscera
  - Pelvic fractures or vertebral (Chance) fractures

CLINICAL ISSUES

- Other signs/symptoms
  - Abdominal wall or perineal hematomas

DIAGNOSTIC CHECKLIST

- Look for extravasation of vascular and endoluminal contrast media
- Look for ectopic gas with wide windows on CT

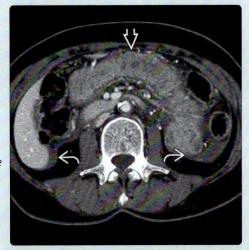
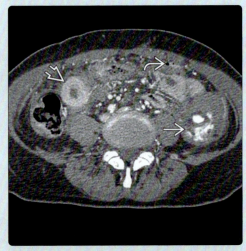

(Left) Axial CECT in a 57-year-old man injured in a high-speed motor vehicle accident shows multiple segments of thick-walled small intestine ⮕ with infiltration of the adjacent mesentery. Higher-than-water-density fluid ⮕ is present within the mesentery and peritoneal recesses. (Right) Axial CECT in the same patient shows more small bowel wall thickening ⮕, free intraperitoneal gas ⮕, and active bleeding ⮕ from the descending colon.

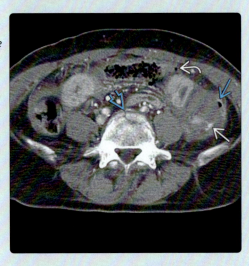
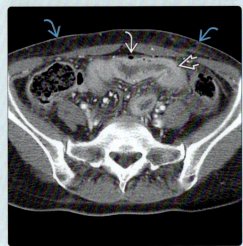

(Left) Axial CECT in the same patient shows bubbles of free air ⮕, sentinel clot, and active bleeding ⮕ adjacent to the descending colon ⮕. Also note the vertebral (Chance) fracture ⮕. At surgery, there were several lacerations of small bowel, and the descending colon had a "degloving" injury with active bleeding. (Right) Axial CECT in the same patient shows free air ⮕, bowel wall thickening ⮕, mesenteric infiltration, and a seat-belt contusion of the abdominal wall ⮕.

Colorectal Trauma

TERMINOLOGY

Definitions

- Blunt or penetrating injury to rectum or colon

IMAGING

General Features

- Best diagnostic clue
  - Colonic wall thickening with adjacent mesenteric hemorrhage or ectopic gas
- Location
  - Transverse and descending colon are most common sites for blunt traumatic injury
  - Rectum is most common for penetrating injury
    - Especially due to insertion of foreign bodies

Imaging Recommendations

- Best imaging tool
  - CECT with multiplanar reformations
- Protocol advice
  - Rectal, oral, and intravenous contrast for penetrating injuries to flank

CT Findings

- Discontinuity or thickening of colonic wall
- Pneumoperitoneum, pericolonic fluid or feces
- Mesenteric stranding, hemoperitoneum
- Active arterial extravasation from colonic vessels
  - Extravasated blood is nearly isodense to vessels
- Extravasation of contrast material inserted via enema
  - Indicates perforation of rectum or colon

DIFFERENTIAL DIAGNOSIS

Pneumoperitoneum From Other Causes

- Pneumomediastinum, pneumothorax, recent peritoneal lavage, or prior laparotomy

Nontraumatic Bowel Wall Thickening

- Colitis, inflammatory bowel disease
- Intramural hemorrhage due to excessive anticoagulation or thrombocytopenia

PATHOLOGY

General Features

- Etiology
  - Depth of laceration varies from serosal tear to full-thickness laceration
  - Seat belt may impale colon between anterior abdominal wall and vertebral column, resulting in colonic injury
  - Pelvic fractures may result in serosal tear from bone fragments
  - Insertion of foreign objects into rectum may result in mucosal or full-thickness injuries
    - Colonoscopy results in colonic perforation in < 1% of procedures
- Associated abnormalities
  - Small bowel and mesenteric injuries
  - Other solid organ injuries
    - Laceration of liver, kidney, spleen, &/or pancreas
  - Pelvic fractures associated with rectal injuries

- "Chance" (transverse) fractures of spine

Gross Pathologic & Surgical Features

- Intramural hematoma
- Hematoma within sigmoid or transverse mesocolon
- Serosal tears
  - "Degloving" injury: Serosa is avulsed from colonic surface
  - Results in ischemic injury of colon if not recognized and repaired at surgery

CLINICAL ISSUES

Presentation

- Other signs/symptoms
  - Abdominal wall contusion from seat belt injury
  - Perineal hematoma in rectal injury

Demographics

- Epidemiology
  - 5% of blunt trauma patients have bowel or mesenteric injuries
  - Colon is 2nd most common organ injured with penetrating trauma

Natural History & Prognosis

- Overall mortality: 10%
- Mortality 50% for missed rectal perforation
- Vascular injury to colonic mesentery may result in delayed rupture

Treatment

- Usually resection of injured colon with diverting colostomy
- Primary repair of damaged segment if deemed feasible at surgery

DIAGNOSTIC CHECKLIST

Image Interpretation Pearls

- Look for
  - Abdominal wall contusion as indirect sign of seat belt injury to colon
  - Ectopic gas with wide windows on CT
  - Active bleeding with high-attenuation focus isodense to adjacent vessels
  - Colorectal perforation with extraluminal extravasation of contrast medium inserted via enema

SELECTED REFERENCES

1. Bortolin M et al: Primary repair or fecal diversion for colorectal injuries after blast: a medical review. Prehosp Disaster Med. 29(3):317-9, 2014
2. Daly B et al: Complications of optical colonoscopy: CT findings. Radiol Clin North Am. 52(5):1087-99, 2014
3. Watson JD et al: Risk factors for colostomy in military colorectal trauma: a review of 867 patients. Surgery. 155(6):1052-61, 2014
4. Bondia JM et al: Imaging colorectal trauma using 64-MDCT technology. Emerg Radiol. 16(6):433-40, 2009
5. Anderson SW et al: Anorectal trauma: the use of computed tomography scan in diagnosis. Semin Ultrasound CT MR. 29(6):472-82, 2008

Colonic Polyps

IMAGING

- **CT "virtual" colonography**
  - Best radiographic alternative to optical colonoscopy
  - Proper technique critical, including utilization of colon-cleansing agent, stool-tagging agent, electronic CO_2 insufflator, and separate supine and prone acquisitions
  - Polyps appear as small or large, sessile or pedunculated, lesions extending into the lumen from colon wall
  - Polyps measuring ≤ 5 mm are generally not reported
  - Polyps measuring ≥ 1 cm referred for polypectomy
  - Management of polyps 5-9 mm in size is debated (follow-up vs. resection)
- **Air- (double-) contrast barium enema**
  - Limited in terms of sensitivity with miss rates as high as 17% (up to 10% miss rate for polyps > 1 cm)
  - Tubular adenomatous polyps
    - Small in size and often pedunculated (on stalk)
  - Tubulovillous adenomatous polyps

  - Medium-sized sessile polyps with fine nodular or reticular surface pattern
  - Villous adenomatous polyps
    - Larger sessile polyps with barium trapped between frond-like projections
  - Hyperplastic polyps
    - Commonly appear as smooth, round sessile nodules measuring < 5 mm
  - Inflammatory polyps
    - Islands of elevated, inflamed, edematous mucosa surrounded by ulceration

PATHOLOGY

- Neoplastic polyps: Adenomatous (tubular, tubulovillous, and villous)
- Nonneoplastic polyps: Hyperplastic, hamartomatous, and inflammatory

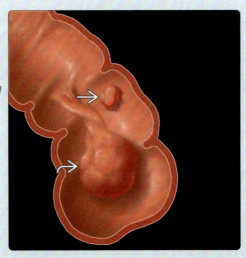
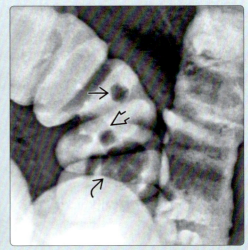

(Left) Graphic shows a tubulovillous adenoma ➤ on a long stalk and a small sessile polyp ➤. (Right) Single-contrast barium enema demonstrates a tubulovillous adenoma with a large head ➤ and a long stalk ➤. A small sessile polyp ➤ is also seen.

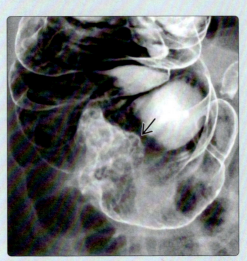
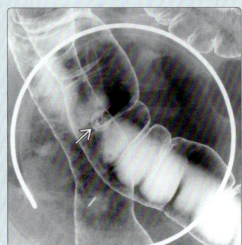

(Left) Air-contrast barium enema shows a large sessile polyp ➤ in the cecum having the typical appearance of a villous adenoma with cauliflower-like surface irregularity. (Right) Air-contrast barium enema shows a small polyp on a short stalk ➤. The outer rim of the "Mexican hat" is the head of the polyp, while the inner ring is the stalk.

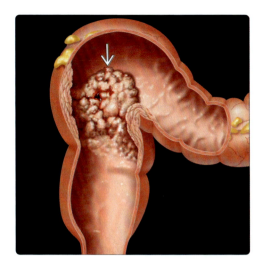

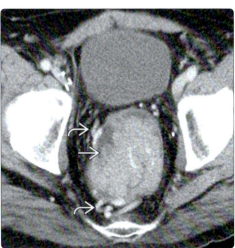

(Left) *Graphic shows a villous adenoma as a polypoid mass* ➡ *in the rectosigmoid colon having a shaggy, nodular surface, sometimes likened to the surface of a cauliflower.* (Right) *This 70-year-old man complained of frequent passage of watery stool but had no symptoms of bowel obstruction. CT shows a large mass* ➡ *that fills the rectum. Note large vessels* ➡ *within and draining the mass. These are typical clinical and CT features of a rectal villous adenoma.*

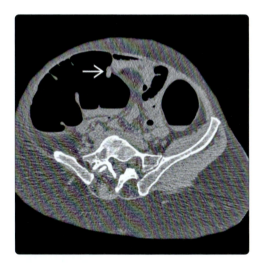

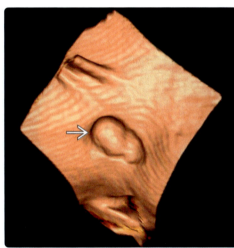

(Left) *Axial CT colonography demonstrates a small sessile adenomatous polyp* ➡ *arising from the cecum.* (Right) *3D endoluminal view in the same patient nicely shows the morphology of the polyp* ➡. *The decision to interpret CT colonography using 2D or 3D reconstructions largely hinges on the comfort level of the interpreting radiologist.*

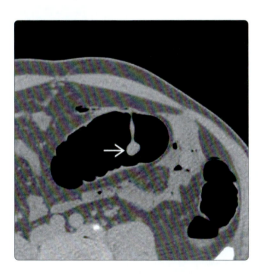

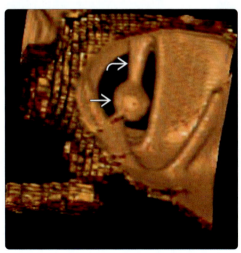

(Left) *Axial CT colonography shows a pedunculated polyp on a long stalk* ➡. (Right) *Endoluminal 3D reconstruction in the same patient demonstrates the polyp* ➡ *and its associated stalk* ➡. *When measuring such a lesion, the reported size should optimally be based on the diameter of the "head" rather than the length of the stalk.*

Colon Carcinoma

IMAGING

- Imaging is critical for detection, diagnosis, staging, and follow-up of colorectal carcinoma (CRC)
- **Detection**: CT colonography, plus stool analysis
  - Complementary role with standard colonoscopy
  - Early cancer: Sessile or pedunculated polyp
  - Advanced cancer: "Saddle" or "apple core" lesion
    - Circumferential narrowing of bowel lumen, overhanging borders, mucosal destruction
- **Staging**: Helical CT ± MR
  - Short segment (< 10 cm) asymmetric mural thickening & luminal narrowing
  - Pericolonic fat infiltration; spread to adjacent organs
  - Metastases to nodes, peritoneum, liver, ovaries
- **Tumor recurrence and surveillance**: PET/CT
  - FDG-avid lesions in chest, abdomen, pelvis

TOP DIFFERENTIAL DIAGNOSES

- Diverticulitis

- Ischemic colitis
- Infectious colitis with TB or ameba
- Ulcerative colitis
- Endometriosis

PATHOLOGY

- Importance of family history
  - CRC in 1st-degree relatives (↑ risk 2-3x)
  - Familial adenomatous polyposis
    - Accounts for < 1% of all colon cancers
  - Hereditary nonpolyposis colorectal carcinoma (Lynch syndrome)
    - Accounts for 5% of all colon cancers

CLINICAL ISSUES

- New treatments for metastatic disease (e.g., resection and ablation) offer hope for cure or prolonged survival
  - Demands accurate staging and surveillance for recurrence

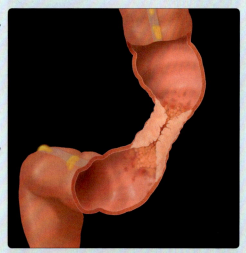
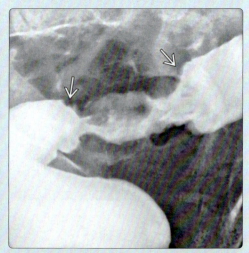

(Left) *Graphic shows an "apple core" constricting tumor of the sigmoid colon with circumferential narrowing of the lumen and a nodular tumor surface, the typical appearance of a left-sided cancer. These patients often complain of constipation and rectal bleeding.* (Right) *Single-contrast barium enema shows a classic "apple core" lesion ➡ of the sigmoid colon. Note the short segment, irregular, circumferential narrowing of the lumen with destroyed mucosa and nodular "shoulders."*

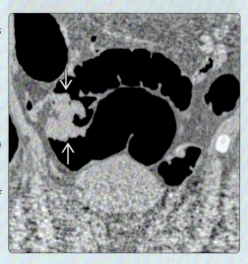
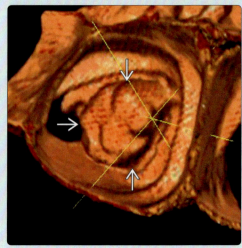

(Left) *Coronal image in 2D from a CT colonography shows a mass ➡ in the sigmoid due to colon cancer. While this mass was sufficiently large enough to prevent passage of the colonoscope, it was possible to both cleanse and distend the colon proximal to the mass using routine CT colonography methods.* (Right) *CT 3D endoluminal view in the same patient shows the mass ➡ and its relationship to the remainder of the colon. One of the accepted indications for CT colonography is to screen the colon proximal to an obstructing lesion.*

Colon Carcinoma

TERMINOLOGY

Abbreviations
- Colorectal carcinoma (CRC)

Definitions
- Malignant transformation of colonic mucosa

IMAGING

General Features
- Best diagnostic clue
  - Short segment colonic wall thickening
- Location
  - Cecum (10%), ascending colon (15%), transverse colon (15%), descending colon (5%), sigmoid colon (25%), rectosigmoid colon (10%), rectum (20%)
- Morphology
  - Early cancer: Sessile or pedunculated polyps
  - Advanced cancer: Annular, semiannular, polypoid, or carpet tumors
- Other general features
  - Radiology is critical for screening, diagnosis, treatment, and follow-up of CRC
  - Screening: **CT "virtual colonoscopy" is comparable to colonoscopy for cancer detection** by experienced observers

CT Findings
- Asymmetric mural thickening of **soft tissue density** ± irregular surface
- Short segment (< 10 cm) of wall thickening & luminal narrowing
- Tumor limited to lumen: Smooth serosal surface
- Extracolonic tumor extension
  - Mass with irregular serosal surface with stranding of pericolonic fat
  - ± loss of tissue fat planes between colon and surrounding muscles
- Metastases to mesenteric nodes, peritoneum, ovaries
- Hepatic metastases are most common (via portal venous drainage)

MR Findings
- MR is more sensitive than CT for evaluation of liver metastases
- Performed with gadoxetate (Eovist, Primovist) enhancement
  - Even better sensitivity (not specificity) than standard MR or CT for liver metastases
  - Metastases are hypointense to avidly enhanced normal liver parenchyma

Nuclear Medicine Findings
- PET
  - Fluorine 18-labeled deoxyglucose uptake is 2x higher in tumors than in normal or nonmalignant lesions
- PET/CT
  - Best combination of morphology and pathophysiology

Imaging Recommendations
- Best imaging tool
  - **Detection: CT colonography**
  - Staging: Multiplanar, contrast-enhanced CECT
  - Tumor recurrence and surveillance: PET/CT

DIFFERENTIAL DIAGNOSIS

Diverticulitis
- CT: Most common in sigmoid colon
  - Bowel wall and fascial thickening; fat stranding; free air and fluid
  - Pericolic inflammatory changes: Abscess, sinuses, fistulas, or strictures
  - Length of involvement > 10 cm
    - Cancer: Short segment involvement ± nodal enlargement

Ischemic Colitis
- Usually seen in watershed areas; splenic flexure and sigmoid colon
  - Thumbprinting: Submucosal gas, edema, or bleeding
  - Stricture: Smooth, tapered margins but no mass effect (chronic)

Infectious Colitis (Unusual Organisms)
- Example: Tuberculosis and amebiasis
- Usually in proximal colon
- Stricture formation may simulate carcinoma
  - May even simulate classic apple core appearance of colon cancer

Ulcerative Colitis
- Significant predisposing factor for colon carcinoma
  - Cancers arise de novo in inflamed mucosa without evolving through polyp stage
- Bowel wall thickening, luminal narrowing, mesenteric hyperemia

Extrinsic Lesions
- CT and MR show extracolonic origin and extent of tumors best
- Endometriosis
- Ovarian cancer
- Direct spread or "drop" metastases (e.g., from gastric cancer)
- Smooth, eccentric, obtuse angles with colonic wall

CLINICAL ISSUES

Presentation
- Most common signs/symptoms
  - Distal colon: Colonic obstruction and hematochezia
    - Abdominal pain and changes in bowel habits
  - Proximal colon: Anemia, weight loss, fever
- Lab data
  - Positive fecal occult blood test
  - ± micro- to normocytic anemia
  - Carcinoembryonic antigen (CEA) > 2.5 µg/L
- Diagnosis: Colonoscopy with mucosal biopsy

DIAGNOSTIC CHECKLIST

Image Interpretation Pearls
- **CT: Short segment circumferential wall thickening with cluster of mesenteric nodes is presumed CRC**

(Left) Axial CECT in a 60-year-old man with right-sided CRC presenting with anemia and liver metastases shows a metastasis ➡ and an incidental cyst ➡. (Right) Axial CECT of the same patient shows a mass ➡ in the ascending colon. Note the ileocolic mesenteric adenopathy ➡. The presence of mesenteric adenopathy adjacent to a colonic mass is strong evidence for lymphatic spread of a primary colon cancer.

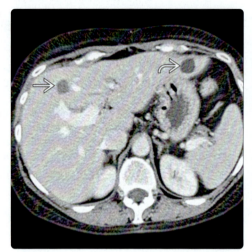
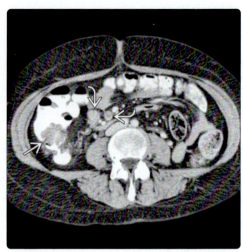

(Left) Axial CECT in a middle-aged man with RLQ discomfort shows multiple nodular omental metastases ➡. (Right) CT in the same patient shows a circumferential soft tissue mass ➡ in the cecum that obstructed the appendix and invaded adjacent mesenteric fat and nodes. Cecal carcinoma may mimic appendicitis with cecal wall thickening, infiltrated fat, and distended appendiceal lumen. The presence of a circumferential cecal mass and omental (or liver) metastases indicates a malignant process.

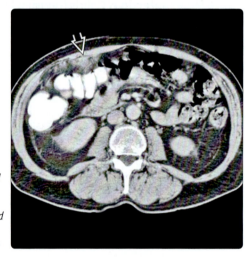
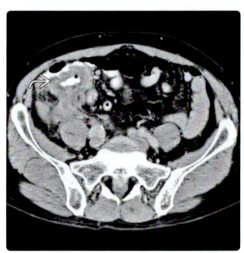

(Left) CT of a 66-year-old man who had prior resection of sigmoid colon cancer and now presents with flank pain and weight loss shows a descending colostomy ➡ and extensive retroperitoneal lymphadenopathy ➡ that enveloped the left ureter and caused hydronephrosis (not shown). (Right) Axial PET/CT in the same case shows large FDG-avid masses ➡ that envelop and obstruct the left ureter, representing recurrent colon carcinoma. In cases of suspected recurrence of CRC, PET/CT is the optimal test.

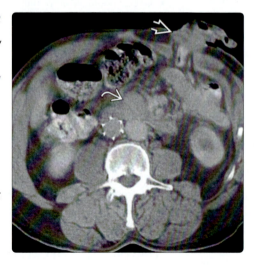
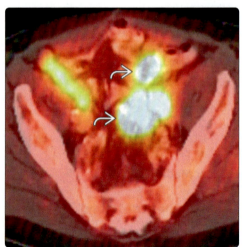

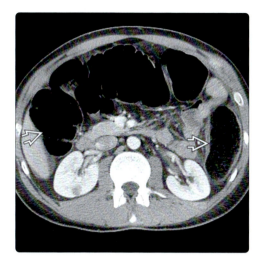
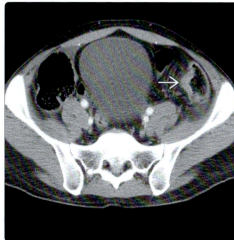

(Left) *Axial CT section of a 31-year-old man presenting with constipation and bright red blood per rectum shows gross dilation of the colon* ➡. (Right) *CECT in the same case shows asymmetric, soft tissue density thickening of the wall of the descending colon* ➡.

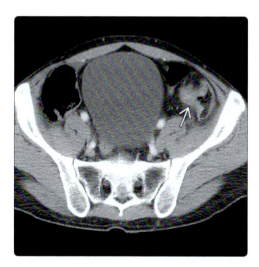
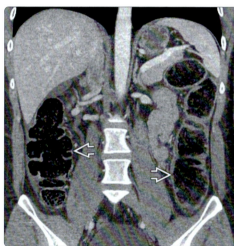

(Left) *Adjacent CECT section in the same case shows an "apple core" lesion* ➡ *at the junction of the descending and sigmoid colon.* (Right) *Coronal reformatted CT in the same case shows gross distention of the colon* ➡ *with stool and gas.*

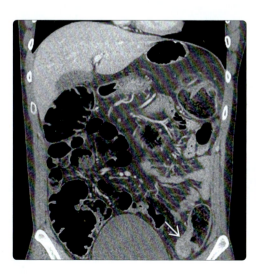
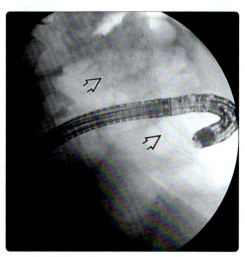

(Left) *Another coronal CT section shows the abrupt narrowing of the colon by the "apple core" lesion* ➡. *Note the abrupt and short thickening of the colonic wall and narrowing of the lumen. The clinical and imaging features are typical of a distal colon cancer, though the patient is younger than most affected patients.* (Right) *In order to overcome the near-complete luminal obstruction and to clean the colon prior to surgical resection, a metallic stent* ➡ *was deployed across the obstructing tumor under endoscopic guidance.*

IMAGING

- Image detection of perirectal tumor spread is vital; requires preoperative radiation ± chemotherapy
- **CT shows tumor extent in pelvis, abdomen, and thorax**
  - Extracolonic tumor extension: Irregular external (serosal) margin of rectum
  - Metastasis to lymph nodes at external iliac and paraaortic chain, inguinal, retroperitoneum, or porta hepatis
  - Metastases to lungs, mediastinal nodes, and bones may precede liver metastases
- **MR is best for depiction of tumor extent in pelvis**
  - Loss of tissue fat planes between rectum and surrounding muscles and organs
  - Strands of soft tissue extending from serosal surface into perirectal fat
- **Transrectal ultrasonography: Excellent for local invasion, pelvic nodes**
- **PET/CT is best for detection of tumor recurrence**
  - Especially valuable in distinguishing scar from tumor in proctectomy site

CLINICAL ISSUES

- Rectal cancer tends to invade locally (lacks serosa)
- Metastases: From upper 2/3 of rectum
  - Superior hemorrhoidal vein → portal vein → liver
  - Batson venous plexus → thoracolumbar vertebrae, periaortic nodes
- Metastases: From lower 1/3 of rectum
  - Middle hemorrhoidal and iliac veins → IVC → lung
- **Pre- and postoperative radiation ± chemotherapy therapy (for locally advanced tumor)**
- Follow-up imaging
  - CT: 3-4 months after surgery, then every 6 months for 2-3 years, then annually for 5 years
  - CEA titer: If elevated, CT is indicated (PET/CT best)
  - Colonoscopy at 1 year following surgery and then every 3-5 years

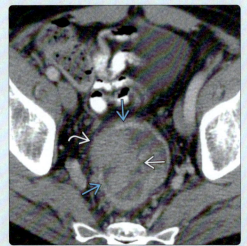 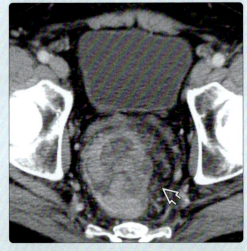

(Left) Axial CECT in a 68-year-old man with frequent passage of small amounts of mucus and stool shows a large rectal mass ➡ that breaks through the rectal wall ⬈, interrupting the otherwise complete rectal mucosal enhancement ➨. There was no colonic obstruction, suggesting the soft nature of this villous carcinoma. (Right) CT in the same patient shows extensive infiltration of the perirectal fat planes ➡, strongly suggesting transmural spread of tumor and the need for neoadjuvant therapy prior to resection.

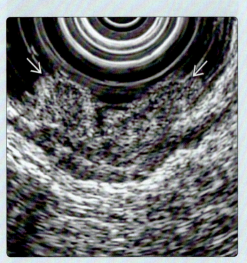 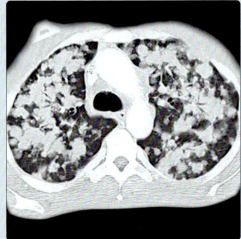

(Left) Transrectal ultrasonography shows a bulky rectal mass ➡ with invasion through the submucosa in this patient with T3 stage rectal carcinoma. (Right) Axial CECT shows extensive pulmonary metastases from rectal carcinoma in a patient with no liver metastases. The dual venous drainage of the rectum (systemic and portal) explains this pattern and results in very different clinical behavior of rectal and colon cancers.

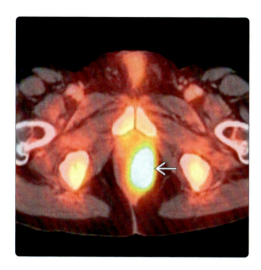
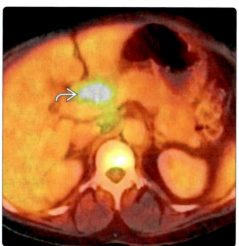

(Left) Axial PET/CT in a 54-year-old man with AIDS shows an FDG-avid mass ➡ in the anal canal, representing a primary anorectal carcinoma. (Right) Axial PET/CT in the same patient shows similar FDG-avid masses in lymph node metastases ➡ in the porta hepatis. This patient had no liver metastases, again emphasizing the unique patterns of spread in rectal vs. colon cancer. Anal cancer is relatively common in homosexual men with AIDS and is related to papilloma viral infection.

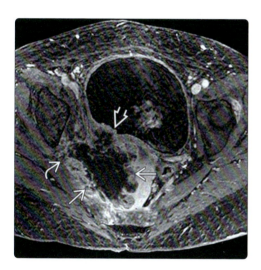
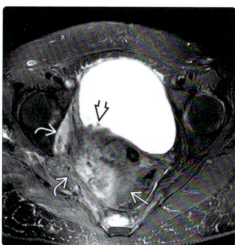

(Left) Axial T1WI MR in a 58-year-old woman with prior low anterior resection of a rectal carcinoma, now returning with right leg sciatica, shows a large irregular mass ➡ that extends into the right sciatic notch ➡ and posterior wall of the bladder ➡. (Right) Axial T2WI MR in the same patient shows the recurrent rectal cancer ➡ and its invasion of the bladder ➡ and pelvic side wall muscles ➡.

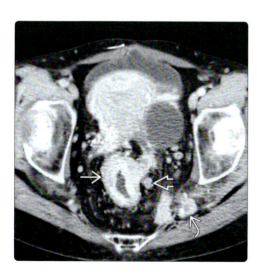
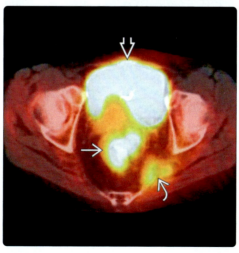

(Left) Axial CECT in a young woman who underwent colectomy for Crohn's colitis shows a circumferential mass ➡ within the rectum that represents carcinoma. Note the adenopathy ➡ adjacent to the rectum and the tumor in the sciatic foramen ➡. (Right) Axial PET/CT in the same patient shows an FDG-avid tumor in the rectum ➡ and in the sciatic foramen ➡. The bladder ➡ is filled with urine containing excreted FDG.

Familial Polyposis and Gardner Syndrome

TERMINOLOGY

- Autosomal dominant genetic disorder characterized by formation of innumerable colonic adenomatous polyps at young age and increased risk for colonic and extracolonic tumors

IMAGING

- **Imaging tests**: Double-contrast barium studies of colon and upper GI tract (may be redundant with endoscopy)
  - CT or MR (for abdominal tumors)
  - Innumerable colonic filling defects or ring shadows ± extraintestinal lesions
- Adenomatous (± malignant) polyps in
  - Colon > stomach > duodenum > small bowel
  - Small (80% < 5 mm) and usually sessile
    - Polyps may carpet colon, stomach, duodenum
- Familial adenomatous polyposis (FAP) coli and Gardner syndrome are expressions of same genetic defect

- Gardner syndrome = FAP + soft tissue tumors, bony osteomas, dental defects, &/or periampullary tumor
  - Soft tissue tumors: Desmoid, mesenteric fibromatosis, lipoma

PATHOLOGY

- Autosomal dominant trait (2/3 of cases) with high penetrance
- Spontaneous mutations (1/3 of cases)

CLINICAL ISSUES

- Mean age at diagnosis: 16 years; 95% have polyps by 35 years
- Colon carcinoma by 34-43 years of age

DIAGNOSTIC CHECKLIST

- Lifetime surveillance for tumors throughout body

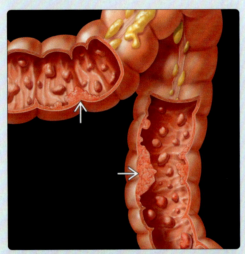

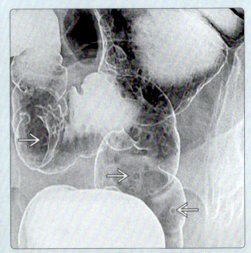

(Left) Graphic shows innumerable small polyps and multifocal carcinomas ⇨ representative of the colonic lesion types seen in patients with familial polyposis coli. (Right) Spot film from an air-contrast barium enema demonstrates multiple small radiolucent filling defects ⇨, which represent sessile adenomatous polyps along the sigmoid colonic mucosa.

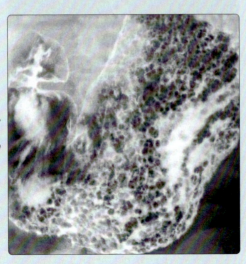

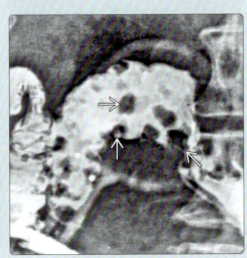

(Left) Upper GI series spot film shows the stomach carpeted with small polyps, all fairly small and uniform in size. While these resemble hyperplastic polyps radiographically, this patient has familial polyposis with adenomatous polyps that have potential for malignant degeneration. (Right) Spot film from an upper GI series in a patient with familial polyposis and Gardner syndrome shows several adenomatous polyps ⇨ in the duodenum.

TERMINOLOGY

Abbreviations
- Familial adenomatous polyposis (FAP) syndrome
- Gardner syndrome may have same genetic mutation
  - Distinction from FAP is largely semantic

Definitions
- Autosomal dominant genetic disorder characterized by formation of innumerable colonic adenomatous polyps at young age and by increased risk for colonic and extracolonic tumors

IMAGING

General Features
- Best diagnostic clue
  - CT or MR showing multiple neoplastic masses of GI tract ± metastases
- Location
  - Adenomatous polyps in
    - Colon > stomach > duodenum > small bowel
- Size
  - Varies from pinpoint to > 1 cm
- Other general features
  - FAP: Rare, but it is most common polyposis syndrome
  - 2 varied expressions of FAP: FAP coli and Gardner syndrome
    - **Gardner syndrome**
      - **Familial polyposis coli, osteomas, epidermoid (sebaceous) cysts**
      - Soft tissue tumors: **Desmoid**, mesenteric fibromatosis, lipoma
      - Dental abnormalities; periampullary, duodenal, and thyroid carcinomas
  - Hundreds or thousands of polyps may carpet colon
  - FAP adenomas: Small (80% < 5 mm) and usually sessile
  - Extracolonic GI tract manifestations of FAP
    - Stomach
      - Fundic gland polyps and adenomas in > 50% of cases
    - Duodenum: Adenomas of 2nd part and periampullary in > 50% of cases
      - **Periampullary cancer**: 2nd most frequent site of cancer outside colon, seen in 12% of FAP patients
    - Jejunum and ileum
      - Adenomas, lymphoid hyperplasia in > 20% of cases
  - Associated with ↑ incidence of malignant CNS tumors

Radiographic Findings
- Fluoroscopic-guided double-contrast barium enema
  - Innumerable variably sized radiolucent filling defects
  - Carpet entire colon, especially rectosigmoid
  - May be widely scattered radiolucent filling defects
- Double-contrast upper GI, small bowel
  - Multiple small filling defects (polyps) in stomach, duodenum, jejunum, and ileum

CT Findings
- CECT
  - Useful for diagnosing and staging colon carcinomas and extracolonic tumors
  - Colorectal cancers are often multiple
  - Look for nodal, peritoneal, hepatic metastases
  - Both desmoid and mesenteric fibromatosis: Higher attenuation than muscle

Imaging Recommendations
- Best imaging tool
  - Double-contrast barium studies of colon and upper GI tract can detect disease but do not replace endoscopic evaluation
  - CT or MR (for abdominal tumors)

PATHOLOGY

General Features
- Etiology
  - FAP is inherited as autosomal dominant trait (2/3 of cases)
  - Occasionally due to spontaneous mutations (1/3 of cases)
  - High penetrance (affected patients will develop signs and symptoms)
- Associated abnormalities
  - Extracolonic malignancies associated with FAP
    - Duodenal ampullary carcinoma (12% lifetime risk)
    - Thyroid cancer
    - Childhood hepatoblastoma
    - Gastric carcinoma
    - CNS tumors (mostly medulloblastoma)
  - Extraintestinal manifestations: Gardner syndrome
    - Epidermoid cyst, lipoma, fibroma, desmoid tumors (3-29%), mesenteric fibromatosis, peritoneal adhesions, retroperitoneal fibrosis
    - Osteomas: Membranous bone (50%), mandible (80%)
    - Teeth: Odontoma, unerupted supernumerary teeth
    - Thyroid cancer: Papillary type more common in girls and young women

CLINICAL ISSUES

Presentation
- Most common signs/symptoms
  - Rectal bleeding and diarrhea (75% of cases)
  - Asymptomatic, pain, mucus discharge
  - Family history of colonic polyps (66-80% of cases)

DIAGNOSTIC CHECKLIST

Consider
- Check for family history: Colonic polyps, abdominal soft tissue tumors, and malignancies at young age

SELECTED REFERENCES

1. Vitellaro M et al: Risk of desmoid tumours after open and laparoscopic colectomy in patients with familial adenomatous polyposis. Br J Surg. 101(5):558-65, 2014
2. Wood LD et al: Upper GI tract lesions in familial adenomatous polyposis (FAP): enrichment of pyloric gland adenomas and other gastric and duodenal neoplasms. Am J Surg Pathol. 38(3):389-93, 2014
3. Zhang Y et al: Adenomatous polyposis coli determines sensitivity to the EGFR tyrosine kinase inhibitor gefitinib in colorectal cancer cells. Oncol Rep. 31(4):1811-7, 2014

(Left) *This 37-year-old man had minimal contact with physicians and presented with rectal bleeding and weight loss. CT shows multiple liver metastases* ⇨. **(Right)** *CT in the same patient shows multiple liver metastases* ⇨ *and a small mass at the duodenal ampulla* ⇨, *subsequently proven to be an adenoma.*

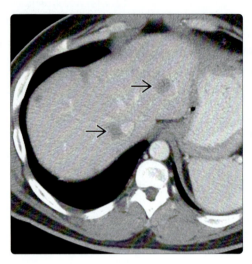
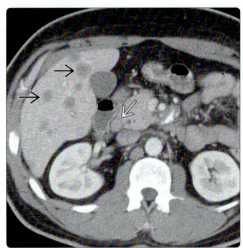

(Left) *CT in the same patient shows a small bowel intussusception* ⇗, *likely induced by small bowel polyps (not visualized).* **(Right)** *CT in the same patient shows a mass* ⇨ *in the buttock and paraspinal region that is higher in attenuation than adjacent muscle and likely represents a desmoid tumor or fibromatosis.*

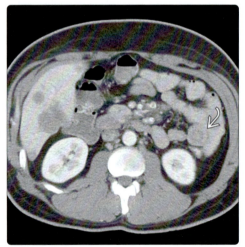
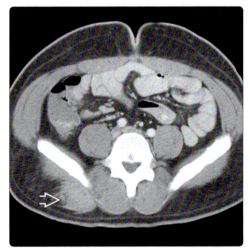

(Left) *CECT in the same patient shows a mass* ⇨ *in the sigmoid colon, subsequently proved to be an adenocarcinoma.* **(Right)** *Following the abdominal CT in the same patient, a CT section through the facial bones reveals cortical thickening and osteomas* ⇗. *All of the highlighted findings are typical features of Gardner syndrome.*

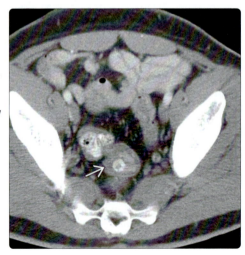
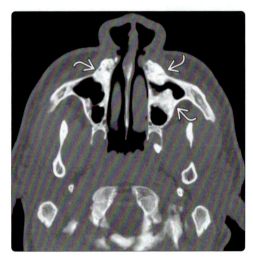

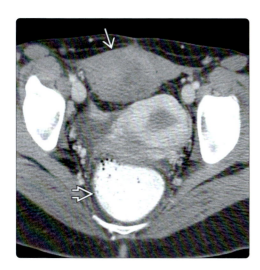

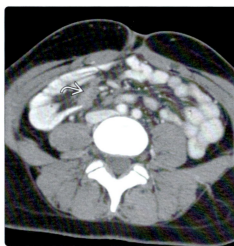

(Left) This 19-year-old woman had known familial adenomatous polyposis and had a total colectomy. She later presented with a hard, palpable abdominal mass. Axial CECT shows evidence of the prior colectomy with an ileal pouch ➡. There is a large mass ➡ in the right rectus muscle that proved to be a desmoid tumor within an incision site. (Right) Axial CECT in the same patient shows a more subtle mass ➡ at the base of the mesentery, also proven to represent desmoid or aggressive fibromatosis.

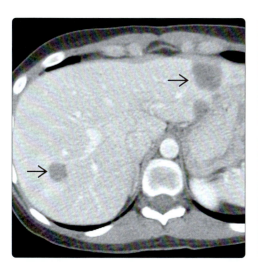

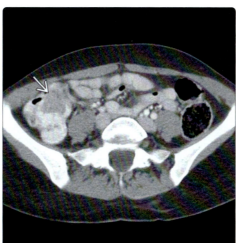

(Left) This young woman presented with weight loss and anemia and had no family history of colon cancer. CECT shows multiple liver metastases ➡. (Right) CECT in the same patient shows a mass ➡ within the ascending colon, subsequently proven to represent primary colon cancer.

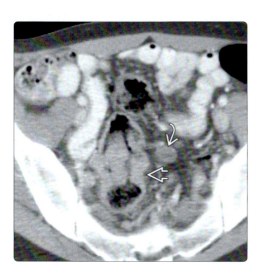

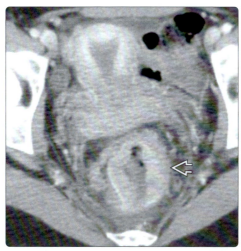

(Left) Another CT section in this patient shows a tumor in the rectosigmoid colon ➡ and extensive spread to the regional nodes ➡. (Right) CECT in the same patient shows the rectal cancer ➡ with extensive infiltration into the perirectal tissues. As with this patient, some cases of familial adenomatous polyposis lack a family history and may result from spontaneous genetic mutation.

Appendiceal Tumors

TERMINOLOGY

- Primary malignant neoplasm of appendix
  - Mucinous cystadenocarcinoma (most common clinically significant type)
  - Colonic-type adenocarcinoma
  - Lymphoma
  - Carcinoid (common, usually incidental at appendectomy)

IMAGING

- Round or oval, cystic or solid mass near tip of cecum
- Mucocele
  - RLQ soft tissue mass with curvilinear mural calcification on radiography is highly suggestive
  - Ovoid cystic mass ± internal echoes (septations) on US
- Mucinous tumor: RLQ cystic mass, usually > 2 cm
  - Mucinous type has strong propensity to form mucocele
  - May have curvilinear calcification in wall
  - Mucinous cystadenocarcinoma is most common cause of pseudomyxoma peritonei

- Lymphoma: Cylindrical, soft tissue-density mass
  - Cannot distinguish from carcinoma on CT
- Carcinoid
  - Rarely diagnosed clinically or by imaging prior to appendectomy
    - May obstruct lumen like other tumor types

TOP DIFFERENTIAL DIAGNOSES

- Mucocele of appendix (other etiologies)
  - Nonneoplastic forms rarely exceed 2 cm in diameter
- Appendicitis (abscess)
  - More inflammatory changes are seen
  - No liver or peritoneal metastases
- Ovarian cystic mass
  - Identify right ovary as source or separate from mass

CLINICAL ISSUES

- Appendiceal tumors are found in 1% of appendectomies (usually carcinoid)

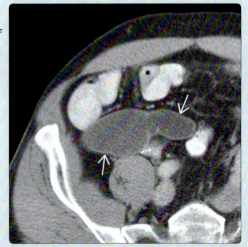
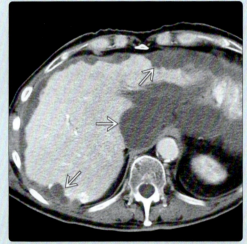

(Left) Axial CECT shows an oval, well-encapsulated cystic mass ➡ arising from the tip of the cecum in this 62-year-old man with mucinous carcinoma of the appendix. With imaging alone, a benign mucocele may not be distinguished from a mucinous carcinoma. (Right) Axial CECT in an 80-year-old man with pseudomyxoma peritonei due to ruptured mucinous carcinoma of the appendix shows the classic scalloped appearance of the surface of the liver ➡ due to peritoneal gelatinous metastases.

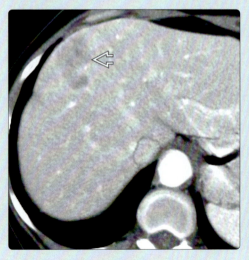
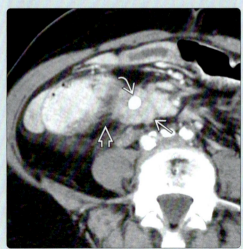

(Left) Axial CECT in a 60-year-old woman with chronic RLQ pain shows a hypodense mass ➡ with a typical appearance of liver metastasis. (Right) Axial CT in the same patient shows a thick-walled appendix ➡ with a calcified appendicolith ➡ within its lumen and infiltration of adjacent fat ➡. While these findings mimic those of appendicitis, there is much more soft tissue density within the wall than would be expected with simple appendicitis. Liver metastases suggest the correct diagnosis of appendiceal carcinoma.

Colonic Metastases and Lymphoma

IMAGING

- Multiplanar, contrast-enhanced CT (or PET/CT) is optimal imaging test
- Lymphoma
  - Bulky colonic mass; without colonic obstruction
  - Preservation of fat planes
- Metastasis
  - May mimic primary adenocarcinoma on imaging

TOP DIFFERENTIAL DIAGNOSES

- Primary colon adenocarcinoma
  - Short, focal, "apple core" lesion < 10 cm in length
  - More likely than lymphoma or metastases to cause colonic obstruction
- Ileocolic tuberculosis
- Gastrointestinal stromal tumor of colon

PATHOLOGY

- Metastatic spread from melanoma or primary tumor of stomach, lung, or breast (rarely, other cancers)
  - Gastric cancer may directly invade transverse colon along gastrocolic ligament
- Lymphoma may arise from and be limited to colon
  - Rare; < 3% of GI tract lymphomas

CLINICAL ISSUES

- Most common signs/symptoms: Rectal bleeding, symptoms of obstruction, especially if intussusception is present
- 50% 5-year survival rate for patients with primary colonic lymphoma
- Prognosis is poor for patients with metastases to colon from melanoma, breast, lung, or gastric cancer

DIAGNOSTIC CHECKLIST

- Colonoscopy may allow diagnosis but can miss lesions limited to outer layers of colon

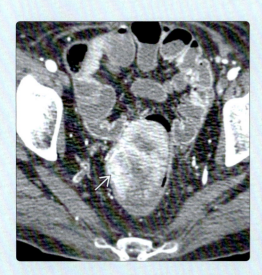
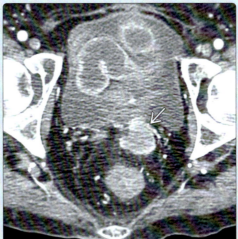

(Left) *Axial CECT in a 67-year-old man presenting with 3 months of intermittent rectal bleeding and clinical symptoms of obstipation shows a bulky, enhancing mass ➡ involving the rectosigmoid colon with no evidence of colonic obstruction.* (Right) *Axial CECT in the same patient reveals an enhancing perirectal nodal metastasis ➡. The patient had a subsequent endoscopic biopsy of the mass, which identified a non-Hodgkin lymphoma.*

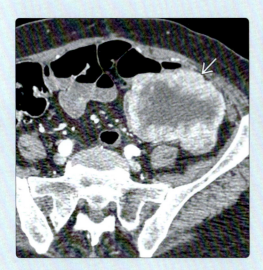
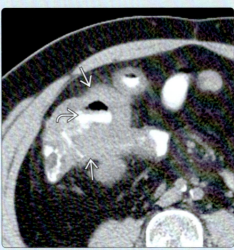

(Left) *Axial CECT in a 71-year-old man with known lung carcinoma presenting with LLQ pain and a palpable mass demonstrates a large heterogeneously enhancing mass ➡ involving the descending colon. This was a colonic metastasis.* (Right) *Axial CECT in a 68-year-old man with weight loss and RLQ pain demonstrates a bulky ileocecal mass with smooth margins ➡. Note the oral contrast filling the lumen of the cecum ➡, indicating the lack of obstruction. Endoscopic biopsy revealed a high-grade B-cell lymphoma.*

SECTION 8
Spleen

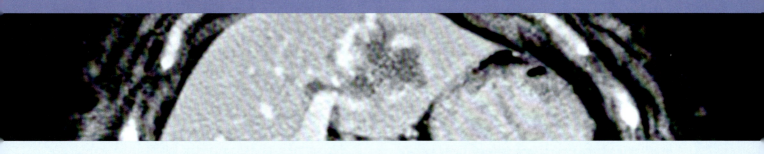

Embryology, Anatomy, and Physiology

The spleen develops from the dorsal mesogastrium and usually rotates to the left, becoming fixed in the left subphrenic location by peritoneal reflections linking it to the diaphragm, abdominal wall, stomach (gastrosplenic ligament), and kidney (splenorenal ligament). It usually develops as 1 "fused" mass of tissue, but variations are common.

One or more **accessory spleens** are found in up to 30% of the general population, usually small spherical structures near the splenic hilum. These can enlarge, especially following splenectomy, and may simulate a neoplastic mass or cause recurrence of hematologic disease.

The spleen may be congenitally absent (**asplenia**) or have many unfused components (**polysplenia**). These are rare splenic anomalies and are associated with cardiovascular anomalies, situs inversus, and other anomalies, often with serious and even life-threatening consequences.

The spleen is rarely on a long mesentery and may be found in any abdominal or pelvic location ("wandering spleen"), placing it at risk for trauma and torsion with infarction.

The spleen is the largest lymphatic organ, the size of which varies among individuals and even in the same person by blood volume, state of nutrition, and hydration. The usual volume range is 100-250 cm³ with a mean of 150 cm³. A calculated splenic index (length x width x breadth) over 480 cm³ is considered splenomegaly. The average length is up to 12 cm with a width and breadth of 7 and 4 cm, respectively.

Imaging Issues

The spleen has a unique histology, consisting of the red and white pulp, which directly affects its appearance on imaging exams. The white pulp is the lymphoid tissue, and the red is composed of the vascular tissue and splenic cords (plates of cells and sinusoids). Because of its vascularity, the red pulp enhances rapidly, giving the spleen a very heterogeneous pattern of enhancement on arterial-phase enhanced CT or MR imaging. This may be mistaken for splenic pathology but is a transient phenomenon not evident on unenhanced or later phases of enhanced imaging.

CT is the imaging modality of choice for the evaluation of the spleen in the acute setting (trauma or pain). MR can be additive in evaluating splenic masses and some metabolic diseases (e.g., hemochromatosis). The spleen has a relatively long T1 and T2 relaxation time. This results in its appearing somewhat hypointense compared to the liver on T1WI and hyperintense on T2WI. With iron deposition, the spleen may show a dramatic loss in signal.

Approach to Abnormal Spleen

Splenomegaly is a very common finding and may result from numerous causes, usually grouped into 5 general etiologies, including congestion, hematologic, inflammatory-infectious, tumor, or infiltrative.

Given its function as a blood filter, it is not surprising that the spleen is a frequent site of metastases on postmortem examination of patients who have died from cancer. However, with the exception of **leukemia and lymphoma**, it is uncommon to make an imaging diagnosis of splenic metastasis.

Many **splenic neoplasms** are benign, either hemangiomas or lymphangiomas, but these have overlapping imaging features, and a specific diagnosis is rarely possible.

One of the most common focal splenic lesions is the **splenic cyst**. It is not possible to distinguish the primary congenital (epithelial-lined) cyst from the acquired cyst by imaging with the latter resulting from prior infarction, infection, or trauma. These are rarely of clinical importance.

Multiple lesions within the spleen are most typically the result of a granulomatous process, which may be either infectious (e.g., histoplasmosis, TB) or noninfectious (sarcoidosis). Splenic granulomata commonly calcify.

The pancreatic tail usually inserts into the splenic hilum through the splenorenal ligament. Inflammatory or neoplastic conditions affecting the pancreatic tail can easily invade the splenic parenchyma, resulting in intrasplenic pseudocyst, for instance. Conversely, splenic tumors or an accessory spleen may mimic a pancreatic tail mass.

Splenic infarction is a relatively common cause of acute left upper quadrant pain. It appears as a sharply defined, often wedge-shaped zone of minimal enhancement abutting the splenic capsule. Patients at risk for infarction include those with sickle cell disease and those with cardiovascular conditions, such as atrial fibrillation. Patients with left ventricular assist devices are especially prone to embolic infarction of the spleen.

The spleen is often injured in blunt and penetrating **trauma**. Most children and adults with splenic lacerations will recover without surgery, but the presence of active extravasation (evident on CT) or clinical instability may demand intervention, either surgery or transcatheter embolization.

Splenosis is the peritoneal implantation of splenic tissue that may follow traumatic rupture of the spleen. This may be mistaken for polysplenia or peritoneal implants of tumor (carcinomatosis). The history of trauma, absence of a normal spleen, and enhancement characteristics identical to spleen usually allow accurate diagnosis.

Differential Diagnosis

Splenomegaly
Common
- Cirrhosis with portal hypertension
- Congestive heart failure
- AIDS
- Splenic metastases and lymphoma
- Hemoglobinopathies
- Leukemia
- Sarcoidosis
- Mononucleosis
- Myeloproliferative disorders
- Splenic trauma

Less Common
- Splenic tumors (primary)
- Systemic infection and abscesses
- Splenic vein occlusion
- Splenic infarction
- Malaria
- Collagen vascular diseases: Rheumatoid arthritis, scleroderma, dermatomyositis, polyarteritis nodosa
- Storage diseases: Amyloidosis, glycogen storage disease
- Peliosis

Multiple Splenic Calcifications

Common
- Histoplasmosis
- Tuberculosis
- Arterial calcification and aneurysm
- *Pneumocystis jiroveci*
- Splenic infarction
- Splenic cyst

Less Common
- Echinococcal (hydatid) cyst
- Healed abscess

Solid Splenic Mass or Masses

Common
- Splenic trauma
- Splenic infarction
- Splenic metastases and lymphoma
- Perfusion artifact

Less Common
- Sarcoidosis
- Splenic infection and abscess
- Splenic tumors

- Peliosis

Cystic Splenic Mass

Common
- Acquired or congenital splenic cyst
- Splenic trauma
- Splenic infarction

Less Common
- Splenic metastases and lymphoma
- Splenic infection and abscess
- Splenic tumors
- Pancreatic pseudocyst

Diffuse Increased Attenuation, Spleen

Common
- Hemochromatosis
- Splenic infarction: Sickle cell anemia

Less Common
- Opportunistic infection
- Thorotrast

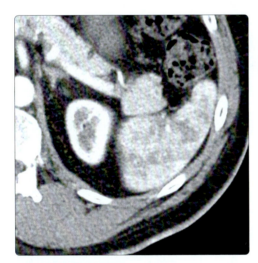
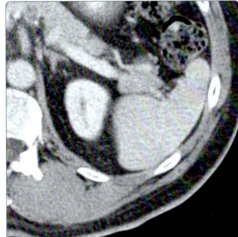

(Left) Arterial-phase axial CECT shows a very heterogeneous spleen caused by rapid enhancement of the vascular sinusoids (red pulp). This should not be mistaken for a pathologic process. (Right) Axial CECT during the venous phase shows the spleen with a homogeneous appearance.

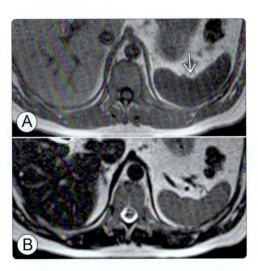
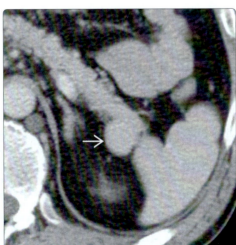

(Left) Axial T1WI MR (A) shows the normal spleen ➡ as slightly hypointense relative to liver. On T2 MR (B), the normal spleen is slightly hyperintense to liver. (Right) Axial CECT shows a "mass" ➡ in the pancreatic tail that is isodense to the spleen and represents an accessory spleen. This could be mistaken for a primary pancreatic mass, such as a neuroendocrine tumor.

Spleen: Imaging Approach and Differential Diagnosis

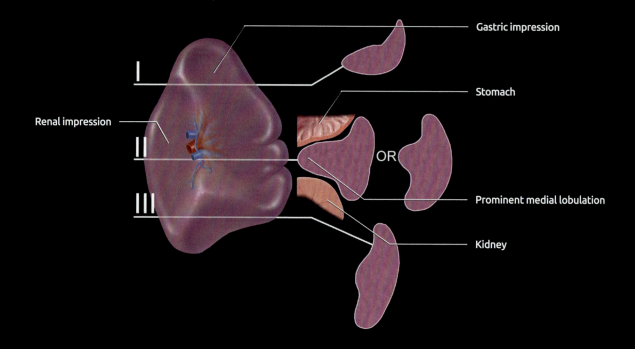

Gastric impression

Stomach

Renal impression

OR

Prominent medial lobulation

Kidney

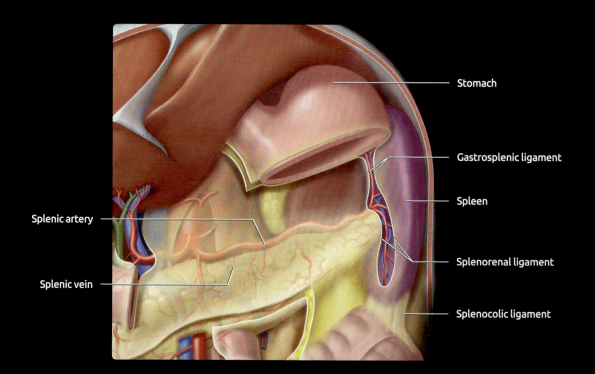

Stomach

Gastrosplenic ligament

Spleen

Splenic artery

Splenorenal ligament

Splenic vein

Splenocolic ligament

(Top) *Graphic shows the medial surface of the spleen and representative axial sections at 3 different levels. The spleen is of variable shape and size, even within the same individual, varying with states of nutrition and hydration. The medial surface is often quite lobulated as it is interposed between the stomach and the kidney.* (Bottom) *The splenic artery and vein course along the body of the pancreas, entering and exiting the spleen via the splenorenal ligament. The tail of the pancreas also inserts into the splenic hilum through the splenorenal ligament. The gastrosplenic ligament carries the short gastric and left gastroepiploic vessels to the stomach and upper portion of the spleen.*

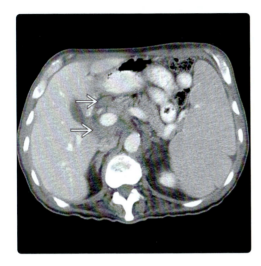

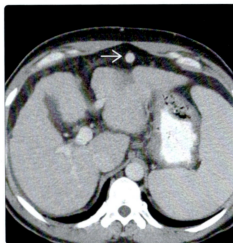

(Left) *Axial CECT in a patient with non-Hodgkin lymphoma shows numerous enlarged upper abdominal lymph nodes ➡. Splenomegaly is a common abnormality and can be caused by congestion, hematologic disorders, inflammatory/infectious conditions, tumors, or infiltrative processes.* (Right) *Axial CECT in a different case of splenomegaly caused by congestion secondary to cirrhosis and portal hypertension shows the recanalized umbilical vein ➡.*

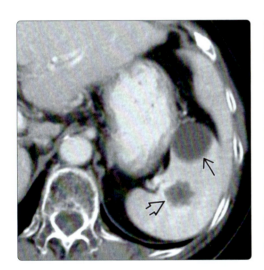

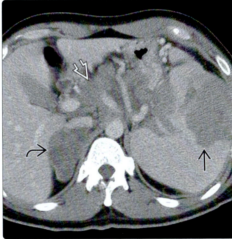

(Left) *Axial CECT shows 2 splenic lesions. The larger lesion ➡ has water density contents and thin, sharp walls, typical of a simple cyst. The smaller lesion ➡ has nodular walls and higher density contents, suggestive of splenic lymphangioma.* (Right) *In this patient with non-Hodgkin lymphoma, the spleen is markedly enlarged with heterogeneous, hypoattenuating, more discrete tumor foci ➡. Lymphomatous infiltration is also present within the adrenal gland ➡ and nodes ➡ throughout the abdomen.*

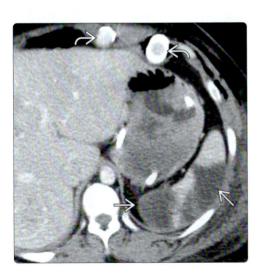

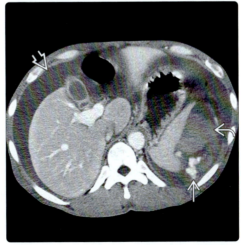

(Left) *Axial CECT in a patient with heart failure and abdominal pain shows a ventricular assist device ➡ and wedge-shaped regions of nonenhancing splenic parenchyma ➡ that extend to the capsular surface, characteristic of acute splenic infarctions.* (Right) *Axial CECT in a patient injured in a motor vehicle crash shows a sentinel clot ➡ adjacent to the spleen and a large hemoperitoneum ➡. Note the active extravasation of blood ➡ that is isodense to enhanced vessels.*

TERMINOLOGY

- Benign ectopic splenic tissue of congenital origin

IMAGING

- Most splenules located in or near splenic hilum or ligaments
  - 20% are near or within pancreatic tail and can mimic pancreatic neuroendocrine tumor
  - May also be in diaphragmatic, pararenal, and gastric sites
- CT: Same enhancement and attenuation as normal spleen
  - Isodense to main spleen on noncontrast images
  - Serpiginous enhancement on arterial phase
  - Homogeneous enhancement on venous/delayed images
- MR: T1WI hypointense and T2WI hyperintense
  - Follows appearance of spleen on all sequences
  - DWI: Isointense to spleen with similar ADC values
- Nuclear medicine: Technetium (Tc-99m) sulfur colloid or Tc-99m heat-damaged red blood cell (RBC) scan
  - Functional uptake in splenic tissue differentiates splenule from other masses

TOP DIFFERENTIAL DIAGNOSES

- Splenosis
- Polysplenia
- Peritoneal metastases and lymphoma
- Visceral mass (especially pancreatic neuroendocrine tumor)
- Splenic artery aneurysm or pseudoaneurysm

PATHOLOGY

- Congenital: Failure of some embryonic splenic buds to unite within dorsal mesogastrium

CLINICAL ISSUES

- Asymptomatic (vast majority of cases)
- May be mistaken for pancreatic or other abdominal mass
- Following splenectomy for lymphoma or ITP, disease may recur if accessory spleen was not removed

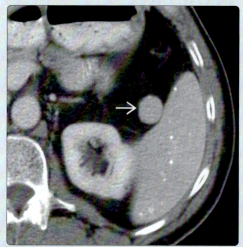

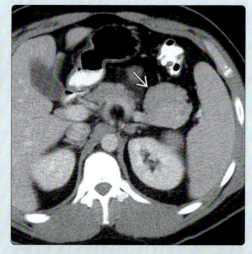

(Left) Axial CECT shows a small spherical accessory spleen ➡ near the splenic hilum. Note the foci of calcification from histoplasmosis in the main and accessory spleen. This appearance is so characteristic as to require no additional evaluation. (Right) Axial CECT demonstrates a large mass ➡ abutting the pancreatic tail and the splenic hilum. The mass was thought to be a neuroendocrine tumor and was resected. Note that the mass is isodense to the spleen. The mass was found to be a splenule at surgery.

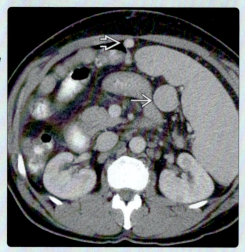

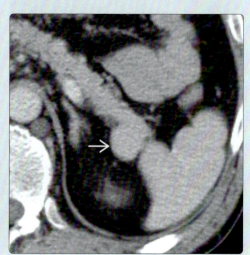

(Left) Axial CECT shows an enlarged spleen due to portal hypertension in this patient with cirrhosis. Note the prominent accessory spleen ➡ as well as the varices ➡. An accessory spleen may enlarge in parallel with the main spleen. (Right) Axial CECT shows a hypervascular mass ➡ within the pancreatic tail that mimics an islet cell tumor. A heat-damaged red blood cell scan (not shown) proved this to be an accessory spleen. Masses in the splenic hilum may arise from or involve the tail of the pancreas or spleen.

TERMINOLOGY

Synonyms
- Splenule, splenunculus

Definitions
- Benign ectopic splenic tissue of congenital origin

IMAGING

General Features
- Best diagnostic clue
  - Small, round, well-marginated nodule in left upper quadrant with same enhancement as normal spleen
- Location
  - In or near splenic hilum or ligaments (most cases)
    - 20% are near or within pancreatic tail
    - Usually left upper quadrant, above renal pedicle
    - Rarely in diaphragmatic, pararenal, and gastric sites
  - Single splenule in vast majority of patients
    - 1 splenule (88%), 2 splenules (9%), > 2 splenules (3%)
    - Multiple splenules usually clustered in 1 location
- Size
  - Varies from 1 mm to a few cm, usually < 2.5 cm

CT Findings
- Same enhancement as normal spleen
  - Isodense to main spleen on noncontrast images
  - Serpiginous enhancement on arterial phase
  - Homogeneous enhancement on venous/delayed images
- Most commonly located near splenic hilum or ligaments
- 2nd most common location is pancreatic tail
  - Usually < 3 cm medial to pancreatic tail
  - Most often along dorsal surface of pancreas
  - Incompletely surrounded by pancreatic parenchyma
- Rare: Torsion of splenule as cause of abdominal pain
  - Nonenhancing mass with surrounding hemorrhage
  - Whorl sign (twisted vascular pedicle) leading to splenule

MR Findings
- T1WI hypointense and T2WI hyperintense
  - Follows appearance of spleen on all sequences
- DWI: Isointense to spleen with similar apparent diffusion coefficient (ADC) values
  - Pancreatic neuroendocrine tumors usually hyperintense on DWI with lower ADC values
- Superparamagnetic iron oxide particles (SPIO) contrast media taken up by splenic tissue (but not tumor)

Nuclear Medicine Findings
- Technetium (Tc-99m) sulfur colloid or Tc-99m heat-damaged red blood cell (RBC) scan
  - Functional uptake in splenic tissue differentiates splenule from other masses
  - Tc-99m heat-damaged RBC scan preferred due to higher specificity and better target to background
- PET/CT
  - FDG-avid mass can mimic tumor

Imaging Recommendations
- Best imaging tool
  - Multiphase CT followed by Tc-99m heat-damaged RBC scan in equivocal cases

DIFFERENTIAL DIAGNOSIS

Splenosis
- Usually result of trauma; portions of disrupted spleen implant anywhere, including abdomen, pelvis, and chest

Polysplenia
- Congenital disorder with multiple small spleens, bilateral left-sidedness of viscera, and cardiovascular anomalies

Peritoneal Metastases and Lymphoma
- e.g., omental or peritoneal metastases

Visceral Mass
- Splenules commonly mistaken for pancreatic neuroendocrine tumors
- Splenules also mistaken for adrenal, gastric, or renal tumors

Splenic Artery Aneurysm or Pseudoaneurysm
- Bright homogeneous enhancement on arterial phase

PATHOLOGY

General Features
- Etiology
  - Congenital: Failure of some embryonic splenic buds to unite within dorsal mesogastrium

Gross Pathologic & Surgical Features
- Structurally normal splenic tissue

CLINICAL ISSUES

Presentation
- Most common signs/symptoms
  - Asymptomatic (vast majority of cases)
- Other signs/symptoms
  - May torse, rupture, and bleed (very rare)
  - May cause recurrence of hematologic disease (e.g., lymphoma or idiopathic thrombocytopenic purpura [ITP]) following prior splenectomy

Demographics
- Epidemiology
  - Incidence: 10-30% of patients at autopsy

Treatment
- In absence of complications (which are extraordinarily rare), no treatment or intervention
- Surgical resection: Only in setting of complications, recurrence of lymphoma, or hypersplenism

DIAGNOSTIC CHECKLIST

Consider
- Accessory spleen is common and can be mistaken for tumor

SELECTED REFERENCES

1. Coquia SF et al: Intrapancreatic Accessory Spleen: Possibilities of Computed Tomography in Differentiation From Nonfunctioning Pancreatic Neuroendocrine Tumor. J Comput Assist Tomogr. ePub, 2014

TERMINOLOGY

- Complex inherited syndromes associated with absence or multiplicity of spleens as well as many other anomalies

IMAGING

- **Asplenia (ASP) syndrome**: Right isomerism or bilateral right-sidedness
  - Absent spleen in virtually all patients
  - Congenital heart disease in ~ 100% of patients
  - Bilateral trilobed lungs
  - Malrotation in most patients
  - Aorta and inferior vena cava (IVC) are frequently ipsilateral (usually right side)
- **Polysplenia (PSP) syndrome**: Left isomerism or bilateral left-sidedness
  - Usually multiple spleens but may have single normal spleen
  - Increased risk of complex cardiac anomalies, although less common with PSP than ASP

- IVC interruption with azygos continuation very common
- Bilateral bilobed lungs
- Truncated/short pancreas or agenesis of dorsal pancreas
  - Increased incidence of diabetes and pancreatitis
- Intestinal malrotation is seen in most patients
- Liver often midline with range of biliary abnormalities
- Aorta usually located to left of midline

TOP DIFFERENTIAL DIAGNOSES

- Splenosis
- Accessory spleen
- Splenectomy

CLINICAL ISSUES

- ASP: Newborn or infant presentation due to cardiac disease with poor prognosis and early mortality
  - ↑ risk of sepsis due to lack of spleen
- PSP: Infant or adult presentation with better prognosis due to lesser incidence of cardiac disease

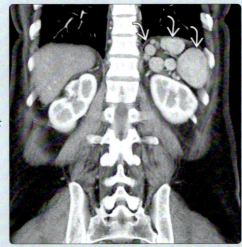
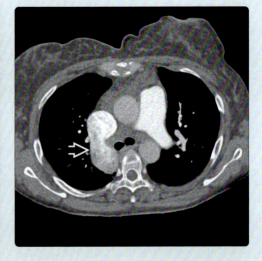

(Left) Coronal volume-rendered CECT in a patient with polysplenia (PSP) syndrome demonstrates multiple spleens ⊅ in the left upper quadrant. The multiple spleens in PSP are typically in the left abdomen and can rarely be on the right. (Right) Axial CECT in the same patient demonstrates a markedly dilated azygous vein ⊳.

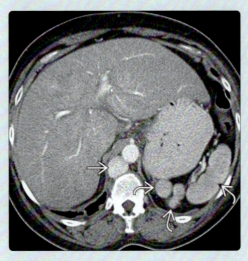
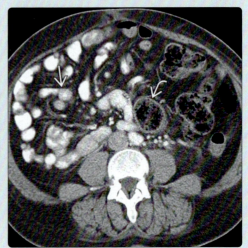

(Left) Axial CECT in the same patient again demonstrates multiple spleens ⊅ and a dilated azygous vein ⊅ to the right of the aorta. Azygous continuation of the inferior vena cava (IVC) is a very common abnormality in PSP syndrome. (Right) Axial CECT in the same patient demonstrates malrotation of the bowel with the small bowel ⊅ abnormally located in the right abdomen and the entirety of the colon ⊅ in the left abdomen. Malrotation is quite common with both asplenia (ASP) and PSP syndromes.

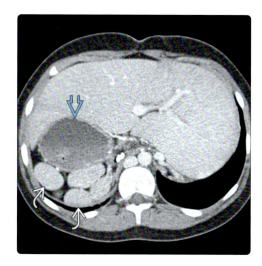

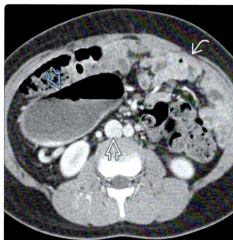

(Left) Axial CECT in a patient with PSP syndrome demonstrates multiple spleens ⇒ located in the right upper quadrant and situs inversus. Note the reversed positions of the liver and stomach ⇒. (Right) Axial CECT in the same patient demonstrates an abnormal right-sided stomach ⇒. Note that the IVC ⇒ is normally located on the right. The majority of the small bowel ⇒ is on one side of the abdomen, in keeping with malrotation.

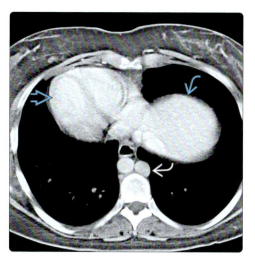

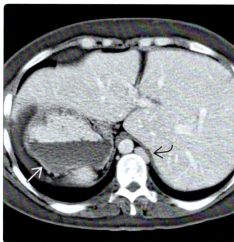

(Left) Axial CECT in a patient with PSP syndrome shows dextrocardia ⇒ and a left-sided IVC ⇒. The liver dome ⇒ is on the left side. (Right) Axial CECT in the same patient shows complete abdominal situs inversus with an otherwise normal-appearing stomach ⇒ on the right-hand side. Note the left-sided IVC ⇒.

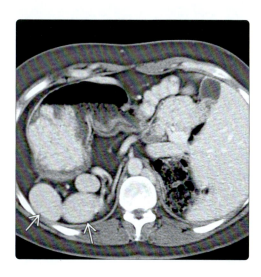

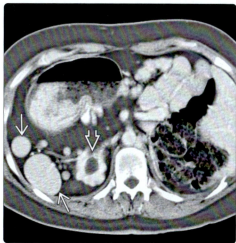

(Left) Axial CECT in the same patient shows multiple splenules ⇒ in the right upper quadrant along with abdominal situs inversus. (Right) Axial CECT in the same patient shows multiple spleens ⇒, situs inversus, and cystic disease of the kidneys ⇒. This patient was 35 years old (patients with PSP are much more likely to reach adulthood than those with ASP).

Splenomegaly and Hypersplenism

TERMINOLOGY

- Splenomegaly: Splenic enlargement caused by a number of different underlying disorders

IMAGING

- Normal spleen is ≤ 13 cm in length
- Splenic index (product of length, breadth, and width of spleen): Normally 120-480 cm³
- Splenic weight (splenic index x 0.55): Normally between 100-250 g
- Splenomegaly: AP diameter > 2/3 distance of AP diameter of abdominal cavity

PATHOLOGY

- Splenomegaly attributable to 5 different general etiologies
  - Congestive
    - Right heart failure, portal hypertension, sickle cell disease (in acute setting), and splenic vein thrombosis
  - Hematologic
    - Polycythemia vera, myelofibrosis, and hemoglobinopathies
  - Inflammatory/infectious
    - Mononucleosis, malaria, and HIV/AIDS most common infections to result in splenomegaly
    - Sarcoid may result in mild splenomegaly with multiple small hypodensities in liver and spleen
  - Space-occupying lesions
    - Space-occupying masses in spleen do not commonly cause splenomegaly and are more likely to replace normal splenic tissue
  - Storage and infiltrative disorders
    - Primary or secondary hemochromatosis, amyloidosis, and glycogen storage diseases

CLINICAL ISSUES

- Complications include splenic rupture and hypersplenism
  - Hypersplenism: Hyperfunctioning spleen removes normal RBC, WBC, and platelets from circulation

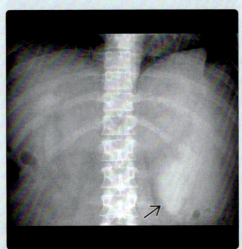
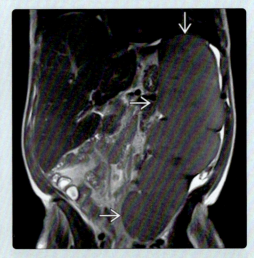

(Left) Frontal radiograph demonstrates "fullness" in the left upper quadrant. The inferior edge ➡ of an enlarged spleen is evident. (Right) Coronal T2 MR demonstrates a markedly enlarged spleen ➡ in a patient with myelodysplastic syndrome. The most common causes of massive splenomegaly are cirrhosis/portal hypertension, lymphoma, chronic myelogenous leukemia, extramedullary hematopoiesis, myelofibrosis, and Gaucher disease.

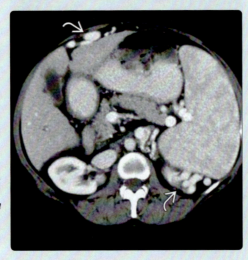
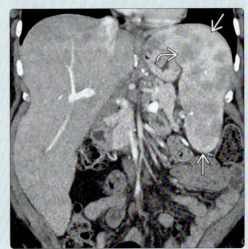

(Left) Axial CECT shows a small, cirrhotic liver with widened fissures and signs of portal hypertension, including splenomegaly and varices ➡. In most patients with splenomegaly, there are clues as to the underlying cause on the imaging study, as in this case. (Right) Coronal CECT in an asymptomatic patient demonstrates a mildly enlarged spleen ➡ with multiple ill-defined hypodense nodules ➡ in a patient with known sarcoidosis. Lymphoma and metastatic disease could have a very similar appearance.

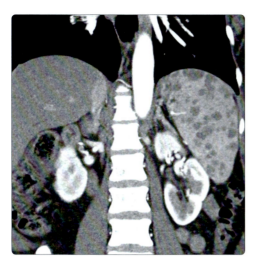
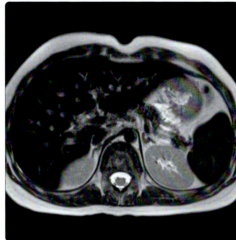

(Left) Coronal CECT demonstrates a mildly enlarged spleen with multiple hypodense nodules. The patient was later found to have thoracic lymphadenopathy, and biopsy showed the spleen to be a manifestation of sarcoidosis. (Right) Axial T2 MR demonstrates marked low signal in the liver, spleen, and bone marrow in a patient with hemosiderosis due to multiple blood transfusions.

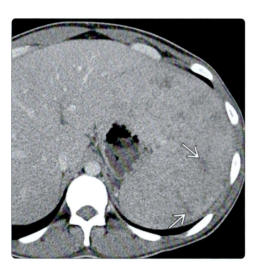
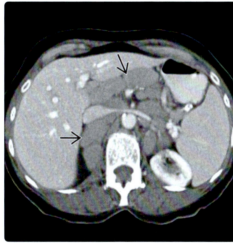

(Left) Axial CECT shows a markedly enlarged spleen with multiple subtle low-density foci ➡ scattered throughout the splenic parenchyma. This was found to be lymphoma, and lymphadenopathy was present elsewhere. (Right) Axial CECT in a patient with non-Hodgkin lymphoma shows splenomegaly and extensive lymphadenopathy ➡. While splenomegaly and lymphadenopathy are characteristic findings in patients with NHL, benign processes, such as sarcoidosis and mononucleosis, may result in similar findings.

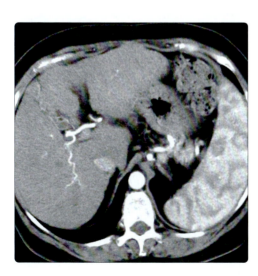
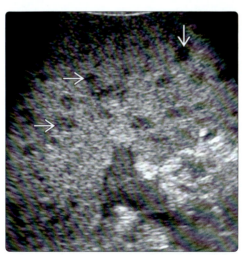

(Left) Axial arterial-phase CECT in a patient with cirrhosis & portal hypertension shows a swirled moiré pattern of splenic enhancement that disappeared on the portal venous phase. This normal variant is often more prominent in patients with cirrhosis and portal hypertension. (Right) US shows splenomegaly with multiple hypoechoic foci ➡ in a patient with granulomatous MAI infection. On US, granulomatous abscesses appear as well-defined, hypoechoic lesions, usually with associated splenomegaly.

TERMINOLOGY

- Global or segmental parenchymal splenic ischemia and necrosis caused by vascular occlusion

IMAGING

- Acute findings on CECT
  - Diagnosis best made on portal venous-phase images due to heterogeneous arterial-phase enhancement
  - Global infarction: Complete nonenhancement of spleen
    - ± cortical rim sign: Preserved enhancement of peripheral rim of spleen in massive infarction
  - Segmental infarction: Wedge-shaped or rounded low-attenuation area usually at periphery of spleen
    - Can be multiple, especially when caused by emboli
- Chronic findings on CECT
  - Most often results in scarring and volume loss
  - Multiple repetitive infarcts in sickle cell disease can lead to small, calcified spleen (autoinfarcted spleen)
  - Infarct can develop into splenic cyst

- Complications (< 20% of patients)
  - Perisplenic fluid/hematoma suggests splenic rupture
  - Development of rim-enhancing fluid collection: Splenic abscess

TOP DIFFERENTIAL DIAGNOSES

- Splenic laceration
- Splenic cyst or abscess
- Heterogeneous arterial-phase enhancement of spleen
- Splenic tumors

CLINICAL ISSUES

- Many different causes but 2 most common are
  - Hematologic disease or hematologic malignancies (sickle cell, myelofibrosis, leukemia, etc.)
  - Embolic conditions (septic emboli, cardiac emboli from atrial fibrillation, etc.)
- Most cases require no treatment but rarely surgery or intervention for pain or complications

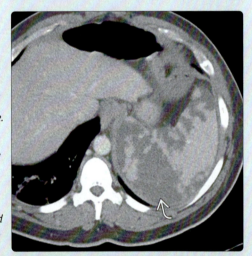
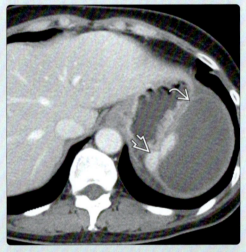

(Left) Axial CECT in a sickle cell patient demonstrates an enlarged spleen with multiple wedge-shaped, acute splenic infarcts ➡. While sickle cell patients can develop a small, calcified autoinfarcted spleen, the spleen may be enlarged in the early stages of the disease. (Right) Axial CECT demonstrates a large, global infarct of the spleen with only a tiny amount of enhancing splenic tissue ➡. Notice the peripheral enhancement (rim sign) ➡ at the margins of the infarct as a result of preserved flow through capsular vessels.

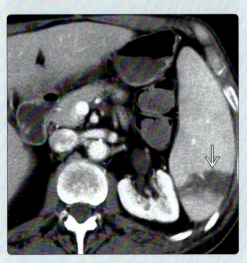
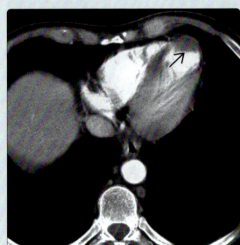

(Left) Axial CECT in a 67-year-old man with a 10-year history of atrial fibrillation, now presenting with acute LUQ pain, demonstrates a peripheral, low-attenuation splenic infarct with straight margins ➡. (Right) Axial CECT in the same patient identifies a left ventricular thrombus ➡ as the source of the arterial embolus to the spleen. Embolic disease is likely the most common cause of splenic infarcts in older patients.

TERMINOLOGY

Definitions

- Global or segmental parenchymal splenic ischemia and necrosis caused by vascular occlusion

IMAGING

General Features

- Best diagnostic clue
  - Peripheral, wedge-shaped, nonenhancing areas within splenic parenchyma on CECT in patients with LUQ pain
- Location
  - Entire spleen may be infarcted or more commonly segmental areas
- Morphology
  - Most commonly wedge-shaped areas of nonenhancement when infarct is segmental
    - Straight margins indicate vascular etiology (rather than mass or fluid collection)
    - May very rarely be rounded (atypical appearance)

Radiographic Findings

- Radiography
  - May be associated with lower left lobe atelectasis and pleural effusion on chest x-ray

CT Findings

- NECT
  - Infarcts may be difficult (or impossible) to visualize without intravenous contrast
  - Areas of hemorrhagic transformation within infarcts appear hyperdense
- CECT
  - Acute findings
    - Diagnosis best made on portal venous-phase images: Heterogeneous enhancement during arterial phase (due to differential enhancement of red and white pulp) makes identification of subtle infarcts difficult
    - Global: Complete nonenhancement of spleen
      - ± cortical rim sign: Preserved enhancement of peripheral rim of spleen in massive infarction due to preserved flow from capsular vessels
      - Mottled higher density areas within infarcted spleen may represent either tiny islands of residual enhancing splenic tissue or hemorrhage
    - Segmental: Wedge-shaped or rounded low-attenuation area usually at periphery of spleen
      - Can be multiple, especially when caused by emboli
      - In some instances, accessory spleens (splenules) may be infarcted
      - Spleen may or may not be enlarged in acute phase
    - Complications (< 20% of patients)
      - Presence of fluid or hematoma surrounding spleen in setting of infarct suggests splenic rupture (most often in setting of large or global infarct)
      - Development of discrete rim-enhancing fluid collection ± internal gas should raise concern for splenic abscess
  - Chronic findings
    - Infarcts should evolve over time, leaving areas of scarring and volume loss in spleen
      - Sites of old infarcts may show calcification
      - Remaining spleen may undergo compensatory hypertrophy
    - Multiple repetitive infarcts in sickle cell disease can lead to small, calcified spleen (autoinfarcted spleen)
    - Infarct can develop into splenic cyst (secondary or acquired cyst)

MR Findings

- T1WI
  - Low signal within area of infarct (can show high T1WI signal due to hemorrhagic infarct)
- T2WI
  - Heterogeneous high signal within area of infarct
- T1WI C+
  - Wedge-shaped area of hypoenhancement

Ultrasonographic Findings

- Grayscale ultrasound
  - Wedge-shaped hypoechoic area(s) within periphery of spleen
    - May rarely be rounded or irregularly shaped at center of spleen (atypical)
  - Bright band sign: Highly echogenic linear bands in area of infarct may be specific sign of infarction
- Color Doppler
  - Diminished or absent flow in areas of infarction

Angiographic Findings

- Conventional angiography: Main splenic artery occlusion or segmental emboli

Imaging Recommendations

- Best imaging tool
  - Portal venous-phase CECT

DIFFERENTIAL DIAGNOSIS

Splenic Laceration

- Hypodense, wedge-shaped defect in spleen in patient with recent history of trauma
- Almost always high-attenuation hematoma adjacent to laceration ± large hemoperitoneum
- May have high-attenuation active arterial extravasation

Splenic Cyst

- Nonneoplastic cysts divided into primary "true" epithelial cysts and secondary "false" cysts (no epithelial lining)
  - Primary cysts most often epidermoid cysts (10-25% of all splenic cysts) but can be parasitic (echinococcal)
  - Secondary cysts result from prior infection, infarction, trauma, or hematoma
- Usually well-defined, rounded fluid attenuation cyst with variable internal complexity and peripheral calcification
- Can result from prior infarct but much better defined, rounded, and water density

Splenic Abscess

- Complex intraparenchymal or perisplenic loculated fluid collection with peripheral enhancement, internal complexity/debris, and possible internal gas
- Unlike infarct, splenic abscess is discrete, rounded fluid collection with adjacent fat stranding/inflammation

- o May develop from evolution of prior infarct
- May appear as multiple small lesions (microabscesses) due to fungal infections in immunocompromised patients

Normal Heterogeneous Enhancement of Spleen in Arterial Phase

- Striated appearance of spleen in arterial phase (due to differential enhancement of red and white pulp) should not be confused with splenic infarcts

Splenic Tumors

- Primary or secondary neoplasms of spleen (whether benign or malignant) should appear focal and mass-like with rounded borders (not wedge-shaped or linear)
- Lymphoma and some metastases (metastatic melanoma or mucinous neoplasms) may appear low density and hypoenhancing, resembling density of infarcts

PATHOLOGY

General Features

- Etiology
  - o Large variety of different causes resulting in occlusion of arterial/venous vasculature supplying spleen
    - **Hematologic disorders**
      - □ Sickle cell hemoglobinopathies: Risk of splenic infarct during high-altitude travel or airplane flight
      - □ Myelofibrosis
      - □ Hypercoagulable states
      - □ Leukemia and lymphoma
      - □ Any cause of hypersplenism/splenomegaly (including mononucleosis and infections)
    - **Thromboembolism**
      - □ Atrial fibrillation
      - □ Aortic atherosclerotic disease with embolization to splenic artery
      - □ Aortic valve emboli from subacute bacterial endocarditis
    - **Anatomic causes**
      - □ Splenic torsion (including torsion due to wandering spleen): Laxity or absence of splenic ligaments results in spleen "wandering" to ectopic locations, increasing incidence of torsion and infarction
    - **Miscellaneous**
      - □ Pancreatitis or pseudocysts
      - □ Portal hypertension
      - □ Any surgical procedure involving upper abdominal organs (particularly pancreatic tail, stomach, left adrenal gland)
      - □ Collagen vascular disease
      - □ Tumors (gastric, pancreatic, adrenal) involving splenic hilum and vessels

CLINICAL ISSUES

Presentation

- Most common signs/symptoms
  - o Many patients can be asymptomatic (1/3 of patients)
    - Most common with small splenic infarcts
  - o Most common symptoms: LUQ pain, fever, chills, malaise, nausea, vomiting

- o May be associated with other infarcts (e.g., kidney and bowel) in patients with splenic infarcts due to emboli
- Lab data: Anemia (53%), leukocytosis (41%), elevated platelet count (7%)

Demographics

- Age
  - o 2-87 years (mean: 54 years)
- Gender
  - o M = F
- Epidemiology
  - o Many different causes but 2 most common causes are
    - Hematologic disease or hematologic malignancies: Sickle cell, myelofibrosis, leukemia, etc; most common causes in younger patients
      - □ Probably caused by congestion and occlusion of splenic vessels by abnormal cells associated with hematologic disorder
      - □ Most common cause of splenic infarcts overall
    - Embolic conditions (septic emboli, cardiac emboli from atrial fibrillation, embolization of ulcerated atherosclerotic plaque); most common cause in older patients

Natural History & Prognosis

- Most cases require no treatment and symptoms cease naturally
- Rarely surgery or intervention for pain or complications
  - o Complications: Abscess, rupture, subcapsular hematoma, hemorrhage, pseudocyst formation

Treatment

- Asymptomatic: Supportive treatment (pain control with analgesics)
- Symptomatic: Splenectomy for intolerable/increasing pain or splenic rupture; image-guided drainage for splenic abscess formation

DIAGNOSTIC CHECKLIST

Image Interpretation Pearls

- Wedge-shaped, peripheral area of nonenhancement on portal venous-phase CECT
- Do not confuse normal striated enhancement pattern on arterial-phase CECT for splenic infarct

SELECTED REFERENCES

1. Gaetke-Udager K et al: Multimodality imaging of splenic lesions and the role of non-vascular, image-guided intervention. Abdom Imaging. 39(3):570-87, 2014
2. Llewellyn ME et al: The sonographic "bright band sign" of splenic infarction. J Ultrasound Med. 33(6):929-38, 2014
3. Lawrence YR et al: Splenic infarction: an update on William Osler's observations. Isr Med Assoc J. 12(6):362-5, 2010

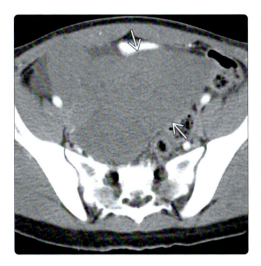

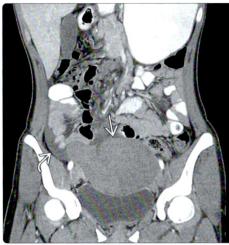

(Left) *Axial CECT in a young child with acute abdominal pain demonstrates a large, hypoenhancing mass* ➡ *in the pelvis.* (Right) *Coronal CECT in the same patient again shows the same mass* ➡ *in the pelvis with fluid in the adjacent right pelvis* ➡ *and no spleen noted in the abdomen. This mass was found at surgery to represent torsion and infarction of a "wandering" spleen. The spleen in such cases is found in ectopic locations due to laxity or absence of the splenic ligaments.*

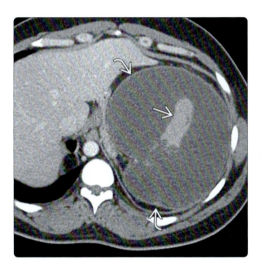

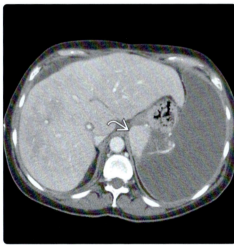

(Left) *A large fluid collection* ➡ *envelops small areas of normal splenic tissue* ➡ *. This was found at surgery to represent a massively infarcted spleen with contained rupture, resulting in the fluid collection.* (Right) *Patient status post embolization for hypersplenism shows severe splenomegaly with no enhancement except for a small portion of the medial spleen* ➡ *. Massive acute infarction is often not desired in splenic embolotherapy, as patients can develop infections of infarcted tissue.*

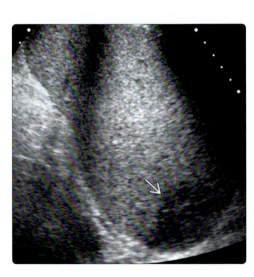

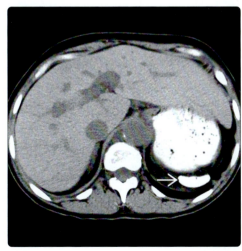

(Left) *Sagittal US in a 48-year-old woman with myelodysplastic syndrome and 1-week history of LUQ pain shows marked splenomegaly and wedge-shaped hypoechoic area* ➡ *in the lower pole of the spleen, consistent with infarction. Patient was placed on analgesics and recovered uneventfully.* (Right) *Axial NECT in a 55-year-old woman presenting with a history of sickle cell anemia demonstrates a spleen that is very small, densely calcified* ➡ *, and nonfunctional, sometimes termed "autosplenectomy."*

TERMINOLOGY

- Dissemination of splenic tissue into ectopic locations following splenic rupture (either traumatic or iatrogenic)

IMAGING

- Can occur in virtually every compartment of body
  - Most common in abdomen/pelvis (65% of cases)
  - Usually located within peritoneal cavity (greater omentum, bowel serosa, parietal peritoneum, undersurface of diaphragm)
  - Less common locations include thorax (usually after diaphragmatic rupture) and subcutaneous soft tissues
- MDCT: Multiple nodules or masses scattered throughout abdomen or pelvis
  - Should follow appearance of spleen on all phases of enhancement
  - Slightly hypoattenuating (5-10 HU less) compared to liver on NECT, striated enhancement on arterial phase, and homogeneous enhancement on venous/delayed phases

- MR: Follows appearance and enhancement of normal spleen on all sequences
- Tc-99m heat-denatured RBC scan: ↑ sensitivity/specificity
  - ↑ uptake within nodules

TOP DIFFERENTIAL DIAGNOSES

- Peritoneal carcinomatosis
- Accessory spleen
- Polysplenia
- Visceral mass or malignancy
- Peritoneal endometriosis

CLINICAL ISSUES

- Can mimic peritoneal carcinomatosis or primary malignancies on CT and PET
- No other clinical significance in most cases
- Most patients are asymptomatic, but rarely, symptoms are due to hemorrhage, rupture, torsion, infarction, or bowel obstruction

(Left) Axial CECT demonstrates absence of the spleen (patient had a history of prior splenectomy for trauma) with small enhancing nodules ➡ in the left upper quadrant. Splenosis is not infrequently seen in close proximity to the splenectomy bed. (Right) Axial CECT in the same patient shows additional splenic implants ➡ along the serosal surface of the left colon and along the posterior margin of the right liver lobe. Splenosis is most commonly seen within the peritoneal cavity, with extraperitoneal splenosis more rare.

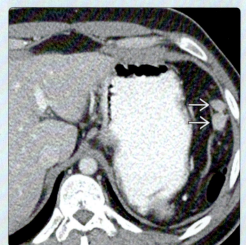
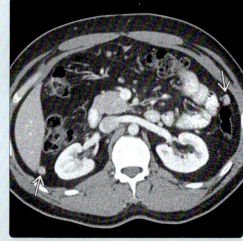

(Left) Axial CECT in a patient with remote history of abdominal trauma shows multiple soft tissue nodules ➡ along the peritoneal surfaces, which might be mistaken for carcinomatosis, but represent splenosis. (Right) Axial CECT shows an enhancing soft tissue nodule ➡ in the left cardiophrenic angle. The patient had a distant history of traumatic splenic injury with diaphragmatic rupture, the most common reason for thoracic splenosis. Thoracic splenosis is quite rare compared to abdominal/pelvic splenosis.

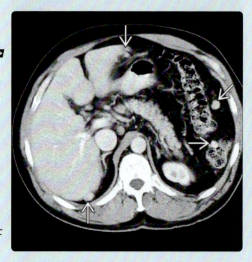
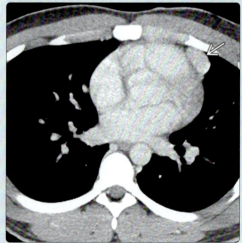

TERMINOLOGY

Definitions

- Dissemination of splenic tissue into ectopic locations following splenic rupture (either traumatic or iatrogenic)

IMAGING

General Features

- Location
  - Most common in abdomen/pelvis (65% of cases)
    - Usually located within peritoneal cavity (greater omentum, bowel serosa, parietal peritoneum, undersurface of diaphragm)
    - Involvement of extraperitoneal spaces uncommon
  - Can occur in virtually every compartment of body
    - Less common locations include thorax (usually after diaphragmatic rupture), subcutaneous soft tissues, and even intracranial cavity

CT Findings

- Multiple nodules scattered throughout abdomen or pelvis
- Nodules follow appearance of spleen on all phases
  - Slightly hypoattenuating (5-10 HU less) compared to liver on NECT, striated enhancement on arterial phase, and homogeneous enhancement on venous/delayed phases

MR Findings

- Follows signal/enhancement of spleen on all sequences
- T1WI: Hypointense to liver; slightly hyperintense to muscle
- T2WI: Hyperintense to liver

Ultrasonographic Findings

- Nonspecific round/oval, homogeneous mass(es)

Nuclear Medicine Findings

- PET
  - Splenosis nodules can be FDG avid and mimic neoplasm
- Tc-99m sulfur colloid
  - ↑ uptake within splenic nodules (similar to native spleen)
- **Tc-99m labeled heat-denatured RBC scintigraphy**
  - ↑ sensitivity/specificity with ↑ uptake within nodules

Imaging Recommendations

- Best imaging tool
  - Tc-99m labeled heat-denatured RBC scan

DIFFERENTIAL DIAGNOSIS

Peritoneal Carcinomatosis

- Usually associated with ascites, omental/peritoneal stranding and nodularity, and known history of underlying malignancy

Accessory Spleen

- Congenital ectopic splenic tissue due to failure in fusion of splenic foci during development
- Most cases are small, solitary, and adjacent to splenic hilum
- May hypertrophy after splenectomy and mimic splenosis

Polysplenia

- Multiple small spleens associated with abdominal situs inversus and cardiovascular anomalies

Visceral Mass or Malignancy

- Splenosis can mimic pancreatic, adrenal, renal, and gastric masses (and vice versa)
  - Splenosis abutting pancreatic tail can mimic neuroendocrine tumor
- CT/MR enhancement characteristics and nuclear scintigraphy helpful in differentiation

Peritoneal Endometriosis

- Soft tissue nodules with variable enhancement usually located in pelvis (uterine ligaments, cul-de-sac, fallopian tubes, etc.)

PATHOLOGY

General Features

- Etiology
  - Blunt traumatic disruption of splenic capsule with seeding of splenic tissue into peritoneal cavity
  - Can occur with elective splenectomy (morselization of spleen; spill into peritoneal cavity)

Gross Pathologic & Surgical Features

- Reddish-blue color; no capsule
- Supplied by small perforating vessels from local tissues
  - Not supplied by splenic artery branches, unlike splenule

Microscopic Features

- May completely resemble normal splenic tissue
  - Cannot differentiate from splenule based on histology

CLINICAL ISSUES

Presentation

- Most are asymptomatic
- Rarely symptomatic due to hemorrhage, rupture, torsion, infarction, or bowel obstruction

Demographics

- Epidemiology
  - Most cases reported in adults; M > F (↑ trauma in men)
  - ~ 70% of patients with splenectomy following trauma
  - Usually detected years after trauma

Natural History & Prognosis

- No clinical significance in most cases
- Recurrent disease after splenectomy with hematologic disorders (idiopathic thrombocytic purpura, lymphoma, etc.)
- No Howell-Jolly bodies, Heinz bodies, or abnormal RBCs on peripheral blood smear despite splenectomy
  - Indicates patient has functioning spleen

Treatment

- In most cases, no treatment is necessary
- Surgical resection only if complications or symptoms are present

SELECTED REFERENCES

1. Diop AD et al: CT imaging of peritoneal carcinomatosis and its mimics. Diagn Interv Imaging. ePub, 2014

Splenic Cyst

IMAGING

- Spectrum of appearances on CT
  - Solitary, well-defined, water density, unilocular cystic lesion
    - Thin wall with sharp interface to normal splenic tissue
    - No peripheral/intracystic enhancement or solid component
  - Some cysts can have septations, trabeculations, thick wall, internal necrotic debris, or calcification
    - May have attenuation greater than simple fluid (due to hemorrhage or protein)
    - Thin eggshell calcification or thick, irregular peripheral calcification
  - Congenital and acquired cysts may be indistinguishable
    - Congenital cysts more likely simple in appearance
    - Acquired cysts often complex with calcification

TOP DIFFERENTIAL DIAGNOSES

- Splenic infection and abscess

- Splenic metastases and lymphoma
- Benign primary splenic tumors
- Intrasplenic pseudocyst

PATHOLOGY

- Congenital epidermoid ("true" cyst)
  - May be due to intrasplenic sequestration of peritoneal mesothelial cells during embryologic development
- Acquired cysts (secondary/"false" cysts or pseudocysts)
  - Due to prior trauma, hematoma, infarction, or infection
  - Arise due to liquefactive necrosis and cystic change

CLINICAL ISSUES

- Most cysts are discovered incidentally on imaging
- Small and asymptomatic: No treatment
- Symptomatic cysts usually treated, with options including percutaneous aspiration/drainage, cyst decapsulation or unroofing, and partial/complete splenectomy
  - Splenectomy for symptomatic large cysts (> 5 cm)

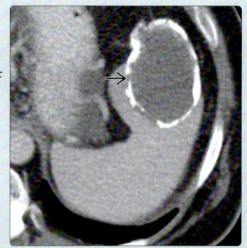
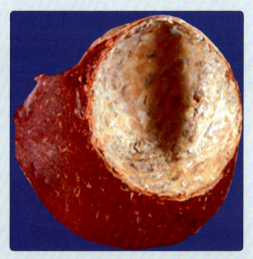

(Left) Axial CECT shows a water density mass with a calcified wall ➡ within the spleen. Note the absence of any enhancing or soft tissue components within this splenic cyst. (Right) Postsplenectomy specimen in the same patient shows the calcified, fibrous wall of the cyst. This was an acquired cyst, probably as a result of prior trauma or infarction.

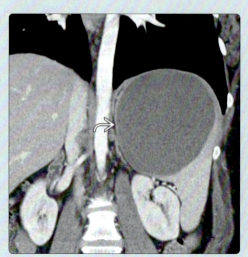
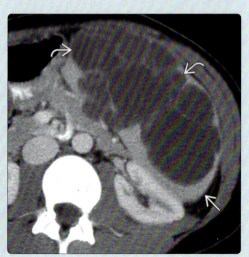

(Left) Coronal CECT in a young woman demonstrates a large, simple-appearing splenic cyst ➡. The patient was symptomatic with pain and early satiety and consequently underwent surgical cyst deroofing. (Right) Axial CECT demonstrates a large, nonenhancing, multiseptated splenic cyst ➡ replacing most of the spleen. Only a posterior sliver of normal spleen remains ➡.

IMAGING

General Features

- Best diagnostic clue
  - Sharply defined, spherical cystic lesion of water density
- Key concepts
  - Classification
    - Congenital epidermoid cysts (primary or "true" cyst)
      □ Demonstrate inner cellular endothelial lining
      □ Account for 10-25% of all splenic cysts
    - Acquired cysts (secondary or "false" cysts)
      □ No inner cellular lining but have fibrous wall
      □ Account for 80% of splenic cysts
      □ Due to prior trauma, hematoma, or infarction

Radiographic Findings

- Curvilinear wall calcification in left upper quadrant

CT Findings

- Spectrum of appearances
  - Solitary, well-defined, water density unilocular cyst
    - Thin wall with sharp interface to normal splenic tissue
    - No peripheral or intracystic enhancement; no solid, nodular soft tissue component
    - Always intraparenchymal (no exophytic component)
  - Some cysts can have septations, trabeculations, thick wall, and internal necrotic debris
    - May have attenuation greater than simple fluid (due to hemorrhage or protein)
  - Cysts may have thin eggshell calcification or thick, irregular peripheral calcification
- Congenital and acquired cysts may be indistinguishable
  - Congenital cysts more likely to be simple in appearance
  - Acquired cysts more likely complex with calcification

MR Findings

- Most cysts are T2 hyperintense and T1 hypointense
- May have ↑ signal intensity on T1WI due to blood products or protein within cyst (especially if ↑ attenuation on CT)

Ultrasonographic Findings

- Anechoic with smooth margins and thin walls
- May have internal echoes, septations, and debris
- Peripheral echogenic calcifications ± acoustic shadowing

DIFFERENTIAL DIAGNOSIS

Splenic Infection and Abscess

- Pyogenic abscess
  - Solitary or multiple, with well-defined irregular borders, peripheral enhancement, and central fluid density
  - ± internal gas due to gas-forming organism
  - Usually clinical history of fever, ↑ WBC, and pain
- Fungal abscess
  - Usually microabscesses with tiny, hypodense nodules throughout spleen
- Parasitic echinococcal or hydatid cyst
  - Complex cyst with internal low-density daughter cysts and thick wall composed of fibrous tissue
  - Often serpiginous, linear densities within cyst due to collapsed parasitic membranes
  - Chronic cysts often demonstrate peripheral or serpiginous, wavy internal calcification
  - May be associated with similar cystic lesions in liver and peritoneal cavity

Splenic Metastases and Lymphoma

- Metastases
  - Homogeneous hypovascular tumors, mucinous neoplasms, and necrotic tumors may mimic cysts
  - Melanoma can appear low density due to necrosis (mimicking cyst)
- Lymphoma
  - Homogeneously enlarged spleen, multiple tiny hypodense nodules, or discrete hypodense mass(es)
  - Discrete masses are hypodense and homogeneous

Benign Primary Splenic Tumors

- Most commonly hemangioma and lymphangioma
- May appear solid or cystic, and can appear completely simple and indistinguishable from splenic cyst
- Hemangiomas may be hypervascular on arterial phase CECT
- Lymphangiomas may be multiloculated with septations

Intrasplenic Pseudocyst

- Pseudocyst developing in pancreatic tail after pancreatitis may invaginate into splenic parenchyma

PATHOLOGY

General Features

- Etiology
  - Congenital epidermoid ("true" cyst)
    - Etiology unclear, but may be due to sequestration of peritoneal mesothelial cells within spleen during embryologic development
  - Acquired cysts (secondary/"false" cysts or pseudocysts)
    - Most often due to prior trauma, hematoma, infarction, or infection (including mononucleosis)
    - Due to liquefactive necrosis and cystic change

CLINICAL ISSUES

Presentation

- Most common signs/symptoms
  - Most cysts discovered incidentally on imaging performed for other reasons
  - Rarely present with pain or palpable mass

Natural History & Prognosis

- Complications are rare and include intracystic hemorrhage, rupture, or superinfection

Treatment

- Small and asymptomatic → no treatment
- Symptomatic cysts usually treated, with options including percutaneous aspiration/drainage, cyst decapsulation or unroofing, and partial/complete splenectomy
  - Splenectomy for symptomatic large cysts (> 5 cm)

SELECTED REFERENCES

1. Rana AP et al: Splenic epidermoid cyst - a rare entity. J Clin Diagn Res. 8(2):175-6, 2014

Spleen

IMAGING

- Benign tumors
  - **Hemangioma**: Most common benign splenic tumor
    - Classic peripheral nodular enhancement seen in hepatic hemangiomas is often not present
    - Like liver hemangiomas, may demonstrate marked hyperintensity on T2 MR and variables degrees of arterial hyperenhancement with persistent delayed enhancement
    - May be multiple as part of generalized angiomatosis (Klippel-Trenaunay-Weber syndrome)
  - **Lymphangioma**: Thin-walled, low-density or cystic lesion (can be solitary or multiple) with sharply defined margins
  - **Hamartoma**: Rare benign tumor of spleen with nonspecific imaging appearance
    - Heterogeneous early enhancement which may persist and become more homogeneous on delayed images
- Malignant tumors
  - **Primary lymphoma**: Most often non-Hodgkin lymphoma (B-cell origin) but much less common than secondary lymphomatous involvement of spleen
    - Imaging patterns including enlarged spleen without discrete mass, solitary dominant hypodense mass, or multifocal hypodense lesions
  - **Angiosarcoma**: Rare, highly aggressive malignant tumor of spleen, with propensity for early, widespread metastases (patients usually die within 1 year)
    - Often multiple lesions with variable enhancement that may superficially resemble hemangiomas

CLINICAL ISSUES

- Most benign splenic tumors are incidental findings on imaging studies performed for other reasons
- Splenic malignancies may present with LUQ pain, palpable mass, splenomegaly, fever, or weight loss
- Suspicious tumors (based on either imaging or clinical scenario) should lead to biopsy ± splenectomy

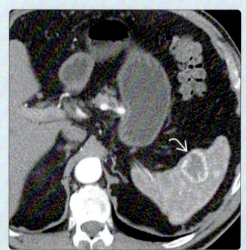 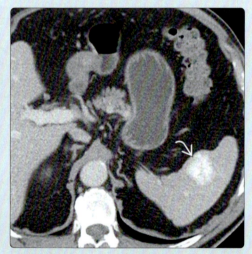

(Left) Axial CECT in the arterial phase demonstrates an incidentally noted splenic mass ➡ with a hypervascular rim of peripheral enhancement. (Right) Axial CECT in the same patient in the venous phase demonstrates that the mass ➡ now shows homogenous enhancement with central fill-in. While the typical nodular, centripetal enhancement seen with hepatic hemangiomas is less common in the spleen; splenic hemangiomas often demonstrate avid enhancement.

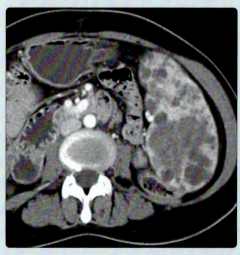 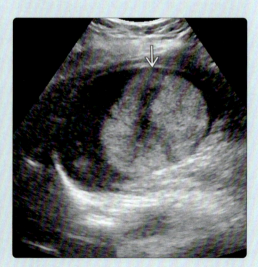

(Left) Axial CECT in a patient with Klippel-Trenaunay-Weber syndrome demonstrates innumerable hypodense lesions in the spleen, compatible with multiple hemangiomas, a classic finding in this disorder. (Right) Ultrasound demonstrates an incidentally identified echogenic mass ➡ arising from the spleen, classic for a splenic hemangioma. Note the central hypoechoic scar, a common feature of larger hemangiomas.

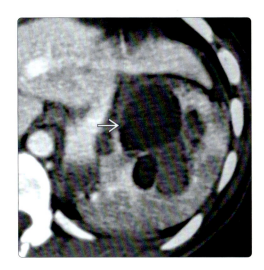

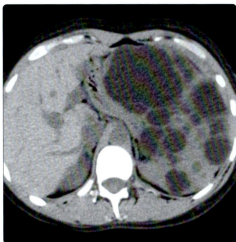

(Left) Axial CECT shows a multiloculated cystic mass ➡ with thin walls and near-water-density contents, a typical appearance for a splenic lymphangioma. (Right) Axial CECT in an 18-year-old girl with splenomegaly shows innumerable near-water-density masses within the spleen, which is markedly enlarged as a result. The lesions have septations and subtle mural nodularity. Resection of the spleen revealed dozens of lymphangiomas.

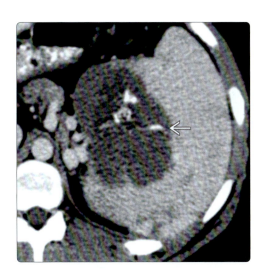

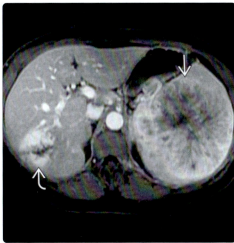

(Left) Axial CECT shows a partially calcified splenic mass ➡ in a patient with left upper quadrant pain. No lymphadenopathy or other extrasplenic pathology was evident. This proved to be primary non-Hodgkin lymphoma. (Right) Axial T1 C+ FS MR demonstrates a large, centrally necrotic, hypervascular mass ➡ in the spleen, ultimately found to be a large splenic angiosarcoma. While the mass ➡ in the liver superficially resembles a hemangioma, the liver lesion was one of multiple metastases in this patient.

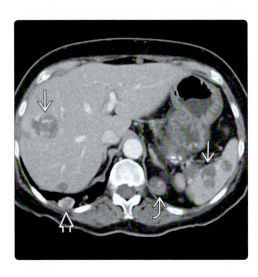

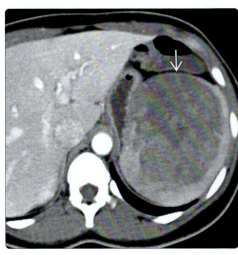

(Left) Axial CECT shows multiple hypodense lesions ➡ in the liver and spleen. Although they resemble hemangiomas with nodular enhancement, these were found to represent metastatic angiosarcoma. Note the additional metastases in the retroperitoneum ➡ and right lung base ➡. (Right) Axial CECT shows a large, hypodense splenic mass ➡. The size of the mass raised concern for malignancy and precipitated splenectomy, where the lesion was found to be sclerosing angiomatoid nodular transformation.

Splenic Metastases and Lymphoma

IMAGING

- **Splenic metastases**
  - Relatively uncommon with autopsy incidence of 7%
  - Most common pathway of spread is hematogenous via splenic artery, but can less commonly spread retrograde via splenic vein or direct splenic invasion
  - Most common primary sites of malignancy: Breast (21%), lung (18%), ovary (8%), stomach (7%), melanoma (6%)
  - Most common multiple lesions (~ 60% of cases)
  - Appearance varies depending on primary malignancy, but most commonly hypoattenuating and solid
    - Some metastases can appear "cystic" and be mistaken for cyst or abscess: Melanoma, breast, ovary, and endometrium
  - Almost always evidence of metastatic disease elsewhere: Isolated metastasis to spleen is extremely rare
- **Splenic lymphoma**
  - Most common malignant tumor of spleen (secondary lymphoma is far more common than primary lymphoma)

  - Several possible imaging patterns, including enlarged spleen without discrete mass, solitary dominant mass, multifocal involvement with several discrete lesions, or innumerable tiny nodules
    - Involved regions of spleen typically appear hypodense, homogeneous, and poorly enhancing
    - Lesions can uncommonly demonstrate necrosis or cystic degeneration (usually after treatment)
    - Splenomegaly alone cannot be used to diagnose splenic involvement
      - 30% of normal-sized spleens harbor tumor in lymphoma patients, and splenomegaly can be present without tumor

TOP DIFFERENTIAL DIAGNOSES

- Primary splenic tumors
- Splenic infarction or infection/abscess
- Sarcoidosis
- Artifact

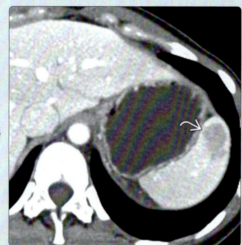
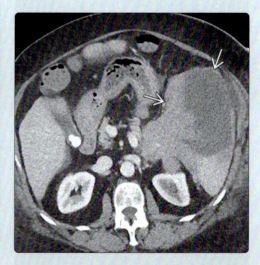

(Left) *Axial CECT demonstrates a solid, hypodense mass ⬈ in the spleen. The lesion was discovered to be lymphoma at biopsy. No other disease was present elsewhere. This was a rare instance of primary splenic lymphoma.* (Right) *Axial CECT demonstrates a mixed cystic and solid mass ➡ centered in the spleen that was found to represent lymphoma. The cystic components within the mass are unusual prior to treatment, as lymphoma usually appears as a solid hypodense mass.*

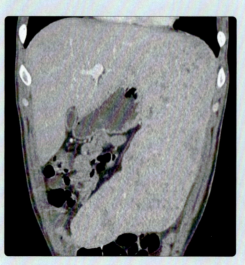
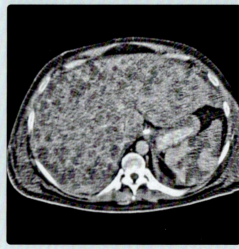

(Left) *Coronal CECT in a patient with known lymphoma demonstrates a markedly enlarged spleen with innumerable tiny hypodense nodules throughout. This "miliary" pattern of disease is a common manifestation of splenic lymphoma.* (Right) *Axial CECT shows innumerable focal lesions in the liver and spleen. Liver biopsy confirmed non-Hodgkin lymphoma. Diffuse involvement of the spleen (or liver) may be difficult to recognize on imaging, often appearing as nonspecific organomegaly.*

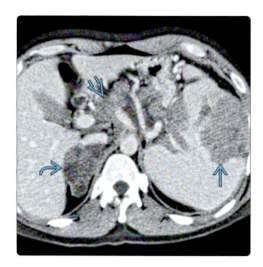

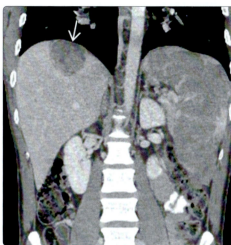

(Left) *Axial CECT in a patient with non-Hodgkin lymphoma shows the spleen to be markedly enlarged with heterogeneous, hypoattenuating, discrete tumor foci ➡. Note the lymphomatous infiltration in the adrenal gland ➡ and nodes throughout the abdomen ➡.* (Right) *Coronal CECT in a patient with melanoma demonstrates innumerable metastases almost completely replacing the spleen, with an additional metastasis to the liver dome ➡.*

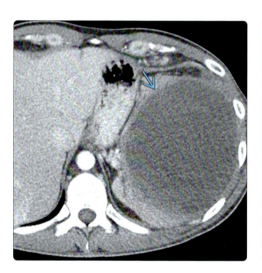

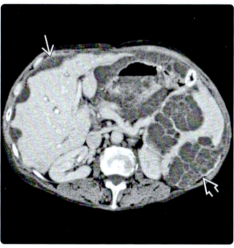

(Left) *Axial CECT demonstrates a large, low-density splenic mass ➡ found to be a melanoma metastasis. Melanoma is one of several tumors which can appear cystic, as in this case, and be misinterpreted as a splenic abscess.* (Right) *Axial CECT in a patient with metastatic ovarian carcinoma shows loculated ascites or cystic peritoneal metastases that indent the surface of the liver ➡ and spleen ➡. Some of the metastases are within the splenic parenchyma.*

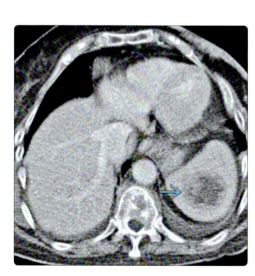

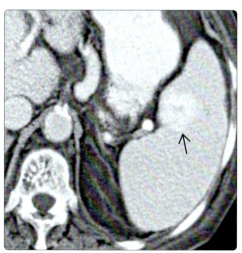

(Left) *Axial CECT in a patient with breast cancer shows a splenic metastasis ➡. Several liver metastases were also present (not shown). In most published reports, breast cancer is the most common primary source for splenic metastases.* (Right) *Axial CECT shows a hypervascular mass ➡ within the spleen that proved to be a metastatic focus from a gastric carcinoid tumor. Tumors arising from the tail of the pancreas or other lower upper quadrant organs should also be considered in the differential diagnosis for splenic tumors.*

SECTION 9
Liver

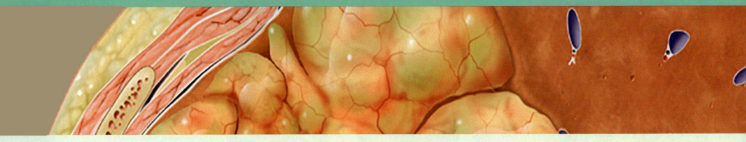

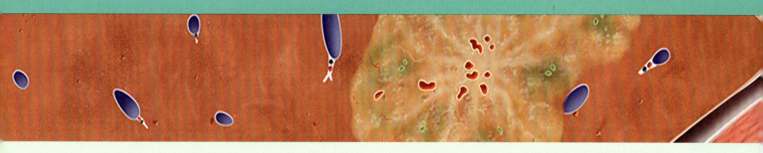

Benign Neoplasms and Tumor-Like Conditions

Malignant Neoplasms

Relevant Anatomy and Embryology

Fibropolycystic Disorders

Anomalies may occur during the embryologic development of the ductal plate that surrounds the portal vein in fetal life. Depending on the stage of fetal development at which these defects occur, a variety of common and uncommon abnormalities of the liver and biliary tree may result, including **congenital hepatic fibrosis, polycystic liver disease, Caroli disease**, and **biliary hamartomas**.

With advancing age, the liver may undergo some loss of volume, resulting in widened fissures and lobulation of its contour. These "senescent" changes may be misinterpreted as evidence of cirrhosis.

Segmental Anatomy of Liver

The Couinaud system of defining liver segmental anatomy divides the liver into 8 segments by vertical planes that extend through the course of the hepatic veins and by a horizontal plane that extends through the right and left portal veins. Understanding this anatomy is particularly important because of recent advances in surgical and interventional therapy for liver disease.

CT and MR Protocols

Scans that are intended to evaluate diffuse or focal hepatic disease must be **multiphasic** with image acquisition at various times during and **following the IV bolus of contrast medium.**

Noncontrast images (NECT or MR): For evaluation of steatosis and hemochromatosis, nonenhanced CT provides the best estimation of liver attenuation. For evaluation by MR, T1W gradient-echo imaging with both in-phase and opposed-phase GRE sequences is essential; selective signal loss on opposed-phase MR is the best noninvasive means of diagnosing steatosis. In patients with hemochromatosis (or lesions with excess iron content, such as cirrhotic regenerative nodules), there is loss of parenchymal signal on the MR with longer echo time, usually the in-phase image. NECT usually shows increased density (attenuation) of the liver in such patients, although effective therapy may reduce liver iron content and restore attenuation to normal.

Early arterial-phase imaging (18-25 seconds): This is the best phase for depicting hepatic arterial anatomy, as it allows multiplanar and 3D reformations as CT or MR arteriography without interference from contrast-opacification of the portal vein. This phase, however, is usually not effective in detecting focal masses, even those that are hypervascular.

Late arterial phase (35-45 seconds): This is usually the optimal phase for depiction of hypervascular hepatic masses, such as hepatocellular carcinoma (HCC), focal nodular hyperplasia, or hypervascular metastases (e.g., those from primary endocrine malignancies).

Portal venous (parenchymal) phase (60-70 seconds): This is usually the optimal phase for depiction of most focal hepatic masses and for visualization of the hepatic and portal veins. It should be obtained in all abdominal and hepatic CT and MR protocols by itself or in addition to other phases.

Delayed phase (5-10 minutes): This is useful to identify washout from hypervascular liver tumors, such as HCC. Conversely, cholangiocarcinoma and certain other lesions become more apparent due to delayed persistent enhancement on this phase.

It is rarely necessary to obtain more than 3 phases of imaging for a particular patient, but the optimal combination of phases should be selected for maximum benefit for the disease process being evaluated.

Hepatobiliary MR Contrast Agents

Most gadolinium-based IV contrast media act as nonspecific vascular and extracellular enhancing agents. They generally have the same effect on MR imaging of vessels and hepatic lesions as iodinated contrast medium for CECT. Therefore, most focal hepatic lesions, which are hypovascular, will be detected as focal hypovascular foci on contrast-enhanced dynamic MR sequences. Hypervascular lesions, such as HCC, will be detected as transiently hyperenhancing lesions on late arterial-phase images with subsequent washout.

Several newer contrast agents have been introduced into clinical imaging, including a heterogeneous group of paramagnetic agents that are taken up in hepatocytes and excreted in bile; these are referred to collectively as **hepatobiliary MR contrast agents**. The 2 most commonly used are gadobenate dimeglumine (MultiHance from Bracco in Milan, Italy) and **gadoxetate** (Eovist from Schering in Berlin, Germany). Gadoxetate (Eovist) has a much greater degree of hepatobiliary excretion (50%) than any other agents. The added benefit of these agents lies in their prolonged retention within functioning hepatocytes, which are present in benign lesions, such as focal nodular hyperplasia, but are absent in metastases and most HCCs. Gadolinium-based hepatobiliary MR agents are incorporated into sequential dynamic and delayed MR imaging with T1WI.

Approach to Hepatic Disease and Hepatic Mass

Almost all detectable focal hepatic lesions appear hypodense relative to enhanced hepatic parenchyma. To render a clinically useful interpretation, it is necessary to characterize the lesion by imaging features and to then consider a list of differential diagnoses of lesions that may have these characteristics.

For example, lesions can be characterized by their size, shape, vascularity, attenuation, or intensity on each phase of contrast enhancement. Hepatomegaly with diffuse low attenuation is usually due to steatosis or other infiltrative processes. A small liver with an enlarged caudate and small right lobe indicates cirrhosis or Budd-Chiari syndrome.

Hepatic vein occlusion is usually the result of **Budd-Chiari syndrome**, a hypercoagulable state, or tumor encasement. **Portal vein occlusion** is usually the result of portal hypertension, septic thrombophlebitis (e.g., diverticulitis), a hypercoagulable state, or tumor encasement or invasion.

A mass that is hypo- or isodense with the liver on NECT and transiently hyperdense (intense) on arterial-phase imaging is a **"hypervascular" lesion** with a limited differential diagnosis. Focal lesions that **washout** to become hypodense (hypointense) on parenchymal or delayed phase are **usually malignant tumors**, while lesions that become isodense (isointense) may be neoplastic or vascular in origin.

A focal lesion that is **hyperdense (hyperintense) only on delayed imaging** has a very limited differential diagnosis, essentially limited to lesions with an **extensive fibrous stroma, such as cholangiocarcinoma**, focal confluent fibrosis, treated tumors, and the central scar of a focal nodular hyperplasia or a fibrolamellar carcinoma. These principles apply to CT and MR using conventional contrast agents as opposed to hepatobiliary contrast-enhanced MR.

Shape is another useful descriptor in determining the nature of a hepatic mass. Most benign and malignant neoplasms are round (spherical), while lesions that have a wedge (pyramidal) shape usually have a vascular etiology, such as a transient hepatic attenuation difference (THAD) or transient hepatic intensity difference. Geographic focal steatosis can also have a wedge shape, often for the same reason, which is focally disordered hepatic metabolism due to altered vascularity.

Differential Diagnosis

Focal Liver Lesion With Hemorrhage
Common
- Hepatic trauma
- Hepatic adenoma
- HCC
- Hepatic cyst
- Autosomal dominant polycystic disease, liver

Less Common
- Coagulopathic hemorrhage, liver
- Hepatic metastases
- HELLP syndrome

Liver "Mass" With Capsular Retraction
Common
- Focal confluent fibrosis
- Cholangiocarcinoma (peripheral)
- Metastases and lymphoma, hepatic
- HCC
- Peritoneal metastases (mimic)

Less Common
- Epithelioid hemangioendothelioma
- Hepatic cavernous hemangioma
- Primary sclerosing cholangitis
- Inflammatory pseudotumor, liver

Fat (Lipid)-Containing Liver Mass
Common
- Steatosis (fatty liver) (mimic)
- Pericaval fat deposition

Less Common
- HCC
- Hepatic adenoma
- Hepatic metastases
- Hepatic angiomyolipoma
- Alcohol-ablated liver tumors (mimic)
- Fat within hepatic surgical defect (mimic)

Rare but Important
- Teratoma or liposarcoma
- Focal nodular hyperplasia
- Xanthomatous lesions in Langerhans cell histiocytosis

Cystic Hepatic Mass
Common
- Hepatic cyst
- Autosomal dominant polycystic disease, liver
- Hepatic pyogenic abscess
- Hepatic amebic abscess
- Biliary hamartomas
- Biloma/seroma
- Steatosis (fatty liver) (mimic)

Less Common
- Hepatic hydatid cyst
- Metastases and lymphoma, hepatic
- Biliary cystadenocarcinoma
- Hepatic candidiasis
- Caroli disease
- Intrahepatic pseudocyst
- Cholangiocarcinoma (mucin-producing variant)

Focal Hypervascular Liver Lesion
Common
- Hepatic cavernous hemangioma
- Focal nodular hyperplasia
- Arterioportal shunt
- THAD (transient hepatic attenuation difference)
- HCC
- Hepatic metastases
- Hepatic adenoma
- Hepatic arteriovenous malformation (Osler-Weber-Rendu)

Less Common
- Nodular regenerative hyperplasia
- Fibrolamellar (hepatocellular) carcinoma
- Superior vena cava obstruction
- Cholangiocarcinoma (peripheral)
- Peliosis hepatis
- Angiosarcoma, liver

Multiple Hypodense Liver Lesions
Common
- Metastases and lymphoma, hepatic
- Simple hepatic cysts
- Hepatic cavernous hemangioma
- Multifocal fatty infiltration
- Hepatic pyogenic abscess
- Autosomal dominant polycystic disease, liver
- HCC
- Hepatic sarcoidosis

Less Common
- Hepatic adenoma
- Hepatic amebic abscess
- Hepatic hydatid cyst
- Hepatic candidiasis
- Biliary hamartomas
- Nodular regenerative hyperplasia

Rare but Important
- Hepatic angiomyolipoma
- Epithelioid hemangioendothelioma
- Caroli disease

Widespread Low Attenuation Within Liver
Common
- Steatosis (fatty liver)

Less Common
- Hepatitis
- Toxic hepatic injury
- Hepatic infarction
- Hepatic metastases and lymphoma
- Hepatic sarcoidosis
- Opportunistic intestinal infections
- HCC
- Wilson disease
- Radiation hepatitis
- Budd-Chiari syndrome
- Glycogen storage disease

(Left) This graphic shows 4 sections that depict the 8 segments of the liver, which are separated by vertical planes through the hepatic veins and horizontal plane through the portal vein. (Right) The sections in this axial CECT correspond to levels in the previous graphic. The liver segments are numbered. The falciform ligament plane separates the medial (segment 4) from the lateral (segments 2 and 3) left lobe. Segment 3 is not shown.

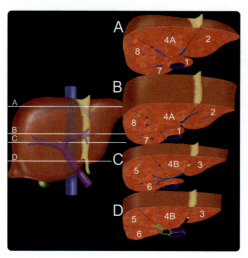

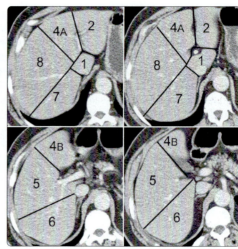

(Left) CT arteriogram shows conventional hepatic arterial anatomy. This coronal reformation shows both hepatic arteries arising from the proper hepatic artery ➡, which in turn arises from the common hepatic artery ➡. (Right) MR angiogram in the venous phase shows the hepatic ➡ and portal vein ➡ branches. Some of the intravenously injected contrast medium is still circulating through the arteries, resulting in enhancement of the aorta ➡.

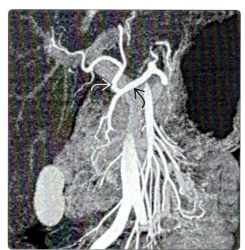

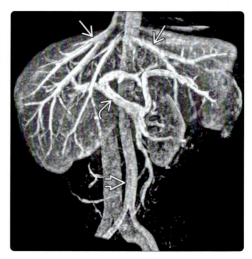

(Left) In this previously healthy young woman with right upper quadrant pain and hypotension, CECT shows a brightly enhancing mass ➡ that has ruptured, causing massive hemorrhage with a sentinel clot ➡. This is essentially diagnostic of a hepatic adenoma. (Right) This man with known cirrhosis presented with acute pain and hypotension. Coronal CECT shows an encapsulated mass ➡, ascites, and sentinel clot ➡ indicating rupture of the mass, essentially diagnostic of hepatocellular carcinoma in this setting.

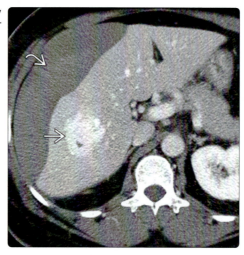

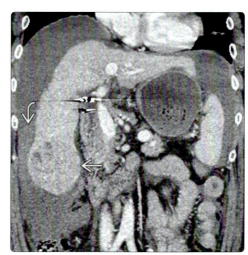

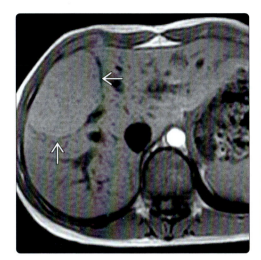 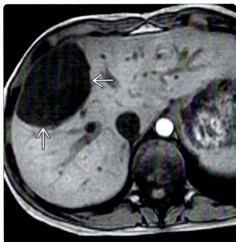

(Left) A hepatic mass in this 18-year-old girl was discovered incidentally on CT. In-phase T1WI MR shows a uniformly hyperintense mass with a thin capsule ➡. (Right) Opposed-phase T1WI MR in the same patient shows signal dropout from the mass ➡, indicating the presence of lipid within the lesion. This, along with the presence of a capsule in a young, otherwise healthy woman is essentially diagnostic of hepatic adenoma.

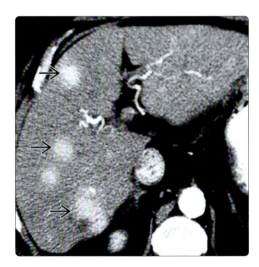 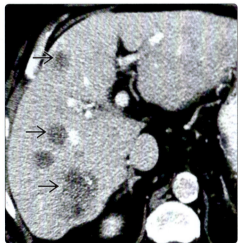

(Left) Arterial-phase CECT shows multiple foci of hypervascularity ➡ within a cirrhotic liver in this patient with multifocal hypervascular hepatocellular carcinoma. (Right) Portal venous (parenchymal) phase in the same patient shows washout of enhancement ➡, typical of hypervascular malignant hepatic tumors. Metastases could have an identical appearance but are rare within a cirrhotic liver.

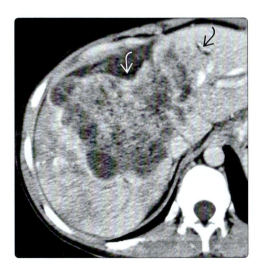 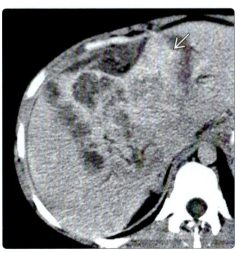

(Left) Portal venous-phase CECT shows a large mass in the liver with heterogeneous enhancement, capsular retraction ➡, and obstruction of the intrahepatic bile ducts ➡ in this patient with intrahepatic (peripheral) cholangiocarcinoma. (Right) Delayed-phase CECT in the same patient shows persistent hyperdense enhancement of most of the tumor ➡. The combination of findings is essentially diagnostic of cholangiocarcinoma.

Liver

TERMINOLOGY

- Part of spectrum of congenital abnormalities resulting in variable degrees of fibrosis and cystic anomalies of liver, bile ducts, and kidneys (fibropolycystic disease)

IMAGING

- **Hepatobiliary signs of fibropolycystic disease**
  - Dysmorphic liver with cysts, abnormal ducts, supernumerary and enlarged hepatic arteries, signs of portal hypertension
  - Variants: Biliary hamartomas, polycystic liver disease, choledochal cyst, and Caroli disease
    - T2WI bright lesions: Hepatic cysts, biliary hamartomas, dilated bile ducts (Caroli disease)
    - Often coexist in same patient
- **Renal signs of congenital fibropolycystic disease**
  - Autosomal recessive (less commonly, dominant) polycystic kidney disease (PKD)
  - Tubular ectasia, cysts, and fibrosis

- All patients with autosomal recessive PKD (ARPKD) have findings of hepatic fibrosis on biopsy
- Not all patients with hepatic fibrosis have ARPKD

TOP DIFFERENTIAL DIAGNOSES

- Isolated polycystic liver disease
- Primary sclerosing cholangitis
- Caroli disease (isolated)
- Biliary hamartomas (isolated)

CLINICAL ISSUES

- Usually have portal hypertension by adolescence
- Often have renal failure as well

DIAGNOSTIC CHECKLIST

- Dysmorphic liver with cysts, abnormal ducts, + signs of portal hypertension
- Similar changes within kidneys (cysts, fibrosis, abnormal ducts)

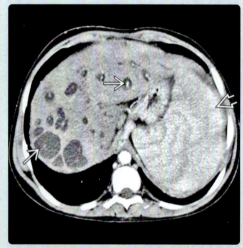
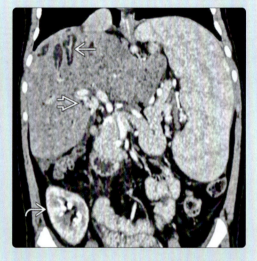

(Left) Axial CECT in a 40-year-old woman shows numerous cysts within the liver, many with the central dot sign ➡ that represents the portal vein branches around which the biliary cystic spaces of Caroli disease are wrapped. This patient had biopsy-proven congenital hepatic fibrosis, which results in hepatic failure and accounts for the splenomegaly ➡. (Right) Coronal CECT in the same patient shows the cystic bile ducts of Caroli disease ➡ with large supernumerary hepatic arteries ➡ and a renal allograft ➡.

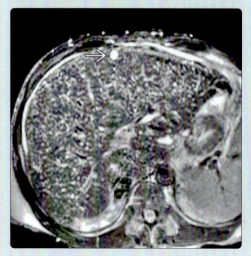
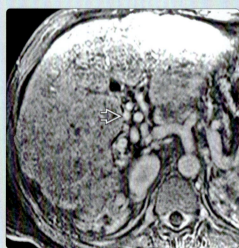

(Left) Axial T2WI MR shows innumerable tiny bright foci throughout the liver, representing biliary hamartomas. Note one of the larger lesions ➡. (Right) Axial T1WI C+ MR in the same patient shows enlarged and supernumerary hepatic arteries ➡ feeding a dysmorphic liver, a common sign of congenital hepatic fibrosis.

Polycystic Liver Disease

TERMINOLOGY
- Autosomal dominant polycystic liver disease (ADPLD)
- Part of fibropolycystic liver (& kidney) disease spectrum

IMAGING
- MR is best modality to show extent & complexity of cysts
  - Shows internal septa & evidence of hemorrhage better than CT
- Extent ranges from scattered cysts to diffuse replacement of liver
  - ± cysts in kidneys & other organs
- Cyst contents often greater than water density/intensity due to hemorrhage (infection less common)
  - Calcification in cyst wall is often seen (due to old hemorrhage)
- Cysts have very low signal intensity on T1WI
  - Higher signal with recent hemorrhage
- Homogeneous high signal intensity on T2WI in some cysts
  - Intracystic hemorrhage: Lower signal intensity in T2WI

- Homogeneous high signal intensity in some cysts
- Intracystic hemorrhage: Lower signal intensity

TOP DIFFERENTIAL DIAGNOSES
- Simple hepatic cysts
- Biliary hamartomas (< 15-mm diameter)
- Cystic metastases
  - Usually appear solid on pretreatment CT or MR

CLINICAL ISSUES
- Dull abdominal pain, abdominal distention, dyspnea, cachexia, early satiety
- Liver progressively enlarges as it is replaced by cysts
- Rarely causes severe hepatic dysfunction

DIAGNOSTIC CHECKLIST
- Isolated ADPLD is underdiagnosed & genetically distinct from PLD associated with ADP kidney disease
- Cannot diagnose ADPLD just by presence of numerous hepatic cysts

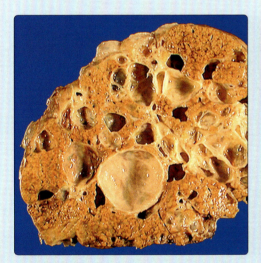
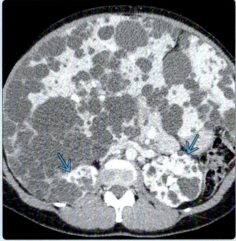

(Left) Gross pathology photograph shows cysts replacing liver parenchyma, ranging in size from microscopic to 5 cm in greatest dimension. This liver, which weighed 9 kg, was resected due to intractable patient discomfort and pressure on other organs. (Right) Axial CECT shows a liver that is nearly replaced with cysts. Note also the involvement of both kidneys ⇗. Most patients with polycystic liver disease also have polycystic kidney disease. Renal but not hepatic failure is a common outcome.

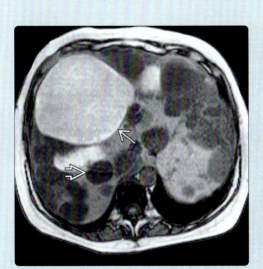
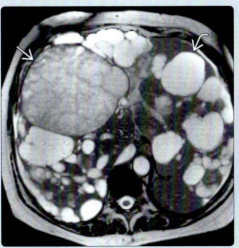

(Left) GRE opposed-phase MR shows numerous hepatic cysts of varying intensity. Some are very low intensity ⇗, as one would expect for simple fluid content, while others are of intermediate intensity. At least 1 has septations and heterogeneous contents ⇗ from prior hemorrhage. (Right) T2 MR in the same patient shows the complex nature of the contents of some of the hepatic cysts with uncomplicated cysts being homogeneously bright ⇗ and complex cysts having heterogeneous contents ⇗.

Hepatic Pyogenic Abscess

IMAGING

- **Multiplanar, contrast-enhanced CT is optimal test**
- CT: Multiseptate mass or cluster of smaller cystic masses
  - Nonliquefied infection may simulate neoplasm
  - Often accompanied by transient hepatic attenuation difference due to hyperemia and pylephlebitis of portal vein branch
  - Gas present in < 20% of pyogenic abscesses
  - Right lower lobe atelectasis and pleural effusion
- US
  - Anechoic (50%), hyperechoic (25%), hypoechoic (25%)
  - ± debris, acoustic enhancement, or shadow

TOP DIFFERENTIAL DIAGNOSES

- Hepatic metastases
  - Multiple; solid or complex
- Hepatic amebic abscess
  - Usually solitary, not multiseptate
- Infarction in liver allograft

- May be indistinguishable from abscess; usually results from hepatic artery thrombosis
- Hepatic hydatid cyst
  - Multiple daughter cysts; calcified wall
- Biliary cystadenocarcinoma
  - Rare; large; solitary; no acute symptoms

CLINICAL ISSUES

- Common causes in Western countries: Postoperative; diverticulitis; cholangitis
- ~ 90% of all liver abscesses are pyogenic
- Fever, RUQ pain, tender hepatomegaly, ↑ WBC
- Treatment: Percutaneous aspiration + parenteral antibiotics (> 90% success)

DIAGNOSTIC CHECKLIST

- Ablation or transarterial chemotherapy of liver tumor may cause necrosis with release of gas, even without infection
  - May be indistinguishable from abscess by imaging alone

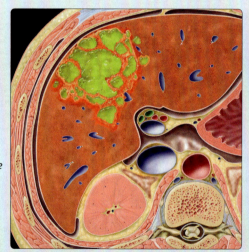
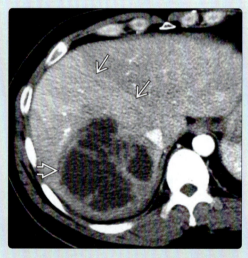

(Left) Schematic illustration shows peripheral multiloculated collections of pus within the surrounding inflamed liver. (Right) Axial CECT in this 33-year-old woman with a pyogenic abscess shows a multiseptate complex mass ➡. Note the straight line ➡ demarcation of the hyperenhancing right hepatic lobe, a transient hepatic attenuation difference due to the hyperemic wall of the abscess, and occlusion of the posterior right portal vein by thrombophlebitis (not shown).

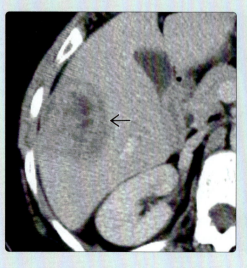
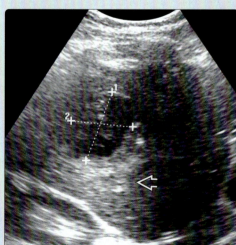

(Left) CECT shows a liver mass ➡ with rim enhancement and central necrosis. The findings are compatible with neoplasm or abscess. (Right) Sonography in the same patient shows a complex fluid-containing mass (cursors) with acoustic enhancement ➡. A US-guided needle aspiration yielded a small amount of pus, and a catheter was placed over a guidewire into the abscess. A repeat CT scan 2 months later showed substantial resolution of the abscess (not shown).

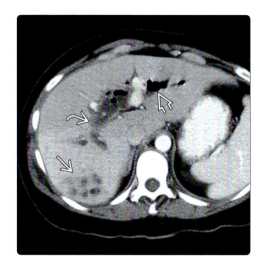
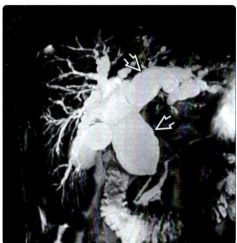

(Left) *Axial CECT in a 37-year-old woman who presented with a history of recurrent episodes of cholangitis demonstrates considerable dilation of the intrahepatic ducts ➡, which also contain gas ⮞. A multiloculated pyogenic abscess is also noted ⮞.* (Right) *Coronal MRCP in the same patient reveals massive dilation of the intrahepatic and proximal extrahepatic bile ducts ⮞, a type 4 choledochal cyst, responsible for the ascending cholangitis and abscess.*

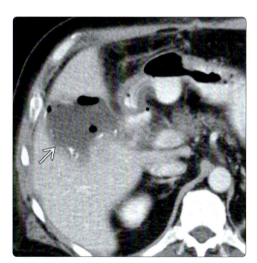
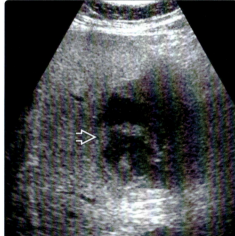

(Left) *Axial CECT in a 46-year-old man who had a recent cholecystectomy shows an abscess ⮞ containing gas and fluid within the liver and the gallbladder bed.* (Right) *Transverse US in the same patient shows a complex fluid collection ⮞, which yielded pus from a US-guided pigtail catheter drainage. Two weeks later, the patient was clinically well and required no further treatment, though a residual liver mass was still present.*

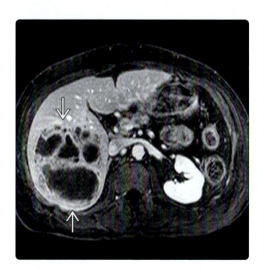
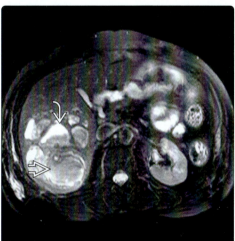

(Left) *Axial contrast-enhanced T1WI MR shows a complex multiseptate mass ⮞ with hypointense contents and enhancing septa.* (Right) *Axial T2WI MR in the same patient shows a multiloculated abscess with heterogeneous fluid content that is variably hyperintense ⮞ with other foci of lower intensity ⮞ reflecting the proteinaceous nature of the pus.*

Hepatic Mycobacterial and Fungal Infections

IMAGING

- Multiple well-defined, rounded **microabscesses (1-4 mm)** in liver ± spleen
- **Ultrasound**
  - Uniformly hypoechoic or echogenic
  - "Wheel within wheel" (early stage) or "bull's eye" (as WBC returns to normal)
- **CT**
  - Biphasic CT more accurate than venous phase only
  - Nonenhancing hypodense centers ± peripheral rim enhancement
  - Healed lesions often calcify
- **MR**: T2WI = multifocal, hyperintense, small lesions
  - Enhanced T1WI: Hypointense lesions ± enhancing rim
  - Detects more lesions

TOP DIFFERENTIAL DIAGNOSES

- Metastases (larger; less numerous; spleen rarely involved)
- Lymphomatous/leukemic foci in liver (less well defined, less numerous, larger)
- Biliary hamartomas (no splenic lesions; occur in healthy patients)
- Caroli disease (central dot sign; communicates with bile ducts)

CLINICAL ISSUES

- Clinical profile: Immunocompromised patient recovering from neutropenia
  - High incidence in transplant patients with fungal colonization
  - *Candida albicans*: Most common cause of fungal microabscesses

DIAGNOSTIC CHECKLIST

- Biopsy specimen for histology/microbiology

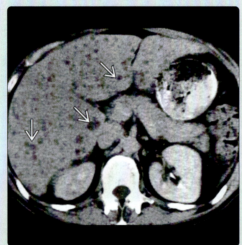
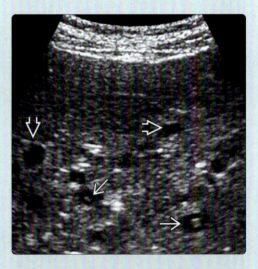

(Left) *Axial CECT in a patient undergoing chemotherapy for acute leukemia, now presenting with a fever, demonstrates fungal abscesses due to Candida. Note the multiple small (< 1-cm) lesions* ➡ *in all lobes of the liver.* (Right) *Transverse grayscale sonogram of hepatic candidiasis shows multiple small, "target" lesions* ➡ *as well as slightly larger hypoechoic abscesses* ➡.

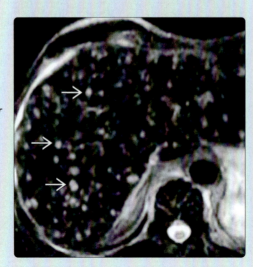
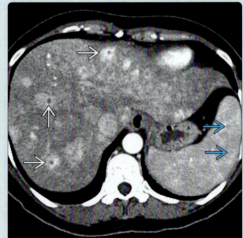

(Left) *Axial T2 MR in an immunosuppressed patient reveals innumerable high-signal fungal (Candida) abscesses* ➡. (Right) *Axial CECT of a 40-year-old man with fever and night sweats shows innumerable focal liver (and possibly splenic* ➡*) lesions, most of which have a brightly enhancing rim and hypodense center* ➡. *Biopsy proved hepatic tuberculosis.*

Hepatic Amebic Abscess

KEY FACTS

IMAGING

- CT: Solitary, peripheral, round or ovoid mass
  - Higher than water density, nonenhancing contents
  - Rim or capsular enhancement
  - Often see transient hepatic attenuation difference due to thrombophlebitis of portal vein and hyperemia of abscess capsule
- US: Abuts liver capsule with hetero- or homogeneous internal echoes, distal acoustic enhancement
- Associated right-sided atelectasis and pleural effusion

TOP DIFFERENTIAL DIAGNOSES

- Posttreatment metastases (cystic or necrotic)
- Hepatic pyogenic abscess
  - Cluster sign: Small abscesses coalesce into single septate cavity
- Hepatic hydatid cyst
  - Numerous peripheral "daughter" cysts
- Biliary cystadenocarcinoma

- No surrounding inflammatory changes

CLINICAL ISSUES

- RUQ pain, tender hepatomegaly, diarrhea with mucus
- Serum indirect hemagglutination positive in > 90% of cases
- High-risk groups in Western countries
  - Recent immigrants
  - Institutionalized
  - Homosexuals
- > 90% respond to antimicrobial therapy
- < 10% require aspiration or drainage

DIAGNOSTIC CHECKLIST

- **Imaging, clinical features, and serology allow diagnosis in almost all cases**
  - Aspiration and drainage are rarely necessary for diagnosis or treatment

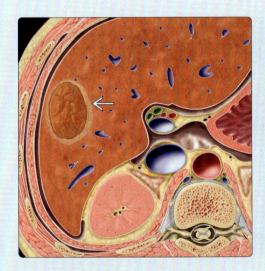
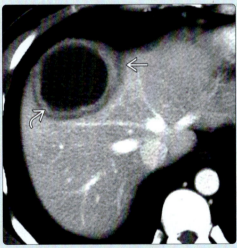

(Left) Graphic demonstrates a unilocular encapsulated mass ➡ with "anchovy paste" consistency of contents. (Right) Axial CECT obtained in a 27-year-old man, who presented with a fever and RUQ pain on returning from a vacation to Mexico, illustrates an abscess with a zone of peripheral low-density edema ➡ surrounding the hyperdense capsule ➡, characteristic findings for a hepatic amebic abscess.

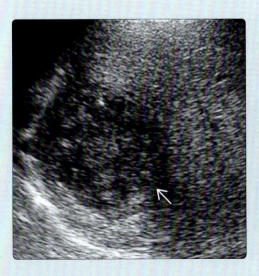
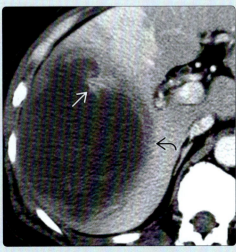

(Left) Longitudinal grayscale ultrasound of the right lobe of the liver in a 41-year-old woman who presented with a fever and RUQ pain demonstrates a hypoechoic mass with diffuse low-level echoes ➡. (Right) Axial CECT in the same patient illustrates a large amebic abscess with a "shaggy" internal wall ➡ and a peripheral zone of edema ➡. As in this case, most (85%) amebic abscesses are solitary and in the right hepatic lobe.

Hepatic Hydatid Cyst

TERMINOLOGY

- Echinococcal (*Echinococcus granulosus*) or hydatid disease

IMAGING

- **Best imaging tool: Multiplanar MR**
  - **Although CT findings are usually diagnostic**
  - Mother and daughter cysts have bright intensity on T2WI; dark on T1WI
  - Shows morphology of lesions better than CT or US
- CT: Shows mural calcification and complete extent of abdominal disease better than MR
  - In up to 60% of cases, cysts are multiple
    - May involve other organs and peritoneal cavity
  - Curvilinear, ring-like calcification of pericyst (wall)
  - Calcified wall usually indicates no active infection if completely circumferential
  - Contains multiple daughter cysts, usually of lower density than mother cyst (hydatid matrix)

- Dilated intrahepatic bile ducts: Due to compression or rupture of cyst into bile ducts
- US: Multiseptate cyst with daughter cysts and echogenic material between cysts
  - Water lily sign: Cyst with floating, undulating membrane and detached endocyst
  - Densely calcified mass (echogenic and shadowing)

TOP DIFFERENTIAL DIAGNOSES

- Biliary cystadenocarcinoma: Rare, solitary, multiseptate, water-density cystic mass, in older women
- Hepatic pyogenic abscess: "Cluster of grapes": Confluent complex cystic lesions
- "Cystic" metastases: Thicker wall; mural nodularity
- Hemorrhagic or infected cyst

CLINICAL ISSUES

- Clinically silent; symptomatic with ↑ in size or cyst rupture
  - Rupture into biliary tree, peritoneal or pleural cavity is not rare

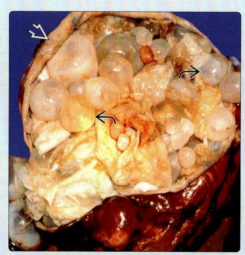
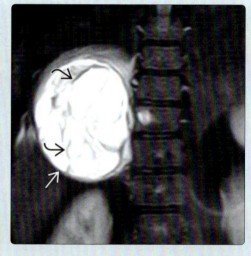

(Left) *Gross photograph of the liver shows an hydatid cyst containing multiple daughter cysts ⊿. The fibrous rim ⟶ can be seen surrounding the cyst. (Courtesy K. Caradine, MD.)* (Right) *Coronal T2WI MR shows a large, complex cystic hepatic mass ⟶. Note the presence of numerous septa ⊿ within the mass, representing scolices, or daughter cysts within the larger endocyst.*

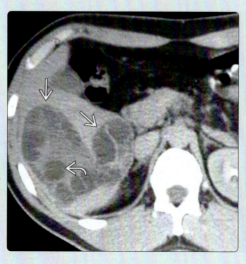
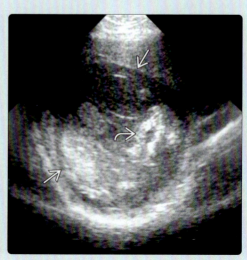

(Left) *Axial CECT shows an oblong, hypodense cystic mass ⟶ with peripheral daughter cysts ⊿ of lower attenuation. These findings are essentially pathognomonic of an hydatid cyst with viable organisms present.* (Right) *Longitudinal sonogram shows a complex echogenic mass ⟶ with enhanced transmission as evidence of fluid content. A curvilinear echogenic scolex ⟶ and highly echogenic debris attest to the complex nature of the cyst contents.*

Hepatic Schistosomiasis

TERMINOLOGY

- Hepatic parasitic infestation by *Schistosoma* species
- a.k.a. bilharziasis, blood fluke

IMAGING

- **CT (or MR) best imaging tool**: Tortoise shell or turtle back appearance
  - Markedly dysmorphic liver with peripheral atrophy, caudate hypertrophy
  - Periportal fibrotic bands and widened fissures
  - Capsular and septal calcification (parallel or perpendicular to liver surface)
  - Portal hypertension in advanced disease
    - Splenomegaly and varices
- US: Bull's-eye lesion: Represents anechoic portal vein surrounded by echogenic mantle of fibrous tissue
  - Hyperechoic and thickened walls of portal venules
  - Mosaic pattern: Network of echogenic septa outlining polygonal areas of normal-appearing liver

- Colonic involvement: Ulceration of mucosa; calcification of colonic wall

TOP DIFFERENTIAL DIAGNOSES

- Hepatic cirrhosis
  - Often has widened fissures but not as much periportal fibrosis or calcification as with schistosomiasis

CLINICAL ISSUES

- Most common cause of hepatic fibrosis in world
  - Over 200 million persons, mostly in tropics
- Different *Schistosoma* species affect urinary tract more than liver
- Oral praziquantel for treatment

DIAGNOSTIC CHECKLIST

- Exclude other causes of hepatic fibrosis or cirrhosis
- Hepatic mosaic tortoise shell pattern of fibrosis and calcification is characteristic

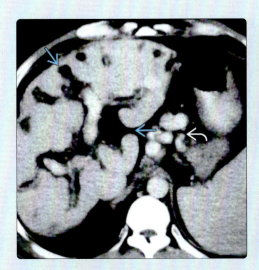
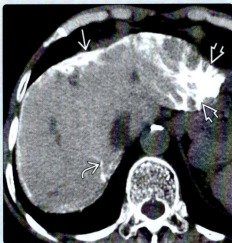

(Left) Axial CT shows signs of portal hypertension, including large varices ⮞ and splenomegaly. Note the widened hepatic fissures ⮞ deeply dividing the segments of the liver along the portal vein branches. The appearance of the liver has been described as that of a tortoise shell. (Right) Axial NECT of the liver shows extensive calcification and peripheral fibrosis in patterns such as thin curvilinear ⮞, subcapsular band-like ⮞, and confluent ⮞, all due to schistosomiasis.

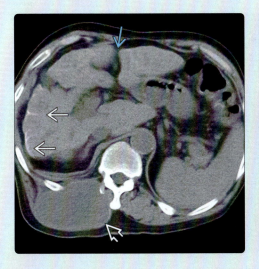
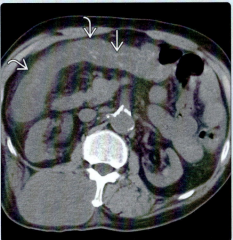

(Left) Axial NECT of a 66-year-old male immigrant from the Philippines with known metastatic sarcoma shows shows widened fissures ⮞ and a small distorted liver. Note branching bands of calcification in parenchyma and capsule ⮞, typical for hepatic schistosomiasis. The mass in the right paraspinal muscle ⮞ is the sarcoma. (Right) Axial NECT in the same patient shows diffuse thickening ⮞ of the wall of the transverse colon with calcification of the mucosa or submucosa ⮞, due to schistosomiasis.

TERMINOLOGY

- Acute hepatitis: Hepatocyte necrosis and inflammation resulting from acute viral infection

IMAGING

- In medical practice, hepatitis usually refers to viral infection
  - Hepatitis B and C are the major ones
  - Only hepatitis B and C cause chronic disease
  - Hepatitis C is leading cause of cirrhosis and hepatocellular carcinoma (HCC) in USA
- **Role of imaging in cases of viral hepatitis**
  - Exclude biliary obstruction or neoplasm (especially HCC)
  - Evaluate parenchymal damage noninvasively
- **US: Sufficient for initial imaging surveillance for HCC of patients with hepatitis C**
  - Prior to development of heterogeneous, nodular, fibrotic, cirrhotic liver
  - US has poor sensitivity and specificity for detection of HCC in cirrhotic liver

- Acute viral hepatitis: Decreased echogenicity of hepatic parenchyma
- Starry-sky appearance: Increased echogenicity of portal venous walls
- **Multiphasic (arterial, venous, delayed phase) CT or MR for cirrhotic patients or those with chronic hepatitis B**
  - Acute hepatitis imaging: Hepatomegaly, periportal edema, gallbladder wall thickening, lymphadenopathy
  - Fulminant hepatic failure
    - Focal or global volume loss of liver, diffuse hepatocellular necrosis (low density) + ascites
  - Cirrhosis
    - Volume loss in medial and anterior segments
    - Widened hepatic fissures
    - Signs of portal hypertension (splenomegaly, ascites, varices)
    - Increased echogenicity of liver and coarsening of parenchymal texture on US

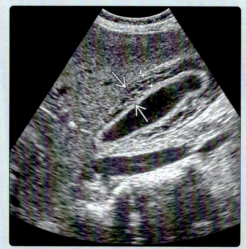

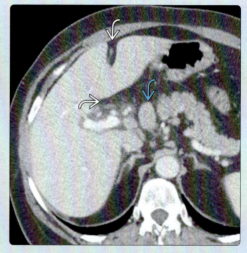

(Left) *Ultrasound in a patient with acute viral hepatitis shows a markedly thickened gallbladder wall ➡, but no calculi, a typical imaging sign.* (Right) *Axial CT in a patient with chronic active viral hepatitis shows lymphadenopathy ➡ in the porta hepatis. The hepatic fissures ➡ are widened, suggesting that the disease has progressed to cirrhosis, which was confirmed on liver biopsy. MR showed additional evidence of cirrhosis, including fibrosis on imaging and elastography.*

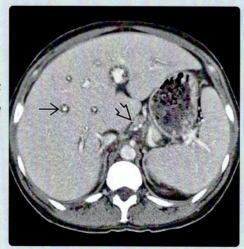

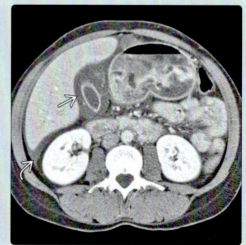

(Left) *Axial CECT in a patient with acute viral hepatitis shows hepatomegaly, periportal edema ➡, and porta hepatis lymphadenopathy ➡.* (Right) *Axial CECT in the same patient shows massive gallbladder wall thickening ➡ and a small amount of ascites ➡. There is nothing specific about these findings to indicate the exact etiology of this case of hepatitis. Imaging helps to exclude other causes of acute abdominal pain and liver dysfunction, such as biliary obstruction.*

TERMINOLOGY

- Chronic hepatitis of unknown etiology characterized by hyperglobulinemia, circulating autoantibodies, & inflammatory changes on hepatic histology

IMAGING

- Autoimmune hepatitis (AIH) is not diagnosed specifically by imaging criteria
- Patients with AIH should be in surveillance program for cirrhosis & hepatocellular carcinoma
  - **Imaging: US is 1st line; CT or MR in more advanced disease or for evaluation of focal mass**
  - US & MR elastography provide assessment & monitoring for hepatic fibrosis & cirrhosis
- Dysmorphic liver with prominent periportal fibrosis, ± signs of portal hypertension, ± irregular intrahepatic ductal dilation
  - MRCP best for detecting irregular dilation of intrahepatic ducts in AIH/PSC overlap disease

TOP DIFFERENTIAL DIAGNOSES

- Primary biliary cirrhosis (PBC)
- Primary sclerosing cholangitis (PSC)
- Hepatitis, viral
- Hepatitis, alcoholic

CLINICAL ISSUES

- Diagnosis based on exclusion of other forms of liver disease
- Exclusion of viral, alcoholic, or toxic hepatic injury
- ~ 20% of patients have overlap syndrome with other autoimmune diseases, especially PBC & PSC
- May have many other autoimmune diseases, including lupus, rheumatoid arthritis, ulcerative colitis, polyglandular autoimmune disease, etc.

DIAGNOSTIC CHECKLIST

- Role of imaging is to detect signs of acute or chronic liver injury, portal hypertension, associated abnormalities (e.g., biliary ductal disease)

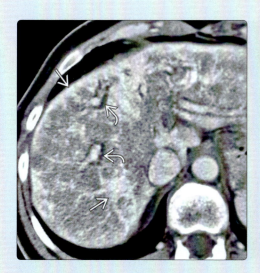
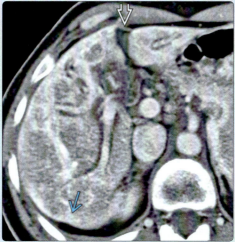

(Left) Axial CECT in a patient with autoimmune hepatitis shows a heterogeneous liver parenchyma and periportal edema ➡ with subcapsular and parenchymal hyperdense bands ➡ that represent fibrosis. (Right) Axial CECT in the same patient shows peripheral fibrosis with retraction of the overlying hepatic capsule ➡, a finding usually associated with confluent fibrosis and indicative of chronic liver injury. Also note the widened fissures ➡, typical of cirrhosis but not specific for autoimmune hepatitis.

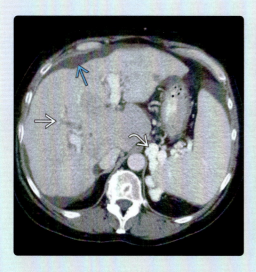
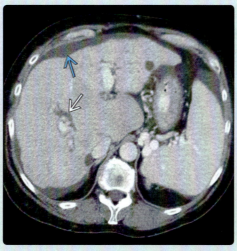

(Left) Axial CECT in a patient with an autoimmune hepatitis/primary sclerosing cholangitis overlap shows a nodular, cirrhotic liver with signs of portal hypertension, including splenomegaly, ascites ➡, and varices ➡. The intrahepatic ducts ➡ are dilated with an abnormal arborization, suggestive of primary sclerosing cholangitis. (Right) Axial CECT in the same patient shows dysmorphic liver, ascites ➡, varices, and dilated, irregular intrahepatic bile ducts ➡ typical of sclerosing cholangitis.

TERMINOLOGY

- Hepatocyte injury + inflammation that results from chronic alcohol consumption

IMAGING

- **Contrast-enhanced MR is most comprehensive imaging modality**
- Alcoholic steatohepatitis (diffuse fatty infiltration)
  - Diffuse hypodensity (on CT) in liver (due to fatty infiltration)
  - T1WI out-of-phase GRE: Decreased signal intensity of liver (due to lipid in liver)
    - MR sequences can be used to quantitate fat content of liver
  - Diffusely increased echogenicity on US
- Acute fulminant hepatitis
  - Volume loss of liver; ascites; high mortality
- Chronic alcoholic hepatitis
  - Mixture of steatosis and early cirrhotic changes

- Widened fissures, ↑ caudate:right lobe ratio
- Cirrhosis due to alcoholic liver disease (ALD)
  - Indistinguishable by imaging from cirrhosis resulting from chronic viral hepatitis
  - Small nodular liver with signs of portal hypertension (ascites, splenomegaly, varices)
    - Right lobe volume loss; widened fissures; bridging fibrosis and regenerative nodules (best seen on MR)
- Protocol advice
  - **Once cirrhosis has developed, sonography is of less value in surveillance**
  - **Need multiphasic, contrast-enhanced CT or MR to detect hepatocellular carcinoma**

CLINICAL ISSUES

- ALD is clinical spectrum from asymptomatic, to chronic progressive, to acute hepatic failure

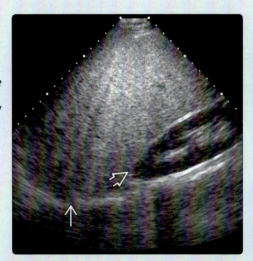
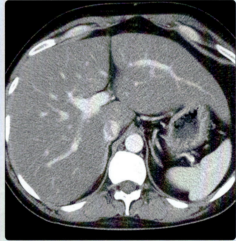

(Left) This 36-year-old man with acute abdominal pain and abnormal liver functions was 1st evaluated with US, which showed an enlarged, diffusely echogenic liver. Note the increased echogenicity of the liver relative to the kidney ➡ and the poor penetration of the sound waves with poor definition of the right hemidiaphragm ➡. (Right) Axial CECT from the same patient confirms hepatomegaly and steatosis with the liver being substantially lower in attenuation than the spleen on the venous-phase CECT.

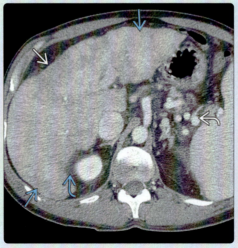
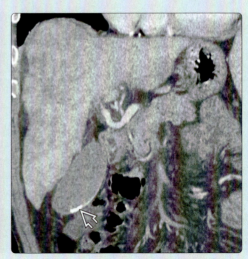

(Left) Axial CECT of a 40-year-old man with chronic alcohol abuse shows a nodular hepatic surface, volume loss of the anterior and medial segments ➡, and signs of portal hypertension (including varices ➡, splenomegaly, and a small amount of ascites ➡). Also noted is patchy low density ➡ representing steatosis and fibrosis. (Right) This coronal reformatted image of the same patient highlights the heterogeneity and nodularity of the liver and shows gallstones ➡, a common occurrence in cirrhosis.

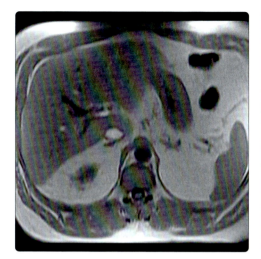
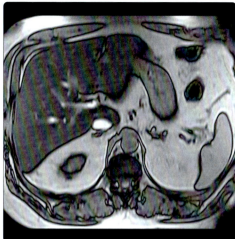

(Left) *Axial gradient-echo (GRE) in-phase MR shows homogeneous signal throughout the liver.* (Right) *In the same patient, axial opposed-phase GRE MR shows "signal dropout" throughout the liver, diagnostic of diffuse steatosis. By imaging criteria, including MR, the etiology of steatosis cannot be determined, nor can steatosis be distinguished from steatohepatitis.*

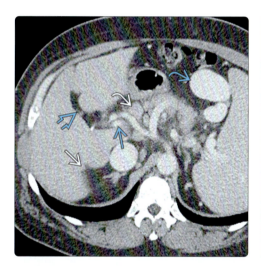
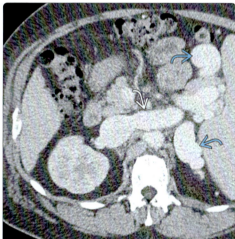

(Left) *Axial CECT of a 48-year-old man with chronic alcoholism shows a small liver with typical cirrhotic morphology, including wide fissures, a deep gallbladder fossa ➡, and a "notch" on the undersurface of the liver ➡. Porta hepatic lymphadenopathy is noted ➡. There are huge perisplenic varices ➡ and a very small, but patent, portal vein ➡.* (Right) *Axial CECT of the same patient shows varices ➡ and a spontaneous splenorenal shunt resulting in marked enlargement of the left renal vein ➡.*

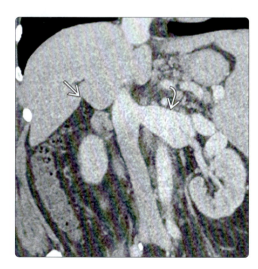
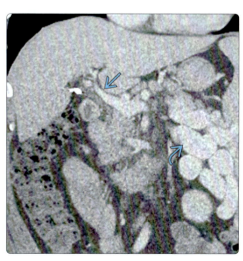

(Left) *Coronal CT of the same patient shows the splenorenal shunt/left renal vein ➡ and the cirrhotic liver with a notched inferior surface ➡.* (Right) *Coronal CT of the same patient shows the small portal vein ➡ and the huge varices ➡. Portal vein size has no correlation with the degree of cirrhosis or portal hypertension.*

Steatosis and Steatohepatitis

TERMINOLOGY

- Steatosis is metabolic complication of variety of toxic, ischemic, and infectious insults to liver
- Characterized by accumulation of increasing amounts of triglycerides within hepatocytes

IMAGING

- **Diagnosis can be suggested by US or CT**
  - **MR is definitive**: Steatotic liver shows signal loss on opposed-phase GRE sequence
- Diffuse (more common) or focal fatty infiltration
  - Often lobar, segmental, or wedge-shaped
  - Along hepatic vessels, ligaments, and fissures
  - Presence of normal vessels coursing through "lesion" (fatty infiltration)
- CT: Liver attenuation (density) less than spleen
- US: ↑ echogenicity, ↑ attenuation of sound beam
- Nonalcoholic steatohepatitis looks similar to simple steatosis and alcoholic steatohepatitis on imaging

TOP DIFFERENTIAL DIAGNOSES

- Lymphoma or metastases
  - Diffuse or multifocal lesions can be seen with steatosis or tumor
  - Can be distinguished by MR or PET/CT
- Hepatitis: Viral or other toxic etiologies
  - May simulate or cause steatosis
- Opportunistic infection, hepatic

PATHOLOGY

- Focal steatosis or focal sparing: Most commonly due to variations in hepatic venous drainage

CLINICAL ISSUES

- Most common cause of chronic liver disease in Western countries
  - Increasing in prevalence with epidemic of obesity and metabolic syndrome

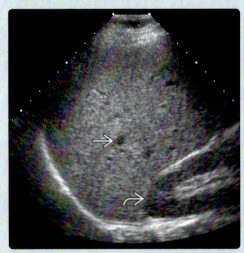
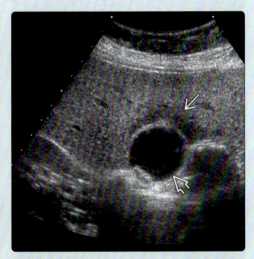

(Left) Ultrasound of a 37-year-old woman with RUQ pain shows diffuse, increased, coarse hepatic echogenicity in comparison with the right kidney ⟹ due to steatosis. Vessel walls ⟹ are less well seen than normally. (Right) In the same patient, there is a zone of less echogenic tissue ⟹ abutting the gallbladder ⟹ that has the typical location and appearance of focal sparing (normal liver in the setting of diffuse steatosis).

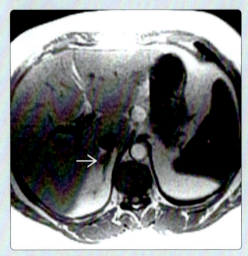
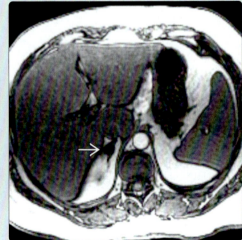

(Left) Axial T1 GRE in-phase MR of diffuse steatosis shows no apparent hepatic abnormality. Note the small right adrenal nodule ⟹. (Right) Axial T1 GRE opposed-phase MR in the same patient shows selective drop out of signal from the liver, indicating the presence of excess lipid within the liver and also within an adrenal adenoma ⟹ (which also contains excess lipid). The most specific imaging test to detect hepatic steatosis is MR, especially GRE in- and opposed-phase images.

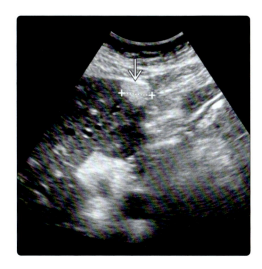

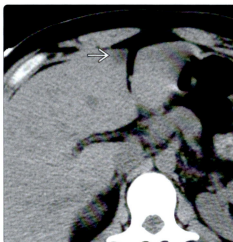

(Left) *Axial US shows a focal hyperechoic lesion* ➡ *in the left lobe of the liver near the falciform ligament.* **(Right)** *Axial NECT in the same patient shows a small, hypoattenuating lesion* ➡ *in the same area, a typical CT and US appearance and location for focal steatosis.*

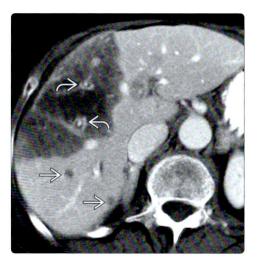

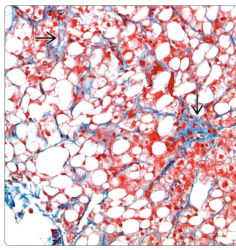

(Left) *Axial CECT of multifocal and geographic steatohepatitis shows a geographic area of low attenuation throughout the anterior and medial segments. In addition, there are spherical and oval lesions* ➡ *in other segments of the liver. Blood vessels* ➡ *course through the zone of fatty infiltration without displacement.* **(Right)** *Photomicrograph of a biopsy specimen shows nonalcoholic steatohepatitis with features of perivenular/pericellular fibrosis* ➡. *(Courtesy M. Yeh, MD, PhD.)*

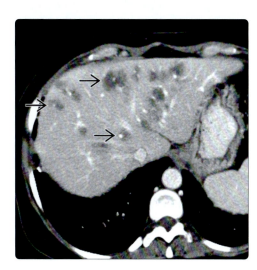

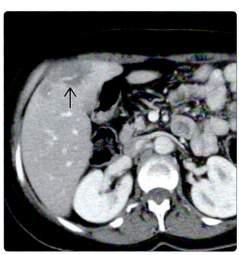

(Left) *Axial CECT of perivascular multifocal steatosis shows multiple hypodense "masses"* ➡ *throughout the liver that may be mistaken for metastases. Note the tendency for the lesions to surround, but not obstruct, blood vessels and to occur near fissures in the liver.* **(Right)** *Axial CECT in the same patient shows other foci of steatosis* ➡ *that surround but do not distort or displace enhanced vessels.*

TERMINOLOGY

- Injury to liver induced by exogenous toxins, either through direct hepatotoxicity or idiosyncratic reaction

IMAGING

- CT is imaging modality of choice
  - Findings may be normal in very acute injury
  - Hepatomegaly with heterogeneous enhancement is most common finding
  - Areas of hypodensity may represent steatosis &/or hepatocellular necrosis
  - Periportal and gallbladder wall edema are common
  - May see volume loss of liver (segmental or global) ± ascites
  - Amiodarone toxicity has different appearance
    - Diffusely increased density, best seen on nonenhanced CT
    - Due to iodine content of amiodarone
- Ultrasound
  - Sonography: Liver may show ↓ or ↑ echogenicity
  - Periportal and gallbladder wall edema

TOP DIFFERENTIAL DIAGNOSES

- Hepatitis (alcoholic, viral, autoimmune)
  - Imaging cannot distinguish among causes of acute hepatitis
- Steatosis (fatty liver)

CLINICAL ISSUES

- **Acetaminophen** (paracetamol or Tylenol)
  - **Most common cause of severe toxic injury** in USA and Europe (40-50% of cases)
- Acute abdominal pain, nausea, vomiting
- May quickly progress to complete hepatic failure
- Usually leads to complete recovery or liver failure within 72 hours

DIAGNOSTIC CHECKLIST

- Global or focal liver volume loss ± ascites = bad prognosis

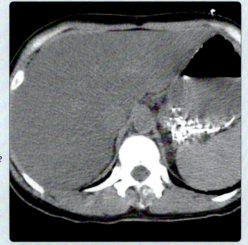 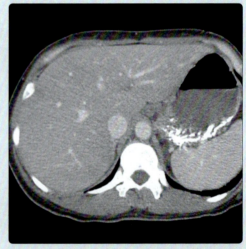

(Left) Axial NECT of a 41-year-old woman who developed acute liver failure after taking an excessive dose of acetaminophen shows diffuse low attenuation throughout the liver, which is due to acute massive hepatocellular necrosis rather than steatosis (although the imaging features are indistinguishable). (Right) Axial CECT section of the same patient shows only diffuse hypoattenuation throughout the liver and ascites (on lower sections). Within 24 hours of this scan, the patient developed hepatic failure.

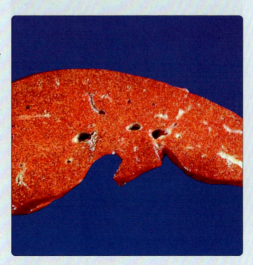 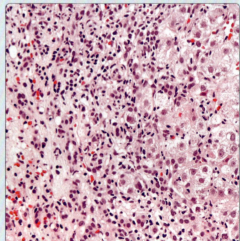

(Left) This same patient required urgent liver transplantation. The explanted liver shows signs of massive hepatocellular necrosis and acute inflammation. (Right) H&E of acute liver failure shows confluent necrosis with lymphoplasmacytic inflammation (left). Swelling and inflammation are seen in the remaining parenchyma (right). (Courtesy S. Kakar, MD.)

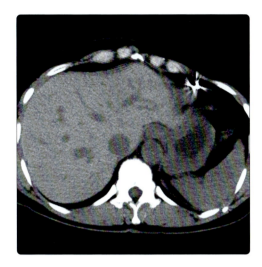

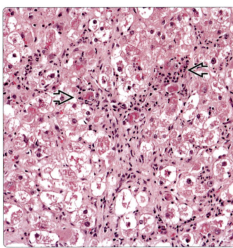

(Left) In this patient with refractory arrhythmias, nonenhanced CT shows diffuse increased density within the liver due to amiodarone deposition, an iodine-containing antiarrhythmic drug with known hepatic and lung toxicity. (Right) Ballooned hepatocytes containing abundant Mallory hyaline are surrounded by neutrophils, known as satellitosis ⊟. This is a frequent feature of amiodarone toxicity. Steatosis may or may not be present. (Courtesy L. Lamps, MD.)

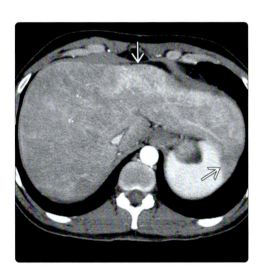

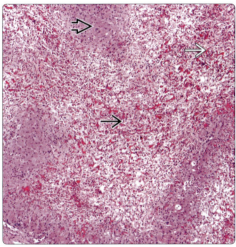

(Left) Axial arterial-phase CECT in a 29-year-old man with acute severe hepatic dysfunction shows an enlarged heterogeneous liver ⊟. Ascites was noted on more caudal sections. The cause was acute alcohol and acetaminophen toxicity. (Right) Multiacinar hemorrhagic necrosis ⊟, congestion ⊟, and lack of inflammation with sparing of periportal hepatocytes ⊟ are typical of acetaminophen toxicity but can also be seen in acute ischemia and acute Budd-Chiari syndrome. (Courtesy S. Kakar, MD.)

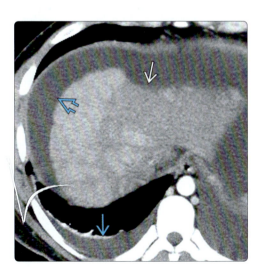

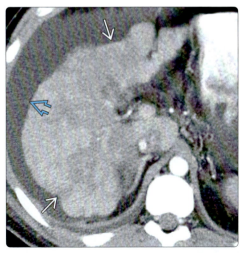

(Left) Axial CT in a 24-year-old man with acute hepatic failure probably due to alcohol and drugs shows a heterogeneous liver with evidence of volume loss (capsular retraction) ⊟. A large amount of ascites ⊟ and pleural effusions ⊟ are also noted. These are ominous findings, usually associated with death or requiring urgent transplantation. (Right) Lower CT section in the same patient shows more of the damaged liver with volume loss ⊟ and ascites ⊟. This patient died of acute hepatic failure.

Cirrhosis

TERMINOLOGY

- Chronic liver disease characterized by diffuse parenchymal injury, extensive fibrosis, and conversion of liver architecture into structurally abnormal nodules

IMAGING

- **US, CT, and MR all play important role** in detection of cirrhosis and surveillance for development of hepatocellular carcinoma (HCC)
- Nodular contour, widened fissures, and enlarged caudate lobe with ascites, splenomegaly, and varices
  - **Caudate: Right lobe ratio often > 1.0 in cirrhosis**
- Classification by etiology and severity is more useful than by morphology
- Siderotic regenerative nodules
  - Hyperdense on nonenhanced CT, isodense on CECT
  - Hypointense on T2 and GRE MR (more sensitive)
  - 3-10 mm in size
- Vascular derangements

- Arterioportal and portovenous shunts
  - Usually peripheral, wedge-shaped, small; seen only on arterial phase
- Varices (gastroesophageal, caput medusae, etc.)
- Fibrosis: Diffuse, lace-like, thick, or confluent foci
  - Hypointense on T1W; hyperintense on T2W MR
  - Delayed, persistant enhancement on contrast-enhanced CT or MR
- Cirrhosis-induced HCC
  - Heterogeneous enhancement on arterial phase; usually hypodense on venous and delayed-phase CT + MR
  - Hyperintense on T2W MR
  - Bright on DWI MR
  - ± capsule, fat, venous invasion, metastases

DIAGNOSTIC CHECKLIST

- MR: Best for detection & characterization of focal nodules within cirrhotic liver

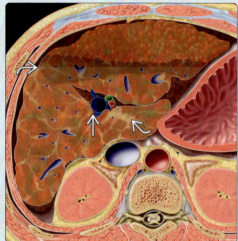
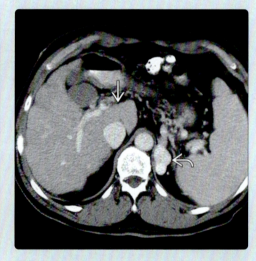

(Left) Graphic shows a cirrhotic liver with a nodular surface contour and an increase in the caudate:right lobe ratio, measured from the branch point of the right portal vein ➡ to the edges of the caudate and right lobes, respectively. Note the bands of fibrosis ➡ and ascites. (Right) Axial CECT shows a cirrhotic liver and large varices ➡. Note the enlarged caudate lobe ➡, which is as wide as the right lobe, although the caudate lobe is normally no more than 60% of the width of the right lobe.

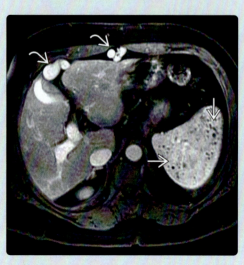
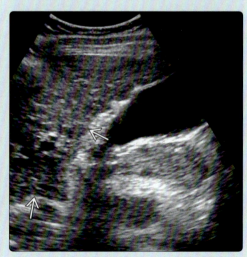

(Left) T1 C+ MR shows obvious signs of cirrhosis with widening of the fissures, right lobe atrophy, and large varices ➡. Within the spleen are innumerable small lesions that are especially evident as hypointense foci ➡, representing Gamna-Gandy bodies. (Right) Sagittal US shows a coarse echotexture of the liver ➡ that is typical, but not diagnostic, of cirrhosis. In the heterogeneous, cirrhotic liver, it can be difficult to diagnose or exclude hepatocellular carcinoma (HCC) by US alone.

TERMINOLOGY

Definitions

- Chronic liver disease characterized by diffuse parenchymal injury, extensive fibrosis, and conversion of liver architecture into structurally abnormal nodules

IMAGING

General Features

- Key concepts
  - Common end response of liver to variety of insults and injuries
  - Classification by **morphology** (not very useful)
    - Micronodular (Laennec) cirrhosis (usual cause: Alcohol abuse)
    - Macronodular (postnecrotic) cirrhosis (usually hepatitis)
  - Classification by **etiology** and **severity** more useful

CT Findings

- Atrophy of right lobe and medial segment of left lobe
- Enlarged caudate lobe and lateral segment of left lobe
  - Caudate is normally < 60% width of right lobe
- Widened fissures between segments/lobes
- Deep gallbladder fossa
- Vascular derangements
  - Varices (gastroesophageal, caput medusae, etc.)
  - Arterioportal (AP) and portovenous shunts
    - AP shunts are usually peripheral, wedge-shaped, small; seen only on arterial phase
    - Small AP shunt difficult to distinguish from very small hepatocellular carcinoma (HCC)
      - □ Follow-up imaging (CT or MR) in 3-6 months is sufficient for surveillance
  - "Corkscrew" hepatic arterial branches
    - Enlarged and displaced around regenerative nodules
- Splenomegaly
- Nodular liver contour (not apparent in all)
- Siderotic regenerative nodules
  - Hyperdense on nonenhanced CT, isodense on CECT
  - Most regenerative nodules are not detected by CT
- Fibrotic and fatty changes
  - Fibrosis: Diffuse, lace-like, thick bands or confluent "masses"
  - Fatty changes: Diffuse or geographic areas of low attenuation
    - Usually limited to alcoholic hepatitis with early cirrhosis
- Peribiliary cysts
  - Cystic dilation of peribiliary gland in wall of large bile ducts
  - Resemble string of pearls or grapes on stem
- Cirrhosis-induced HCC
  - CECT
    - Heterogeneous enhancement on arterial phase; usually iso- to hypodense on venous and delayed-phase scans
    - ± capsule, portal or hepatic venous invasion, metastases

MR Findings

- Siderotic regenerative nodules: Paramagnetic effect of iron within nodules
  - T1WI: Hypointense
  - T2WI: Increased conspicuity of low signal intensity
  - Gamna-Gandy bodies (siderotic nodules in spleen)
    - T1WI and T2WI: Hypointense
- Dysplastic regenerative nodules
  - T1WI: Hyperintense; T2WI: Hypointense
  - Minimal vascularity
  - Take up and retain hepatobiliary MR contrast agents on delayed phase
    - Most specific test to distinguish from HCC
- HCC nodule
  - T2WI: Hyperintense
  - T1WI C+: Increased enhancement on arterial phase
    - Washes out to hypointense on venous and delayed phases
  - Diffusion-weighted imaging
    - Restricted diffusion (bright signal) within HCC
  - Rarely take up or retain hepatobiliary MR contrast agents
- Fibrotic and fatty changes
  - T1WI: Fibrosis = hypointense; fat = hyperintense
  - T2WI: Fibrosis = hyperintense; fat = hypointense
- MR elastography
  - Shows promise in noninvasive evaluation of extent of liver fibrosis

Ultrasonographic Findings

- Grayscale ultrasound
  - Nodular liver contour and parenchyma
  - Increased and coarsened liver echogenicity
- Color Doppler
  - Used to determine portal vein patency and direction of flow
    - Hepatofugal is sign of severe portal hypertension
- **Ultrasound is of most value and accuracy in screening patients with less advanced chronic liver disease**
  - Less accurate in detecting or characterizing nodules within cirrhotic liver
  - Presence of fibrosis, fat, regenerative nodules makes detection of HCC very difficult

Imaging Recommendations

- Best imaging tool
  - **Multiphasic contrast-enhanced CT or MR**
- Protocol advice
  - US is suitable for screening until cirrhosis is established
  - CECT is preferable in acutely ill patients or those with ascites
  - MR is preferable in alcoholic cirrhosis and for detection/distinction of hepatic nodules
    - Include delayed-phase MR or CT (5-10 minutes)
    - Hepatobiliary MR contrast agents may aid in detection of HCC
      - □ Gadoxetate (Eovist, Primovist) is retained in normal liver, variably in cirrhotic liver, rarely in HCC

(Left) Arterial-phase CT shows one of several peripheral hypervascular lesions ➡. Also note the corkscrew enlarged hepatic arterial branch ⬈ and the widened fissures, all typical of cirrhosis. **(Right)** Delayed-phase CT of the same patient shows no sign of washout from the site of the shunt. AP shunts are common within the cirrhotic liver. Imaging features that favor AP shunt over HCC include peripheral and subcapsular location, small size, wedge shape, and no corresponding lesion on venous or delayed-phase imaging.

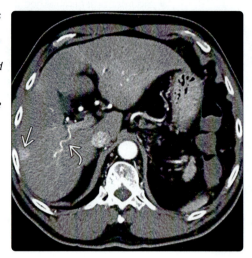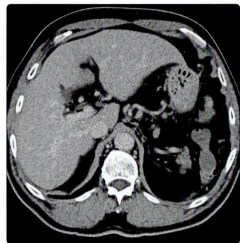

(Left) Axial CECT in a patient with autoimmune hepatitis and primary sclerosing cholangitis shows a nodular, cirrhotic liver with splenomegaly, ascites ➡, and varices ➡. The intrahepatic ducts ➡ are dilated with an abnormal arborization due to PSC. **(Right)** On a venous-phase CT, there is a heterogeneous focus of parenchymal scarring ➡ with retraction of the hepatic capsule ➡, typical signs of focal confluent fibrosis. Also noted are ascites ➡, varices ➡, and splenomegaly ➡.

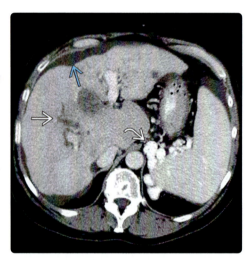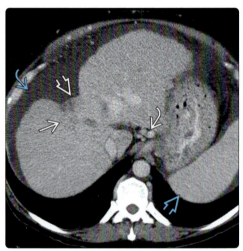

(Left) Axial T2 FS MR shows a small cirrhotic liver ➡ and ascites ➡. Also shown are water-intensity lesions in the portal triads ➡ that do not arborize (branch) as bile ducts and are spherical in shape, representing peribiliary cysts. **(Right)** CT of a patient with cirrhosis shows that the portal vein branches ➡ are surrounded by a collar of low density, some of which probably represent periportal edema. However, there are also discrete, low-density focal lesions ➡ that represent periportal cysts.

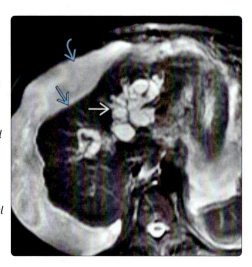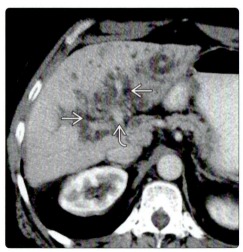

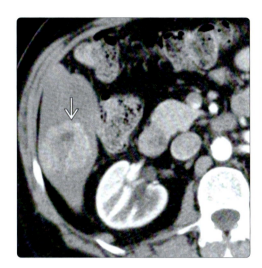
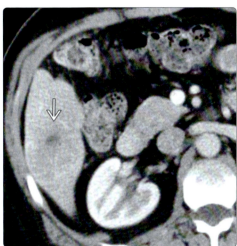

(Left) On this arterial-phase CECT in a patient with cirrhosis and HCC, the mass is heterogeneously hyperdense and hypervascular ➡. (Right) On portal venous (hepatic)-phase CECT in the same patient, the mass ➡ is iso- to hypodense to the liver. These are typical features of HCC, particularly for a tumor detected as part of a surveillance program for patients with known cirrhosis who are at risk for developing HCC.

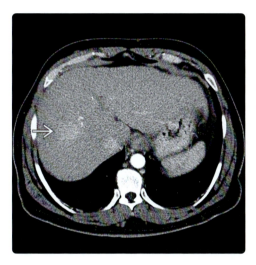
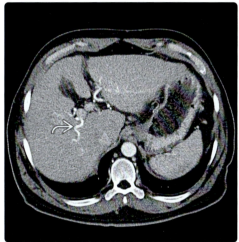

(Left) Arterial-phase CECT of a 56-year-old man with chronic viral hepatitis shows a subtle hypervascular mass ➡. This proved to be HCC. (Right) A more caudal CECT section in the same patient shows signs of cirrhosis, including widened fissures, a big caudate lobe, and an enlarged "corkscrew" hepatic artery ➡.

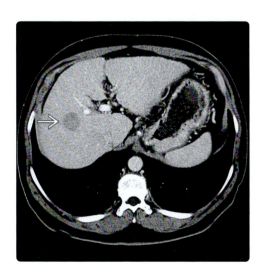
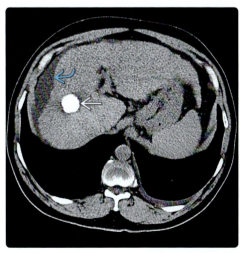

(Left) Portal venous (hepatic)-phase image in the same patient shows the mass ➡, an HCC, much more clearly due to washout of contrast medium from the lesion. (Right) In the same patient, the tumor was treated with intraarterial chemotherapy mixed with Ethiodol, an oily iodinated contrast medium that results in dense, very persistent enhancement of the tumor ➡. The tumor responded well to treatment, but liver function deteriorated, as evidenced by volume loss and development of ascites ⟳.

KEY FACTS

TERMINOLOGY

- Diffuse micro- or macronodular transformation of hepatic parenchyma without fibrous septa between nodules
- Larger focal lesions are called multiacinar (large) regenerative nodules (LRNs)
- Benign lesions: No potential for malignant transformation

IMAGING

- **Gadoxetate (Eovist)-enhanced, multiphasic MR is best imaging test for diagnosing large regenerative nodules**
- Diffuse nodular regenerative hyperplasia (NRH) and focal LRNs have different etiologies and imaging features
- Diffuse NRH
    o Associated with other diseases and drugs (e.g., myeloproliferative; immunosuppressives)
    o Signs of portal hypertension are common (> 50%)
- LRNs
    o Multiple focal liver masses or nodules 0.5-5.0 cm with persistent enhancement on hepatobiliary-enhanced MR [Gadoxetate (Eovist, Primovist)]
    o Hypervascular on arterial-, portal venous-f, and delayed-phase imaging (**no washout**)
    o May have central scar ± perinodular halo
    o Hyperintense on T1WI (75%)
    o Isointense or hypointense nodules on T2WI
    o With signs of underlying disease (e.g., Budd-Chiari: Thrombosed hepatic veins &/or inferior vena cava)

TOP DIFFERENTIAL DIAGNOSES

- **Imaging features are more diagnostic than histologic**
- Multifocal hepatocellular carcinoma
    o Can be differentiated by MR features and clinical setting
- Focal nodular hyperplasia
    o Imaging and histologic features may be identical to NRH
    o Different clinical setting; FNH usually isolated lesion in healthy young woman

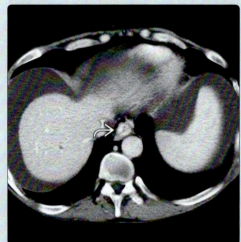

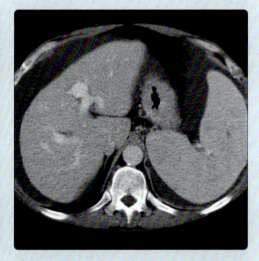

(Left) Axial CECT in a 52-year-old man with a renal transplant shows massive ascites and esophageal varices ⟶. (Right) Axial CT section of the liver in the same patient shows no evidence of fibrosis or focal lesions; liver biopsy showed no cirrhosis but diffuse nodular regenerative hyperplasia. This is a recognized cause of liver failure in the absence of cirrhosis and a known complication of solid organ transplantation, among many other etiologies.

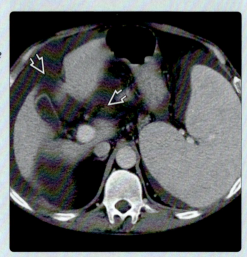

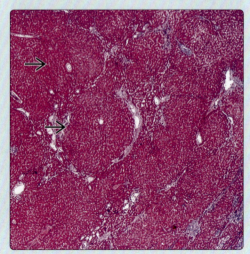

(Left) Another CT section in the same renal transplant patient shows widened hepatic fissures ⟶, suggestive of cirrhosis. Liver biopsy showed no cirrhosis but diffuse nodular regenerative hyperplasia. (Right) Trichrome stain highlights the nodules ⟶. By definition, there are no fibrous septa between the nodules in nodular regenerative hyperplasia. (Courtesy S. Kakar, MD.)

TERMINOLOGY

Definitions

- Nodular regenerative hyperplasia (NRH): Uncommonly recognized entity characterized by diffuse monoacinar (micronodular) transformation of liver parenchyma without fibrous septa between nodules
- Large regenerative nodules (LRNs): Larger focal lesions are called multiacinar (large) regenerative nodules
- Both NRH and LRN categorized as benign regenerative nodules

IMAGING

General Features

- Best diagnostic clue
  - NRH: Diffuse liver lesions are often not visible at all
  - LRNs: Multiple hypervascular nodules up to 5 cm with **delayed enhancement on hepatobiliary-enhanced MR**
- Size
  - Monoacinar lesions in NRH are only ~ 1 mm in diameter with clusters of lesions up to 10 mm
  - LRNs: 0.5-5.0 cm in diameter
- Key concepts
  - Diffuse NRH and focal LRNs have different predisposing conditions and different imaging features

CT Findings

- CECT
  - Diffuse NRH
    - No focal masses; liver may look normal or dysmorphic
    - Signs of portal hypertension are common (> 50% of reported cases)
  - LRNs
    - Multiple focal liver masses or nodules (2 to hundreds)
      - Homogeneously hypervascular on arterial- and portal venous-phase imaging (**no washout**)
      - May have central scar ± perinodular hypo-/hyperdense halo
      - Along with signs of underlying disease (e.g., for Budd-Chiari: Thrombosed hepatic veins &/or inferior vena cava, central hepatic hypertrophy, and peripheral atrophy)
      - Signs of portal hypertension in > 50%

MR Findings

- T1WI
  - LRNs: Hyperintense (75%)
- T2WI
  - Isointense or hypointense nodules; fewer detected
  - Halo sign: Nodule surrounded by peliosis
- Multiphasic enhanced MR
  - Bright homogeneous enhancement on arterial and portal venous phase
  - ± ring (halo) enhancement; ± central scar
- MR with gadoxetate: Uptake and delayed clearance (prolonged enhancement)
  - Confirms benign hepatocellular nature of lesions
  - Bright uniform or peripheral enhancement
  - Mimics appearance of focal nodular hyperplasia (FNH) (as does histology)

DIFFERENTIAL DIAGNOSIS

Multifocal Hepatocellular Carcinoma

- Imaging features are distinct from NRH
- Heterogeneously hyperdense on arterial phase with rapid washout (CT and MR)
- Hypointense on T1WI, hyperintense on T2WI
  - LRNs are hyperintense on T1WI; iso- or hypointense on T2WI
- Usually no uptake or retention of hepatobiliary MR contrast agents

Focal Nodular Hyperplasia (Multiple)

- Imaging and histology may be identical to LRNs
- Different clinical setting: FNH usually isolated lesion in healthy young woman

PATHOLOGY

General Features

- Associated abnormalities
  - NRH: Many associated diseases
    - Solid organ and bone marrow transplantation, myeloproliferative disorders, chemotherapy, autoimmune disease
  - LRNs
    - Budd-Chiari syndrome (accounts for > 70% of cases), heart disease, chronic portal vein thrombosis, cirrhosis

Microscopic Features

- LRNs: Multiacinar nodules, consist of different-sized hepatocytes 1-2 plates wide and narrow sinusoids organized to form LRNs
  - Between nodules are areas of centrilobular atrophy with curvilinear areas of sinusoidal dilation, marked congestion, and paucity of fibrosis
- NRH: Monoacinar lesions present in liver that is neither fibrotic nor cirrhotic
- Both forms of disease have obliteration of small portal ± hepatic veins
  - Leads to ischemic atrophy with secondary hyperplastic response in areas of favorable blood flow
  - Relatively mild and diffuse ischemia → diffuse form of NRH

DIAGNOSTIC CHECKLIST

Consider

- LRNs in dysmorphic liver are easily confused with other masses, such as hepatocellular carcinoma (HCC)
  - Important to recognize underlying liver disorder (e.g., Budd-Chiari) and characteristic appearance of LRNs
- Diffuse NRH may cause variceal bleeding in absence of cirrhosis

Image Interpretation Pearls

- LRNs: Imaging and path appearance almost identical to FNH
- Multiple focal hypervascular masses without washout in Budd-Chiari patient = LRNs, **not** HCC

(Left) *T1 C+ MR in a 63-year-old man with a myeloproliferative disorder shows marked splenomegaly, likely due to extramedullary hematopoiesis. The liver shows no apparent diffuse or focal abnormality, but biopsy revealed diffuse nodular regenerative hyperplasia, a known complication of myelodysplasia and the medications used to treat it.* **(Right)** *Another T1 MR in the same patient again shows no apparent hepatic lesion in this case of biopsy-proven nodular regenerative hyperplasia.*

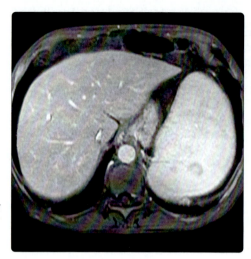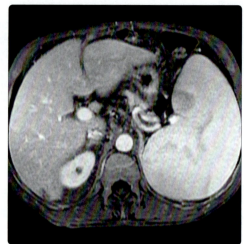

(Left) *Axial T1 C+ MR shows numerous 2-cm hyperintense lesions in a patient with Budd-Chiari syndrome. Note the hypointense "halo" around some of these large regenerative nodules (LRNs) ➡, a characteristic but not common feature.* **(Right)** *Axial T2 MR in the same patient demonstrates fewer and much less evident hypointense foci ➡ of the focal multiacinar form of nodular regenerative hyperplasia in the right hepatic lobe.*

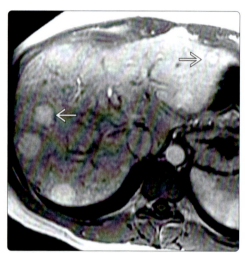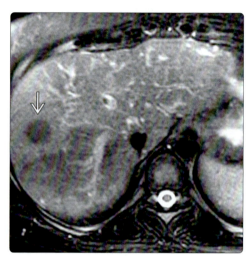

(Left) *Gross pathology section of an explanted dysmorphic liver from a patient with Budd-Chiari syndrome shows caudate hypertrophy ➡, lateral segment atrophy ➡, and multiple large, orange, discolored regenerative nodules ➡.* **(Right)** *Axial CECT in a man with chronic Budd-Chiari syndrome shows multiple hypervascular LRNs ➡, the macroscopic form of nodular regenerative hyperplasia.*

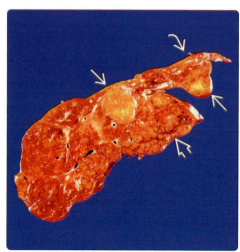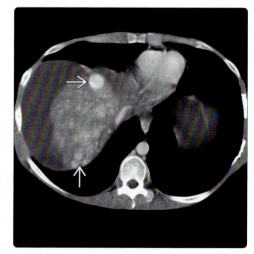

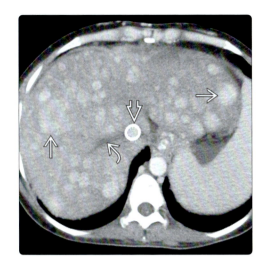

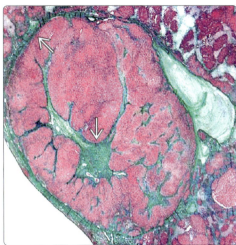

(Left) *Axial CECT shows classic findings of Budd-Chiari and multiacinar LRNs. Note the inferior vena cava stent ➡, an occluded right hepatic vein ➡, and innumerable LRNs ➡ that are persistently hyperdense on this portal venous-phase image.* (Right) *Photomicrograph shows a resected LRN that has a reticulin stain (in green) ➡ that highlights the peripheral and central "scar" that is seen in some LRNs, very similar to that found in focal nodular hyperplasia.*

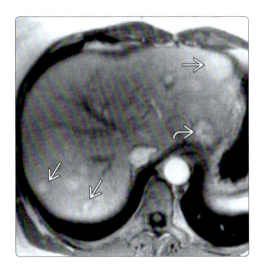

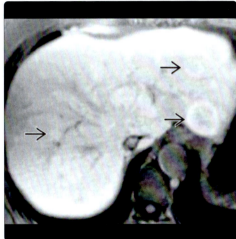

(Left) *Arterial phase of a contrast-enhanced T1 MR shows multiple hypervascular foci. Some of the lesions seem to have a hypointense rim ➡, while others have a hypointense central scar ➡, findings that can be seen with FNH.* (Right) *A delayed MR scan in the same patient after IV administration of a hepatobiliary contrast agent shows persistent uptake and retention of the contrast within the nodules ➡, indicating functional hepatocytes and a benign etiology.*

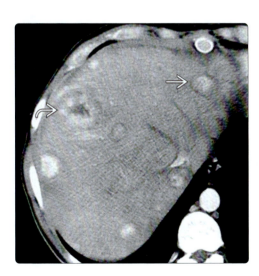

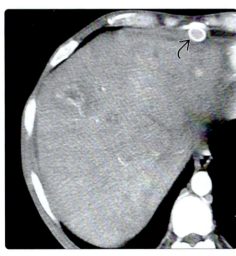

(Left) *Arterial-phase CECT in a 35-year-old man with Budd-Chiari syndrome shows multiple enhancing LRNs, including some with peripheral "halos" ➡ and others with central "scars" ➡.* (Right) *Additional LRNs are noted on this CECT section from the same patient. Note the extrahepatic venous graft ➡.*

TERMINOLOGY

- Localized proliferation of liver parenchyma within cirrhotic liver in response to liver injury
  - May progress to become dysplastic or even malignant [hepatocellular carcinoma (HCC)]

IMAGING

- **Multiphasic gadoxetate (Eovist, Primovist)-enhanced MR, plus diffusion-weighted imaging is optimal imaging tool**
  - Regenerative: Innumerable nodules in cirrhotic liver with decreased signal intensity on T2WI or GRE
    - Hypovascular without washout or capsule
    - Typically < 2 cm; retain Eovist on delayed phase (brighter than liver)
  - Dysplastic: Fewer, larger, hypovascular, hyperintense (bright) on T1WI and hypointense (dark) on T2WI
    - Usually 2-4 cm in diameter; retain Eovist (bright) on delayed-phase imaging

- Lesion may have imaging features of both dysplastic and malignant (HCC) nodule; this nodule-in-nodule pattern often suggests malignant degeneration of dysplastic nodule
  - Malignant (HCC): Solitary or several; bright on T2WI and diffusion-weighted imaging
    - Hypervascular with washout on venous and delayed phase; encapsulated
    - Minimal uptake and retention of Eovist (usually)
- **CT: Effective in surveillance; detection and characterization of cirrhosis and HCC**
  - Regenerative nodules (RNs): May be seen on NECT as hyperattenuating to surrounding liver
    - CECT: RNs enhance slightly less than liver; disappear
  - Dysplastic nodules: Iso-/hyperattenuating in arterial phase; not hypervascular
  - HCC
    - Hypervascular on arterial phase; washout ± capsule on venous or delayed phase

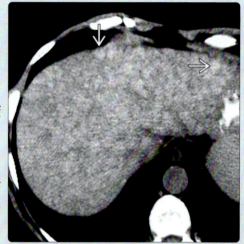
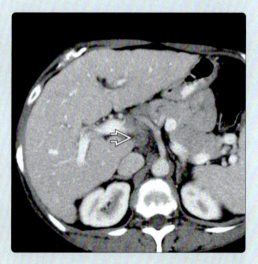

(Left) Axial NECT in a 54-year-old woman with primary biliary cirrhosis shows innumerable small, hyperdense, regenerative nodules ➡ surrounded by lace-like fibrosis. (Right) Axial CECT in the same patient demonstrates that the nodules disappear into the background cirrhotic liver, owing to minimal enhancement of the nodules and persistent enhancement of the fibrotic bands. Also noted is prominent porta hepatis lymphadenopathy ➡, another typical feature of primary biliary cirrhosis.

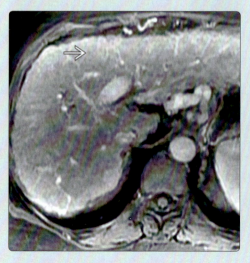
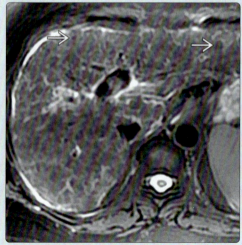

(Left) Axial contrast-enhanced T1WI MR in a 61-year-old woman with cirrhosis shows a nodular liver with widened fissures, typical for cirrhosis. There are innumerable small, hypointense, cirrhotic regenerative nodules ➡, but these are not very evident. (Right) Axial T2WI MR in the same patient shows the cirrhotic nodules more clearly, as subcentimeter, hypointense ("dark") lesions ➡, a characteristic appearance of benign regenerative nodules.

Regenerative and Dysplastic Nodules

TERMINOLOGY

Synonyms
- Cirrhotic nodules

Definitions
- Localized proliferation of liver parenchyma within cirrhotic liver in response to liver injury
  - May progress to become dysplastic or even malignant

IMAGING

General Features
- Best diagnostic clue
  - Regenerative: Multiple nodules in cirrhotic liver with ↓ signal intensity on T2WI or GRE
  - Dysplastic: Fewer, larger, hyperintense on T1WI and hypointense on T2WI; hypovascular
  - Malignant [hepatocellular carcinoma (HCC)]: Usually solitary, hyperintense on T2WI and diffusion-weighted imaging; hypervascular with washout ± capsule
- Size
  - Regenerative nodules (RNs) are commonly < 2 cm
    - Dysplastic nodules usually 2-4 cm in diameter
    - HCC can be any size (usually 2-10 cm)

Imaging Recommendations
- Best imaging tool
  - **Multiphasic gadoxetate (Eovist, Primovist)-enhanced MR plus diffusion-weighted imaging**
- Protocol advice
  - Need T1WI and T2WI, plus contrast-enhanced T1WI, to evaluate vascularity
  - Gadoxetate (Eovist, Primovist) may help distinguish among nodules
    - Expect uptake and retention on delayed-phase imaging for regenerative and dysplastic nodules
    - Minimal uptake or retention within HCC nodules
      - Some HCC show patchy uptake and retention

CT Findings
- NECT
  - RNs: May be seen on NECT as hyperattenuating to surrounding liver
    - Due to increased iron or glycogen content
    - Or surrounding "halo" of low-attenuation fibrosis
- CECT
  - **CT: Effective in surveillance; detection and characterization of cirrhosis and HCC**
  - RNs: Enhance slightly less than liver
    - Results in disappearance of RNs on CECT
  - Dysplastic nodules: Iso-/hyperattenuating in arterial phase
    - Most are not hypervascular
    - Hypervascularity raises concern for development of HCC
  - HCC: Heterogeneously hypervascular on arterial phase with washout on venous and delayed
    - Capsule; venous invasion; multiplicity increase confidence in diagnosis of HCC

MR Findings
- T1WI
  - RNs
    - Variable signal intensity, usually isointense to liver (undetected)
  - Dysplastic nodules
    - Variable signal intensity
    - Usually iso-/hyperintense to liver (bright on T1WI)
- T2WI
  - RNs
    - ↓ signal intensity (dark) compared to liver (due to iron content)
  - Dysplastic nodules
    - Low-grade nodules tend to have lower signal intensity compared to liver (dark on T2WI)
    - High-grade nodules tend to have slightly higher signal intensity compared to liver
      - ↑ signal intensity corresponds to ↑ dedifferentiation and concern for HCC
- T2* GRE
  - RNs: ↓↓ signal intensity compared to liver
    - **Blooming** (appearing larger) due to ↑ susceptibility effect of iron
- T1WI C+
  - RNs
    - Isointense to liver (undetected) or slightly hypointense
  - Dysplastic nodules
    - Variably hyperintense to adjacent liver
      - Increasing vascularity increases concern for malignant degeneration of dysplastic nodule
- MR with gadobenate dimeglumine or gadoxetate (Eovist, Primovist): Avid uptake and retention
  - Indicates functioning hepatocytes
  - Favors benign etiology (regenerative or low-grade dysplastic nodule)
    - High-grade dysplastic nodules and HCC lack functioning hepatocytes and biliary excretion
      - → no uptake (hypointense on delayed imaging)

Ultrasonographic Findings
- Nodules may appear as hypo-, iso-, or hyperechoic
  - Most regenerative and dysplastic nodules are not apparent on US

DIAGNOSTIC CHECKLIST

Image Interpretation Pearls
- Some overlap in imaging appearance of regenerative and dysplastic nodules and even HCC
  - MR is best imaging modality, especially with hepatobiliary contrast media [e.g., gadoxetate (Eovist or Primovist)]
  - Imaging allows confident diagnosis of lesions ≥ 2 cm
  - RNs have similar appearance as low-grade dysplastic nodules; high-grade dysplastic nodules have similar appearance to some HCCs (true on histology as well)

Reporting Tips
- Characterize appearance of focal nodules in cirrhotic liver by density or intensity on all phases of imaging
  - Assess vascularity and washout

(Left) *In this 50-year-old man with cirrhosis, there is a well-defined spherical mass ➡️ that is hyperintense (bright) on T1WI MR and showed no signal loss on opposed-phase T1WI GRE MR (not shown).* **(Right)** *In the same patient, the lesion ➡️ is hypointense (dark) on T2WI MR, typical of a dysplastic nodule (and atypical for hepatocellular carcinoma).*

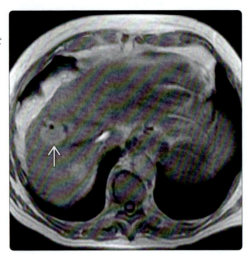 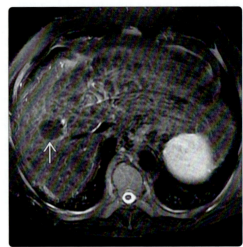

(Left) *The lesion ➡️ shows minimal vascularity or enhancement on this late arterial-phase T1WI C+ MR of the same patient, typical of a dysplastic nodule.* **(Right)** *Venous phase T1WI MR in the same patient shows the lesion (dysplastic nodule) ➡️ as hypointense to background liver, more likely due to increased enhancement of the background liver than washout of contrast from the lesion. The lesion is nonencapsulated.*

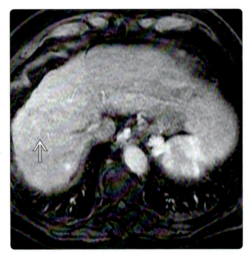 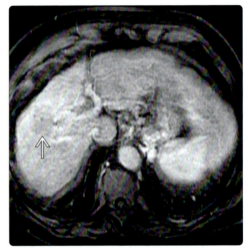

(Left) *Axial T1WI MR in a 61-year-old woman with cirrhosis shows a well-defined hyperintense (bright) lesion in the lateral segment that proved to be a dysplastic nodule ➡️.* **(Right)** *Another axial T1WI MR in the same patient shows a hypointense (dark) lesion in segment 6 that proved to be a hepatocellular carcinoma ➡️.*

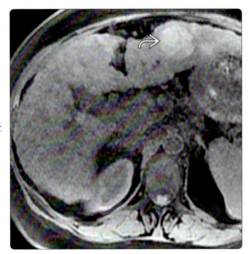 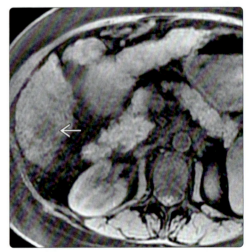

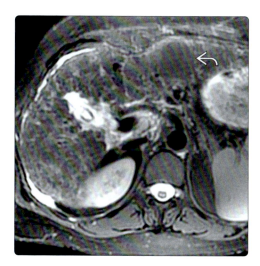
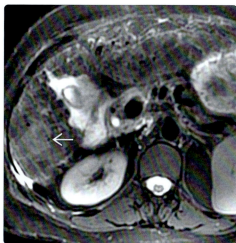

(Left) Axial T2WI MR in the same patient shows the dysplastic nodule ⮕ to be relatively hypointense (dark), a characteristic appearance of a dysplastic nodule. (Right) Another axial T2WI MR in the same patient shows the hepatocellular carcinoma ⮕ to be relatively hyperintense, a typical feature of a malignant nodule or mass (hepatocellular carcinoma).

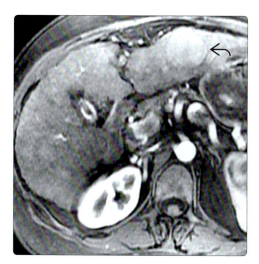
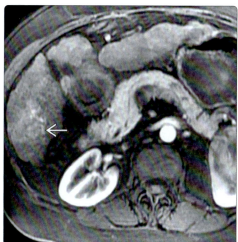

(Left) Axial T1WI C+ MR in the arterial phase shows minimal enhancement of the dysplastic nodule ⮕, a characteristic appearance of this lesion. (Right) Another T1WI C+ MR in the arterial phase in the same patient shows heterogeneous, hypervascular enhancement of the hepatocellular carcinoma ⮕, a typical appearance of this lesion.

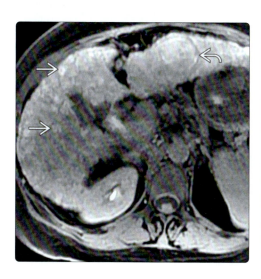
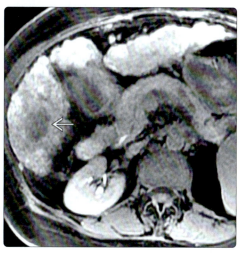

(Left) Axial delayed (hepatobiliary)-phase T1WI MR in the same patient shows enhancement and retention of gadoxetate (Eovist) by the dysplastic nodule ⮕ and within many of the regenerative nodules ⮕, typical features of benign hepatocellular lesions. (Right) Axial delayed-phase T1WI MR in the same case shows no retention of contrast within the hepatocellular carcinoma ⮕. On DWI, the dysplastic nodule was dark, and the hepatocellular carcinoma was bright, additional corroborative features.

TERMINOLOGY

- Communication between branch of hepatic artery and portal venous system

IMAGING

- Best diagnostic clue
  - Wedge-shaped area of hyperattenuation with straight margins seen during arterial phase of CECT or MR
  - Becomes isodense to hepatic parenchyma during portal venous phase of CECT or gadolinium-enhanced MR
- Usually located peripherally in liver
- Usually ≤ 1.5 cm [e.g., cirrhotic arterioportal (AP) shunts]
  - Larger in some cases of postbiopsy AP shunts
  - Early enhancement of peripheral portal vein (PV) branches prior to visualization of main PV

TOP DIFFERENTIAL DIAGNOSES

- Hypervascular liver mass [e.g., hepatocellular carcinoma (HCC)]

- Usually round or oval, not wedge-shaped
- Usually shows washout on venous phase
- Hemangioma
  - Attenuation tracks blood pool on all phases
- Focal sparing with fatty liver
  - Not really hypervascular foci
  - Relatively high-attenuation areas of "normal" liver surrounded by low-attenuation fatty liver

PATHOLOGY

- Small AP shunts are not amenable to biopsy
  - Too small; invisible on nonenhanced CT, MR, and US

DIAGNOSTIC CHECKLIST

- **Small (< 1.5 cm) AP shunts are common in cirrhosis**
  - **If unassociated with focal lesion on MR, probably insignificant**
  - Follow-up in ~ 6 months is indicated and adequate
- Do not mistake multiple small AP shunts for multifocal HCC

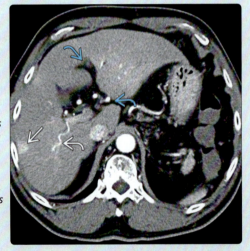 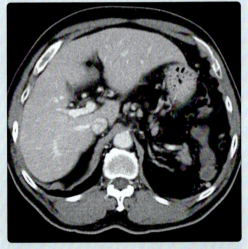

(Left) *Axial arterial-phase CECT in a patient with cirrhosis shows multiple peripheral, wedge-shaped, hypervascular foci ➡. Also note the large, "corkscrew" hepatic arterial branch ➡, a typical feature of cirrhosis. The liver has a cirrhotic morphology with wide fissures ➡. (Right) Axial venous-phase CT in the same patient shows none of the peripheral hypervascular lesions, which have become isodense to liver, typical for arterioportal shunts in cirrhosis. At the follow-up CT in 6 months, the lesions had disappeared.*

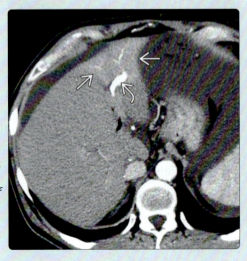 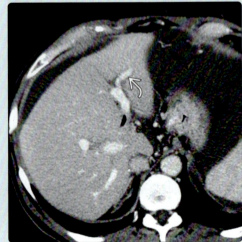

(Left) *Arterial-phase CECT in a 46-year-old man with cirrhosis and a history of a prior US-guided liver biopsy shows hyperenhancement of a portion of the lateral segment of the liver ➡ and early enhancement of the portal vein branch that drains this segment ➡, representing an arterioportal shunt, probably due to the prior liver biopsy at this site. (Right) Portal venous-phase CECT in the same patient shows enhancement of the portal vein branch ➡ but otherwise appears normal.*

Passive Hepatic Congestion

TERMINOLOGY

- Stasis of blood within liver parenchyma as result of impaired hepatic venous drainage

IMAGING

- **Diagnosis can be made or suggested on color Doppler US or contrast-enhanced CT or MR**
  - **Echocardiography can be definitive**
  - CT and MR also show extent of liver injury
- **Ultrasonography**
  - Diameter of hepatic vein: Normal: 5.6-6.2 mm
    - Mean: 8.8 mm (in passive congestion)
    - Increases up to 13 mm with constrictive pericarditis
  - Loss of normal triphasic flow pattern in dilated hepatic veins and inferior vena cava (IVC)
  - "Cardiac cirrhosis": Flattening of Doppler waveform in hepatic veins
    - To-and-fro motion in hepatic veins and IVC
- **Contrast-enhanced CT or MR**

- Early retrograde enhancement of dilated IVC and hepatic veins
- Heterogeneous, mottled, reticulated, mosaic parenchymal pattern
- Periportal low attenuation (perivascular lymphedema)
- Hepatomegaly and ascites
- Chest findings vary by etiology
  - Pleural effusions; cardiomegaly
  - Small heart with pericardial thickening

CLINICAL ISSUES

- Passive hepatic congestion usually secondary to
  - Congestive heart failure
  - Constrictive pericarditis
  - Tricuspid insufficiency
  - Right heart failure
- Characteristic sign on physical exam
  - Hepatojugular reflux

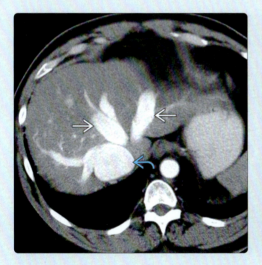

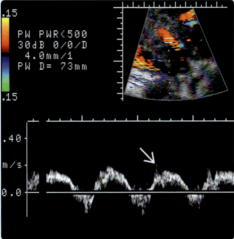

(Left) Axial CECT in the arterial phase shows early retrograde opacification of dilated hepatic veins ➡ and the IVC ➡ due to reflux of injected contrast medium through the heart, a sign of impaired antegrade hepatic venous drainage. (Right) Increased pulsatility of portal vein Doppler signal is demonstrated ➡ in this patient with passive hepatic congestion secondary to tricuspid insufficiency. The hepatic veins and IVC were markedly dilated.

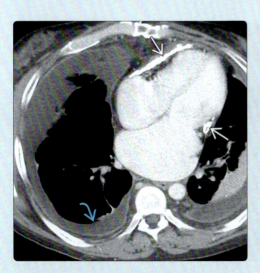

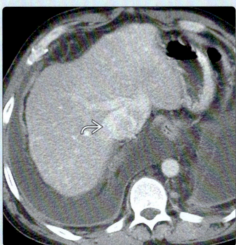

(Left) Axial venous-phase CECT shows bilateral pleural effusions ➡ and a thickened, calcified pericardium ➡ that compresses and distorts both the right and left ventricles, consistent with constrictive pericarditis. (Right) Venous-phase CECT in the same patient shows dilation of the IVC ➡. The liver is diminished in size with a nodular surface, suggesting the presence of "cardiac cirrhosis."

TERMINOLOGY

- Acute, chronic, or neoplastic occlusion of portal vein (PV) due to thrombosis, thrombophlebitis, or tumor invasion
- Chronic PV occlusion with numerous periportal collaterals is referred to as "cavernous transformation"

IMAGING

- **Color Doppler US initially**: Accurate and cost effective
  - Periportal collaterals may be mistaken for patent PV
  - Tumor vessels may be evident within PV mass
- **Multiphasic, multiplanar enhanced CT or MR**
- Contrast-enhanced CT of **acute PV thrombosis**
- Arterial phase (25-40 seconds post bolus injection)
  - High attenuation/intensity within involved hepatic lobe or segment due to arterioportal shunting
  - Transient hepatic attenuation difference (THAD)
- Venous phase (60-70 seconds post bolus injection)
  - Equilibration of hepatic contrast enhancement
  - Visualization of low-density thrombus

- CECT of **chronic PV thrombosis**
  - Numerous periportal collateral veins along usual course of PV
  - Peripancreatic and gallbladder wall varices are common
  - Nonvisualization of PV &/or splenic vein
- **CECT of PV tumor invasion**
  - Lumen of vein may be expanded by thrombus
  - Variable degree of contrast enhancement of intraluminal tumor thrombus
  - Contiguity of parenchymal tumor with PV thrombus

CLINICAL ISSUES

- Primary PV thrombosis may mimic cirrhosis
  - Results in dysmorphic and malfunctioning liver
  - Often results from prothrombotic condition
- Thrombosis or fibrosis of extrahepatic PV may complicate or preclude liver transplantation

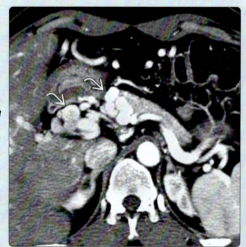
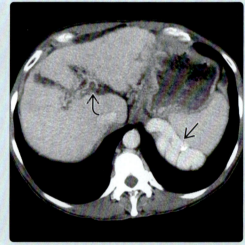

(Left) Axial CECT in a 55-year-old man with hepatitis B who presented for routine CT screening to rule out hepatocellular carcinoma (HCC) shows cavernous transformation of the portal vein with numerous small collateral veins ⇨ in the porta hepatis and hepatoduodenal ligament. The main portal vein cannot be identified. (Right) Axial CECT of a 55-year-old man with cirrhosis and bleeding gastric varices shows "bland" (not malignant) thrombosis of the portal vein ⇨, a cirrhotic liver, and huge upper abdominal varices ⇨.

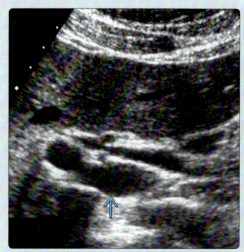
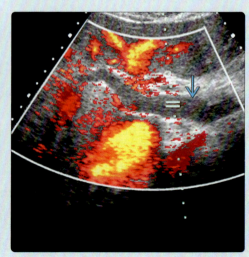

(Left) Longitudinal grayscale ultrasound obtained through the porta hepatis in a 51-year-old woman presenting with vague right upper quadrant pain and a recent elevation of liver function tests reveals no apparent abnormalities of the portal vein ⇨. (Right) Longitudinal power Doppler ultrasound obtained in the same patient in the same field of view reveals an acute thrombosis ⇨ of the portal vein with a complete absence of flow, which was undetectable with grayscale sonography alone.

Portal Vein Occlusion

TERMINOLOGY

Synonyms
- Portal vein (PV) thrombosis

Definitions
- Acute, chronic, or neoplastic occlusion of PV due to thrombosis or tumor invasion
- Chronic PV occlusion with numerous periportal collaterals is referred to as "cavernous transformation"

IMAGING

General Features
- Best diagnostic clue
  - Low-attenuation thrombus in PV on CECT
  - On MR and power Doppler: Absence of blood flow or flow void in PV
    - May be caused or simulated by slow flow in portal hypertension
    - Nonvisualization of PV (chronic occlusion)
    - Cavernous transformation of PV (collateralization in porta hepatis)

CT Findings
- Contrast-enhanced CT of acute thrombosis
  - Arterial phase (25-40 seconds post bolus injection)
    - High attenuation within involved hepatic lobe or segment due to arterioportal shunting
      - Transient hepatic attenuation difference
  - Venous phase (60-70 seconds post bolus injection)
    - Equilibration of hepatic contrast enhancement
    - Visualization of low-density (if bland) thrombus
  - Nonocclusive thrombosis: Low-density thrombus partially filling PV lumen
  - Occlusive thrombosis: Low-density thrombus filling PV lumen
    - Extent variable: May include major intrahepatic branches, splenic vein, superior mesenteric vein
    - Congested (nonoccluded) mesenteric veins upstream from thrombus, mesenteric edema, bowel wall thickening, ischemia from venous congestion
    - Ileus, ascites, and splenomegaly may be seen
- CECT of chronic PV thrombosis
  - Chronic occlusion (cavernous transformation) of PV
    - Numerous periportal collateral veins along usual course of PV
    - Peripancreatic and gallbladder wall varices are common
  - Nonvisualization of PV &/or splenic vein
    - Thrombosed vein becomes fibrotic "cord" not visible on imaging
  - Well-developed portosystemic collaterals
    - e.g., splenorenal shunt; esophageal, periumbilical varices
  - Associated findings
    - Splenomegaly
    - Liver: Atrophy/hypertrophy complex
      - Usual pattern is hypertrophy of central (deep) segments, atrophy of peripheral segments
      - May impart lobulated or rounded contour to liver

- Increased hepatic artery size &/or flow
- CECT of PV tumor invasion
  - Lumen of vein may be expanded by thrombus
    - Main PV > 23-mm diameter
  - Variable degree of contrast enhancement of intraluminal tumor thrombus
    - Linear enhancing "threads and streaks"
      - Best seen on arterial phase of biphasic CECT
    - Primary tumor usually visible in hepatic parenchyma or pancreas, often in direct contiguity with thrombus
    - Commonly seen in hepatocellular carcinoma and pancreatic neuroendocrine tumors

MR Findings
- T1WI
  - High-signal filling defect
- T2WI
  - High-signal acute or tumor thrombus
  - Absence of usual flow void
- T1WI C+ FS
  - Liver parenchyma supplied by thrombosed veins may enhance avidly in arterial phase due to increased hepatic artery flow
    - Transient hepatic intensity difference
  - Subacute thrombus hyperintense on T1 and T2 due to methemoglobin
  - Tumor thrombus on enhanced MR
    - Analogous to CECT (expanded lumen, enhancing thrombus, contiguous with tumor)

Ultrasonographic Findings
- Grayscale ultrasound
  - Acute
    - Echogenic or anechoic clot
  - Subacute
    - Isoechoic clot
- Color Doppler
  - Lack of flow within PV more evident on color Doppler
  - Tumor vessels usually visible within tumor thrombus
  - Partial thrombosis
    - Filling defect within PV
  - Cavernous transformation
    - Numerous venous collaterals in porta hepatis
    - Large collaterals may be mistaken for patent PV
  - Neoplastic invasion of PV
    - Pulsatile arterial waveforms with reversed flow

Imaging Recommendations
- Best imaging tool
  - Color Doppler US initially: Accurate and cost effective
  - Contrast-enhanced CT or MR for comprehensive evaluation
- Protocol advice
  - Color and spectral Doppler US
  - Contrast-enhanced CT or MR

DIAGNOSTIC CHECKLIST

Consider
- Distinguish between tumor and bland thrombus in setting of cirrhosis

(Left) *Axial CECT of a 59-year-old man with cirrhosis shows heterogeneous hepatic enhancement, and as a result, an occluded portal vein ➡️ with cavernous transformation of the portal vein and extensive varices ➡️.* (Right) *CT section in the same patient shows extensive varices ➡️ within the hepatoduodenal ligament and gallbladder wall ➡️.*

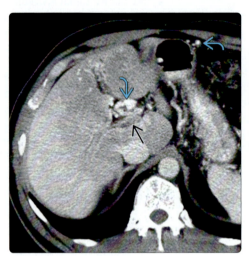
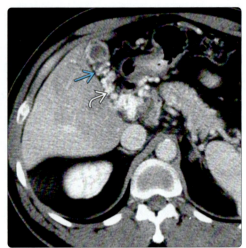

(Left) *Axial CECT in a young woman with right upper quadrant pain and fever shows a large, pyogenic abscess ➡️ and hyperenhancement of the right lobe of the liver ➡️, both due to pylephlebitis and occlusion of the right portal vein from diverticulitis.* (Right) *Axial arterial-phase CECT of a young man recovering from a gunshot wound to the abdomen shows hyperenhancement of the anterior right lobe of the liver, a perfusion anomaly ➡️ due to pylephlebitis and occlusion of the anterior branch of the right portal vein ➡️.*

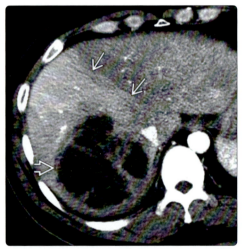
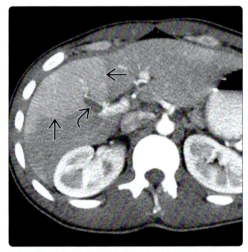

(Left) *In this 32-year-old woman with bleeding esophageal varices but no history of liver disease, CT shows an occluded portal vein ➡️ and large collateral veins ➡️. Note the dysmorphic liver with hypertrophy of the central liver and atrophy of the periphery, giving it rounded contours. The spleen is surgically absent.* (Right) *CT in the same patient shows more of the collateral veins ➡️ in the mesentery due to primary portal vein thrombosis. This patient was subsequently found to have a prothrombotic condition.*

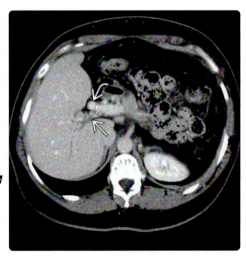
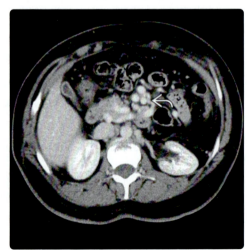

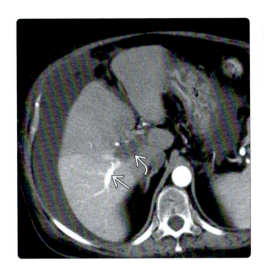

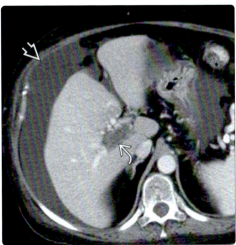

(Left) *Arterial-phase CECT of a 59-year-old woman with portal vein thrombosis due to a prothrombotic condition shows thrombus ⟰ of the posterior branch of the right portal vein. Compensatory increased flow through the hepatic artery ⟰ accounts for the transient hepatic attenuation difference in the posterior right lobe.* (Right) *Portal venous-phase CECT in the same patient shows uniform enhancement of the liver, the thrombosed right portal vein ➔, and ascites ➔.*

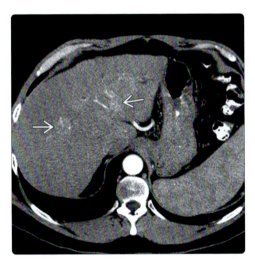

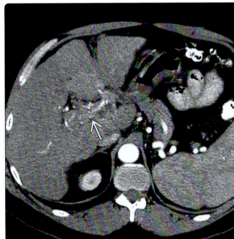

(Left) *Arterial-phase CECT of a 63-year-old man with hepatitis C and HCC shows distention of the left and right portal veins by enhancing tumor thrombus ➔. The primary hepatic tumors are difficult to identify since most of the tumor is within the portal veins rather than the parenchyma.* (Right) *Arterial-phase CECT in the same patient shows the diameter of the veins is increased, and tumor vascularity is evident within the thrombus, particularly within the more central right portal vein ➔.*

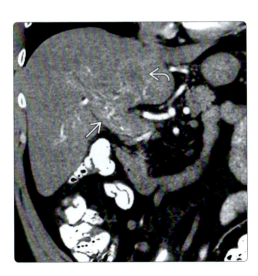

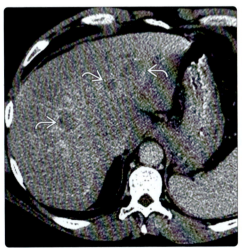

(Left) *The parenchymal ➔ and portal vein ➔ tumors are somewhat easier to recognize as contiguous structures on this coronal reformatted arterial-phase CECT in the same patient.* (Right) *Axial venous-phase CECT in the same patient shows the parenchymal tumors ➔ as hypodense structures relative to hepatic parenchyma due to contrast washout from the HCC, a characteristic feature of this tumor. Tumor within the portal veins showed the same finding on other sections (not shown).*

TERMINOLOGY

- Hepatic injury due to global or segmental hepatic venous outflow or inferior vena cava (IVC) obstruction

IMAGING

- Multiphasic CT or MR [± gadoxetate (Eovist) enhancement]
  - Characteristic findings: Nodular regenerative hyperplasia in dysmorphic liver with venous collateral and ascites
  - Hypertrophied caudate lobe with atrophy and necrosis of peripheral liver ("pseudotumor")
  - Intrahepatic and systemic venous collaterals bypass obstructed hepatic veins and IVC
    - Spider web pattern of hepatic venous collaterals on CT, MR, angiography
  - Large regenerative nodules (form of nodular regenerative hyperplasia) are characteristic of chronic Budd-Chiari syndrome (BCS)
    - Imaging and histology are similar to FNH

- May have peripheral halo and central scar
- Hypervascularity persists into venous phase, usually without washout
- Uniform or peripheral delayed retention (bright) on gadoxetate-enhanced MR
- US
  - Absent, reversed, or flat flow in hepatic veins; reversed flow in IVC on color Doppler US
  - Venovenous collaterals
  - Heterogeneous liver parenchyma

DIAGNOSTIC CHECKLIST

- Do not mistake BCS for cirrhosis
  - Pathogenesis, imaging findings, prognosis, and treatment are very different
- Do not mistake caudate hypertrophy or large regenerative nodules for hepatocellular carcinoma
- Check for hypercoagulable conditions (most common cause)

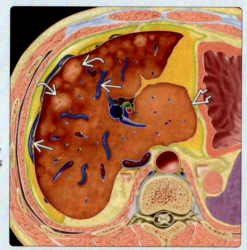

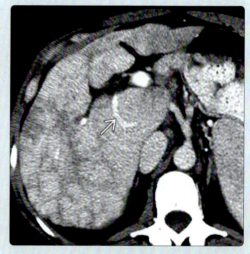

(Left) *Axial anatomic illustration of Budd-Chiari syndrome demonstrates ascites, venous collaterals* ➡, *heterogeneous hepatic parenchyma due to centrilobular necrosis, and hypervascular regenerative nodules* ➡. *Note the sparing of the caudate lobe with hypertrophy* ➡ *as well as the thrombosed inferior vena cava (IVC).* (Right) *Axial CECT shows caudate hypertrophy, a large caudate collateral vein* ➡, *and peripheral atrophy and heterogeneity. The hepatic veins were occluded.*

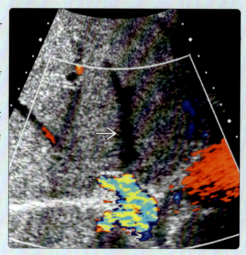

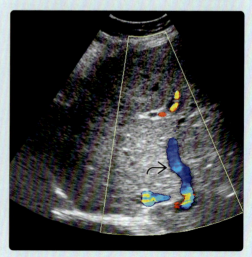

(Left) *Transverse color Doppler ultrasound of the liver in a 48-year-old woman with known polycythemia vera, RUQ pain, and elevated liver function tests reveals a lack of flow within the right hepatic vein* ➡. (Right) *Color Doppler ultrasound in the same patient demonstrates a large intrahepatic collateral vein* ➡ *bypassing the occluded hepatic veins.*

Budd-Chiari Syndrome

TERMINOLOGY

Abbreviations
- Budd-Chiari syndrome (BCS)

Synonyms
- Hepatic venous outflow obstruction

Definitions
- Global or segmental hepatic venous outflow obstruction
  - At level of large hepatic veins or suprahepatic segment of inferior vena cava (IVC)

IMAGING

General Features
- Best diagnostic clue
  - Caudate hypertrophy, peripheral atrophy, ascites, and collateral veins bypassing occluded IVC
- Location
  - Hepatic veins, IVC, or centrilobular veins
- Characteristic finding: Nodular regenerative hyperplasia in dysmorphic liver

CT Findings
- NECT
  - Acute phase
    - Diffusely hypodense, enlarged liver
    - Narrowed IVC and hepatic veins; ascites
    - Hyperdense IVC and hepatic veins (due to increased attenuation of thrombus)
  - Chronic phase
    - Heterogeneous hypodensity and atrophy of peripheral liver
      □ Hypertrophy of caudate lobe, which is spared
      □ Caudate often greater in diameter than right lobe
      □ Normal caudate to right lobe is ≤ 0.6 (60%)
    - Nonvisualization of IVC and hepatic veins
- CECT
  - Acute phase
    - Classic flip-flop pattern seen
      □ Early enhancement of caudate lobe and central portion around IVC, decreased peripheral liver enhancement
      □ Later decreased enhancement centrally with increased enhancement peripherally
    - Narrowed hypodense hepatic veins and IVC with hyperdense walls
  - Chronic phase
    - Total obliteration of IVC and hepatic veins
    - Venovenous collateral veins
    - **Large regenerative nodules: Focal, multiacinar form of nodular regenerative hyperplasia**
      □ Enhancing 1- to 4-cm hyperdense nodules, ± hypodense ring, ± central scar
      □ Usually multiple

MR Findings
- T1WI
  - Normal intensity of liver centrally with peripheral heterogeneity and hypointensity
  - Narrowed or absent hepatic veins and IVC
  - Hyperintense regenerative nodules and enlarged caudate lobe
- T2WI
  - Nonvisualized hepatic veins and IVC
  - Peripheral fibrotic liver is higher in signal intensity
  - Iso- or hypointense regenerative nodules
- T2* GRE
  - No demonstrable flow in hepatic veins or IVC
- T1WI C+
  - Occlusion of IVC or hepatic veins, plus collaterals
  - Tumor thrombus (rare) may show enhancement
  - Acute phase
    - Damaged parenchyma, mostly peripheral, enhances < central liver
  - Congested liver with increased water content
    - Peripheral liver enhances < central liver, secondary to ↑ parenchymal pressure, ↓ blood supply
  - Chronic phase
    - Enhancement is more variable, may be increased
    - **Nodules**: Intense enhancement that persists into venous phase (usually no washout)
    - Uniform or peripheral delayed retention, **bright on gadoxetate-enhanced MR**

Ultrasonographic Findings
- Grayscale ultrasound
  - Hepatic veins narrowed, nonvisualized, or filled with thrombus
  - Hypertrophied caudate lobe
- Color Doppler
  - Hepatic veins and IVC
    - Absent or flat flow in hepatic veins
    - Reversed flow in hepatic veins or IVC
    - "Bicolored" hepatic veins due to intrahepatic collateral pathways
    - Sensitivity: 87.5%
  - Portal vein
    - Slow hepatofugal flow ≤ 11 cm/second
  - Hepatic artery: Resistive index ≥ 0.75

Angiographic Findings
- Inferior venacavography or hepatic venacavography
  - Spider web pattern of hepatic venous collaterals
  - Thrombus in hepatic veins or IVC
  - Long segmental compression or stenosis of IVC
    - Acute phase: Due to diffuse hepatomegaly
    - Chronic phase: Hypertrophy of caudate lobe
  - Hepatic arteries
    - Acute phase: Narrowing, stretching, bowing
    - Chronic phase: Dilated with arterioportal shunts

DIAGNOSTIC CHECKLIST

Consider
- Distinguish BCS from cirrhosis; do not mistake focal, large regenerative nodules of BCS for hepatocellular carcinoma

Image Interpretation Pearls
- Recognize large, benign regenerative nodules and caudate pseudotumor

(Left) Axial CECT shows thrombosis of the major hepatic veins ⇨ and a heterogeneous liver. (Right) Axial CECT in the same patient shows striking hypertrophy of the caudate lobe ➡ but normal enhancement relative to the spleen ⇨. The peripheral liver is atrophic and enhances minimally. This is a classic example of the caudate pseudotumor of Budd-Chiari syndrome, in which the caudate is so enlarged and different in attenuation than the remainder of the liver that it might be mistaken for a neoplasm.

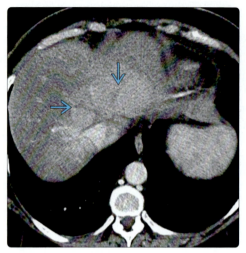 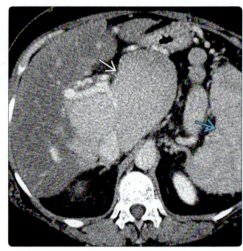

(Left) Axial arterial-phase CECT of a 45-year-old woman with ascites and lower extremity swelling shows one of multiple hypervascular masses ⇨. (Right) Arterial-phase CECT in the same patient shows another hypervascular mass ⇨, with a central scar, resembling a focal nodular hyperplasia (FNH). These large (multiacinar) regenerative nodules, also called focal nodular regenerative hyperplasia, occur commonly in Budd-Chiari syndrome and resemble FNH on both imaging and histology.

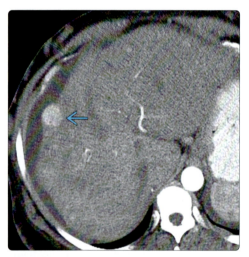 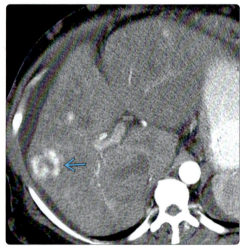

(Left) Axial venous-phase CECT in the same patient shows an intrahepatic collateral vein ⇗, a large azygous vein ➡, and subcutaneous collaterals ➡ bypassing the occluded IVC. (Right) Venous-phase CECT in the same patient shows occlusion of the retrohepatic IVC ⇗. The liver is dysmorphic and enhances heterogeneously, especially in the periphery. Ascites ⇨ is present.

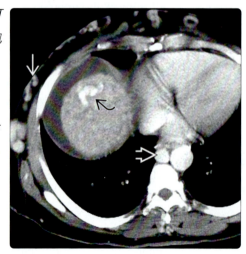 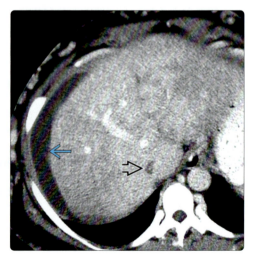

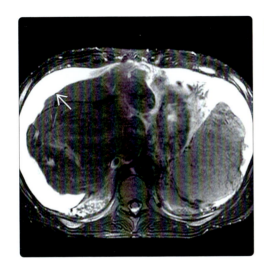
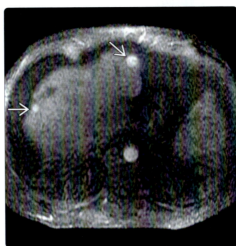

(Left) *Axial T2 MR of a 25-year-old man with liver malfunction shows ascites ➡ and a dysmorphic (abnormally shaped) liver with central hypertrophy and peripheral atrophy.* (Right) *Axial arterial-phase T1 C+ FS MR in the same patient shows 2 of several focal nodules ➡ that are hyperintense on this sequence. These are large regenerative nodules, the focal multiacinar form of nodular regenerative hyperplasia, that occur in Budd-Chiari syndrome and other conditions that cause chronic hepatic ischemia.*

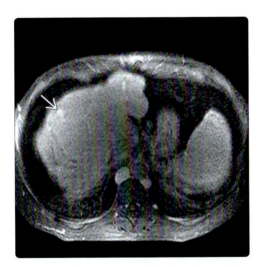
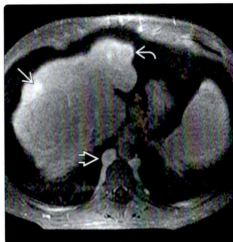

(Left) *Axial venous-phase T1 MR in the same patient shows persistent enhancement (no washout) of a focal regenerative nodule ➡.* (Right) *Axial delayed-phase enhanced T1 C+ MR in the same patient shows persistent enhancement of one of the nodules ➡, while another shows peripheral ring or halo enhancement ➡. The IVC is occluded, and large azygous collaterals are seen ➡.*

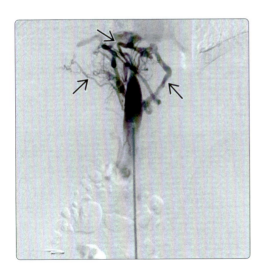
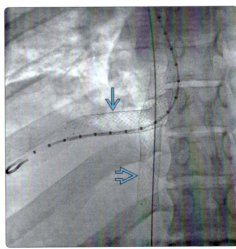

(Left) *Film from an inferior vena cavogram shows occlusion of the intrahepatic IVC and numerous collateral veins ➡ resembling a spider web.* (Right) *Subsequent film from the same procedure shows deployment of metallic stents within the IVC ➡ and right hepatic vein ➡ following balloon dilation of these vessels. This patient was diagnosed as having Budd-Chiari syndrome due to a hypercoagulable condition, the most common etiology in western countries.*

Sinusoidal Obstruction Syndrome

TERMINOLOGY

- Hepatic sinusoidal obstruction syndrome (**SOS**) (preferred term)
  - "Hepatic venoocclusive disease" was term previously used
- Hepatic venous outflow obstruction due to occlusion of terminal hepatic venules and sinusoids

IMAGING

- Ultrasound is preferred initial imaging tool
  - Sensitivity and specificity are low (overlap those of graft-vs.-host disease)
  - US provides suggestive evidence of SOS; helps exclude other diagnoses (e.g., opportunistic infection)
    - Hepatosplenomegaly; ascites; periportal edema
    - Hepatofugal flow on Doppler; ↑ resistive index (> 0.75)
    - Abnormal portal vein waveform; small-caliber hepatic veins

- MR may be most specific imaging tool
  - On hepatobiliary (delayed-) phase gadoxetate-enhanced (Eovist) MR
    - Diffuse reticular pattern of low intensity relative to normal background parenchyma
    - Reported to be specific finding of SOS
- CT: Neither sensitive nor specific
  - May show peripheral heterogeneous hypoenhancement of liver parenchyma

CLINICAL ISSUES

- Acute onset of painful hepatomegaly, jaundice, ascites, peripheral edema within 3 weeks following hematopoietic or stem cell transplantation (most common etiology)
  - Other causes: Chemotherapy (especially oxaliplatin for colorectal cancer metastases); liver transplantation
  - Exposure to various toxic agents
- May coexist in patients with peliosis hepatis (same risk factors)

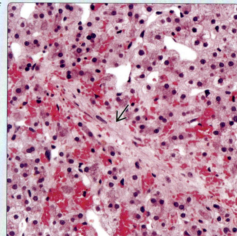
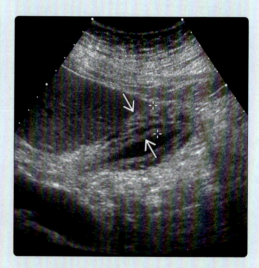

(Left) Complete obliteration of the central vein ➡ accompanied by centrizonal sinusoidal congestion is seen in venoocclusive disease. (Courtesy S. Kakar, MD.) (Right) Sonography shows gallbladder wall edema ➡ as well as ascites and periportal edema on other images (not shown). These imaging findings are nonspecific but consistent with venoocclusive disease, which was established by clinical and biopsy evaluation.

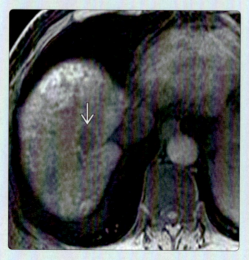
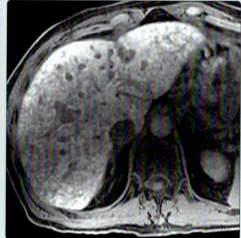

(Left) This man with hepatic metastases from colon cancer developed jaundice while receiving oxaliplatin chemotherapy. A 20-minute delayed gadoxetate-enhanced (Eovist) MR shows 1 of 2 small metastases ➡ and peculiar enhancement of liver parenchyma. (Right) Another image from the delayed-phase MR shows diffuse, reticulated hypodensity throughout the liver, representing sinusoidal obstruction syndrome due to the oxaliplatin chemotherapy.

Peliosis Hepatis

TERMINOLOGY

- Rare benign disorder characterized by sinusoidal dilation and presence of multiple blood-filled lacunar spaces within liver

IMAGING

- Multiphasic CECT or MR is best imaging tool
  - Larger cavities communicating with sinusoids have same attenuation or intensity as blood vessels
    - Multiple small accumulations of contrast; hyperdense in center or periphery of lesion
    - Thrombosed cavities appear as nonenhancing nodules
    - Fluid collection with enhancing rim represents hematoma
  - Arterial phase: Early globular, vessel-like enhancement
    - Portal phase: Centrifugal or centripetal enhancement without mass effect on hepatic vessels
    - Delayed phase: Late, diffuse, homogeneous hyperattenuation
  - Hyperintense on T2WI
    - Multiple foci of ↑ signal due to presence of subacute blood (hemorrhagic necrosis)
  - If peliotic cavities are < 1 cm in diameter, CT and MR findings may appear normal

PATHOLOGY

- Most cases are idiopathic and asymptomatic
- Associated with chronic wasting diseases and other chronic illnesses, steroid medications, and oral contraceptives
- After renal or cardiac transplantation (usually small foci not detected by imaging)
- Bacillary peliosis hepatis caused by *Bartonella* infection in patients with AIDS

CLINICAL ISSUES

- Regression after drug withdrawal, cessation of steroid therapy, resolution of associated infectious disease
- Consider clinical setting (e.g., AIDS, chronic illness, medications)

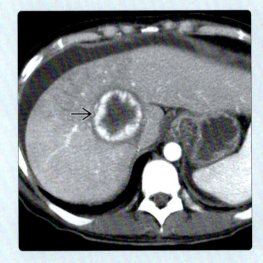

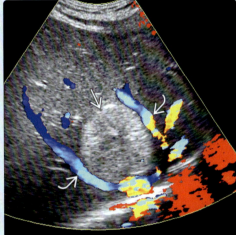

(Left) Axial arterial-phase CECT in a 42-year-old woman with diabetes and a failed renal transplantation shows a solid peripheral ring of bright enhancement ⇨ unlike the nodular, discontinuous pattern that is typical of hemangiomas. The lesion showed centripetal "fill in" of contrast on venous phase (not shown). (Right) Transverse color Doppler ultrasound in the same patient shows a hyperechoic liver mass ⇨ without prominent vascularity. The hepatic veins ⇒ are not compressed.

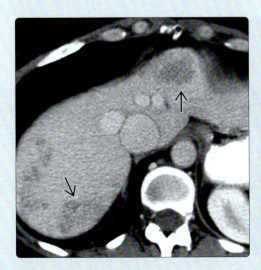

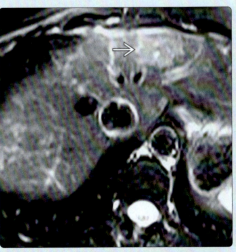

(Left) Axial venous-phase CECT in a 42-year-old woman with a 25-year history of oral contraceptive use shows multiple hypodense lesions ⇨ with enhanced periphery. (Right) Axial T2WI MR in the same patient shows a hyperintense lesion in the left lobe ⇨ corresponding to one of the lesions seen on CT. The other liver lesions had a similar appearance and partially resolved after discontinuation of contraceptives. Ultrasound-guided biopsy proved peliosis hepatis.

Hepatic Infarction

IMAGING

- Contrast-enhanced MR or CT is optimal imaging test
  - Peripheral, wedge-shaped, low-attenuation areas with absent or heterogeneous enhancement
  - Lesions may have geographic segmental distribution with straight margins
  - Lesions more conspicuous after enhancement (as perfusion defects)
  - CT or MR angiography can obviate diagnostic catheter angiography in some cases
    - Catheter angiography may be necessary for treatment
- Gadoxetate (Eovist, Primovist)-enhanced scan
  - Heterogeneous, patchy enhancement represents ischemic parenchyma
  - May see accumulation of contrast-opacified bile within infarcted tissue on delayed imaging

TOP DIFFERENTIAL DIAGNOSES

- Focal steatosis: (Can be diagnosed by selective signal loss on opposed-phase MR sequences)
- Hepatic abscess
- Hepatic trauma

CLINICAL ISSUES

- Hepatic infarction is rare due to dual blood supply from hepatic artery and portal vein, extensive collateral pathways
- Serious complication of liver transplantation
  - May be due to occlusion of hepatic artery &/or portal vein

DIAGNOSTIC CHECKLIST

- New focal liver lesion with branching pattern in transplant patient with deteriorating function suggests infarction
- Preservation of portal tracts helps differentiate infarction from abscess, biloma, or postbiopsy hematoma

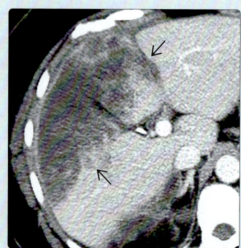
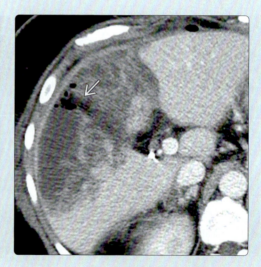

(Left) Axial CECT obtained in a 64-year-old woman who presented with RUQ pain and fever for 3 days after hemicolectomy for cecal carcinoma demonstrates a large, wedge-shaped area of nonenhancement ⇒ due to infarction. (Right) Axial CECT in the same patient shows gas ⇒ within infarcted liver tissue. The gas in the infarcted tissue was secondary to nitrogen gas release, not infection.

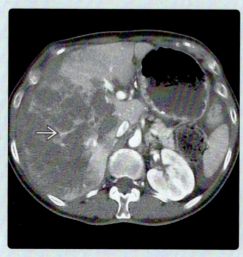
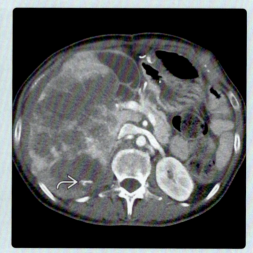

(Left) Axial CECT of a 63-year-old woman with autoimmune "connective tissue disease" and sudden RUQ pain shows a massive hypodense lesion throughout the right lobe of the liver with normal hepatic blood vessels ⇒ coursing through it, suggesting that this is not a tumor. (Right) Axial CECT in the same patient shows active bleeding ⇒ on arterial phase. At surgery, a necrotic right lobe of liver was resected. No tumor or other specific lesion was found, and the infarction was attributed to hypercoagulability and vasculitis.

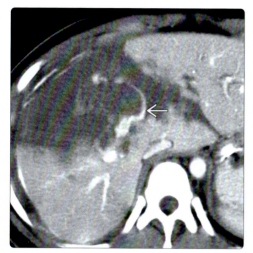 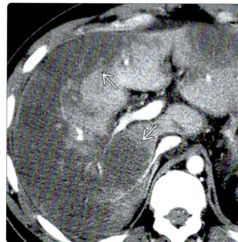

(Left) Axial CECT following blunt trauma shows no enhancement of the anterior right lobe of the liver. The hepatic artery to this segment was transected with acute extravasation ➡. (Right) Axial CECT of a 72-year-old man who developed severe RUQ pain and abnormal liver function on awakening from cardiac surgery shows massive foci of nonenhancement of the liver parenchyma ➡ involving all lobes of the liver. This patient died soon after the CT scan.

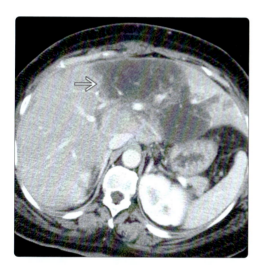 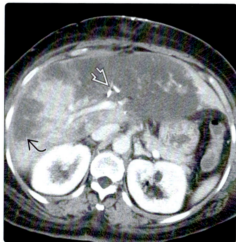

(Left) Axial CECT in a 57-year-old man 1 week post cholecystectomy shows an hepatic infarction due to the surgical disruption of hepatic arterial flow. Note the hypoattenuation of the left lobe of the liver with a linear, geographic distribution ➡. (Right) Axial CECT at a more inferior level in the same patient shows surgical clips within the course of the left hepatic artery ➡ and patchy hypoattenuation in the right hepatic lobe ➡.

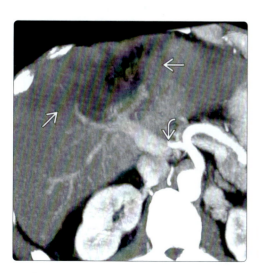 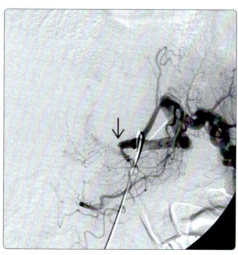

(Left) Thick, axial reconstructed CECT following liver transplantation shows the hepatic artery is thrombosed at the anastomosis ➡ with a large liver infarction ➡ of the allograft. The rest of the allograft is presumably still perfused by the portal vein, but biliary and hepatic necrosis developed soon afterward. (Right) Celiac arteriogram in the same patient shows the lack of arterial blood supply to the allograft with occlusion of the hepatic artery ➡ at the anastomosis.

Hereditary Hemorrhagic Telangiectasia

TERMINOLOGY

- Osler-Weber-Rendu syndrome
- Hereditary multiorgan disorder resulting in fibrovascular dysplasia with development of telangiectasias and AVMs
  - Skin, lungs, liver, mucus membranes, GI tract, and brain are all potentially involved

IMAGING

- **CECT (or MR) with multiplanar and angiographic reconstructions depict complex hepatic (and multiorgan) vascular alterations typical of HHT**
  - Large, tortuous extrahepatic ± intrahepatic arteries with early filling and enlargement of hepatic ± portal veins
  - Heterogeneous enhancement of hepatic parenchyma
  - Telangiectasias: Small vascular spots; more readily recognizable on reconstructed multiplanar images
  - Large, confluent vascular masses; appear as larger vascular pools (1-3 cm) with early and persistent enhancement during arterial phases

- **US**: Good screening modality for hepatic involvement
  - Dilated hepatic arteries, multiple AVMs
  - High-velocity flow in hepatic arteries (> 150 cm/sec)
  - Pulsatile flow in hepatic &/or portal veins
- **Catheter angiography**
  - Not necessary for diagnosis if CTA or MRA is available

CLINICAL ISSUES

- May be asymptomatic or anemic due to recurrent bleeds
- Multiple mucocutaneous telangiectasias with multiorgan involvement, including
  - Nasal mucosa: Recurrent epistaxis
  - Gastrointestinal: GI bleeding and angiodysplasias
  - Pulmonary: Hemoptysis, cyanosis, polycythemia, dyspnea on effort, clubbing, bruit
- Complications: High-output congestive heart failure, hepatic failure, portal hypertension

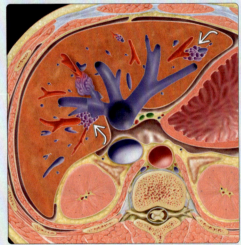
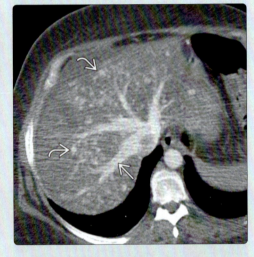

(Left) Graphic shows dilated hepatic veins and arteries with direct intraparenchymal communication through tortuous vascular channels ➡. (Right) Axial CECT shows early filling of dilated hepatic veins ➡ and innumerable small tangles of telangiectatic vessels ➡, findings diagnostic of hereditary hemorrhagic telangiectasia (HHT).

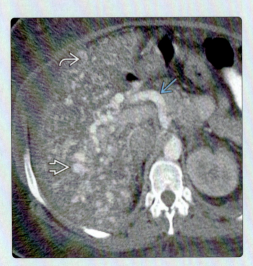
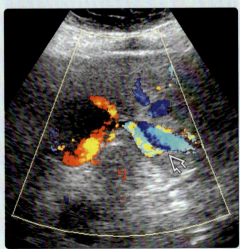

(Left) CT section in the same patient shows an enlarged hepatic artery ➡, innumerable small tangles of telangiectatic vessels ➡, and larger vascular masses or pools ➡. These findings are diagnostic of HHT (Osler-Weber-Rendu syndrome). (Right) Color Doppler sonography shows tangled masses of enlarged arteries and veins with vascular malformations ➡ bypassing the hepatic sinusoids.

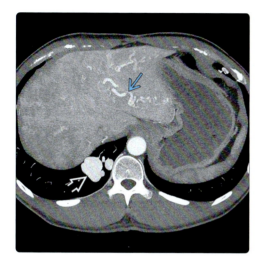

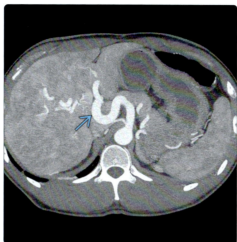

(Left) Arterial-phase CECT of a 31-year-old man with hepatic dysfunction, nosebleeds, and hemoptysis shows 1 of several large arteriovenous malformations (AVMs) ⇗ in the right lung base. The liver has a mottled enhancement pattern and enlarged, tortuous hepatic arterial branches ⇒. (Right) CT section in the same patient shows massive enlargement of the hepatic artery ⇒ and mottled enhancement of the hepatic parenchyma.

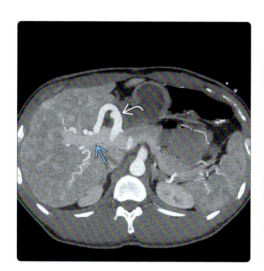

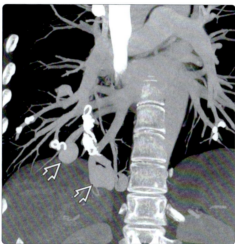

(Left) More caudal CT section in the same patient shows the huge hepatic artery ⇒ and premature filling of the portal vein ⇒. (Right) Coronal volume-rendered reconstruction of the CT in the same patient demonstrates the pulmonary AVMs ⇗. HHT (Osler-Weber-Rendu syndrome) is a hereditary disorder that results in fibrovascular dysplasia with the potential to develop telangiectasias and AVMs within many organs, most commonly the skin, lungs, liver, and GI tract.

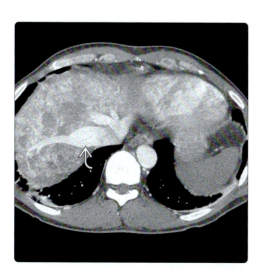

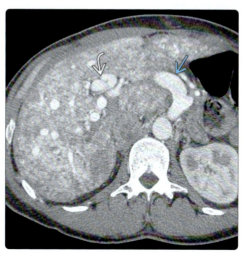

(Left) Axial CECT of a 47-year-old man with high-output heart failure due to HHT shows that the liver has a very mottled enhancement with enormous dilation of the hepatic veins ⇒, which are opacified prematurely. (Right) CT section in the same patient shows a huge hepatic artery ⇒ and diffuse telangiectasias and AVMs ⇒ throughout the liver, bypassing the sinusoids and accounting for the poor enhancement of the parenchyma.

Transjugular Intrahepatic Portosystemic Shunt (TIPS)

TERMINOLOGY

- Shunt between main portal vein and hepatic vein created with balloon-expandable metallic stent

IMAGING

- **US is primary imaging tool following transjugular intrahepatic portocaval shunt (TIPS)**
  - Goal of US: Detect stenosis before shunt occludes or symptoms recur
  - Echogenic stent is easily seen on US but does not block sound transmission
  - Color Doppler shows patency and flow direction within TIPS, portal vein, hepatic veins, and their branches
- **Shunt malfunction**
  - Hepatofugal or bidirectional flow within TIPS
  - Continuous flow (no pulsatility or respiratory change) within TIPS
  - **TIPS velocity < 90 or > 250 cm/s** at any point

- Flow away from shunt (hepatopetal) in right and left portal branches
- **Focal severe turbulence** (post stenosis)
- Absence of flow: Occlusion
- **CT and MR angiography**
  - Indicated if US is technically compromised or equivocal
  - Offers global view; including depiction of neoplastic occlusion of TIPS
- **Portal venography via jugular vein catheterization**
  - Definitive test for TIPS stenosis or occlusion
  - May allow balloon dilation of TIPS lumen or placement of new shunt within stenotic TIPS

CLINICAL ISSUES

- **Candidates for TIPS**
  - Cirrhosis with intractable ascites or variceal bleeding
  - Budd-Chiari syndrome
  - Temporizing measure, preceding liver transplantation

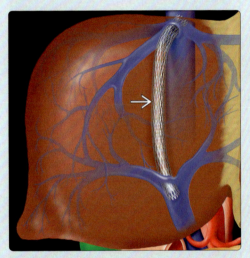
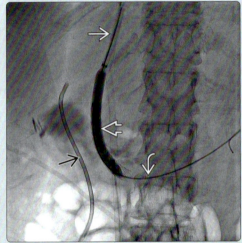

(Left) Graphic of transjugular intrahepatic portocaval shunt (TIPS) creation shows the hepatic vein punctured within 2 cm of the inferior vena cava (IVC). The metallic wire TIPS ➡ extends to the right portal vein, adjacent to its junction with the main portal vein. (Right) Image from a TIPS procedure shows the IV catheter ➡ proceeding down the IVC then penetrating the liver parenchyma to enter the portal vein ➡. The intraparenchymal tract is dilated with a balloon ➡. Incidentally noted is a plastic biliary stent ➡.

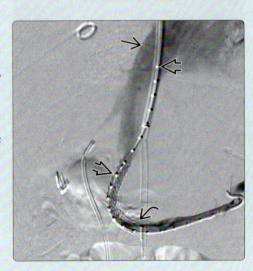
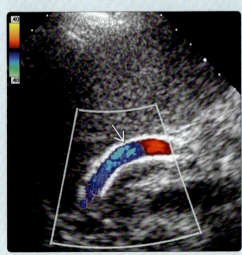

(Left) Film from the same procedure shows the TIPS itself ➡ deployed with its distal end in the hepatic vein ➡ and its proximal end in the main portal vein ➡. (Right) Longitudinal color Doppler ultrasound shows the mid portion of a normally patent TIPS ➡. Although the stent is highly echogenic, it does not obstruct sonographic visualization. Color Doppler indicates brisk flow toward the heart, the expected finding.

TERMINOLOGY

Abbreviations

- Transjugular intrahepatic portocaval shunt (TIPS)

Definitions

- Shunt between main portal vein (PV) and hepatic vein (HV) created with balloon-expandable metallic stent

IMAGING

General Features

- Location
  - Most common route: Right HV → right PV → main PV

Ultrasonographic Findings

- Grayscale ultrasound
  - Echogenic stent easily seen on grayscale images but does not block sound transmission
    - Fabric-covered stent may cause acoustic shadowing soon after placement
      □ Probably due to gas bubbles trapped in fabric
      □ May preclude US evaluation of TIPS patency for a few days
      □ Usually resolves, allowing subsequent US surveillance for TIPS stenosis
  - Stent is typically curved but not kinked
  - Hepatic and portal ends "squarely" within veins (best seen on grayscale US)
- Pulsed Doppler
  - Portal vein, satisfactory function
    - Hepatopetal flow toward heart
    - Flow toward shunt in right and left portal branches (occasionally away in left branch)
  - Shunt malfunction
    - Hepatofugal or bidirectional flow within TIPS
    - Peak velocity in portal vein < 35 cm/s
    - Flow away from shunt (hepatopetal) in right and left portal branches
  - Within shunt, malfunction
    - Continuous flow (no pulsatility or respiratory change)
    - **Shunt velocity < 90 or > 250 cm/s** at any point
    - Temporal drop in velocity ≥ 50 cm/s
    - Point-to-point increase in velocity ≥ 50 cm/s indicates focal stenosis
    - **Focal severe turbulence** (post stenosis)
    - Absence of flow: Occlusion
      □ Always confirm angiographically
- Color Doppler
  - Within shunt, malfunction
    - Visible stenosis, focal or diffuse
    - Focal color change indicates high velocity
    - Focal severe flow disturbance (post stenosis)
    - Absence of flow: Occlusion
      □ Check with spectral Doppler (more sensitive); always confirm angiographically

Other Modality Findings

- CTA, MRA
  - Anatomic depiction of stenosis, occlusion, or collateralization
  - IV contrast administration is essential for CTA; generally required for MRA

Imaging Recommendations

- Best imaging tool
  - **US is primary TIPS surveillance tool**
  - CT or MR angiography
    - Indicated if US is technically compromised or equivocal
    - Offers global view; including depiction of neoplastic occlusion of TIPS

Angiographic Findings

- Portal venography via jugular vein catheterization
  - Definitive test for TIPS stenosis or occlusion
  - May allow balloon dilation of TIPS lumen or placement of new shunt within stenotic TIPS

CLINICAL ISSUES

Presentation

- Most common signs/symptoms
  - Signs of failing TIPS
    - Recurrence of ascites, variceal hemorrhage
- Clinical profile
  - Candidates for TIPS
    - Cirrhosis with intractable ascites or variceal bleeding
    - Budd-Chiari syndrome
    - Temporizing measure, pre liver transplantation

Natural History & Prognosis

- Causes of TIPS shunts failure
  - Technical problems: Malposition, kinks, incomplete deployment, hepatic perforation with hemoperitoneum, or bile leak
  - Venous trauma during stent insertion: HV stenosis often precedes PV fibrosis or stenosis
  - Neointimal hyperplasia (may be ameliorated by covered stents but insufficient data)
  - Thrombosis
  - Hepatic arterial injury and arteriovenous fistula
  - Gallbladder injury
- Guarded prognosis
  - Maintaining shunt patency is difficult
  - Inevitable liver disease progression
  - High risk of cirrhosis-related HCC
  - 7-45% 30-day mortality

SELECTED REFERENCES

1. Orloff MJ: Fifty-three years' experience with randomized clinical trials of emergency portacaval shunt for bleeding esophageal varices in Cirrhosis: 1958-2011. JAMA Surg. 149(2):155-69, 2014
2. Kirby JM et al: Image-guided intervention in management of complications of portal hypertension: more than TIPS for success. Radiographics. 33(5):1473-96, 2013
3. Qin JP et al: Clinical effects and complications of TIPS for portal hypertension due to cirrhosis: a single center. World J Gastroenterol. 19(44):8085-92, 2013
4. Micol C et al: Contrast-enhanced ultrasound: a new method for TIPS follow-up. Abdom Imaging. 37(2):252-60, 2012
5. Wu X et al: Favorable clinical outcome using a covered stent following transjugular intrahepatic portosystemic shunt in patients with portal hypertension. J Hepatobiliary Pancreat Sci. 17(5):701-8, 2010
6. Kim MJ et al: Technical essentials of hepatic Doppler sonography. Curr Probl Diagn Radiol. 38(2):53-60, 2009

TERMINOLOGY

- Orthotopic liver transplantation (OLT)

IMAGING

- Allograft rejection
  - No reliable imaging findings to suggest or confirm diagnosis
- Biliary leak
  - From entry of T-tube: Easily treated
  - From biliary anastomosis: Requires revision
  - From intrahepatic ducts: Biliary necrosis; catastrophic
- Biliary obstruction
  - Responds to balloon dilation & stenting
- Hepatic artery (HA) stenosis
  - US: Damped waveform in HA distal to stenosis: Slow systolic upstroke; decreased resistive index (RI) (< 0.5)
  - Narrowing at HA anastomosis with turbulent flow, focally increased velocity (> 0.3 min/sec)
  - CT (or MR) angiography for detailed analysis

- HA thrombosis
  - Accompanied by biliary necrosis; catastrophic
- Hepatic arterial pseudoaneurysm
  - From biopsy or surgical error
- Portal vein (PV) stenosis
  - Uncommon: Treated by angioplasty & stent
- Recurrent disease within allograft
  - Primary sclerosing cholangitis: Tends to recur
  - Hepatocellular carcinoma (HCC)
  - Recurrent viral hepatitis or primary biliary cirrhosis
- Extrahepatic complications
  - Abdominal fluid collections
  - Posttransplant lymphoproliferative disorder

DIAGNOSTIC CHECKLIST

- Selection & interpretation of imaging studies demand close interactions among hepatologists, transplant surgeons, diagnostic & interventional radiologists

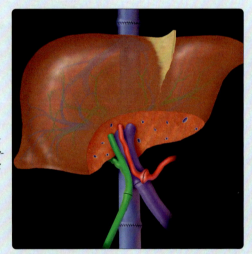
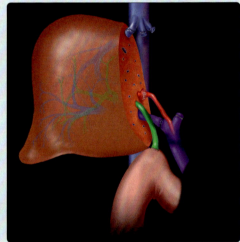

(Left) *Graphic shows the typical anatomy for whole-liver transplantation. Some liver is cut away to show anastomoses more clearly, as there are a number of common variations for vascular and biliary anastomoses.* (Right) *Graphic shows the typical anatomy of an adult partial-liver recipient (living donor). Note the biliary-enteric anastomosis to a Roux limb. Complications are more common than for whole-liver allografts due to the many transected vessels and ducts and the small size of the structures for anastomosis.*

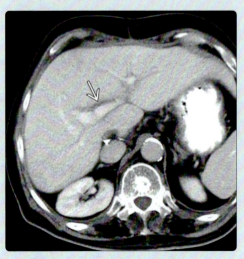
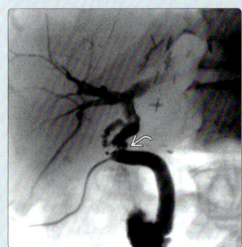

(Left) *Axial CECT shows a "halo" of low density ➡ surrounding some of the portal veins. This is a typical feature of periportal lymphedema, which is common and of no clinical concern in the early posttransplantation setting.* (Right) *T-tube cholangiogram shows a mild waist-like narrowing at the biliary anastomosis ➡ without dilation of the upstream bile ducts. This is the normal appearance of a duct-to-duct anastomosis.*

TERMINOLOGY

Definitions

- Whole-liver allograft (cadaver donor)
  - Orthotopic liver transplantation (OLT)
  - Included from donor
    - Intact inferior vena cava (IVC)
      □ Anastomosed end to end or as "piggyback" side to side
    - Hepatic artery (HA)
      □ Anastomosed end to end, sometimes with aortic (Carrel) patch
    - Portal vein (PV)
      □ End-to-end anastomosis
    - Bile duct
      □ Anastomosed end to end with recipient duct (70%) or to Roux limb
- Cadaver split liver (2 halves to separate recipients)
  - Right lobe to adult recipient (IVC, HA, PV, bile duct)
  - Left lobe to child recipient (complex anastomoses)
- Living-donor transplant
  - Child recipient: Generally receives lateral segment of donor liver
  - Adult recipient: Receives right lobe of donor
  - Complex biliary & vascular anastomoses

IMAGING

"Normal" (Common) Posttransplantation Findings

- Right pleural effusion (usually resolves spontaneously)
- Right adrenal hematoma
  - Adrenal veins injured or ligated during OLT
  - No clinical importance
- Periportal lymphedema
  - Lucent "halo" around PVs & IVC on CT, MR, US
  - No significance; resolves spontaneously as lymphatics reform
- Vascular & biliary anastomoses may show waist-like narrowing
  - But should not have functional narrowing with obstructed flow
  - Normal indices on US: HA
    - Resistive index (RI): 0.5-0.7
    - Rapid systolic acceleration time (< 80 ms)
    - Flow velocity at anastomosis < 200-300 cm/sec
  - PV
    - Mild phasicity with respiration; no turbulent flow
  - Hepatic veins (HV), IVC
    - Triphasic waveforms reflective of cardiac contractility
- Biliary anastomosis
  - Expect waist-like narrowing without dilation of upstream ducts
  - Duct-duct anastomosis may be stented with T-tube for several months
    - Allows access for cholangiography
      □ Performed in early post-OLT period & repeated as indicated
- Liver parenchyma
  - Normal texture by all imaging modalities with normal flow in all vessels

- Partial liver recipients
  - Liver regenerates to near normal volume within several months of OLT

Pretransplantation Evaluation

- Imaging & clinical evaluation of severity of cirrhosis & portal hypertension
  - Size & morphology of liver
  - Ascites, splenomegaly, extent of varices
  - Presence & stage of hepatocellular carcinoma (HCC)
    - Size, number, presence of vascular invasion, extrahepatic spread
    - Early-stage HCC may be good candidate for transplantation [↑ model for end-stage liver disease (MELD) points]
  - MELD
    - Based on etiology of cirrhosis, plus serum creatinine, bilirubin, & INR
- Detailed evaluation of hepatic vessels
  - Note any anomalies (e.g., "replaced" HA)
    - Check for severe atherosclerosis, median arcuate ligament compression of celiac axis
  - PV: Check for thrombosis, mural calcification, diminutive size
  - HVs: Check for thrombosis (Budd-Chiari)

Allograft Rejection

- No reliable imaging findings to suggest or confirm diagnosis
- Clinical suspicion leads to image-guided biopsy of allograft
  - US is best modality for guidance
    - Safest, least expensive, least discomfort

Biliary Complications

- Biliary leak
  - Leak from entry of T-tube
    - Often encountered after removal of T-tube after several months
    - Recognized by cholangiography, biliary scintigraphy, or aspiration of fluid collection identified by US or CT
    - Easily confirmed by ERCP & treated by placement of temporary biliary stent
  - Leak from biliary anastomosis
    - Usually due to surgical error
    - Often requires surgical revision of anastomosis
  - Leak from intrahepatic ducts
    - May be due to biopsy (resolves spontaneously)
    - Usually due to biliary necrosis
      □ Catastrophic result of HA stenosis or thrombosis
    - Usually requires retransplantation in adults
  - Strictures or irregularity of intrahepatic ducts
    - Nonspecific
    - Possible etiologies include incomplete distention (artifact), infection, rejection, ischemia, recurrent primary sclerosing cholangitis
- Biliary filling defects
  - Stones: Usually late complication
  - Debris: May reflect cholangitis, infection, rejection, ischemia
  - May respond to endoscopic sweeping of debris from duct ± temporary stent

- Biliary obstruction
  - Anastomotic
    - Complete obstruction usually requires surgical intervention
  - Partial
    - Usually responds to balloon dilation & stenting

Vascular Complications

- HA stenosis
  - Clinical signs: Worsening liver function
  - US: Usually 1st imaging study to suggest diagnosis
    - Examine artery in porta hepatis & within liver (main, right, & left HA)
    - Damped ("tardus parvus") waveform in HA distal to stenosis
      - Slow systolic upstroke; decreased RI (< 0.5)
    - Narrowing at HA anastomosis with turbulent flow, focally ↑ velocity (> 0.3 min/sec)
  - CT (or MR) angiography can confirm stenosis, occlusion, redundancy, kinking, or other abnormalities of HA
  - Catheter angiography usually reserved for intervention (balloon angioplasty ± stent)
- HA thrombosis
  - Usually marked by liver dysfunction, fever, malaise
  - Imaging shows no flow within HA beyond anastomosis
  - Often accompanied by **biliary necrosis** (bile ducts totally dependent on arterial supply)
    - Focal hypodense lesion or fluid collection within liver
      - May have branching pattern along portal/biliary branches
    - Can be confirmed by needle aspiration & percutaneous drainage of biloma
    - Adults: Usually fatal or requires retransplantation
    - Children: May develop sufficient collateral HA flow to preserve allograft function
- Hepatic arterial pseudoaneurysm
  - Intrahepatic: Usually due to liver biopsy
    - May resolve spontaneously or require embolic therapy
  - At HA anastomosis
    - May be due to technical error or infection
    - May respond to stent across aneurysm site or require surgical revision
- PV stenosis
  - Relatively uncommon
  - Can be suggested by US (turbulent, rapid flow across anastomosis; loss of respiratory phasicity), CT, or MR
  - Confirmed by transhepatic portography
    - Can be treated by angioplasty & stent
- IVC anastomotic stenosis
  - Relatively uncommon
  - Can be suggested by US (anastomotic narrowing, turbulent, rapid flow across anastomosis), CT, or MR
    - US
      - Loss of respiratory & cardiac phasicity (should be triphasic)
    - May see echogenic clot within IVC caudal to anastomosis
  - Presence of intraluminal pressure gradient across anastomosis confirms physiologically significant stenosis
    - Can be treated by angioplasty & stent

Recurrent Disease Within Allograft

- Primary sclerosing cholangitis
  - Tends to recur several years after OLT
- HCC
  - Relatively uncommon with proper selection of OLT candidates with early-stage HCC (according to Milan or UCSF criteria)
  - Appearance is similar to HCC in native liver
    - Heterogeneous hypervascular mass with washout; tendency toward venous invasion
- Recurrent viral hepatitis or primary biliary cirrhosis
  - Detected by imaging with return of cirrhotic morphology
    - Widened fissures, ascites, varices
  - Hepatitis B rarely recurs after transplantation due to effective antiviral prophylaxis
  - Hepatitis C recurs more frequently, as prophylaxis is less effective

Extrahepatic Complications

- Abdominal fluid collections
  - Loculated ascites ± infection; abscess; biloma
  - Easily identified by CT
  - Usually amenable to image-guided aspiration & drainage
- Posttransplant lymphoproliferative disorder
  - Caused by Epstein-Barr viral infection & immunosuppression
  - Clinical spectrum
    - Polyclonal proliferation of lymphocytes
      - Treated with antiviral medication
    - High-grade monoclonal lymphoma (non-Hodgkin)
  - Soft tissue density masses in lymph nodes, bowel, hepatic allograft, & other organs & structures throughout body
    - Recurrence within hepatic allograft
      - Soft tissue density mass(es) with tendency toward periportal distribution

CLINICAL ISSUES

Natural History & Prognosis

- Prognosis is good for properly selected patients
- Depends largely on patient's overall health at OLT
  - Varies somewhat by etiology of liver disease
    - e.g., better for patients with alcoholic cirrhosis than patients with chronic viral hepatitis
  - 1-year patient survival: 80-90%; 5 year: 75-88%

DIAGNOSTIC CHECKLIST

Image Interpretation Pearls

- US is good surveillance tool for most causes of allograft dysfunction
  - Interrogate all arteries & veins separately
- Selection & interpretation of imaging studies demands close interactions among hepatologists, transplant surgeons, diagnostic & interventional radiologists

SELECTED REFERENCES

1. Liu YI et al: Multidetector computed tomography triphasic evaluation of the liver before transplantation: importance of equilibrium phase washout and morphology for characterizing hypervascular lesions. J Comput Assist Tomogr. 36(2):213-9, 2012

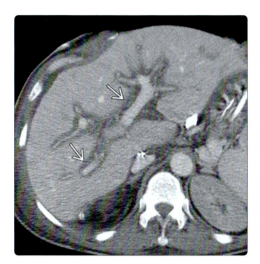 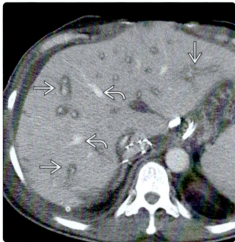

(Left) Axial CECT of a 57-year-old man with pain following recent transplantation shows a "halo" of low density ➡ surrounding the portal veins. (Right) Axial CT shows more of the periportal edema ➡, while the space around the hepatic veins ➡ is less affected. This is a common finding in the early posttransplantation setting and results from the transection of lymphatics and accumulation of lymph along the portal tracts. It generally resolves as lymphatic connections reform.

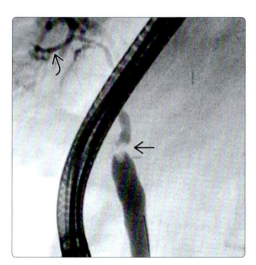 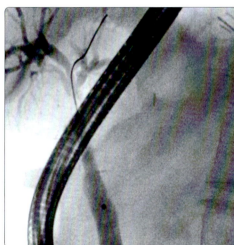

(Left) ERCP shows narrowing at the biliary anastomosis ➡ and a filling defect within the duct, which may represent some debris. There is only mild dilation of the intrahepatic (donor) ducts ➡. (Right) This same patient was treated with an endoscopic balloon sweep, dilation of the stricture, and placement of a temporary plastic stent with good results.

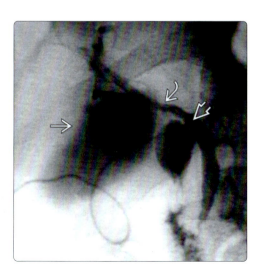 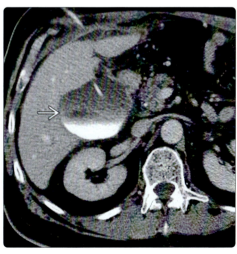

(Left) Film from a T-tube cholangiogram shows a collection of extraluminal contrast medium ➡ that originated from the site of entry of the T-tube into the recipient bile duct ➡ just distal to the anastomosis ➡. (Right) Axial CECT in the same patient reveals an extravasated collection of bile ➡ that was drained by US-guided placement of a pigtail catheter. The patient recovered uneventfully with removal of the T-tube several months later.

(Left) Color Doppler US shows a classic damped "tardus parvus" wave pattern ➡ of the right hepatic artery with a slowed systolic upstroke. Also note the decreased resistive index of 0.46 ➡. These findings are usually indicative of hepatic artery stenosis. (Right) CT angiography in the same patient demonstrates marked tortuosity of the hepatic artery ➡ and at least 1 stenotic focus at the arterial anastomosis ➡. Balloon angioplasty and stent were successful in relieving the stenosis.

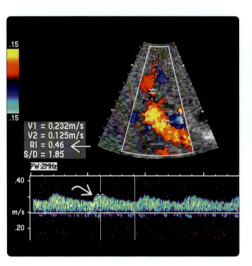
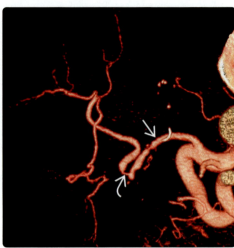

(Left) Oblique pulsed Doppler US 1 day after transplant shows a normal hepatic artery Doppler waveform ➡ at the porta hepatis. Resistive index ➡ is 0.59, which is normal. (Right) Color Doppler US in the same patient 1 day later shows a dampened flow within the hepatic artery with a tardus parvus waveform ➡ and a prolonged acceleration time (86 ms) ➡.

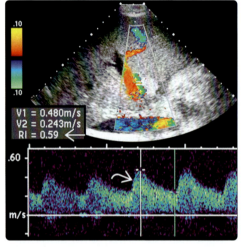
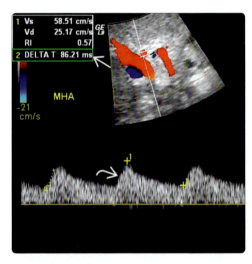

(Left) Oblique pulsed Doppler US in the same patient 2 days post transplant shows damped hepatic arterial Doppler waveforms due to hepatic arterial stenosis. Peak systolic velocity is 30 cm/sec, and the resistive index ➡ has fallen to 0.41. (Right) CT angiography in the same patient confirms a stricture at the hepatic artery anastomosis ➡. Hepatic arterial anastomotic stenosis or thrombosis is a common cause of allograft dysfunction and may lead to biliary necrosis and failed transplantation.

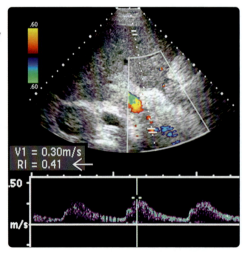
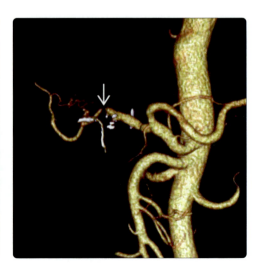

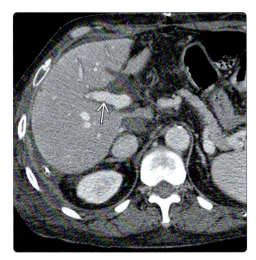

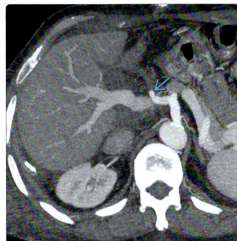

(Left) *Axial CECT of a 61-year-old man with allograft dysfunction shows an opacified portal vein* ➡ *but no hepatic artery.* **(Right)** *Thick-plane axial CT reconstruction in the same patient shows occlusion of the hepatic artery near its anastomosis* ➡. *This requires urgent revascularization by angioplasty or surgery, which is often unsuccessful. If this is the case, retransplantation is often required.*

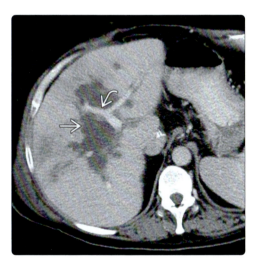

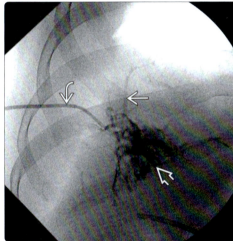

(Left) *Axial CECT shows a patent portal vein* ➡ *but no hepatic artery. There is a low-density lesion* ➡ *in the liver with a branching configuration that parallels the portobiliary tracts. This is a biloma resulting from hepatic artery thrombosis.* **(Right)** *A percutaneous catheter* ➡ *was introduced to decompress the biloma. Injection of the catheter opacifies nondilated ducts* ➡, *but many of the duct walls are necrotic and are surrounded by an amorphous collection* ➡ *of bile and contrast medium.*

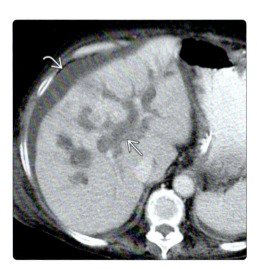

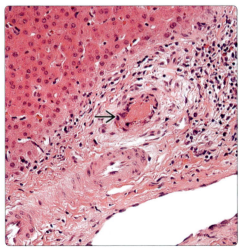

(Left) *In this patient with deteriorating allograft function, CT shows a large, low-density lesion* ➡ *that has linear, branching, and rounded components, which represent the spectrum of findings from biliary ischemia in the allograft, due to hepatic artery thrombosis. Also note the ascites* ➡. **(Right)** *This example of hepatic artery thrombosis shows ischemic bile duct injury with an eosinophilic bile cast* ➡. *(Courtesy L. Yerian, MD.)*

(Left) Color Doppler US of the portal venous anastomosis shows turbulent rapid flow ➡, suggesting stenosis. (Right) In the same patient, transhepatic cannulation of the portal vein and injection of contrast medium confirms a tight stenosis at the portal vein anastomosis ➡. This was treated with balloon dilation with good results.

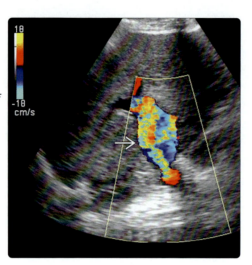
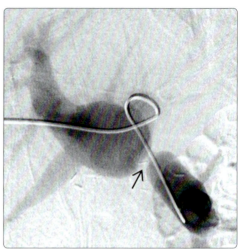

(Left) Axial CECT of a 60-year-old man with lower extremity edema following transplantation shows a normal-caliber suprahepatic inferior vena cava ➡. (Right) Axial CECT in the same patient at the level of the anastomosis ➡ shows marked narrowing of the lumen. The inferior vena cava was distended on more caudal sections.

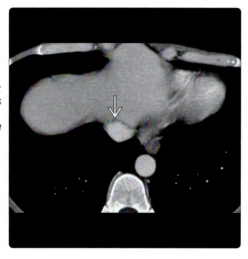
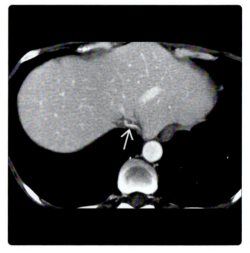

(Left) Axial CT in the same patient shows dilation of the inferior vena cava just caudal to the anastomosis ➡ of the donor and recipient inferior vena cava. (Right) Inferior vena cavagram in the same patient confirms tight stenosis at the anastomosis ➡. At least 1 collateral vein ➡ is opacified. Balloon dilation relieved the stricture with normalization of intraluminal pressure across the anastomosis.

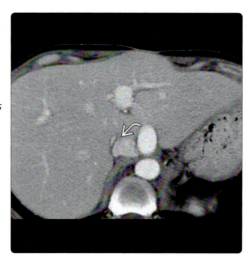
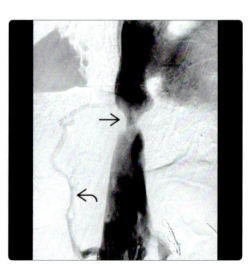

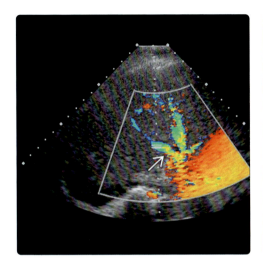

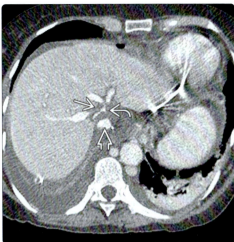

(Left) In this patient who had hepatic dysfunction and leg swelling following a recent liver transplantation, color Doppler US suggests narrowing of the hepatic veins near their confluence ➡. (Right) Axial CECT in the same patient shows evidence of a "piggyback" anastomosis of the donor inferior vena cava ➡ to the recipient inferior vena cava ➡. The donor inferior vena cava and confluence of hepatic veins appear to be strictured ➡.

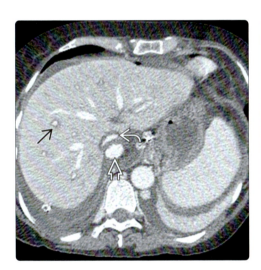

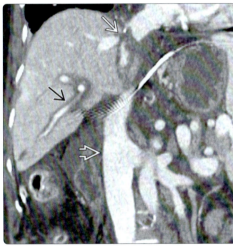

(Left) A more caudal section in the same patient shows a narrowed donor inferior vena cava ➡, dilated recipient inferior vena cava ➡, and periportal edema ➡ within the liver allograft. (Right) Coronal reformatted CT from the same patient shows distention of the recipient inferior vena cava ➡, stricture at the inferior vena cava anastomosis ➡, and periportal edema ➡. This patient had allograft dysfunction and leg edema.

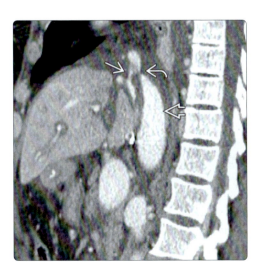

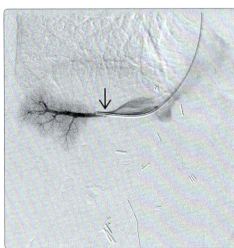

(Left) CT reformation in the same patient shows the strictured "piggyback" anastomosis ➡ to the recipient inferior vena cava ➡ and narrowing of at least 1 of the hepatic veins ➡. (Right) Catheter hepatic venogram confirms stenosis of the hepatic veins at the inferior vena cava anastomosis ➡. These strictures were balloon dilated with improvement of symptoms and liver function.

(Left) *In this 52-year-old man who had received a multivisceral transplant (liver, pancreas, and small bowel), axial CECT shows the anastomotic site between the donor and recipient aorta ➡ with this vessel feeding the small bowel, liver, and pancreatic ➡ allografts, all of which appear normal.* **(Right)** *Axial CT in the same patient shows a normal appearance of the infrarenal aortic anastomosis ➡ and the pancreatic allograft ➡.*

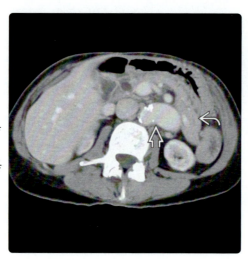
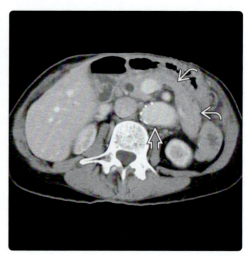

(Left) *Lower axial CT in the same patient shows a normal appearance of the small bowel allograft ➡. All 3 transplanted organs functioned normally, and the patient no longer required parenteral nutrition nor insulin.* **(Right)** *Coronal reformatted CT in the same patient shows the end-to-side aortic anastomosis ➡, which supplied blood to all 3 allografts.*

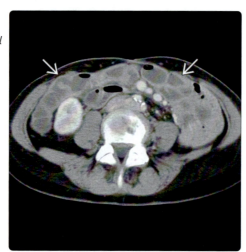
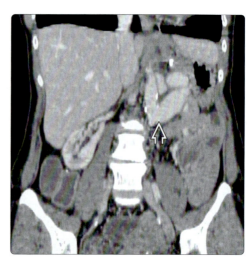

(Left) *In this 54-year-old woman with a multivisceral transplant, axial CT shows the pancreatic ➡ and liver allografts. The small bowel allograft was normal in appearance on more caudal sections (not shown). The aortic anastomosis is noted ➡.* **(Right)** *On this 3D reconstruction of the same CT scan, the donor aorta is redundant and acutely kinked ➡, causing luminal narrowing and requiring surgical revision. The anastomosis with the native aorta is seen ➡.*

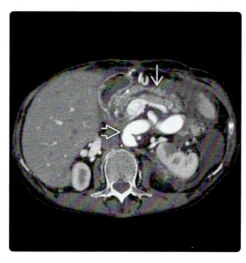
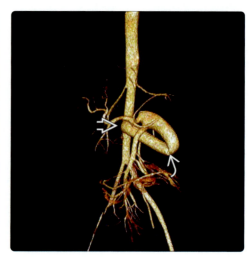

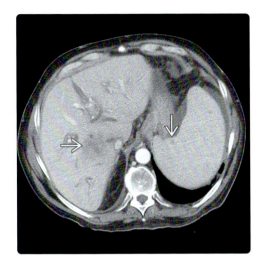

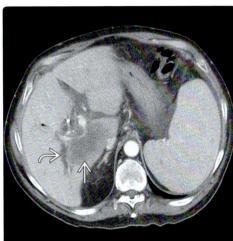

(Left) Axial CECT of a 55-year-old man with fever and weight loss months after transplantation due to posttransplant lymphoproliferative disorder (PTLD) shows hepatosplenomegaly with poorly defined, hypodense masses ➡ within both organs. (Right) Axial CT in the same patient also shows obstruction of intrahepatic bile ducts ➡ due to a combination of the hepatic tumor ➡ and porta hepatic adenopathy (better shown on the following images).

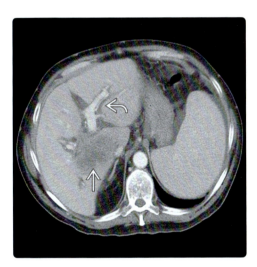

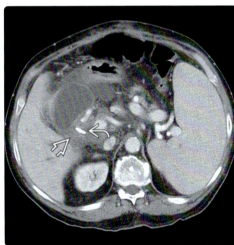

(Left) Axial CT in the same patient shows more of the hepatic tumor (PTLD ➡) and the obstructed bile ducts ➡. (Right) CT in the same patient shows porta hepatic adenopathy ➡ that contributed to the biliary obstruction. This was partially relieved by a biliary stent ➡. All of these features are typical of PTLD following hepatic transplantation.

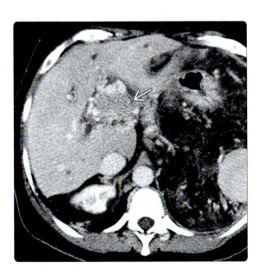

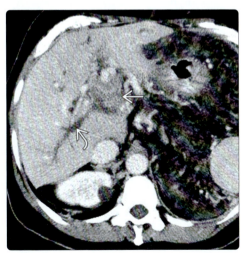

(Left) In a patient with PTLD, axial CECT shows dilation of the intrahepatic bile ducts and a hypovascular mass ➡ in the hilum that compresses the portal vein and central bile ducts. Biopsy of the mass proved PTLD within the hepatic allograft. (Right) A more caudal section in the same patient shows the central hilar mass of PTLD ➡ that compresses and partially obstructs the portal vein and common hepatic duct with dilated ducts upstream ➡.

Liver

TERMINOLOGY

- Iatrogenic changes to hepatic morphology that may cause or simulate pathologic conditions

IMAGING

- **Gas collection** in hepatic or perihepatic lesion or portal vein
  - Consider iatrogenic infarction of hepatic mass or liver parenchyma
  - Consider retained absorbable oxidized cellulose (Surgicel, Gelfoam)
    - Sponge-like appearance of gas bubbles
    - Little or no fluid nor capsule
  - Not always indicative of infection
- Embolized, iodinated, poppyseed oil (Ethiodol, Lipiodol)
  - May mimic calcified or hypervascular mass on plain radiography or CT, respectively
- Treated tumor often undergoes progressive volume loss and fibrosis

- May simulate focal confluent fibrosis, peripheral cholangiocarcinoma, or cirrhosis
  - Hepatic mets from breast cancer often result in pseudocirrhosis appearance
- Treated, nonviable tumor on MR
  - Often bright on nonenhanced T1WI, dark (hypointense) on T2WI
  - Opposite typical appearance of viable tumor
- Consider prior resection of portions of liver
  - May have similar appearance to congenital absence or hypoplasia of hepatic segments
- Iatrogenic arterioportal (AP) fistula
  - Complication of percutaneous liver biopsy
  - May simulate other vascular lesions, including tumor
- Small peripheral AP shunts are common, spontaneous findings in cirrhotic liver

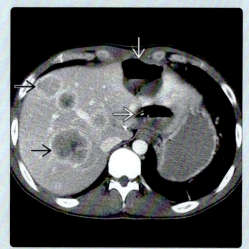
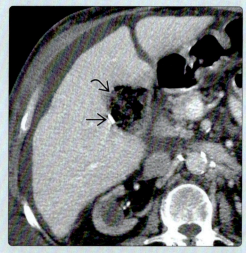

(Left) Axial CECT shows several viable enhancing liver metastases ⇲ and 2 masses with gas and necrotic debris ⇲ that are the result of percutaneous radiofrequency ablation. (Right) Axial CECT shows a collection of gas ⇲ but very little fluid in the cholecystectomy bed, mimicking an abscess. Note the surgical clips ⇲. This is bioabsorbable oxidized cellulose (Surgicel), which was used as a hemostatic agent to control bleeding from the operative bed during cholecystectomy.

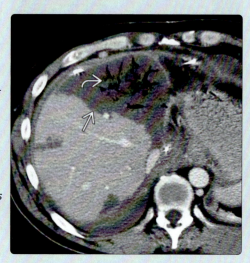
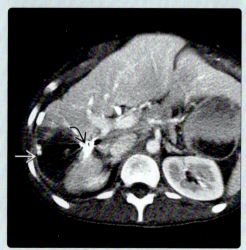

(Left) Axial CECT shows an absence of enhancement of the left lobe with a straight line of demarcation ⇲ and portal venous gas ⇲, all due to hepatic arterial ligation during attempted resection of a peripheral cholangiocarcinoma. (Right) Axial CECT shows a metallic coil ⇲ in the right hepatic artery, with a wedge-shaped collection ⇲ of gas and fluid "downstream." Needle aspiration and drainage of this collection showed an infected hepatic infarction.

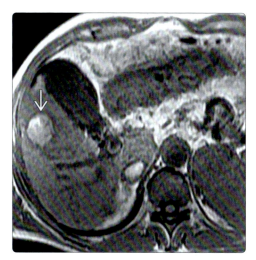

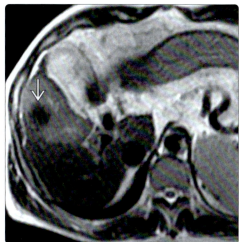

(Left) *Axial T1WI MR of a hepatocellular carcinoma (HCC) following arterial chemoembolization shows the mass* ⇒ *as hyperintense, which would be unusual for a viable HCC. No viable tumor is present.* (Right) *In the same patient, the nonviable HCC lesion* ⇒ *is hypointense on T2WI, which would be atypical for a viable HCC.*

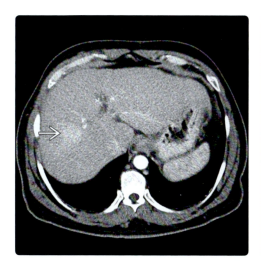

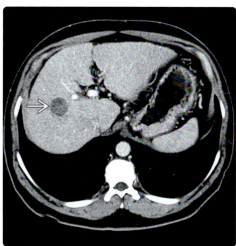

(Left) *Arterial phase CECT of HCC shows a subtle, hypervascular, 2-cm nodule* ⇒ *in the right lobe along with signs of cirrhosis (widened fissures, etc.).* (Right) *Portal venous phase image in the same patient shows classic washout of contrast medium from the nodule* ⇒*, essentially diagnostic of HCC in this setting. The patient was treated with transarterial chemoembolization, including Lipiodol.*

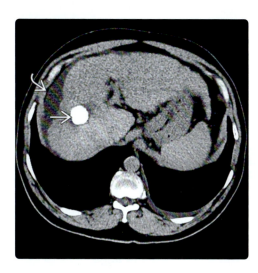

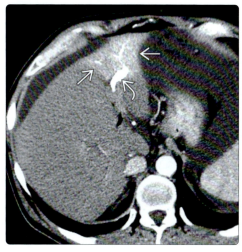

(Left) *Follow-up NECT in the same patient shows retention of the iodinated Lipiodol* ⇒ *within the tumor. Note the indirect evidence of hepatic injury, with volume loss of the right lobe and ascites* ⇒*.* (Right) *Arterial phase CECT shows hyperenhancement of a portion of the lateral segment of the liver (THAD)* ⇒ *and early enhancement of the portal vein branch* ⇒ *that drains this segment. This represents an arterioportal shunt and is probably the result of a prior biopsy of the liver at this site.*

Liver

IMAGING

- Simple, uncomplicated cyst
  - Often multiple (usually < 10), of variable size
- **US**: Anechoic mass, accentuated through transmission
  - Smooth borders; thin or invisible wall
  - Usually no or few thin septations
- **CT**: Contents: Water density (-10 to +10 HU)
  - No mural nodularity or wall calcification
- **MR**: Contents
  - T1WI: Hypointense (dark)
  - T2WI: Hyperintense (very bright)
- **Hemorrhage into or infection of cyst may simulate tumor**
  - Thickened wall ± calcification
  - Mural nodularity ± fluid-debris level
  - No enhancement of "solid" material or cyst contents
  - Varied MR signal intensity (due to mixed blood products)
- Cyst aspiration may be helpful in confirming infected or hemorrhagic cyst

TOP DIFFERENTIAL DIAGNOSES

- Polycystic liver disease: More numerous cysts ± cysts in other organs
- Cystic or necrotic metastases: Usually show complexity on careful image analysis
- Biliary cystadenocarcinoma: Solitary, large, complex, in middle-aged woman
- Biliary hamartomas: Multiple, all < 15 mm, variably echogenic on US
- Cavernous hemangioma: May simulate cyst on T2WI
- Hepatic pyogenic abscess: More complex; in febrile patient
- Hydatid (echinococcal) disease: Invariably more complex with daughter cysts ± calcified wall

DIAGNOSTIC CHECKLIST

- Sonography shows cyst morphology better than CT
- Hepatic metastases from gastrointestinal stromal tumor
  - Respond to chemotherapy so well that they simulate simple cysts on follow-up exams

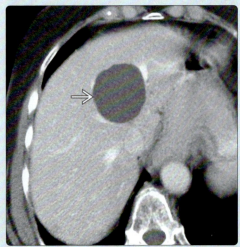
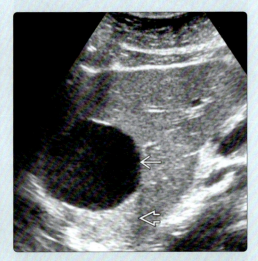

(Left) Axial CECT shows a spherical hepatic mass ⇨ with water density and homogeneous contents. No internal debris or wall irregularities are present. This is a classic simple cyst. (Right) US in the same patient shows an anechoic mass ⇨ with accentuated through transmission ⇨. Either CT or US would have been sufficient to establish the diagnosis in this patient.

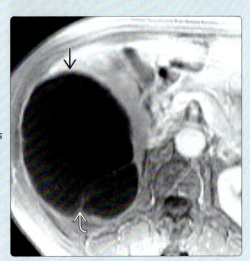
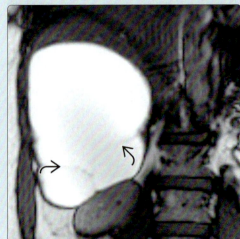

(Left) Axial T1WI MR shows a large, cystic hepatic mass ⇨ that has homogeneous low intensity and several thin septa ⇨. (Right) Coronal T2WI MR shows uniform high intensity and the septa ⇨. The cyst has remained stable for years, and no other evaluation or intervention was performed.

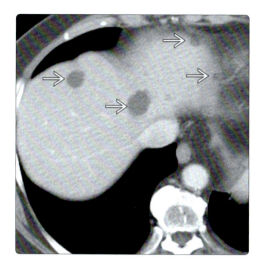

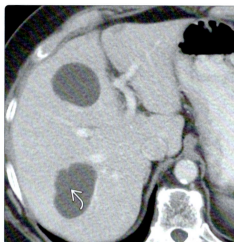

(Left) Axial CECT shows multiple water density hepatic lesions ➡ with no discernible walls. (Right) Axial CECT section in the same patient shows that one of the larger cysts has a thin septum ➡. Simple hepatic cysts are commonly multiple, and this is not necessarily evidence of autosomal dominant polycystic disease, which usually results in many more and larger cysts. Biliary hamartomas can also cause an appearance of multiple "cysts," but these are rarely > 15 mm in diameter.

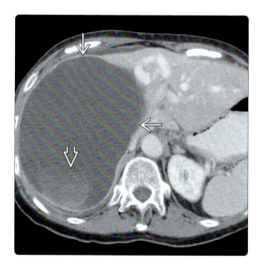

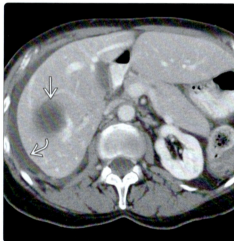

(Left) Axial CT section in this patient shows a heterogeneous focus of higher attenuation ➡ within a large cyst ➡, suggestive of acute hemorrhage. (Right) Axial CT section in the same patient shows ascites ➡ that had an attenuation of ~ 15 HU, suggesting intraperitoneal rupture of the cyst ➡. These findings were confirmed at surgery, and the cyst was resected.

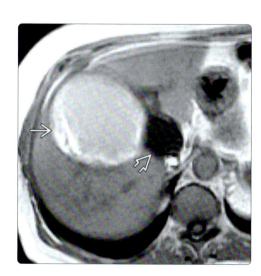

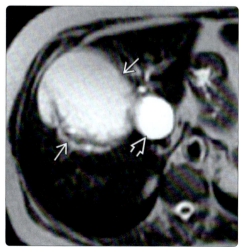

(Left) Two masses are seen in the liver of this 70-year-old woman with RUQ pain with the larger cyst having contents that are bright ➡ on T1WI MR, while the smaller cyst's contents are low in signal ➡. (Right) Axial T2WI MR in the same patient shows very bright, uniform signal within the smaller (simple) cyst ➡, while the larger cyst's contents are more heterogeneous with mural irregularity and debris evident ➡. Aspiration of the larger cyst yielded hemorrhagic fluid with no sign of infection or neoplasm.

Hepatic Cavernous Hemangioma

IMAGING

- Best imaging modality: **Multiphasic MR** (though most can be diagnosed confidently on **multiphasic CT**)
  - **Hemangiomas are nearly as bright as CSF on T2WI**
  - **Follow blood pool on contrast-enhanced images**
  - Small hemangiomas ("capillary"): < 2 cm
    - Arterial and venous phases: Usually show homogeneous enhancement ("flash-filling")
  - Typical hemangiomas: 2-5 cm in diameter
    - Arterial phase: Early peripheral, nodular or globular, discontinuous enhancement
    - Venous phase: Progressive centripetal enhancement, still isodense (isointense on MR) to vessels
    - Delayed phase: Persistent complete "filling in"
  - Giant hemangioma: > 5 cm in diameter
    - Arterial phase: Typical peripheral, nodular, cloud-like, or globular enhancement

- Venous and delayed phases: Incomplete centripetal filling of lesion (scar does not enhance)
  - Scar is even more intense (brighter) than rest of lesion on T2WI
- **Ultrasonography**
  - Hemangiomas are typically uniformly or peripherally echogenic
  - Small, uniformly echogenic lesion in healthy, young patient is almost always hemangioma

DIAGNOSTIC CHECKLIST

- Hepatocellular carcinoma and hypervascular metastases may mimic hemangioma on arterial phase but usually "wash out" on delayed phase
- Cholangiocarcinoma may show delayed enhancement
  - But other features are distinctive (e.g., biliary obstruction)

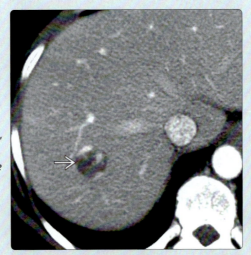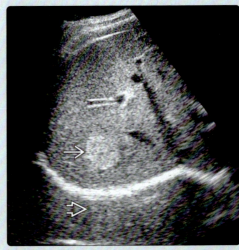

(Left) *Axial venous/parenchymal-phase CECT shows a spherical mass ➡ with nodular, discontinuous, peripheral enhancement that is nearly isodense to blood vessels. The lesion was also isodense with blood on an unenhanced CT (not shown) and showed progressive centripetal "fill in" on delayed CECT.* (Right) *Sagittal sonogram in the same patient shows a uniformly hyperechoic lesion ➡ in the peripheral right lobe with possible acoustic enhancement ➡, typical features of hemangioma.*

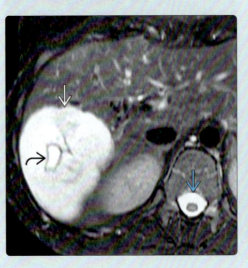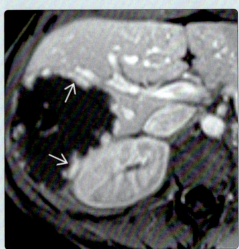

(Left) *Axial T2WI MR demonstrates a mass ➡ with marked hyperintensity, similar to that of CSF ➡. A central scar ➡ within the mass is even more hyperintense, a typical feature of a large or giant hemangioma.* (Right) *Axial arterial-phase T1WI MR in the same patient shows nodular, discontinuous, peripheral enhancement ➡ of the hemangioma, isointense to hepatic vessels, that persisted and progressed on subsequent phases (not shown).*

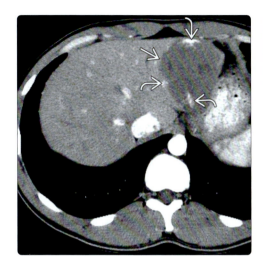
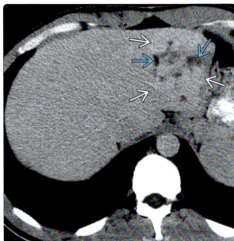

(Left) *In this man with an hepatic mass discovered on a prior US, arterial-phase CECT shows nodular, peripheral, cloud-like enhancement ⮞ of the mass ➡. Venous-phase CT (not shown) showed centripetal enhancement with the enhanced portions of the mass remaining isodense with blood pool.* (Right) *In the same patient, a 10-minute delayed CECT shows almost complete "fill in" of the mass ➡ , except for a few foci of scar or necrosis ➡ typical of larger hemangiomas. The enhanced portions of the mass remain isodense with blood pool.*

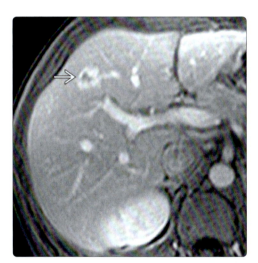
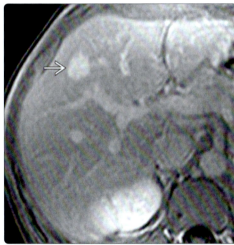

(Left) *Axial late arterial-phase T1WI contrast-enhanced MR shows a small mass ➡ with solid ring enhancement, an unusual feature for cavernous hemangioma.* (Right) *The hemangioma ➡ in the same patient demonstrates rapid and complete fill in on this portal venous-phase image and remained isointense to blood pool on delayed-phase images rather than washing out, as would be expected for most malignant hepatic masses.*

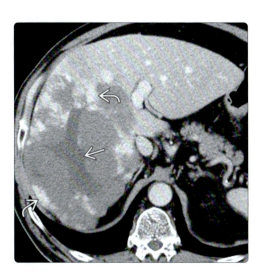
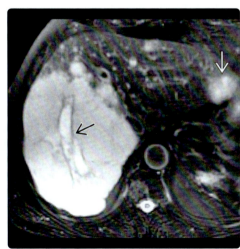

(Left) *Axial venous/parenchymal-phase CECT in a 55-year-old man with a palpable RUQ mass shows a large mass with nodular or cloud-like peripheral enhancement ⮞ and a nonenhancing central scar ➡. This was a proven "giant" hemangioma.* (Right) *Axial T2WI MR in the same patient shows a large, diffusely hyperintense "giant" hemangioma with a central scar ➡ that is even more intense. Several other hemangiomas were also noted ➡.*

Focal Nodular Hyperplasia

TERMINOLOGY

- Benign hepatic mass caused by hyperplastic response to localized vascular abnormality
- 2nd most common benign tumor, usually in young women
  - Was considered rare until multiphasic CT and MR became widespread

IMAGING

- **Multiphasic CT or MR with conventional contrast media**
  - **Bright, homogeneously enhancing mass on arterial phase with small, T2WI (bright), central scar is diagnostic** of focal nodular hyperplasia (FNH)
  - Portal venous phase scan
    - Hypodense or isodense to normal liver
  - Delayed scans
    - Mass: Isodense to normal liver
    - Central scar: Hyperdense or hyperintense (due to fibrous tissue)
- **Gadoxetate-enhanced (Eovist) MR**

- Prolonged enhancement of entire FNH (except scar) on hepatobiliary phase, ≥ liver
- **Most specific test to diagnose FNH** (but not always necessary)

TOP DIFFERENTIAL DIAGNOSES

- Hepatic adenoma
  - Rarely retains gadoxetate on hepatobiliary-phase MR
- Fibrolamellar carcinoma
  - Heterogeneous mass; large, calcified scar; no retention of gadoxetate on MR
- Hypervascular metastases
  - Often multiple; no retention of gadoxetate

DIAGNOSTIC CHECKLIST

- Imaging is more reliable than histology in making diagnosis of FNH
- Classic FNH resembles cross section of orange
  - (Homogeneous, central "scar," radiating septa)

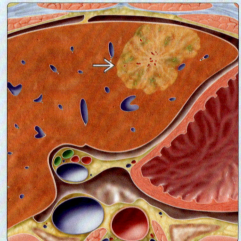
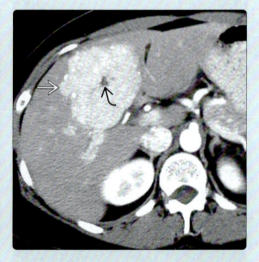

(Left) Graphic shows a homogeneous, vascular, nonencapsulated mass ➡ with a central scar and thin radiating septa dividing the mass into hyperplastic nodules. Note the cluster of small arteries near the central scar. (Right) Axial arterial-phase CECT shows bright, homogeneous enhancement of a mass ➡ with a central scar ➡ in an asymptomatic young woman who had a mass found on ultrasound. The CT findings in this case are diagnostic of focal nodular hyperplasia (FNH) and require no further evaluation.

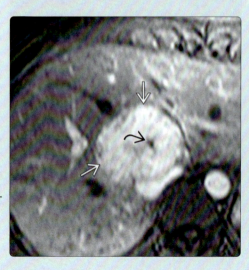
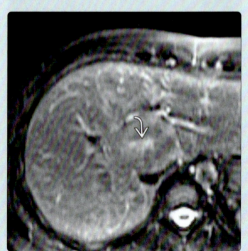

(Left) Axial arterial-phase T1WI MR using conventional contrast media of a young woman shows bright, homogeneous enhancement of the FNH ➡ with no early enhancement of the scar ➡. (Right) Axial T2WI MR in the same patient shows the FNH as isointense to the liver, whereas the central scar is hyperintense ➡. The near isointensity of the mass to the liver on both T1WI and T2WI MRs would be very unusual for any mass other than FNH.

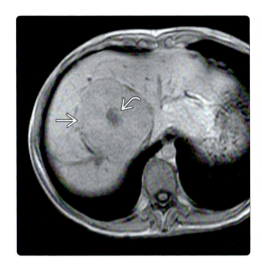
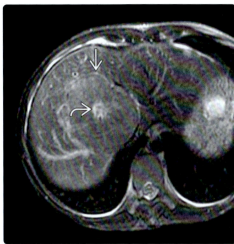

(Left) Axial T1WI MR of a 28-year-old woman with a mass detected on US performed for right upper quadrant pain shows the mass ➡ as nearly isointense to the liver with a hypointense central scar ➚. (Right) Axial T2WI MR of the same patient shows the mass ➡ is also nearly isointense to the normal liver, whereas the scar is hyperintense ➘.

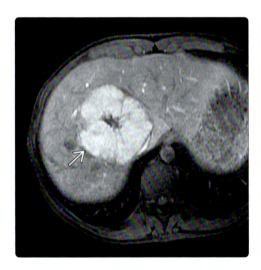
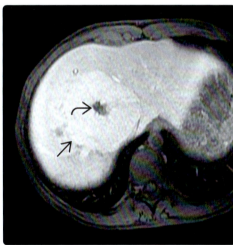

(Left) On arterial-phase axial T1WI MR following bolus injection of gadoxetate (Eovist) in the same patient, the FNH ➡ enhances brightly and homogeneously, except for the central scar. (Right) On venous-phase axial T1WI MR of the same patient, the mass ➡ has returned to near isointensity with background liver, and the central scar ➘ remains hypointense.

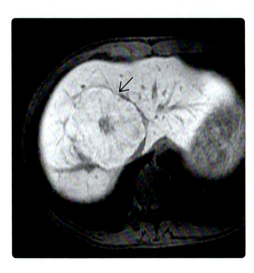
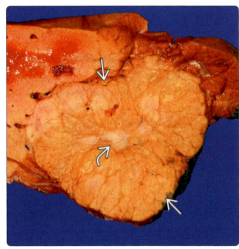

(Left) On hepatobiliary (20-minute delayed)-phase T1WI MR, the FNH ➘ retains gadoxetate and is now homogeneously hyperintense to background liver (except for the central scar), a feature indicating the presence of functioning hepatocytes and delayed biliary clearance. These MR features are diagnostic of FNH. (Right) Gross photograph of the bisected, resected specimen shows the circumscribed FNH ➡ and the central fibrous scar ➘. The FNH was resected because it was causing pain.

IMAGING

- Key features (not always present): Hypervascular, fat-containing, hemorrhagic, encapsulated
- **MR shows some elements better than CT (lipid & hemorrhage)**
  - T1WI: Mass: Heterogeneous signal intensity
    - Increased signal intensity (due to fat or recent hemorrhage)
    - Decreased signal intensity (necrosis, calcification, old hemorrhage)
  - T2WI: Mass: Heterogeneous signal intensity
    - Increased signal intensity (old hemorrhage, necrosis)
    - Decreased signal intensity (fat, recent hemorrhage)
- **Gadoxetate-enhanced MR (Eovist, Primovist)**
  - Adenoma shows no substantial uptake or retention
  - Key distinction from focal nodular hyperplasia (FNH)

PATHOLOGY

- **New classification based on genetics, pathology, & tumor biology**
- Inflammatory hepatic adenoma (HA) (most common; 40%)
  - Occur in young women on oral contraceptives & obese women
  - Likely to show MR (& clinical) evidence of hemorrhage (up to 30%)
  - 10% estimated likelihood of malignant degeneration to hepatocellular carcinoma (HCC)
- *HNF-1α*-mutated HA (30-40%)
  - Least aggressive subtype (rare bleeding or HCC)
  - Exclusively in women; 90% have history of oral contraceptive use
- *β-catenin*-mutated HA (10-15%)
  - Most likely to occur in men, those taking androgenic steroids, & in patients with glycogen storage disease
  - Highest risk of malignant transformation (> 10%)

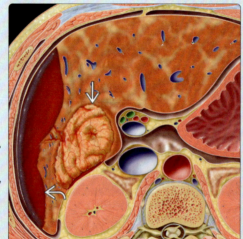
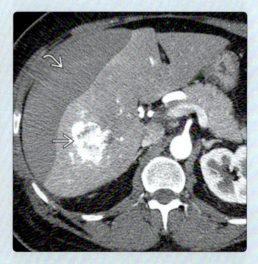

(Left) *Graphic shows a hypervascular mass ➡ in the right lobe and spontaneous subcapsular bleeding ➡.* **(Right)** *Axial CECT of a 40-year-old woman with sudden RUQ pain and syncope shows an intensely enhancing mass ➡ in the right lobe of the liver. A lentiform, heterogeneous collection of fluid indents the surface of the liver, and within this collection is a focus of higher density ➡ likely representing a "sentinel" clot. A ruptured "inflammatory" hepatic adenoma was resected.*

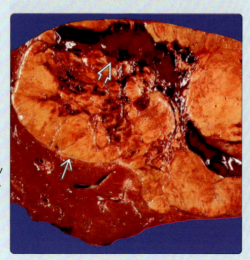
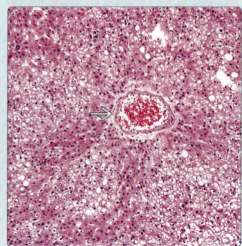

(Left) *Gross photograph of a resected specimen shows a large adenoma ➡ with central areas of rupture and hemorrhage ➡. (Courtesy M. Yeh, MD, PhD.)* **(Right)** *Photomicrograph of a hepatic adenoma features a thin-walled unpaired vessel ➡ surrounded by neoplastic hepatocytes with abundant steatosis. Imaging often reveals these features, directly or indirectly. (Courtesy M. Yeh, MD, PhD.)*

TERMINOLOGY

Synonyms
- Hepatocellular adenoma, liver cell adenoma

Definitions
- Heterogeneous group of benign hepatocellular neoplasms with distinctive genetic, pathologic, & clinical features

IMAGING

General Features
- Best diagnostic clue
  - Heterogeneous, hypervascular mass with foci of fat or hemorrhage in young woman
- Location
  - Subcapsular region of right lobe of liver (75%)
  - Intraparenchymal or pedunculated (10%)
- Size
  - Varies from 6-30 cm
- Key concepts
  - Very uncommon relative to focal nodular hyperplasia (FNH) & hepatocellular carcinoma (HCC)
  - 3 distinct subtypes with different genetics, pathology, clinical features

CT Findings
- Depending on hepatic adenoma (HA) subtype
  - Encapsulation seen in ~ 20%, best on delayed-phase CECT
  - Hemorrhage within tumor, best seen on NECT as hyperdense foci
  - Intratumoral lipid, best seen on NECT as hypodense foci
  - Hypervascularity
    - Most intense & persistent in inflammatory subtype of HA
  - Calcification: Focal, present in ~ 5%

MR Findings
- T1WI
  - Mass: Heterogeneous signal intensity
    - Increased signal intensity (due to fat & recent hemorrhage), more evident on MR than CT
    - Decreased signal intensity (necrosis, calcification, old hemorrhage)
  - Rim (fibrous pseudocapsule): Hypointense
- T2WI
  - Mass: Heterogeneous signal intensity
    - Increased signal intensity (old hemorrhage, necrosis)
    - Decreased signal intensity (fat, recent hemorrhage)
  - Rim (fibrous pseudocapsule): Hypointense
- T1WI C+
  - Gadolinium, arterial phase
    - Heterogeneous hypervascular enhancement (especially in inflammatory subtype)
  - Delayed phase
    - Pseudocapsule: Hyperintense to liver & adenoma
- Gadoxetate-enhanced MR (Eovist, Primovist)
  - Hepatocellular-specific contrast agent
  - Adenoma shows no substantial uptake or retention on delayed imaging
    - Key distinction from FNH

Ultrasonographic Findings
- Grayscale ultrasound
  - Well-defined, solid, echogenic mass
  - Complex, hyper-/hypoechoic, heterogeneous mass with anechoic areas
    - Due to fat, hemorrhage, necrosis, & calcification
    - Capsule may be seen

Imaging Recommendations
- Best imaging tool
  - Gadoxetate-enhanced MR, including multiphasic & delayed imaging
  - In- & opposed-phase GRE

DIFFERENTIAL DIAGNOSIS

Hepatocellular Carcinoma
- May be hard to distinguish on imaging or pathology
- Biliary, vascular, nodal invasion & metastases = malignancy
- HCC typically occurs in older, cirrhotic men
  - Adenoma occurs in young, healthy women

Fibrolamellar Hepatocellular Carcinoma
- Large, lobulated mass with scar & septa
- Vascular, biliary invasion & metastases common

Focal Nodular Hyperplasia
- Arterial phase
  - FNH is **homogeneously** enhancing mass
- All other phases: Isodense to normal liver
- T2WI: Scar is typically hyperintense

Hypervascular Metastases
- Usually multiple; look for primary tumors
  - Breast, thyroid, kidney, & endocrine
- Arterial phase: Heterogeneous enhancement
- Portal & delayed phases: Iso-/hypodense washout

PATHOLOGY

General Features
- Etiology
  - ↑ risk in oral contraceptive & anabolic steroid users
  - Pregnancy increases growth rate & risk of rupture
  - Hepatic steatosis ↑ growth & number of adenomas
  - Diabetes mellitus
  - von Gierke type I glycogen storage disease
    - Multiple adenomas in 60% of affected patients

Staging, Grading, & Classification
- Proposed **new classification based on genetics, pathology, & tumor biology**
- 3 distinct subtypes
  - Inflammatory HA
    - Most common subtype (40-50%)
    - Includes those previously called "telangiectatic HA"
    - Occur in young women on oral contraceptives & obese women
    - 60% have mutation of *IL6ST* gene with altered glycoprotein metabolism

- MR: No excessive fat or lipid within masses; persistent hypervascularity through arterial & venous phases due to sinusoidal dilation, peliotic areas, & abnormal vessels
  □ Bright on T2WI
  □ Likely to show MR (& clinical) evidence of hemorrhage (up to 30%)
  □ 10% estimated likelihood of malignant degeneration to HCC
- *HNF-1a*-mutated HA
  – 2nd most common subtype (30-35% of HAs)
  – Association with diabetes & familial hepatic adenomatosis
  – Exclusively in women; 90% have history of oral contraceptive use
  – Mutated *HNF-1a* gene promotes lipogenesis & hepatocellular proliferation
  – MR: Diffuse lipid deposition within HAs
    □ Most evident as signal dropout on opposed-phase GRE T1WI
    □ Macroscopic fat deposits are less common
    □ Only moderate enhancement on arterial phase; no persistent enhancement on venous & delayed
  – Least aggressive subtype
    □ HAs of this subtype < 5 cm rarely bleed & have minimal risk of HCC
- *β-catenin*-mutated HA
  – Least common subtype (10-15% of HAs)
  – Subtype most likely to occur in men, those taking androgenic steroids, & in patients with glycogen storage disease
    □ Also associated with metabolic syndrome
  – Mutation of *β-catenin* disrupts hepatocyte proliferation, growth, adhesion, etc.
  – This subtype carries highest risk of malignant transformation (> 10%)
  – MR features: No distinctive pattern established
    □ Usually hypervascular with evidence of hemorrhage or necrosis within tumor
- Unclassified HA subtype
  – Does not fit other profiles of HA subtypes

Gross Pathologic & Surgical Features

- Well-circumscribed mass within noncirrhotic liver
  - Soft, pale, or yellowish tan
  - Frequently bile-stained nodules
  - Foci of fat, hemorrhage, infarction
  - "Pseudocapsule" & occasional "pseudopods"
- **Adenomatosis**
  - No strict definition (generally > 10 adenomas)
  - Associated with glycogen storage disease, steatosis, & diabetes
  - May number > 100 adenomas
    – May cause hepatic dysfunction, hemorrhage

Microscopic Features

- Sheets or cords of hepatocytes
- Absence of portal & central veins & bile ducts
- Increased amounts of glycogen & lipid
- Scattered, thin-walled, unpaired, vascular channels
- Few scattered Kupffer cells

CLINICAL ISSUES

Presentation

- Most common signs/symptoms
  - RUQ pain (40%): Due to hemorrhage
  - Asymptomatic (20%)
    – Especially those with *HNF-1a* type
  - No elevation of serum α-fetoprotein
- Diagnosis: Biopsy & histology

Demographics

- Age
  - Young women in childbearing age group
  - Predominantly in 3rd & 4th decades
- Gender
  - 98% seen in females
    – Not seen in males unless on anabolic steroids or with glycogen storage disease

Natural History & Prognosis

- Complications
  - Hemorrhage: Intrahepatic or intraperitoneal (40%)
  - Rupture: Increased risk in pregnancy
  - May regress on withdrawal of oral contraceptives
- **Risk factors for degeneration into HCC**
  - Male gender (10x more frequent than in women on per case basis)
  - Concomitant glycogen storage disease
  - Anabolic steroid use
  - *β-catenin*-mutated subtype of HA
  - HA mass size > 5 cm
- Prognosis
  - Usually good
    – After discontinuation of oral contraceptives
    – After surgical resection of large or symptomatic HAs
  - Poor
    – Intraperitoneal rupture
    – Rupture during pregnancy
    – Malignant transformation
    – Adenomatosis (> 10 adenomas)
      □ May hemorrhage, impair hepatic function

Treatment

- Adenoma < 5 cm
  - Observation & discontinuation of oral contraceptives or other steroids
- Adenoma > 5 cm & near surface
  - Surgical resection
  - Consider transcatheter embolization
- Pregnancy should be avoided due to ↑ risk of rupture
- Transplantation for some cases of adenomatosis

DIAGNOSTIC CHECKLIST

Image Interpretation Pearls

- Spherical, well-defined, hypervascular, & heterogeneous mass due to hemorrhage & fat; most evident on MR
- Gadoxetate-enhanced MR is most specific imaging test

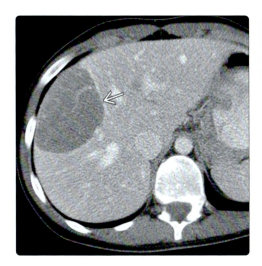

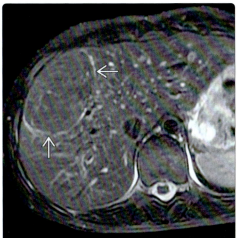

(Left) *Axial venous-phase CECT of an 18-year-old girl injured in a vehicle crash shows a subcapsular, encapsulated mass* ➡ *that is not very vascular, a typical (but not diagnostic) feature of the HNF-1a-mutated subtype of hepatic adenoma.* (Right) *Axial T2WI FS MR in the same patient shows the mass as almost isointense to background liver with a thin hyperintense capsule* ➡, *typical features of an HNF-1a-mutated subtype of hepatic adenoma.*

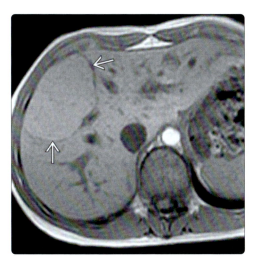

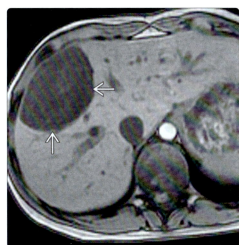

(Left) *Axial in-phase T1WI MR in the same patient shows a uniform iso- to slightly hyperintense peripheral liver lesion with a thin, low-intensity capsule* ➡. (Right) *Axial opposed-phase T1WI GRE MR in the same patient shows marked signal loss from the mass* ➡, *which indicates the presence of diffuse lipid, another typical feature of this subtype of hepatic adenoma.*

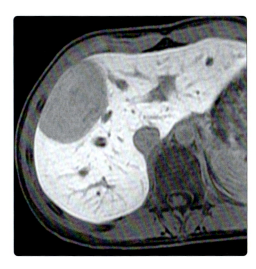

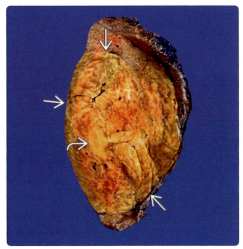

(Left) *On this delayed-phase image in the same patient, obtained after IV administration of gadoxetate (Eovist, Primovist), the normal liver enhances brightly, whereas the mass shows no retained contrast, indicating that it lacks functioning bile ductules and differentiating it from an focal nodular hyperplasia.* (Right) *Gross photograph of the resected specimen, an HNF-1a-mutated subtype of hepatic adenoma, shows an encapsulated, pale, tan mass* ➡ *with diffuse and focal lipid* ➡.

(Left) *In this 54-year-old woman who had a liver mass detected on CT, an axial T1WI GRE in-phase MR shows the mass ➡ as slightly hyperintense to a normal-appearing liver. On opposed-phase GRE MR (not shown), there was no signal dropout from the lesion, indicating no lipid content.* **(Right)** *On T2WI MR in the same patient, the mass ➡ is slightly hyperintense to the liver, and a central scar ➡ is quite hyperintense.*

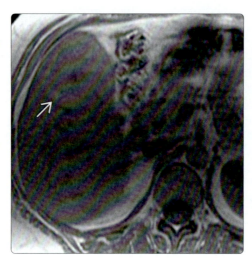
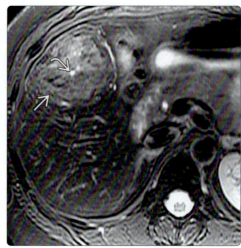

(Left) *On MR section taken after the bolus injection of gadoxetate (Eovist) in the same patient, the mass is hypervascular ➡, whereas the central scar is hypointense ➡. The mass and central scar were nearly isointense on the venous-phase images (not shown).* **(Right)** *On a 20-minute delayed image in the same patient, the mass ➡ retains less contrast material than normal liver. Because there was concern that the lesion was not a typical focal nodular hyperplasia, it was resected.*

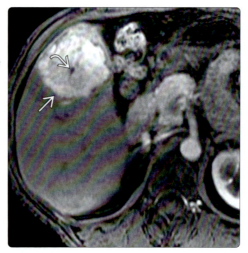
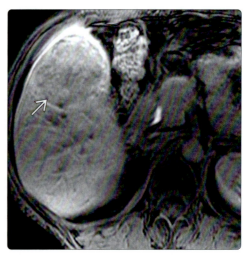

(Left) *Gross photo of the pathology specimen shows an encapsulated mass with blood pooling and foci of hemorrhage.* **(Right)** *Histologic specimen in the same patient shows disorganized hepatocytes with abundant eosinophilic nuclei on H&E staining, unpaired blood vessels ➡ distributed haphazardly throughout the lesion, and foci of chronic inflammation ➡. The final diagnosis was hepatic adenoma of the inflammatory subtype. (Courtesy T. Longacre, MD.)*

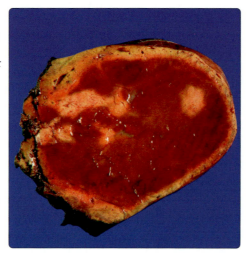
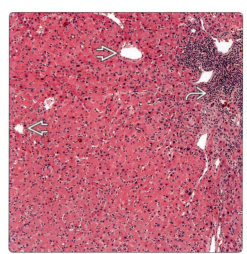

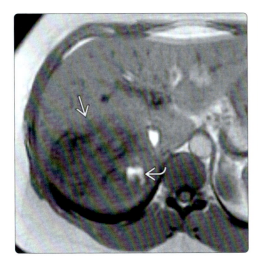
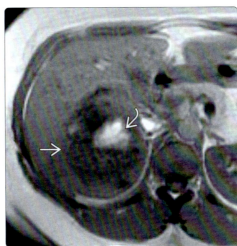

(Left) Axial T1WI MR of a 35-year-old woman with RUQ pain shows a hepatic mass ➡ containing several hyperintense foci ➡ that represent hemorrhage. (Right) Axial T1WI MR shows more hyperintense foci ➡ of hemorrhage within the hypointense mass ➡.

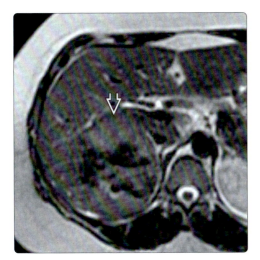
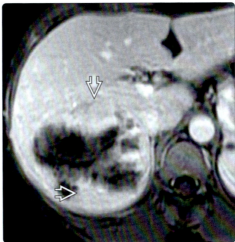

(Left) Axial T2WI MR in the same patient shows a heterogeneous mass with some foci of slight hyperintensity ➡ that represent lipid. (Right) Axial portal venous-phase T1WI MR in the same patient shows persistent hypervascular enhancement ➡ in the nonnecrotic and nonhemorrhagic portions of the mass, typical features of the inflammatory subtype of hepatic adenoma, which was confirmed on resection.

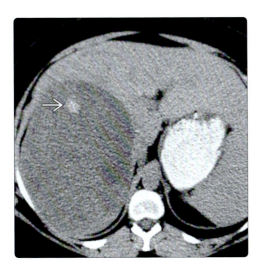
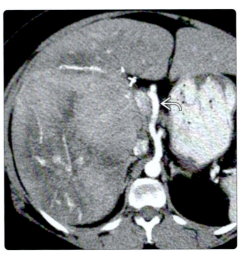

(Left) Axial NECT shows a very large, sharply demarcated, mostly homogeneous mass with a small focus of hemorrhage ➡. (Right) Axial arterial-phase CECT in the same patient shows hypervascularity with enlarged vessels within and on the surface of the tumor. Note the large hepatic artery ➡. The inflammatory subtype of hepatic adenomas are usually heterogeneously hypervascular and often encapsulated with focal hemorrhage, as in this patient.

(Left) *Axial opposed-phase T1WI GRE MR shows an encapsulated mass* ➡ *with hyperintense foci* ➡ *representing hemorrhage or fat. The in-phase images showed increased signal within the mass.* (Right) *Axial T2WI FS MR in the same patient shows that the mass is nearly isointense to the liver with a central focus of hyperintensity* ➡ *(hemorrhage). Fat content would have shown signal dropout on this sequence. A capsule or pseudocapsule is seen in ~ 20% of adenomas.*

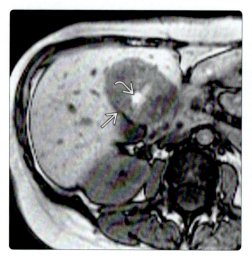
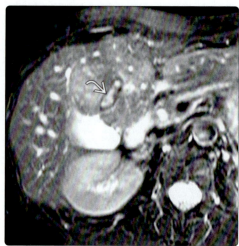

(Left) *Axial CT during the arterial phase of enhancement shows a brightly enhancing mass* ➡ *with a focal calcification* ➚*, the latter being a less common feature of adenomas.* (Right) *Ultrasound in the same patient confirms the solid mass with calcification* ➡ *and shows a capsule* ➡ *around the mass. The capsule is a common feature and the focal calcification a less common feature of adenomas, as was proven in this case.*

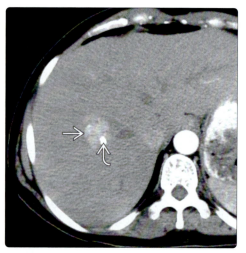
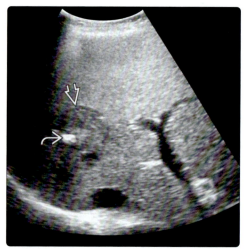

(Left) *Axial arterial-phase T1WI C+ MR of a 32-year-old woman who had been using oral contraceptives for 14 years shows 1 of about 10 encapsulated, enhancing focal masses* ➡. (Right) *More adenomas* ➡ *are seen on this section. In the absence of chronic liver disease or a known malignancy, these findings were considered diagnostic of adenomas. Following cessation of oral contraceptive use, these adenomas decreased in size and number within 4 months.*

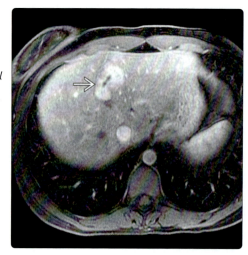
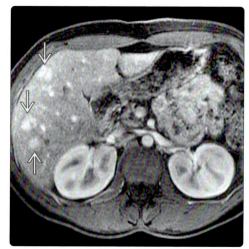

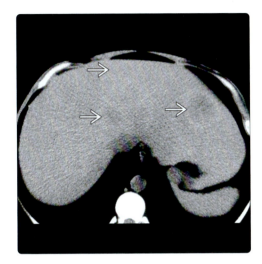
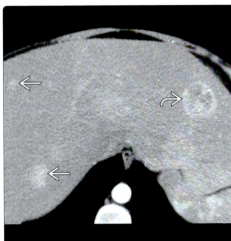

(Left) *Axial NECT of a 37-year-old man with type I glycogen storage disease and multiple adenomas shows hepatomegaly and low-attenuation masses ➡ within the liver. The low attenuation is due to intratumoral lipid. These are foci of the β-catenin-mutated subtype of hepatic adenoma.* (Right) *Hepatic arterial-phase CECT in the same patient shows that some lesions are hypervascular ➡, whereas others ➡ show heterogeneous enhancement.*

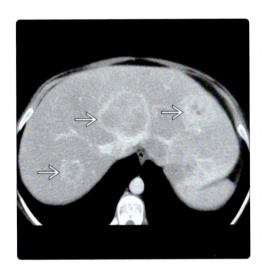
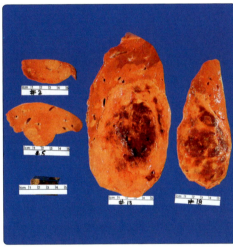

(Left) *Axial portal venous-phase CECT in the same patient shows capsular enhancement or compressed hepatic parenchyma around most of the adenomas ➡. Adenomas are usually multiple in the setting of type I or III glycogen storage disease and carry a high risk of malignant degeneration, especially those > 5 cm in diameter and those in men.* (Right) *Gross photograph of the resected specimens in a case of hepatic adenomatosis shows multiple adenomas with hemorrhage and necrosis. (Courtesy M. Yeh, MD, PhD.)*

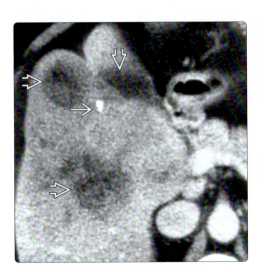
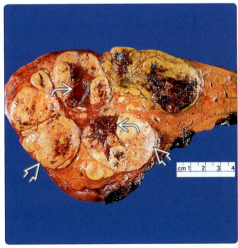

(Left) *Axial CECT shows a large, heterogeneous hepatic mass with several foci ➡ measuring < water attenuation, indicating fat content. Also noted are foci of calcification ➡. Serial CT scans had shown slow growth of the mass over 7 years.* (Right) *Gross pathology from the same patient shows the mass with foci of fat ➡ and hemorrhage ➡. Histology revealed foci of hepatocellular carcinoma within this adenoma, which had the β-catenin mutation, as did the foci of hepatocellular carcinoma.*

Biliary Hamartomas

TERMINOLOGY

- Uncommon (~ 3% of general population), congenital, benign malformations of biliary tract
- a.k.a. von Meyenburg complex; biliary microhamartomas

IMAGING

- **Imaging protocols: Multiphasic, multiplanar CECT or MR with MRCP**
- Multiple, near water-density/-intensity liver lesions < 1.5 cm in diameter
  - Irregularly spherical; markedly hyperintense on T2WI
  - No communication with biliary tree
- US: Small and well-circumscribed lesions
  - US shows much more echogenicity and fewer "cystic lesions" than anticipated based on prior CT or MR
  - Fibrotic parts of lesions are very echogenic

TOP DIFFERENTIAL DIAGNOSES

- Autosomal dominant polycystic liver disease
  - Larger, more variable, more numerous hepatic cysts
  - Plus cysts in other organs; family history
- Multiple simple hepatic cysts
  - Usually fewer cysts of varying size
- Caroli disease
  - Central dot sign on CECT and MR
  - ERCP and MRCP: Communicating bile duct abnormality
- Multiple/solitary, small metastatic lesions
  - More complex and varied in size
- Opportunistic infection, hepatic
  - Must be considered in immunosuppressed patient with fever

DIAGNOSTIC CHECKLIST

- Should be considered as likely diagnosis in setting of innumerable small, mildly complex "cysts" in healthy patient
- These are of no clinical significance
  - Must not be mistaken for metastases or other lesions

(Left) Axial CT in a healthy young man shows innumerable small "cystic lesions" throughout the liver with some nodularity and irregularity of the "cyst" walls ➡; the latter being a typical finding for biliary hamartomas. (Right) Transverse US of the same patient shows 1 of many echogenic foci ➡ and many more "cystic lesions" ➡. Smaller biliary hamartomas are often echogenic due to the fibrous nodularity in their walls.

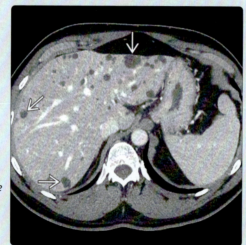
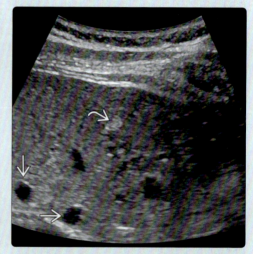

(Left) Axial T2 MR shows innumerable tiny bright foci throughout the liver ➡, representing biliary hamartomas. This patient also had evidence of congenital hepatic fibrosis on imaging and liver biopsy, both part of the congenital hepatic and renal fibropolycystic disease spectrum. (Right) MRCP shows small spherical "cysts" ➡ that do not communicate with the (normal) biliary tree. This feature helps to distinguish biliary hamartomas from Caroli disease.

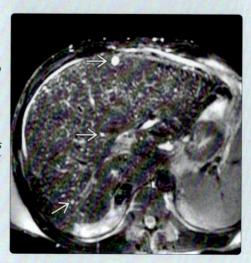
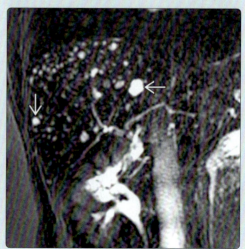

Hepatic Angiomyolipoma and Lipoma

TERMINOLOGY

- Benign mesenchymal tumor containing variable amounts of smooth muscle (myoid), fat (lipoid), and proliferating blood vessel (angioid) components

IMAGING

- **Best imaging tools: Multiphasic MR**, although CECT allows diagnosis in many cases
- Well-circumscribed hepatic mass with variable fat and vascular content
  - Only 50% of hepatic angiomyolipomas have substantial fat component
- MR detects fat component better than CT
  - Fatty component of tumor results in hyperintense (high-signal) foci on T1WI and T2WI
  - Opposed-phase GRE imaging may show signal dropout from lipid
- Arterial phase: Prominent enhancement of nonfatty portion of lesion
  - Central vessels within lesion if mass is large

TOP DIFFERENTIAL DIAGNOSES

- Hepatocellular carcinoma (~ 5% of hepatocellular carcinomas contain macroscopic fat)
- Focal steatosis
- Hepatic adenoma (~ 10-20% have fat component)
- Metastases (from teratoma or liposarcoma)

PATHOLOGY

- Associated with tuberous sclerosis in < 10% of cases

DIAGNOSTIC CHECKLIST

- Small, fat-density hepatic mass in patient with tuberous sclerosis is benign
- Angiomyolipoma that is primarily myeloid or angioid may be indistinguishable on imaging from other hepatic tumors, including hepatocellular carcinoma

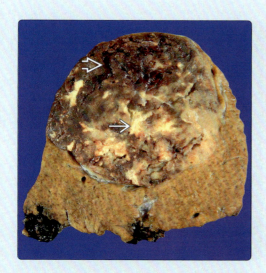

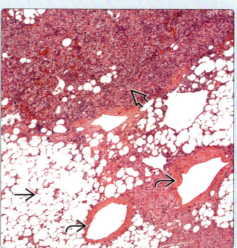

(Left) Gross photograph of a fixed specimen shows a heterogeneous, mottled, tan, yellow, and brown tumor with areas of hemorrhage and degeneration ➡. Note that the background liver is not cirrhotic. The yellow component ➡ is fat. (Courtesy J. Misdraji, MD.) (Right) Hematoxylin and eosin-stained section shows a tumor composed of 3 elements: Adipose tissue ➡, vessels ➡, and plump spindle cells ➡. (Courtesy J. Misdraji, MD.)

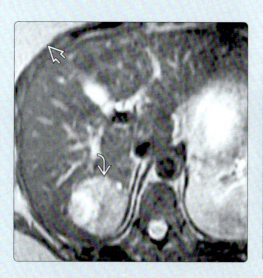

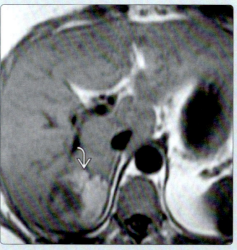

(Left) Axial T2 MR shows a heterogeneously bright mass with a fatty component ➡ that is nearly isointense to subcutaneous fat ➡. The rest of the tumor has the moderate hyperintensity typical of most neoplasms on T2 MR. (Right) Axial T1 MR in the same patient shows that most of the mass ➡ is hyperintense, an unusual feature of most neoplasms and generally indicative of the presence of fat or hemorrhage within the mass. This tumor was resected and proved to be an isolated angiomyolipoma.

TERMINOLOGY

- Heterogeneous group of lesions occurring in liver and bile ducts (among other organs) characterized by fibroblastic and myofibroblastic proliferation with inflammatory infiltrate

IMAGING

- **Multiphasic, multiplanar CT or MR**
  - 2 main types that mimic cholangiocarcinoma
    - Large, solitary, peripheral mass, often with heterogeneous & delayed contrast enhancement
    - Mass in hepatic hilum appearing identical to Klatskin tumor (short stricture with dilated ducts upstream)
- **Direct cholangiography, transhepatic or ERCP**
  - Useful for depiction and treatment of biliary variant

TOP DIFFERENTIAL DIAGNOSES

- IgG4-related sclerosing disease (IgG4-RD)

- Probable cause of many reported cases of inflammatory pseudotumor
- Peripheral hepatic mass
  - Cholangiocarcinoma (peripheral)
  - Hepatocellular carcinoma
  - Hepatic metastases and lymphoma
- Hilar biliary stricture or mass
  - Cholangiocarcinoma (hilar cholangiocarcinoma)

CLINICAL ISSUES

- Core biopsy or resection is needed for definite diagnosis
  - May suffice for peripheral hepatic type; not biliary type
- May respond to steroids and other antiinflammatory medications
  - Especially if due to IgG4-related sclerosing disease

DIAGNOSTIC CHECKLIST

- Look for imaging, clinical, and laboratory (serum IgG4 levels) evidence of IgG4-related sclerosing disease

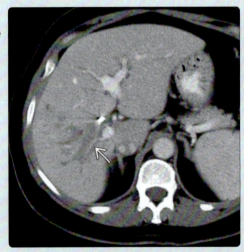
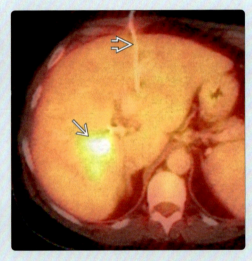

(Left) CECT in the portal venous-parenchymal phase shows an infiltrating tumor ➡ that encases and narrows the right portal vein. (Right) Axial PET/CT in the same patient shows an FDG-avid mass ➡ in the hilum, extending along the right portal vein. The bile ducts were obstructed at the hilum, requiring a biliary stent ➡. This was interpreted as a cholangiocarcinoma, but surgical resection (right hepatectomy) showed only inflammatory pseudotumor of the liver and bile ducts.

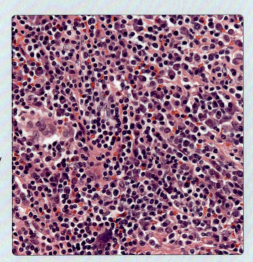
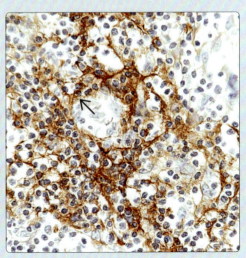

(Left) High-power H&E micrograph shows plasma cells and lymphocytes with occasional histiocytes in this inflammatory pseudotumor specimen. (Courtesy T. Longacre, MD.) (Right) Histochemical staining of an inflammatory pseudotumor specimen shows CD21(+) spindle cells ➡, which are present in some inflammatory pseudotumors. This specimen also shows an inflammatory infiltrate of lymphocytes and plasma cells. (Courtesy T. Longacre, MD.)

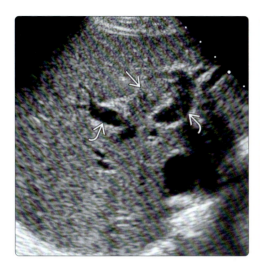 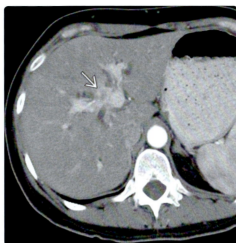

(Left) Sonography in a 48-year-old woman with jaundice shows dilated intrahepatic ducts ⇗ and a subtle mass ⇨ at the common duct bifurcation. (Right) Arterial phase CECT in the same case shows dilation of intrahepatic ducts and a poorly defined, small, enhancing mass ⇨ at the duct bifurcation.

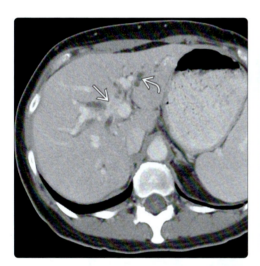 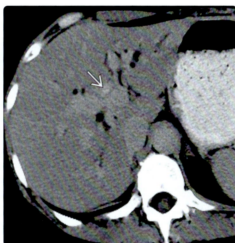

(Left) Portal venous phase CT in the same case shows the ductal obstruction ⇗ and the mass ⇨ at the confluence of the main right and left ducts. (Right) Delayed-phase CT in the same case shows persistent, increased retention of contrast material within the hilar mass ⇨, findings considered very suggestive of a hilar (Klatskin) cholangiocarcinoma.

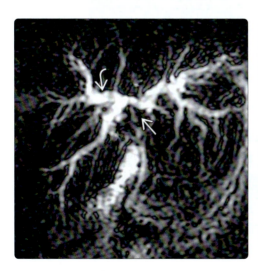 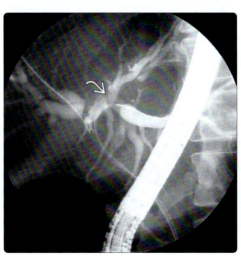

(Left) Thick-slab MRCP in the same case shows biliary obstruction at the bifurcation ⇨ and dilation of intrahepatic ducts ⇗. (Right) ERCP in the same case shows the same high-grade short stricture at the hilum ⇗. All imaging findings were considered to indicate a Klatskin tumor, but surgery proved this was an inflammatory pseudotumor. In cases such as this, only detailed analysis of resected specimens may allow distinction of inflammatory pseudotumor from cholangiocarcinoma.

IMAGING

- **Patients with chronic liver disease must be in surveillance program (clinical & imaging)**
  - Small, curable hepatocellular carcinomas (HCCs) can be diagnosed by CT & MR
  - Criteria for HCC are often specific enough to guide therapy without tissue confirmation
- **Multiphasic contrast-enhanced CT or MR is definitive imaging study**
- Key imaging features
  - Hypervascular mass on arterial phase (CT or MR) with "washout" on venous & delayed phases
  - Presence of capsule or fat content
  - Evidence of portal or hepatic vein invasion
  - Bright lesion on T2WI & diffusion-weighted MR
  - Hypointense lesion on hepatobiliary phase of gadoxetate-enhanced (Eovist, Primovist) MR
- **Multiphasic CT** accurately detects great majority of HCC ≥ 2 cm in diameter

- CT is widely available, less operator & interpreter dependent, better tolerated by patients than MR
- Disadvantages: Slightly lower sensitivity & specificity than MR
  - Exposes patients to ionizing radiation & iodinated contrast media
- **MR in experienced hands using current protocols is more sensitive & specific than CT for diagnosis of HCC**
  - MR allows more confident diagnosis of arterioportal shunts
  - MR distinguishes among focal nodular lesions more accurately than CT
  - More operator & interpreter dependent

CLINICAL ISSUES

- Radiologists must use approved CT or MR protocols
  - Should characterize focal nodular lesions using LI-RADS or Organ Procurement & Transplantation Network classification scheme

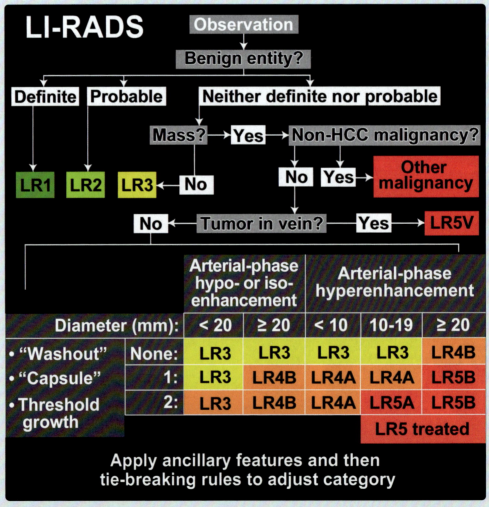

The Liver Imaging Reporting and Data System is endorsed by the American College of Radiology for categorization of focal nodular lesions found on CT or MR in the cirrhotic liver. It is designed to standardize the interpreting and reporting of findings so that these are more uniform, accurate, and useful to referring physicians.

TERMINOLOGY

Abbreviations

- Hepatocellular carcinoma (HCC)

IMAGING

General Features

- Best diagnostic clue
  - Hypervascular mass with "washout" of contrast enhancement & capsule on delayed-phase CT or MR
- Key concepts
  - **Patients with chronic liver disease must be in surveillance program, including**
    - Regularly scheduled history physical exam
    - Laboratory markers (liver function & tumor markers)
    - Imaging studies (US, CT, &/or MR, as detailed below)
    - Evaluate extent of cirrhosis & portal hypertension
    - Screen for development of HCC
  - Important to detect & stage HCC accurately
    - Small tumors are curable with resection, ablation, or transplantation
    - Multiple or large tumors, or those with venous invasion, can be palliated with chemo- or radioembolization
- **Multiphasic contrast-enhanced CT or MR is definitive imaging study**
  - **Findings are often specific enough to guide therapy without tissue confirmation**

CT Findings

- CECT
  - Multiphasic CT accurately detects great majority of HCCs ≥ 2 cm in diameter
    - MR offers improved distinction among different types of focal nodules within cirrhotic liver
    - MR is often used in "problem-solving" for hepatic lesions initially discovered on US or CT
  - Advantages of CT
    - Widely available
    - Less operator & interpreter dependent than for MR or US
    - Fast exam time is well tolerated by patients
  - Disadvantages include
    - Exposes patients to ionizing radiation & iodinated contrast media
      - Though radiation & contrast dose are reduced with newer protocols & CT scanners
  - **Mandatory to perform multiphasic enhanced imaging**
    - Arterial phase: ~ 25-35 seconds after start of bolus infusion of contrast medium
    - Portal venous phase: ~ 60- to 70-second delay
    - Delayed phase: ~ 3- to 5-minute delay
  - Hepatic arterial-phase (HAP) scan
    - Heterogeneous hypervascular enhancement (for moderately & poorly differentiated HCC)
      - Well-differentiated HCC may be hypodense to liver on all phases of enhancement
    - Wedge-shaped areas of ↑ parenchymal density on HAP: Perfusion abnormality due to portal vein occlusion by tumor thrombus & ↑ arterial flow

  - Portal venous-phase scan
    - HCC is often nearly isodense to surrounding liver
  - Delayed scan: HCC hypodense to surrounding liver
    - "Washout" of contrast enhancement is key finding
      - Helps to distinguish HCC from regenerative nodules & arterioportal shunts (both common in cirrhosis)
  - Associated findings
    - Presence of capsule (circumferential rim around mass)
      - Best seen on delayed phase; hyperdense to HCC & liver
    - Satellite tumors near primary HCC mass
    - Macroscopic fat within hepatic mass (in cirrhotic liver)
    - Signs of cirrhosis ± portal hypertension
      - Dysmorphic, nodular liver with widened fissures, small right lobe
      - Splenomegaly, varices, ascites
  - Signs of **portal or hepatic vein invasion** by HCC
    - Expansion of vein lumen
    - Enhancement of tumor within vein
    - Contiguity of tumor & vein

MR Findings

- **MR in experienced hands using current protocols is more sensitive & specific than CT for diagnosis of HCC**
  - Advantage is mostly limited to tumors < 2 cm & fewer false-positive exams
    - MR allows more confident diagnosis of arterioportal shunts
    - MR distinguishes among focal nodular lesions more accurately than CT
  - Disadvantages of MR relative to CT
    - More operator & interpreter dependent
    - More expensive & less widely available
    - Longer exam time makes it less attractive for some patients
- T1WI
  - Variable intensity depending on degree of vascularity, fibrosis, necrosis, steatosis
  - HCC may be hypo-, iso-, or hyperintense to liver
  - Tumors with fat or hemorrhage are hyperintense
- T2WI
  - Usually hyperintense to liver
    - Regenerative nodules are hypointense on T2WI
  - HCC arising within dysplastic nodule
    - Nodule-within-nodule pattern
    - HCC appears as small focus of increased signal intensity within decreased signal intensity nodule
- T1 C+ (with conventional gadolinium agents)
  - Heterogeneously hyperintense with "washout" on portal venous & delayed phase
  - Rapid "washout" with residual capsular enhancement = HCC, **not** arterioportal shunt
- Hepatobiliary contrast agent [gadoxetate (Eovist, Primovist)]
  - On 20-minute delayed (hepatobiliary) phase
    - Normal liver (& some portions of cirrhotic liver) enhance brightly
    - Most HCCs are seen as hypointense focal masses
    - Rare for well-differentiated HCC to show delayed persistent enhancement with gadoxetate

- o Increases sensitivity of MR in diagnosing small HCC
- Diffusion-weighted MR (DWI)
  - o Restricted diffusion within HCC is often detected as bright signal within focal lesion
  - o Adds sensitivity & specificity to MR detection of HCC
- Gradient-echo (GRE) MR
  - o Signal dropout on opposed-phase GRE sequence indicates presence of intracellular fat (lipid)
  - o This finding in focal mass within cirrhotic liver is very suggestive of HCC

Ultrasonographic Findings

- Grayscale ultrasound
  - o Highly operator & interpreter dependent
  - o Lower sensitivity & specificity than CT or MR in diagnosing HCC
    - – Especially within nodular, fibrotic, cirrhotic liver
  - o Mass with mixed echogenicity due to tumor necrosis & hypervascularity
  - o Hypoechoic: Due to solid tumor
  - o Hyperechoic: Due to fatty metamorphosis
    - – Small hyperechoic HCC can simulate hemangioma
  - o Capsule
    - – Thin hypoechoic band around mass
- Color Doppler
  - o Shows hypervascularity & tumor shunting in some cases
  - o Small HCC: Indistinguishable from regenerative & dysplastic nodules

Angiographic Findings

- Conventional
  - o Hypervascular tumor
    - – Marked neovascularity & arteriovenous shunting
    - – Large hepatic artery & vascular invasion
  - o Threads & streaks sign
    - – Sign of tumor thrombus in portal vein
- Not generally used for diagnosis
  - o Commonly used for transarterial chemo- or radioembolization of nonresectable tumors

Surveillance for Hepatocellular Carcinoma

- Goal is to detect early, small HCC at curable stage
- Who should be screened
  - o All patients with proven cirrhosis (any etiology)
  - o Hepatitis B carriers who also have cirrhosis or
    - – Are Asian or African American
    - – Have family history of HCC
    - – Have high viral loads
- Which imaging modality should be used
  - o Sonography
    - – Usually repeated at ~ 6-month intervals
    - – Effective in expert hands in examining thin patients with relatively nonfibrotic livers
  - o Multiphasic CT or MR
    - – To evaluate any focal lesion > 1 cm detected by US
    - – To evaluate liver that is distorted by fat, fibrosis, nodularity
    - – To evaluate patient considered at high risk for HCC even with normal US
    - – Usually repeated at ~ 12-month intervals as problem-solving test

Distinguishing Hepatocellular Carcinoma From Other Nodular Lesions Within Cirrhotic Liver

- Regenerative nodules: Small (often < 1 cm), hypovascular
  - o Very hypointense on T2WI & GRE MR sequences
  - o Retain gadoxetate (Eovist) on delayed-phase MR
  - o Not bright on DWI
- Dysplastic nodules: Often larger (2.0-3.5 cm), hypovascular
  - o Hyperintense on T1WI, hypointense on T2WI MR (opposite of HCC)
  - o Not bright on DWI
  - o Usually retain gadoxetate on delayed-phase MR
- Arterioportal shunts
  - o Common in cirrhotic liver
  - o Usually ~ 1 cm in size, wedge-shaped, subcapsular in location
  - o Evident only on arterial-phase CT or MR (no "washout" or capsule)
  - o Not present on unenhanced T1- or T2WI nor on DWI

Liver Imaging Reporting & Data System

- Endorsed by American College of Radiology for categorization of focal nodular lesions found on CT or MR in cirrhotic liver
- Designed to standardize interpretation & reporting of findings so that these are more uniform, accurate, & useful to referring physicians
- Liver Imaging Reporting & Data System (LI-RADS) "5" classification indicates confident diagnosis of HCC
  - o Identical to Organ Procurement & Transplantation Network category 5 lesion
  - o Criteria: Lesion 1-2 cm that shows arterial-phase hyperenhancement & "washout" with peripheral rim (capsule) enhancement or growth by > 50% within 6-month period of follow-up
  - o Or hypervascular lesion > 2 cm & either "washout" or capsule or interval growth > 50%

Imaging Recommendations

- Best imaging tool
  - o In cirrhotic patient, multiphasic CT or MR
  - o Triphasic CT or MR (arterial, venous, & delayed phases)
    - – MR with gadoxetate enhancement has greater sensitivity & specificity

DIAGNOSTIC CHECKLIST

Image Interpretation Pearls

- Within cirrhotic liver
  - o Encapsulated or fat-containing mass is likely HCC
  - o Mass with restricted diffusion or no uptake of gadoxetate is likely HCC

Reporting Tips

- **Use LI-RADS classification system**
  - o Provides standardized criteria for interpreting findings of CT & MR examinations in patients with chronic liver injury

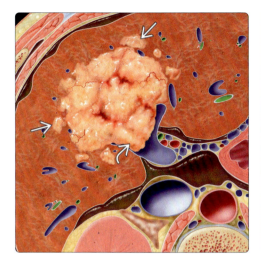

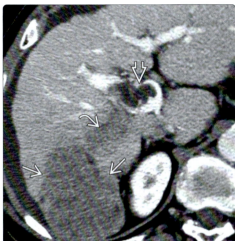

(Left) *Graphic shows a heterogeneous hypervascular mass invading the portal vein ➡. The surrounding liver is cirrhotic with a nodular contour, and there is ascites. Satellite nodules of HCC ➡ surround the dominant mass.*
(Right) *Axial CECT in the venous phase shows a hypodense mass ➡ in a cirrhotic liver invading and occluding the posterior branch of the right portal vein ➡. Nonocclusive thrombus ➡ is present within the main portal vein. This HCC was hypervascular on arterial-phase CECT.*

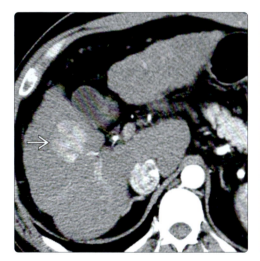

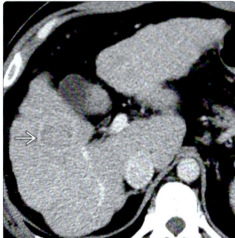

(Left) *Axial CECT in the arterial phase shows a hypervascular mass ➡ in the right lobe of a cirrhotic liver, the latter marked by surface nodularity, widened fissures, and a shrunken right lobe.*
(Right) *Axial CECT in the portal venous phase in the same patient shows "washout" of contrast from the mass ➡ and a hyperdense capsule, findings diagnostic of HCC.*

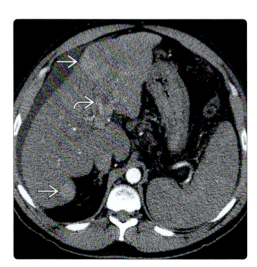

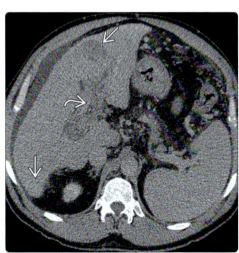

(Left) *In this patient with cirrhosis, surveillance US showed a single hepatic mass. Arterial-phase CT shows 2 hypervascular masses ➡ with tumor invasion of the left portal vein ➡.* (Right) *Portal venous-phase CT shows "washout" from the 2 HCCs ➡ and from the portal vein tumor thrombus ➡.*

(Left) *Multifocal HCC may simulate metastases, as in this case. Axial arterial-phase CECT shows multiple hypervascular foci* ➡ *and expansion of the left portal vein* ➡ *by enhancing tumor thrombus.* **(Right)** *Axial portal venous-phase CECT in the same patient shows "washout" of contrast from the HCC foci* ➡ *as well as the portal vein tumor thrombus* ➡*. The presence of the tumor thrombus is useful in distinguishing HCC from metastases, which rarely invade the portal vein.*

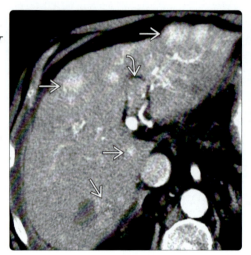
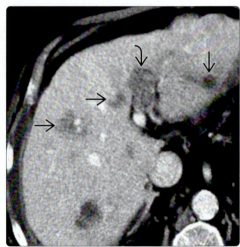

(Left) *Arterial-phase CECT in an 80-year-old man with no known liver disease shows a large mass with a mosaic pattern of enhancement and a thin rim or capsule* ➡*. These are typical features of HCC that arise in a noncirrhotic liver, such as someone with chronic hepatitis B infection.* **(Right)** *Catheter angiogram in the same patient shows that the "capsule" is comprised of large feeding arteries* ➡ *along the periphery of the mass. Transarterial chemoembolization was performed.*

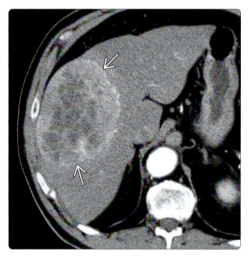
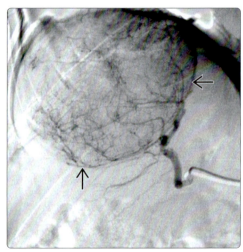

(Left) *(A) T2WI MR shows a focal mass* ➡ *that is slightly hyperintense to background liver. (B) The same lesion* ➡ *is hypervascular on arterial-phase T1WI C+ MR.* **(Right)** *(A) In the same patient, on delayed-phase T1WI MR, the mass* ➡ *demonstrates contrast "washout" and a capsule, very typical signs of HCC. (B) DWI shows bright signal* ➡ *representing restricted diffusion, another typical feature of HCC.*

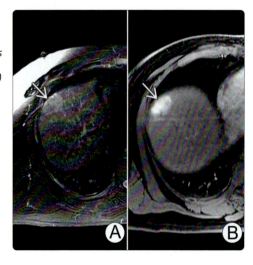
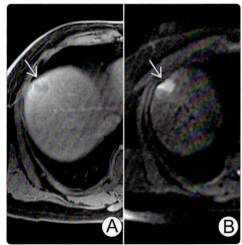

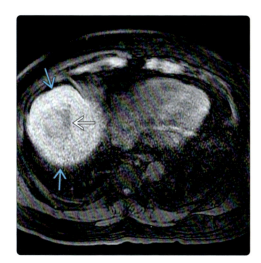

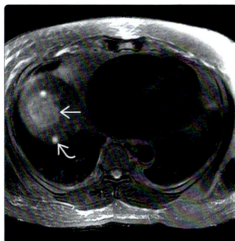

(Left) In this 66-year-old man with chronic hepatitis B, nonenhanced T1WI FS MR shows a mass ➡ as hypointense relative to surrounding liver ⇨. (Right) In the same patient, axial nonenhanced T2WI MR shows a moderately hyperintense spherical mass ➡ in the hepatic dome, along with 2 smaller cysts ➡.

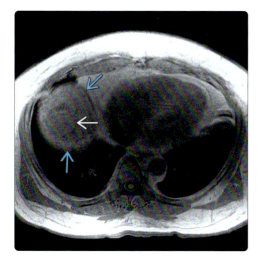

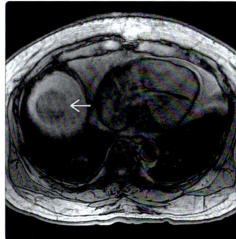

(Left) Nonenhanced in-phase T1WI GRE MR in the same patient shows the mass ➡ as slightly hypointense to liver ⇨. (Right) Opposed-phase T1WI GRE MR in the same patient shows signal dropout from the mass ➡, indicating lipid content. The presence of microscopic fat (as in this case) or macroscopic fat is a very suggestive sign of HCC in a mass within a cirrhotic liver.

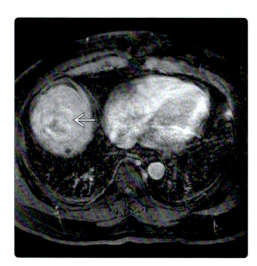

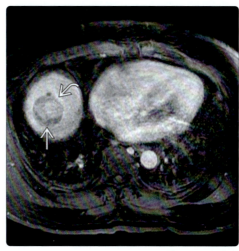

(Left) Arterial-phase contrast-enhanced T1WI MR in the same patient shows heterogeneous hypervascularity within the mass ➡, which is essentially diagnostic of HCC in this setting. (Right) Delayed-phase contrast-enhanced T1WI MR in the same patient shows "washout" of contrast from the mass ➡ and a suggestion of a capsule ➡, another characteristic sign of HCC.

TERMINOLOGY

- Tumor arising from intrahepatic bile ducts

IMAGING

- **Multiphasic CT or MR with delayed-phase imaging (~ 10 minutes)**
- Mass-forming intrahepatic cholangiocarcinoma
  - Homogeneous or heterogeneous mass with irregular borders and "**satellite**" nodules
- T1WI MR: Heterogeneous hypointense mass
- T2WI MR: Hyperintense periphery (cellular tumor) + large central hypointensity (fibrosis)
- Arterial-phase C+ (enhanced) CT or MR
  - Thin or thick, rim-like enhancement frequently seen around periphery of tumor
- Venous-phase C+ CT or MR
  - Progressive, gradual, and concentric filling-in (centripetal enhancement)

- Usually not isodense to vessels (unlike cavernous hemangioma)
- Delayed-phase C+ CT or MR
  - Substantial **delayed enhancement** (i.e., > that of liver parenchyma) is common (~ 74%)
  - Entire mass may be enhanced only on delayed-phase images
  - Regions of fibrosis display delayed enhancement (delayed), while those of coagulative necrosis and mucin show no enhancement
- **± capsular retraction** (frequent) with parenchymal atrophy of liver segments peripheral to tumor
- **Bile ducts will be dilated upstream** from tumor
  - May not be evident in very peripheral CCA
- **Ultrasonography**
  - Hyperechoic (75%); iso- &/or hypoechoic (14%) mass
  - Intrahepatic bile ducts of involved hepatic segment may contain calculi or intraductal mass (echogenic): Mucin is echo-free

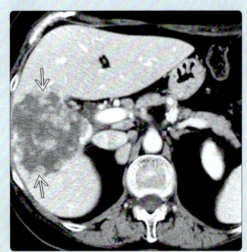
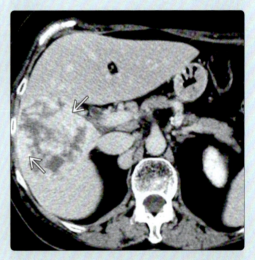

(Left) Axial CECT of a 67-year-old woman shows heterogeneous enhancement of a mass ➡, but not the nodular, peripheral pattern, isodense with blood vessels, which is characteristic of hemangioma. (Right) Axial CT in delayed phase of the same patient shows foci of hyperdense persistent enhancement ➡, but the lesion does not fill in from the periphery as would be expected of a hemangioma, and the enhanced foci are hyperdense to blood pool (proven cholangiocarcinoma).

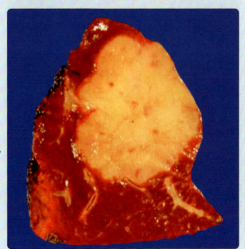
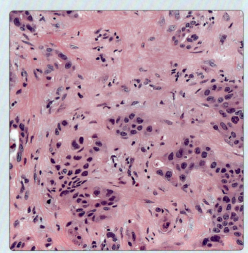

(Left) Intrahepatic cholangiocarcinomas generally arise in noncirrhotic livers. This gross photograph shows a white-tan, firm, and distinct mass in a background of noncirrhotic liver. (Courtesy M. Yeh, MD, PhD.) (Right) Desmoplastic stroma is a common finding in intrahepatic cholangiocarcinoma. (Courtesy M. Yeh, MD, PhD.)

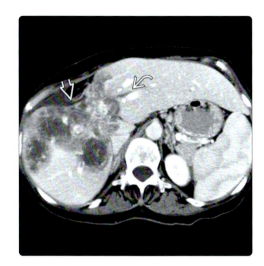
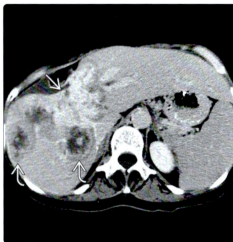

(Left) Axial CECT in the portal venous phase shows a heterogeneous infiltrative mass with intrahepatic biliary obstruction ➡ and volume loss with capsular retraction ⮕. (Right) Axial CECT in the delayed phase of the same patient shows increased and persistent enhancement of the tumor ➡ due to its fibrous stroma. Hepatocellular carcinoma would typically show washout on this phase. Other tumor foci have the target pattern of enhancement ➡ of other types of adenocarcinomas.

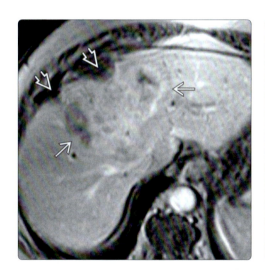
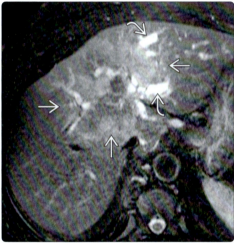

(Left) Axial T1WI C+ MR in the venous phase shows a large but subtle heterogeneous mass ➡. Capsular retraction ⮕ is also noted. This tumor showed persistent enhancement on 10-minute delayed images (not shown). (Right) Axial T2WI MR shows mild hyperintensity within the hepatic mass ➡. Dilated intrahepatic ducts ➡ are noted upstream from the mass. These are typical features of cholangiocarcinoma but may be seen with other tumors.

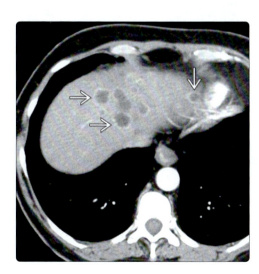
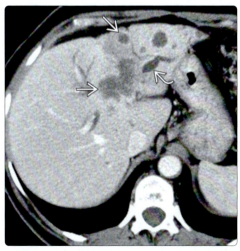

(Left) Axial CECT in arterial phase of a 55-year-old woman with jaundice shows multifocal masses with continuous peripheral ring enhancement ⮕. (Right) The portal venous phase in the same patient shows little enhancement of the tumors ➡. The intrahepatic bile ducts are dilated ➡, and the left lobe of the liver is atrophic. Parenchymal atrophy of liver segments affected by peripheral cholangiocarcinoma is common and may be evident as lobar atrophy or capsular retraction.

Epithelioid Hemangioendothelioma

IMAGING

- **Multiple or coalescent peripheral hepatic nodules with target appearance and capsular retraction on enhanced CT or MR**
- Target-like enhancement pattern of tumor
  - Delayed or nonenhancing central part of tumor (myxoid and hyalinized stroma)
  - Enhancing (hyperemic) peripheral inner rim (increased vascularity)
  - Nonenhancing peripheral outer rim or "halo" (avascular rim)
- MR: Usually hypointense on T1WI, hyperintense on T2WI
- Spectrum of growth in lesions may be seen
  - Nodular form (more common)
  - Diffuse or extensive form (very rare)

TOP DIFFERENTIAL DIAGNOSES

- Peripheral cholangiocarcinoma
- Treated malignancy

- Focal confluent fibrosis (seen in cirrhotic livers)
- Hemangioma (especially in cirrhotic liver)

PATHOLOGY

- Must not be confused with infantile hemangioendothelioma
  - Benign primary vascular liver tumor
  - Resolves spontaneously in many cases

CLINICAL ISSUES

- Presentation: Abdominal pain, jaundice, hepatosplenomegaly
- Diagnosis: Tumor cells stain positive for factor VIII-related antigen
- Slowly progressing, low-grade, malignant vascular tumor of liver
  - Most patients survive 5-10 years after diagnosis

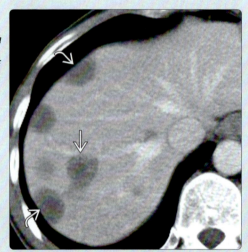
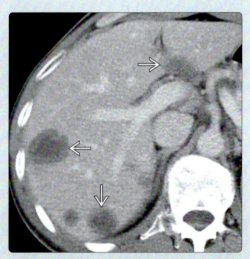

(Left) Axial CECT shows multiple peripheral, hypovascular lesions ➡ with a target appearance (central lucency), typical CT findings of epithelioid hemangioendothelioma. The subcapsular lesions are associated with retraction of the overlying liver capsule ➘. (Right) CT of the same patient shows more of the multicentric target lesions ➡ typical of epithelioid hemangioendothelioma, mostly in a peripheral location within the liver.

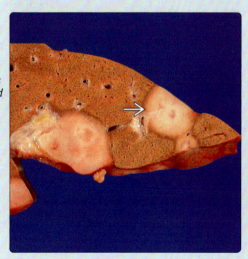
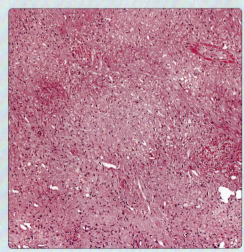

(Left) Gross pathology of the same liver after explantation shows the target appearance of the lesions with necrosis and white fibrous tissue in the center of the lesions as well as a peripheral rim of compressed parenchyma ➡ and tumor. (Right) Central portion of epithelioid hemangioendothelioma is typically hypocellular with loosely arranged spindle cells in a fibromyxoid or sclerotic stroma. The findings can simulate a scar or sclerosed hemangioma. (Courtesy S. Kakar, MD.)

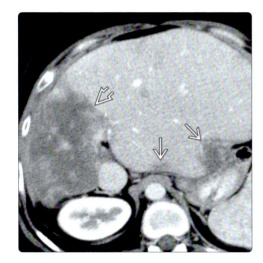

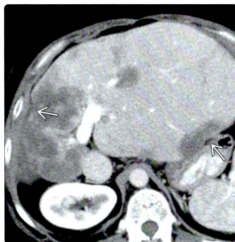

(Left) *Axial CECT in a 30-year-old man with abdominal pain and weight loss shows marked volume loss of the right hepatic lobe, which is essentially replaced by a heterogeneous, hypodense tumor ➡. Other tumors are seen in the left lobe as well ➡.* (Right) *Axial CT in the same patient shows additional tumor foci with capsular retraction evident over at least 2 lesions ➡.*

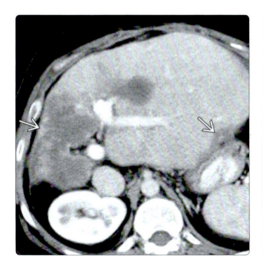

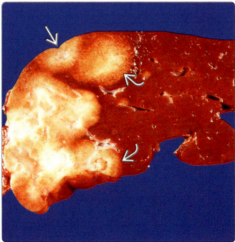

(Left) *Lower CT section in the same patient shows more of the confluent tumors ➡ and volume loss.* (Right) *Gross photograph of the explanted liver shows the yellow-white predominance of fibrotic matrix within the tumors and the peripheral rims of hyperemic tumor and compressed liver ➡. The capsular retraction over one of the peripheral masses is also evident ➡. The liver itself is not cirrhotic.*

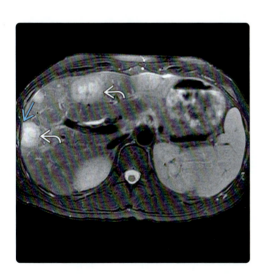

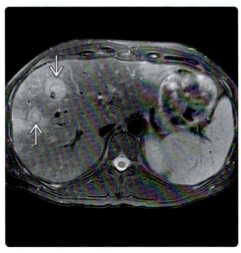

(Left) *In this 38-year-old woman, T2WI MR shows capsular retraction ➡ over one of the multiple peripheral foci of epithelioid hemangioendothelioma ➡. These are typical clinical and imaging features of hepatic epithelioid hemangioendothelioma.* (Right) *An axial T2WI MR in the same patient shows the target appearance and peripheral location of some of the foci of epithelioid hemangioendothelioma ➡ with the myxoid stroma in the center of the tumors being relatively hyperintense.*

Biliary Cystadenocarcinoma

TERMINOLOGY

- Rare, malignant or premalignant, unilocular or multilocular cystic tumor
  - Almost always solitary, in middle-aged women

IMAGING

- Best imaging protocol
  - **Multiplanar, multiphasic CECT or MR**
  - Complex encapsulated, multiloculated cystic mass with septa and mural calcifications
  - MR: Variable signal intensity locules depending on content of cystic fluid (mucinous vs. serous)
  - Enhancement of internal septa, capsule, and nodules suggests malignancy
- Potential to develop into cystadenocarcinoma even after years of stability

TOP DIFFERENTIAL DIAGNOSES

- Hemorrhagic or infected hepatic cyst

- **Cysts have no enhancement** of nodules or septa
- Hepatic pyogenic abscess
  - Cluster sign: Small abscesses aggregate, sometimes coalesce into single large septate cavity
  - Rim of abscess locules will enhance
- Cystic metastases
  - Show debris and mural nodularity
- Hydatid (echinococcal) disease
  - Often has numerous peripheral daughter cysts or scolices of different density or intensity

CLINICAL ISSUES

- **Complete excision is mandatory to prevent malignant transformation and recurrence**

DIAGNOSTIC CHECKLIST

- Large, well-defined, homogeneous or heterogeneous "complex cystic" mass with septations and nodularity
  - Enhancing mural nodules suggest malignancy

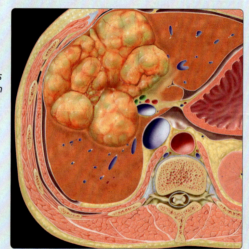
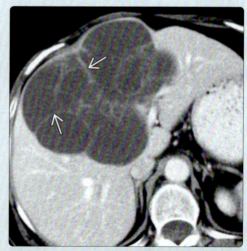

(Left) Graphic shows a lobulated "complex cystic" mass with a vascularized wall and septa. (Right) Axial CECT in a middle-aged woman shows a "complex cystic" mass with lobulated margins and an enhancing wall and septa ➡. These findings in a patient with no other known tumor are probably sufficiently diagnostic of a biliary cystadenoma to warrant resection without further evaluation.

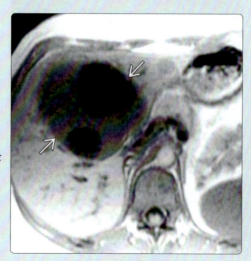
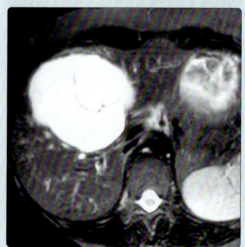

(Left) Axial T1WI MR in a middle-aged woman shows a classic multiseptate, cystic, hepatic mass ➡ with cyst contents having features characteristic of fairly simple fluid. There is slight heterogeneity of the signal that varies between some of the cyst compartments. (Right) Axial T2WI MR in the same patient shows the bright signal of fluid content within the large septate mass.

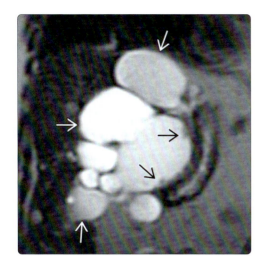

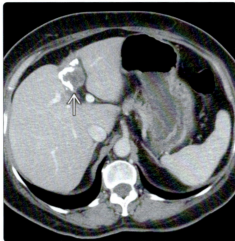

(Left) Coronal T2WI MR shows a large, septate cystic mass ➡️ with mural nodularity ➡️ within 1 of the larger cystic spaces, strongly suggesting a neoplastic etiology, a biliary cystadenoma with foci of cellular atypia in the mucosal lining. (Right) In this 45-year-old woman, CT shows a partially calcified "complex cystic" mass ➡️, which was clearly separate from the gallbladder. This was interpreted as an "indeterminate mass" with a recommendation for follow-up.

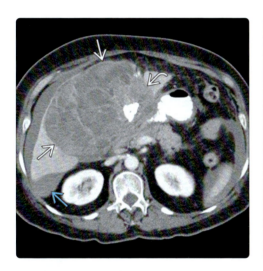

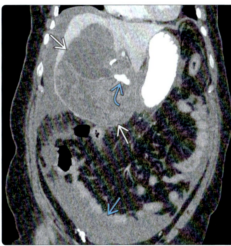

(Left) The same patient returned 5 years later with RUQ pain; axial CT shows marked interval enlargement of the mass ➡️, along with solid mural nodularity ➡️, calcification, and exudative or hemorrhagic ascites ➡️. (Right) Coronal reformatted CT of the same patient shows the large, septate, encapsulated mass ➡️ with its mural nodularity and coarse calcification ➡️, along with complex ascites ➡️ due to spontaneous rupture of the cystic tumor. This biliary cystadenocarcinoma proved fatal.

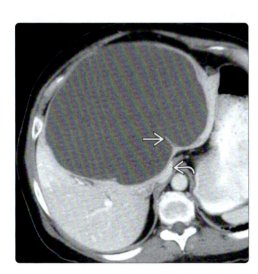

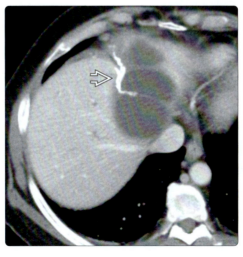

(Left) Initial CT scan of this 56-year-old man shows a large cystic mass with septa ➡️. Note the proximity to and mass effect on the inferior vena cava ➡️ and hepatic veins. (Right) Repeat CT scan in the same patient 1 year after resection of the mass shows recurrence of a septate cystic mass. Portions of the radiopaque staple line ➡️ are visible. Resection of the entire lining of a cystadenoma is necessary to prevent recurrence.

Fibrolamellar Carcinoma

KEY FACTS

TERMINOLOGY

- Uncommon malignant hepatocellular tumor
  - Distinct clinical, histopathologic, and imaging features differentiate it from conventional hepatocellular carcinoma

IMAGING

- **Multiphasic CT or MR with gadoxetate (Eovist) as contrast medium**
- Heterogeneously enhancing, large, lobulated mass with hypointense central scar and radial septa
  - Calcification and necrosis are common (> 50%)
  - Nodal metastases (> 50%)
  - Varies from 5-20 cm (mean: 13 cm) at diagnosis
  - "Satellite" nodules are often present
  - No persistent uptake of gadoxetate (Eovist) on delayed-phase imaging
- Slow-growing tumor that usually arises in normal (noncirrhotic) liver

- Usually diagnosed in adolescent or young adult patients

TOP DIFFERENTIAL DIAGNOSES

- Focal nodular hyperplasia (FNH)
  - Marked **homogeneous** enhancement on arterial phase
  - Nonencapsulated and **no calcification**
  - Homogeneous uptake + delayed retention of gadoxetate (Eovist)
- Conventional hepatocellular carcinoma
  - Heterogeneously hypervascular with washout and capsule
- Peripheral cholangiocarcinoma
  - Often causes hepatic volume loss and capsular retraction
  - Bile duct dilation upstream from mass

DIAGNOSTIC CHECKLIST

- Do not confuse fibrolamellar carcinoma with FNH
  - Distinct imaging features, especially with Eovist-enhanced MR

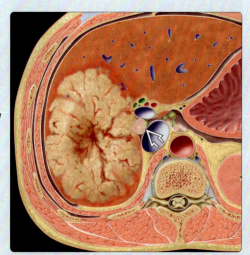
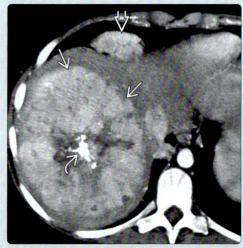

(Left) Axial graphic shows a large, heterogeneous, hypervascular mass with a central scar and porta hepatis lymphadenopathy ➡. (Right) Axial CECT in a 15-year-old boy shows a large, heterogeneous, hypervascular mass ➡ with a large, calcified central scar ➡ and cardiophrenic lymphadenopathy ➡. In a young person, these findings are essentially diagnostic of fibrolamellar hepatocellular carcinoma.

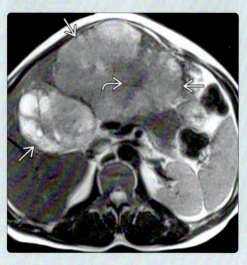
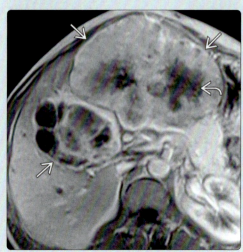

(Left) T2WI MR in a 25-year-old man with early satiety and weight loss shows a large, heterogeneous, bilobed mass ➡ that is hyperintense to the liver. Note the hypointense central scar ➡. (Right) Axial arterial-phase T1WI C+ MR in the same patient shows well-demarcated, lobulated, heterogeneous, and relatively vascular, dominant and "satellite" masses ➡. The fibrous scars ➡ show little enhancement on this phase of imaging but would often demonstrate delayed persistent enhancement, all typical features of FLC.

Hepatic Angiosarcoma

IMAGING

- **Best imaging tool: Multiphasic, multiplanar CT or MR to detect full extent of disease**
- Rare, highly aggressive malignancy with several morphological types
- 3 patterns
  - Multifocal hypervascular masses in liver ± spleen (may have peripheral and delayed enhancement that simulate hemangiomas)
  - Single/multiple hepatic masses with variable necrosis
  - Diffuse infiltration of liver; micronodular
- Often metastatic to spleen, nodes, lungs, bones, kidneys
- PET/CT: FDG-avid tumor(s) and metastases
  - Can help in distinguishing angiosarcoma from hemangioma

TOP DIFFERENTIAL DIAGNOSES

- Hepatic cavernous hemangioma

- Centripetal nodular enhancement that approximates density of blood on all phases
- More homogeneously intense on T2WI than angiosarcoma
- Hepatic metastases and lymphoma
  - Hypervascular metastases: Hyperdense in late arterial phase; usually hypo- or isodense on portal venous and delayed phase (washout)
- Hepatocellular carcinoma
  - Heterogeneous hypervascular mass(es), vascular invasion, cirrhotic liver
- Hepatic adenoma
  - Usually heterogeneously hypervascular with foci of hemorrhage, necrosis, fat, ± capsule

CLINICAL ISSUES

- Rapid and early metastatic spread: Spleen, lung, bone marrow, nodes, etc.
- Prognosis is poor; death within 1 year

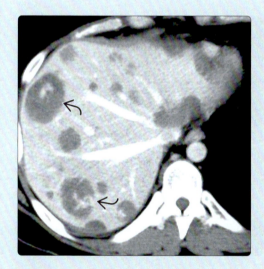
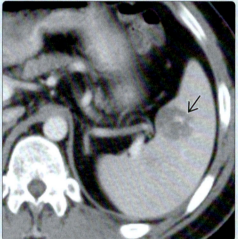

(Left) In this 31-year-old man with abdominal pain and weight loss, axial CECT in the venous phase shows multifocal tumors ⤷, many with central, progressively enhancing channels nearly isodense to vessels. (Right) Axial CT in the same patient shows similar lesions in the spleen ⤷. These lesions simulate some but not all of the imaging features of cavernous hemangiomas; biopsy of one of the masses confirmed angiosarcoma.

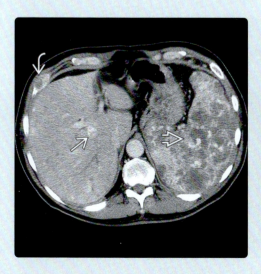
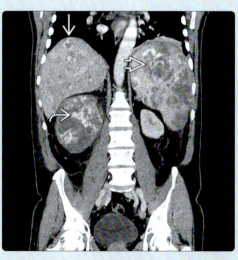

(Left) Axial CECT of a 69-year-old man with abdominal pain and weight loss shows heterogeneous, hypervascular malignancy in multiple sites, including the liver ⤷, spleen ⤷, and an anterior rib ⤷. (Right) Coronal CECT of the same patient shows additional tumors in the liver ⤷, spleen ⤷, and kidney ⤷. The tumors do not fulfill the strict imaging criteria for hemangioma, including nodular peripheral enhancement that is isodense to blood vessels.

IMAGING

- **Multiphasic CT or MR are 1st-line tests**
- **Accuracy: Helical CT (~ 80%), MR and PET (~ 90%)**
- Hepatic lymphoma
  - Diffuse low density on CT may mimic steatosis
    - Easily distinguished from steatosis on MR
  - Multiple well-defined, homogeneous, low-density (CECT) or high-intensity (T2WI) masses
- Liver metastases
  - Hypovascular metastases: Low-density center with peripheral rim or target-like enhancement
  - Hypervascular metastases: Hyperdense (intense) on arterial-phase CECT or CEMR
- Cystic metastases (< 20 HU)
  - Fluid levels, debris, mural nodules
  - Very bright (like cysts) on T2WI MR (but more complex)
- Liver-specific MR contrast agents (e.g., gadoxetate)
  - Metastases: Hypointense lesions become more apparent compared with bright enhancement of liver on delayed-phase imaging
- **CECT is usually best as whole-body screening test**
  - **Even better if combined as PET/CT**
  - Metastases and lymphoma are usually FDG-avid masses
- Decision for thermal ablation or surgical resection
  - May require most sensitive tests (gadoxetate-enhanced MR, PET/CT, or intraoperative US)
- **US**: Hypoechoic metastases; usually from hypovascular tumors
  - Hyperechoic metastases: From GI or hypervascular primaries
  - Cystic metastases: Complex walls and contents

DIAGNOSTIC CHECKLIST

- Multiphasic (arterial- and venous-phase) CT
  - Essential to evaluate for known or suspected hypervascular (e.g., endocrine) primary tumor

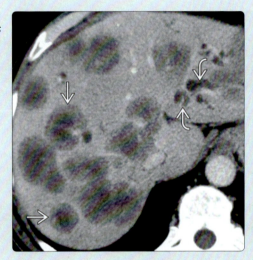
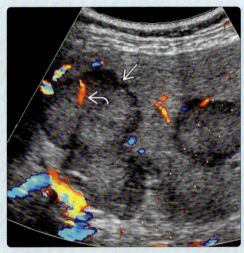

(Left) Axial CECT shows multiple spherical liver lesions ➡ with a target appearance. This is the most typical appearance for liver metastases, especially from colon cancer. Also note the focally dilated bile ducts ➡ due to compression by the metastases. (Right) Color Doppler ultrasound in the same patient shows multiple spherical liver lesions with a target appearance ➡, some containing visible blood vessels ➡. This is the typical appearance of metastatic colorectal carcinoma.

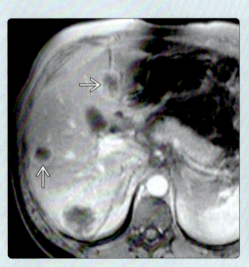
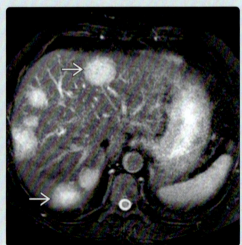

(Left) Axial T1WI C+ MR in a patient with metastatic colon cancer shows multiple liver metastases with several typical features, including a continuous ring of enhancement ➡. (Right) Axial T2WI FS MR in the same patient shows heterogeneous hyperintensity within the hepatic metastases ➡. Most metastases are heterogeneously hyperintense on T2WI and hypovascular and hypointense on T1WI.

IMAGING

General Features

- Key concepts
  - Hepatic lymphoma: Non-Hodgkin lymphoma (NHL) > Hodgkin lymphoma
    - Primary (rare); secondary in up to 50% of patients with NHL
  - Liver metastases
    - Most common malignant tumor of liver
      □ Compared to primary malignant tumors (18:1)
    - Liver is 2nd only to regional lymph nodes as site of metastatic disease
    - Autopsy studies reveal 55% of oncology patients have liver metastases

CT Findings

- CECT
  - Lymphoma
    - Diffuse infiltration and low density
    - Multiple well-defined, homogeneous, low-density masses
  - Hypovascular metastases (most common type)
    - Low-attenuation center with peripheral rim enhancement
    - Indicates vascularized viable tumor in periphery and hypovascular or necrotic center
    - Rim enhancement may also be due to compressed normal parenchyma
  - Hypervascular metastases (usually from endocrine primary tumor)
    - Hyperdense in late arterial-phase images
    - May have internal necrosis without uniform hyperdense enhancement
    - Hypo-/isodense on NECT and portal venous phase
      □ Often washout to become hypodense on delayed-phase CECT
  - Cystic metastases (< 20 HU)
    - Fluid levels, debris, mural nodules

MR Findings

- T1WI
  - Lymphoma and metastases: Hypointense lesions
    - Melanoma metastases: Hyperintense due to melanin
- T2WI
  - Lymphoma: Focal or diffusely hyperintense
  - Metastases
    - Moderate to high signal relative to background liver
    - Very high signal intensity (e.g., cystic and neuroendocrine metastases)
      □ Mimic cysts or hemangiomas but usually with thick wall or fluid level
- T1WI C+
  - Hypovascular metastases
    - Same pattern of enhancement as CECT
    - Low signal in center and peripheral rim enhancement
    - Perilesional enhancement may be tumor vascularity or hepatic edema
  - Hypervascular metastases
    - Hyperintense enhancement on arterial phase

- Hepatobiliary contrast agents [e.g., gadoxetate (Eovist, Primovist)]
  - On delayed scans, normal liver is brightly enhanced
  - Metastases are conspicuous as hypointense focal lesions
  - Most sensitive, but not specific, imaging test for determining presence and number of metastases

Ultrasonographic Findings

- Grayscale ultrasound
  - Hepatic lymphoma
    - Multiple well-defined, hypoechoic lesions
    - Diffuse form: May detect innumerable subcentimeter hypoechoic foci
      □ Otherwise indistinguishable from normal or fatty liver
  - Metastases: Heterogeneously echoic masses
  - Bull's-eye or target metastatic lesions
    - Alternating layers of hyper- and hypoechoic tissue
    - Solid mass with hypoechoic rim or halo
    - Usually from aggressive primary tumors
  - Cystic metastases
    - Almost all show complex walls and contents
  - Calcified metastases
    - Markedly echogenic with acoustic shadowing
- Intraoperative US: Reference standard for hepatic tumors of all kinds

Nuclear Medicine Findings

- PET
  - Lymphoma and metastases
    - 1F-18 FDG-avid focal lesions
    - Excellent staging tool for lymphoma and metastases
      □ High metabolic activity of liver may obscure some lesions

Imaging Recommendations

- Best imaging tool
  - Metaanalysis of sensitivity for detection of colorectal metastases
    - Per patient basis
      □ Helical CT (80%), MR (92%)
      □ PET: 90-95%
    - Per lesion basis (all modalities have lower but similar sensitivity)
      □ All do better for lesions > 1.5 cm
      □ Gadoxetate-enhanced MR much better than CT for lesions < 1.5 cm
  - CECT is usually best as whole-body screening test
    - Even better if combined with PET as PET/CT
  - Decision for thermal ablation or surgical resection
    - May require most sensitive tests (gadoxetate-enhanced MR, PET/CT, or intraoperative US)
- **When to obtain multiphasic (arterial- and venous-phase) CT**
  - Known or suspected hypervascular (e.g., endocrine) primary tumor

SELECTED REFERENCES

1. Abu Hilal M et al: Oncological efficiency analysis of laparoscopic liver resection for primary and metastatic cancer: a single-center UK experience. Arch Surg. 147(1):42-8, 2012

(Left) *Axial arterial-phase CECT in a patient with a metastatic carcinoid tumor shows a hypervascular metastasis ➡ adjacent to inferior vena cava.* **(Right)** *Axial venous-phase CECT in the same patient shows the mass ➡ as nearly isodense to liver and difficult to recognize. For hypervascular tumors, it is critical to obtain both arterial- and venous-phase images through the liver. Hypervascular tumors include primary HCC and adenomas, metastatic endocrine, renal, thyroid, and some melanoma, sarcoma, and breast cancers.*

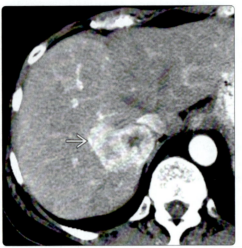 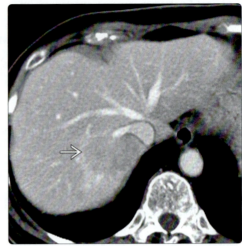

(Left) *Axial CECT in a patient with a metastatic gastric gastrointestinal stromal tumor shows a heterogeneous soft tissue density metastasis ➡.* **(Right)** *Axial CECT in the same patient following treatment shows the metastasis as a near-water-density cystic mass ➡, which could be mistaken for a simple cyst. Cystic metastases can result from a variety of primary tumors, especially sarcomas and cystadenocarcinomas of the ovary. Attention to details, such as mural nodularity and comparison with prior imaging studies, is key.*

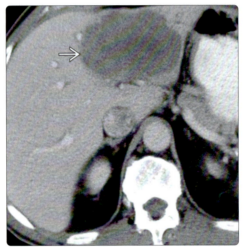 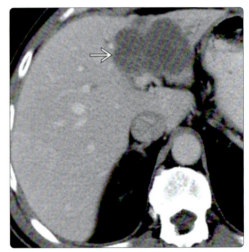

(Left) *Axial T2WI FS MR of a 44-year-old man with colon cancer showed a total of 4 metastases, 3 of which are seen on this section ➡.* **(Right)** *Axial T1WI C+ MR obtained 20 minutes after the IV administration of gadoxetate (Eovist) reveals at least 3 additional metastases ➡. Gadoxetate can make small metastases much more evident than on routine MR or CT evaluation. In this patient, the presence of 6 metastases precluded surgical or ablative therapy.*

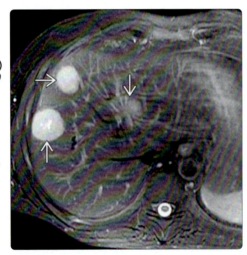 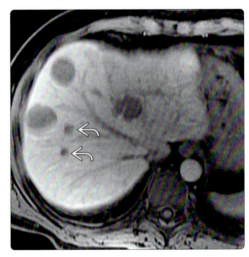

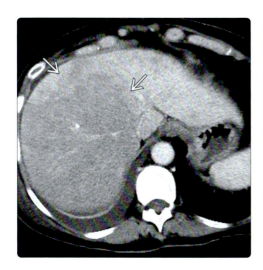

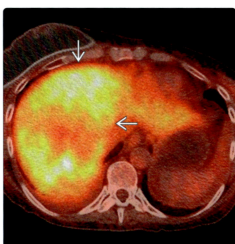

(Left) Axial CECT of a 59-year-old woman with breast cancer and liver disfunction shows poorly defined low density ➡️ replacing most of the right lobe of the liver in a pattern suggesting steatosis or widespread metastases. (Right) One week later, a PET/CT scan was performed. Axial fused PET/CT shows that the abnormal portions of the liver ➡️ are FDG avid, indicating malignant disease (metastases). PET/CT can be valuable in detection of subtle or diffuse liver metastases or lymphoma.

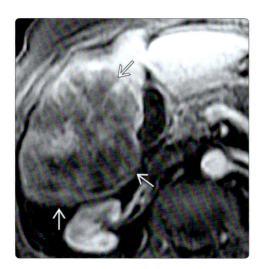

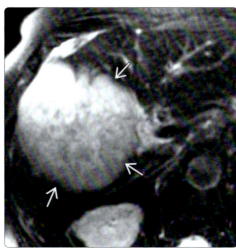

(Left) Axial T1WI C+ MR in a patient with hepatic lymphoma shows a large, heterogeneously hypointense mass ➡️. (Right) Axial T2WI FS MR in the same patient shows that the large solitary mass ➡️ is heterogeneously hyperintense.

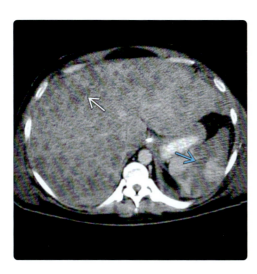

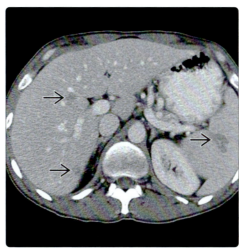

(Left) Axial CECT in a patient with diffuse hepatic lymphoma shows innumerable small foci of tumor in the liver ➡️ and spleen ➡️. On NECT, the liver appeared diffusely enlarged and low in attenuation, resembling benign steatosis. (Right) Axial CECT in a patient with non-Hodgkin lymphoma (NHL) and AIDS shows multifocal hypodense masses ➡️ in the liver and spleen. Similar masses were present in the kidneys and in multiple nodal groups. AIDS patients and transplant recipients are at high risk for developing NHL.

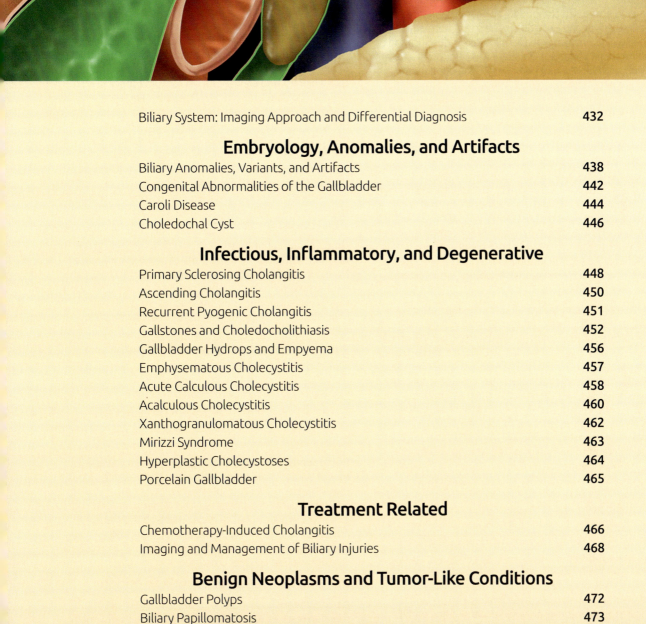

Imaging Indications and Protocols

Oral and IV cholangiography have been supplanted by newer cross-sectional imaging and cholescintigraphy. MR hepatobiliary IV contrast agents may be used to supplement CT or MR cholangiography.

Cholescintigraphy is a nuclear medicine study used to evaluate the morphology and function of the biliary tree. In a "**HIDA scan**," the patient receives an IV administration of Tc-99m iminodiacetic acid compound, an agent that has rapid uptake by the liver and excretion in the bile. A normal study has a hepatic parenchymal phase followed by identification of the radiotracer within the gallbladder (GB), indicating a patent cystic duct, and subsequent passage into the duodenum, indicating a patent common duct. While the anatomic detail of a HIDA scan is limited, the functional information is valuable in diagnosing cystic duct or common duct occlusion or a biliary leak.

Ultrasonography (US) is the primary imaging modality for most GB and biliary abnormalities. US detects gallstones within the GB with almost 100% accuracy. The diagnosis of acute cholecystitis is established with only slightly less accuracy based on the findings of gallstones, GB wall thickening, and focal tenderness over the GB (the sonographic Murphy sign). US may also allow diagnosis of complications of cholecystitis, such as gangrene or perforation, although CT is often better suited for the evaluation of disease beyond the GB wall. GB wall mass lesions, such as polyps and carcinoma, are also well depicted by US.

CT is less sensitive than US in diagnosis of gallstones, because the attenuation of gallstones may vary from less than water to densely calcified. Furthermore, CT detects sludge (the viscous, echogenic layer of material within the GB that is often present in fasting patients and those with GB dysfunction) much less frequently than US. CT is accurate in diagnosing complications of acute cholecystitis and in revealing the mass (biliary, hepatic, or pancreatic), which is the usual cause of painless jaundice. Newer thin-section and multiplanar CT detects more than 70% of stones in choledocholithiasis and shows indirect signs, such as abrupt narrowing of the common bile duct (CBD), in a higher percentage of cases. CT or MR is the primary modality for diagnosis and staging of pancreaticobiliary neoplasms. Multiplanar displays, especially along the course of the biliary and pancreatic ducts and vessels, are especially effective in providing findings that have an impact on diagnosis and management of pancreaticobiliary diseases.

CT cholangiography is a noninvasive alternative to direct or MR cholangiography and is useful for the preoperative evaluation of the biliary anatomy in a potential living liver donor, as some common ductal anomalies may preclude or complicate this procedure. A standard without-and-with IV contrast CT scan is initially performed using the conventional nonionic contrast media. Next, a slow IV drip infusion of iodipamide is performed with delayed CT imaging, and multiplanar reformations of the opacified biliary tree are obtained. Spatial resolution usually exceeds that of MRCP but is less than that of direct cholangiography.

MR cholangiopancreatography (MRCP) has largely supplanted endoscopic retrograde cholangiopancreatography (ERCP) in the diagnosis of lesions affecting the biliary or pancreatic ducts. MRCP is a primary tool in the evaluation of biliary obstruction (from calculi or intrinsic and extrinsic masses), while ERCP is usually reserved for interventions, such

as the placement of a biliary stent to bypass an obstructed bile duct.

MRCP utilizes a variety of heavily T2-weighted sequences to show the bile (and pancreatic duct) as bright signal fluid. While spatial detail is limited, it is usually sufficient to establish the diagnosis and guide management. MRCP can also be combined with other sequences in multiple planes to yield comprehensive evaluation of the liver, biliary tree, and pancreas.

The IV administration of gadoxetate (Eovist or Primovist) allows high-quality MR evaluation of the hepatic parenchyma during the arterial and venous phases of imaging, and delayed imaging can provide unique advantages over the usual gadolinium-based contrast media for some specific indications. Gadoxetate (Eovist) has the unique property of having 50% hepatobiliary excretion. Imaging after a 20-minute delay shows dense enhancement of normal hepatic parenchyma as well as enhancement of the biliary tree. This allows for better quality MR cholangiography for such indications as preoperative evaluation of potential hepatic donation, biliary leaks following trauma or surgery, and biliary obstruction. The presence of hepatic dysfunction (e.g., with elevated serum bilirubin) may impair the quality of the cholangiographic phase of a gadoxetate-enhanced MR scan.

Direct cholangiography retains an important role in the diagnosis and treatment of biliary disease. Percutaneous transhepatic cholangiography is the optimal modality for patients with known or suspected biliary obstruction when ERCP is unavailable (e.g., following prior surgical biliary diversion) or to diagnose, stage, and treat intrahepatic or proximal extrahepatic biliary obstruction (e.g., Klatskin tumor).

ERCP is performed for known or suspected biliary obstruction that may require endoscopic placement of a biliary stent, retrieval of stones, or the acquisition of a biopsy specimen or brush cytology/histology confirmation of malignancy.

ERCP is also the modality of choice for diagnosis and treatment of traumatic or postsurgical bile leaks, which will usually resolve following placement of a biliary stent.

Postoperative (T-tube) cholangiography is a valuable and easy means of evaluating a biliary tree that has been altered by surgery (e.g., liver transplantation, choledochoenterostomy) when the surgeon has left a tube in place within the CBD with an external limb that can be accessed for injection of contrast medium. A T-tube cholangiogram allows for convenient and safe diagnosis of retained stones, leaks, or strictures.

Imaging Evaluation of Jaundiced Patient

A patient who has jaundice or significant elevation of liver function tests, especially alkaline phosphatase or bilirubin, either has biliary obstruction or severe diffuse hepatic disease. The role of imaging in this setting is to determine the presence, level, and cause of biliary obstruction.

Criteria for diagnosing biliary dilation vary somewhat among investigators and according to the age of the patient. As a general rule, the presence of visible continuous arborization (branching) of the intrahepatic ducts indicates dilation. The bile ducts course along the portal triads and should not be > 40% of the diameter of the adjacent portal vein. The common hepatic duct should measure < 6 mm at the porta hepatis and the CBD < 8 mm, although it commonly measures up to 10 mm in elderly patients who have had a prior cholecystectomy. Dilation of the extrahepatic ducts should always be correlated with any clinical or biochemical evidence of obstruction before recommending extensive evaluation.

The character of the transition from a dilated to narrow duct is an important criterion. Abrupt narrowing is usually due to tumor, stone, or iatrogenic injury, while tapered narrowing is more commonly due to inflammation, such as from pancreatitis or cholangitis. Malignant tumors also cause eccentric narrowing of the duct and a mass in or around the duct and may be associated with other signs of "invasiveness," such as vessel encasement.

The **level of the obstruction** is determined by the point of transition from dilated to narrowed ducts.

Intrahepatic causes of obstruction include primary sclerosing cholangitis and liver tumors, usually malignant.

Porta hepatis obstruction is most commonly due to cholangiocarcinoma (Klatskin tumor). Primary sclerosing cholangitis, GB carcinoma, metastases, or iatrogenic injury (usually from a laparoscopic cholecystectomy) are other etiologies that may result in obstruction at the porta hepatis.

Intrapancreatic causes of obstruction include pancreatic carcinoma, chronic pancreatitis, CBD stones, cholangiocarcinoma, and ampullary lesions (dysfunction or tumor).

Differential Diagnosis

Distended Gallbladder
Common
- Cholecystitis
- Prolonged fasting
- Hyperalimentation
- Postvagotomy state
- Anticholinergic medication
- Diabetes mellitus
- Obstruction of CBD
- Alcoholism
- Acute pancreatitis
- Hepatitis

Less Common
- Hydrops and empyema, GB
- Autoimmune (IgG4-related) pancreatitis
- AIDS cholangiopathy
- Choledochal cyst (mimic)

Gas in Bile Ducts or Gallbladder
Common
- Sphincterotomy
- Choledocholithiasis
- Patulous sphincter of Oddi
- Biliary-enteric anastomosis
- Portal vein gas (mimic)

Less Common
- Emphysematous cholecystitis
- Gas within gallstones
- Duodenal diverticulum
- Gallstone ileus
- Crohn's disease
- Duodenal ulcer
- Acute pancreatitis
- Chemotherapy-induced cholangitis
- Recurrent pyogenic cholangitis

- Pancreato-biliary parasites
- Duodenal carcinoma
- Ampullary carcinoma

Focal Gallbladder Wall Thickening
Common
- Hyperplastic cholecystosis
- GB carcinoma

Less Common
- Xanthogranulomatous cholecystitis
- Porcelain GB
- Metastases and lymphoma, GB
- GB wall polyps
- Epithelial polyps, GB
- Mesenchymal tumor, GB
- Intramural hematoma, GB

Dilated Common Bile Duct
Common
- Choledocholithiasis
- Postcholecystectomy
- Pancreatic ductal carcinoma
- Senescent change, CBD
- Chronic pancreatitis

Less Common
- Other pancreatic neoplasms
- GB carcinoma
- Autoimmune (IgG4-related) cholangitis or pancreatitis
- Primary sclerosing cholangitis
- Pancreatic pseudocyst
- Ascending cholangitis
- Biliary trauma
- Small bowel obstruction
- Choledochal cyst

Asymmetric Dilation of Intrahepatic Bile Ducts
Common
- Primary sclerosing cholangitis
- Cholangiocarcinoma
- Ascending cholangitis
- Hepatocellular carcinoma
- Hepatic metastases and lymphoma
- AIDS cholangiopathy

Less Common
- Recurrent pyogenic cholangitis
- Autoimmune (IgG4-related) cholangitis
- Pancreato-biliary parasites
- Chemotherapy cholangitis
- Hepatic hydatid cyst
- Intraductal papillary mucinous neoplasm, biliary

Selected References

1. Chang JH et al: Role of magnetic resonance cholangiopancreatography for choledocholithiasis: analysis of patients with negative MRCP. Scand J Gastroenterol. 47(2):217-24, 2012
2. Drake LM et al: Accuracy of magnetic resonance cholangiopancreatography in identifying pancreatic duct disruption. J Clin Gastroenterol. 46(8):696-9, 2012
3. Frydrychowicz A et al: Gadoxetic acid-enhanced T1-weighted MR cholangiography in primary sclerosing cholangitis. J Magn Reson Imaging. 36(3):632-40, 2012
4. Harbrecht J et al: [Transgastric-, transhepatic endosonography-guided biliary drainage (EUCD) in a patient with locally advanced cholangiocarcinoma.] Z Gastroenterol. 50(1):30-3, 2012
5. Hyodo T et al: CT and MR cholangiography: advantages and pitfalls in perioperative evaluation of biliary tree. Br J Radiol. 85(1015):887-96, 2012
6. Katz DS et al: Imaging of abdominal pain in pregnancy. Radiol Clin North Am. 50(1):149-71, 2012

(Left) *Longitudinal US in a 40-year-old woman with pain shows a distended gallbladder* ➡ *and multiple small, echogenic stones* ➡. **(Right)** *Tc-99m HIDA scan shows flow of the radiotracer from the liver into the common bile duct* ➡ *and bowel* ➡ *but not into the gallbladder. This indicates cystic duct obstruction and suggests acute cholecystitis.*

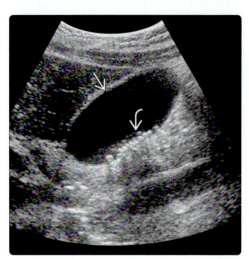
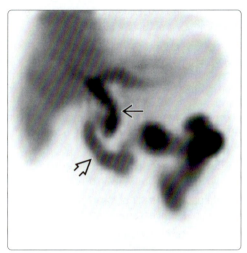

(Left) *Coronal CECT demonstrates a poorly marginated hypodense mass* ➡ *in the pancreatic head/neck, typical of pancreatic adenocarcinoma. Note that the tumor encases the portal vein* ➡, *portal/SMV confluence, and the SMV* ➡. **(Right)** *This 55-year-old man has alcoholic cirrhosis, accounting for the dysmorphic liver with widened fissures. Note the distended, hydropic gallbladder* ➡. *Patients with alcoholic cirrhosis commonly have gallstones and a poorly contractile gallbladder.*

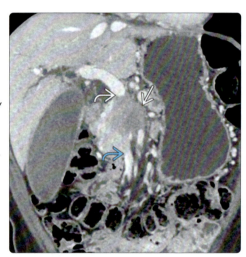
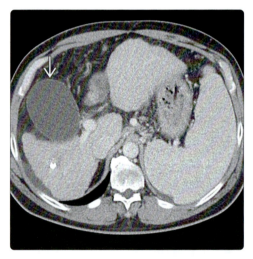

(Left) *In this 36-year-old man, CT shows gas and fluid within the gallbladder* ➡ *and common duct* ➡ *due to the presence of a biliary stent (not shown). The gallbladder wall is normal.* **(Right)** *In this 68-year-old man with diabetes and sepsis, CT shows gas within the lumen* ➡ *and wall of the gallbladder* ➡ *with a hazy margin where the gallbladder abuts the liver. This emphysematous cholecystitis was treated urgently with percutaneous cholecystostomy and later with cholecystectomy.*

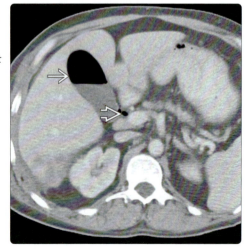
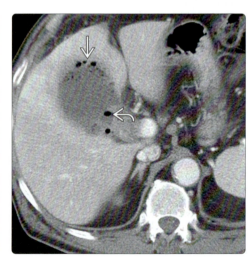

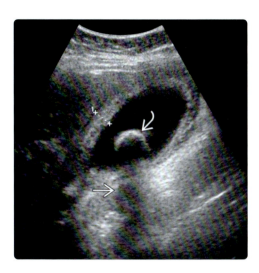

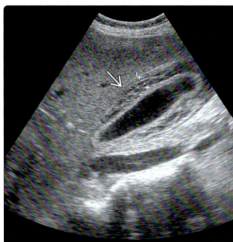

(Left) *In this 50-year-old woman with acute cholecystitis, US shows a large echogenic stone ⟶ with an acoustic shadow ⟶ and a thickened gallbladder wall (calipers). These findings, along with a positive sonographic Murphy sign, are diagnostic of acute cholecystitis.* (Right) *In this 35-year-old man with acute viral hepatitis, sonography shows a markedly thickened wall of the gallbladder ⟶ but no calculi. Acute hepatitis often causes massive gallbladder wall thickening along with periportal edema.*

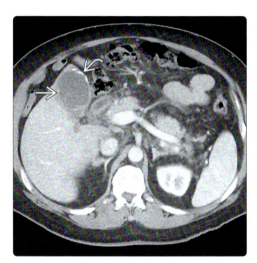

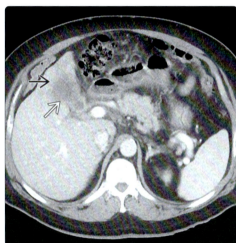

(Left) *In this 68-year-old man, CT shows partial calcification ⟶ of the gallbladder wall. The gallbladder wall ⟶ that is adjacent to the liver is irregularly thickened, and the interface with the liver is quite irregular.* (Right) *Another CT section in the same patient shows tumor invasion of the adjacent liver ⟶ by this gallbladder cancer; the primary mass arises from the gallbladder wall ⟶.*

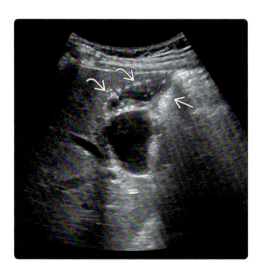

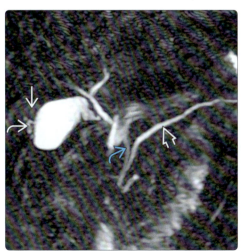

(Left) *In this 42-year-old man, sonography shows a fundal mass ⟶ with cystic components and echogenic foci ⟶.* (Right) *Coronal MRCP in the same patient shows foci of high T2 signal intensity ⟶ within the fundal mass ⟶, representing dilated Rokitansky-Aschoff sinuses. These are characteristic features of fundal adenomyomatosis, a benign, hyperplastic cholecystosis. The common bile duct ⟶ and pancreatic duct ⟶ are marked.*

(Left) In this elderly woman with no acute symptoms, CT shows dilation of the intrahepatic bile ducts ➡. **(Right)** CT in the same patient shows evidence of a prior cholecystectomy with clips ➡ in the gallbladder bed. Both intrahepatic and extrahepatic ducts ➡ are dilated to a degree beyond what is usually seen following cholecystectomy alone, but this patient had no clinical nor biochemical evidence of biliary obstruction.

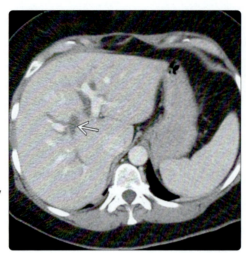
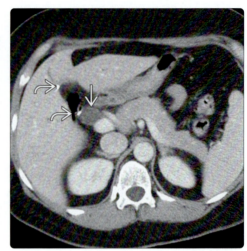

(Left) In this 50-year-old man with chronic alcoholic pancreatitis, CT shows a heavily calcified and atrophic pancreas ➡ with dilation of the intrahepatic bile ducts ➡ and pancreatic duct ➡. **(Right)** More caudal CT section in the same patient shows several intra- and peripancreatic pseudocysts ➡. The pseudocysts and chronic fibroinflammatory scarring caused a stricture of the distal common bile duct.

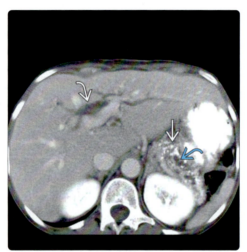
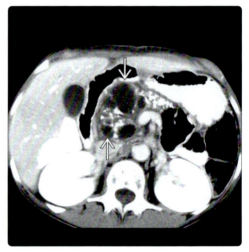

(Left) In this elderly man, CT shows intrahepatic ductal obstruction due to liver metastases ➡ from colon cancer. Note the dilated, arborizing ducts ➡. **(Right)** In this 55-year-old woman, CT shows asymmetric dilation of the intrahepatic bile ducts ➡ due to a multifocal, peripheral (intrahepatic) cholangiocarcinoma ➡.

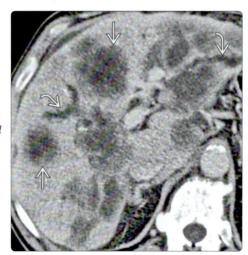
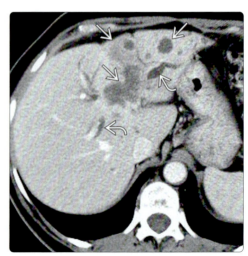

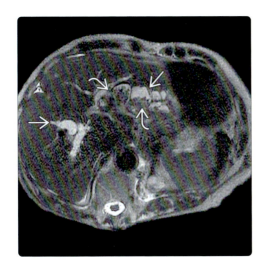

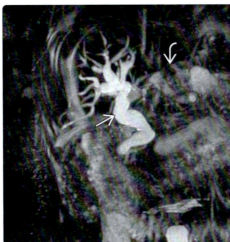

(Left) *In this elderly woman with recurrent pyogenic cholangitis, a T2 FS MR shows dilated intrahepatic bile ducts ➡. Within the dilated left lobe ducts, there are numerous and large filling defects representing calculi ➡. **(Right)** MRCP in the same patient confirms diffuse dilation of the intra- and extrahepatic ducts ➡. The dilated left lobe ducts are less apparent because they are partially filled with stones ➡ and they may be out of the plane of the MR section.*

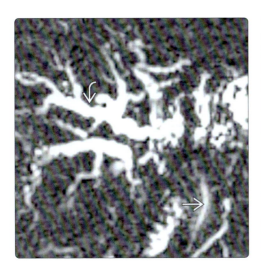

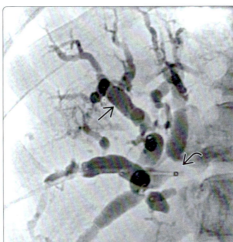

(Left) *MRCP shows markedly dilated intrahepatic ducts ➡ and a normal common bile duct ➡. The presence of severe dilation and abrupt transition at the confluence of the main left and right ducts suggests the diagnosis of Klatskin tumor (cholangiocarcinoma).* **(Right)** *Transhepatic cholangiogram in the same patient shows dilated intrahepatic ducts ➡ and complete obstruction at the confluence of the main ducts ➡ due to a Klatskin tumor.*

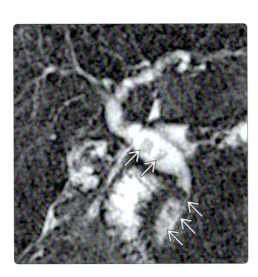

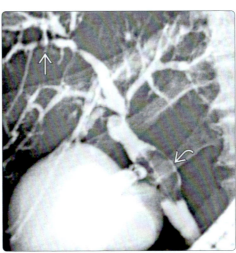

(Left) *MRCP in the coronal plane shows multiple calculi ➡ within the dilated common bile duct.* **(Right)** *ERCP shows irregular arborization of the intrahepatic bile ducts with multiple strictures ➡ due to primary sclerosing cholangitis. The polypoid mass ➡ within the common bile duct is a cholangiocarcinoma.*

Biliary Anomalies, Variants, and Artifacts

TERMINOLOGY

- Variants and artifacts that may simulate pathology or potentially complicate hepatobiliary surgical procedures

IMAGING

- **Congenital anomalies of gallbladder (GB)**
  - Anomalies of number, shape, or position
  - Most are of no clinical significance but may make surgery more difficult
- **Most common biliary variants**
  - Usually aberrant right posterior branch, which can drain into left HD ("crossover anomaly"), common hepatic duct, common bile duct, cystic duct, or GB
    - May complicate or preclude living donor right liver transplantation
    - May result in bile leak or stricture following cholecystectomy
- Anomalous insertion of cystic duct

- Must be recognized at cholecystectomy to avoid iatrogenic biliary injuries
- Persistent postoperative dilation of bile ducts
  - Especially common in patients who had choledocholithiasis and dilated common duct prior to surgery
  - No need for additional evaluation in absence of clinical or laboratory signs of biliary obstruction

CLINICAL ISSUES

- Normal biliary variants are common (42% of population)
- No clinical significance unless surgery is planned
- Risk of injury if surgeon is unaware (especially anomalies of cystic duct and right hepatic duct)

DIAGNOSTIC CHECKLIST

- Pseudocalculi, strictures, and other MR artifacts are common in biliary tree, making familiarity with artifacts critical to avoid unnecessary intervention

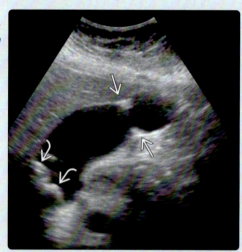
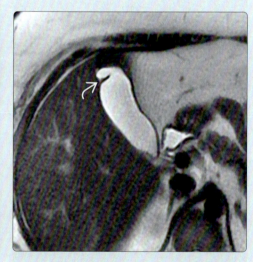

(Left) *Ultrasound of a 51-year-old woman shows a prominent fold ➡ (a phrygian cap) within the gallbladder fundus. Although a congenital abnormality, it is considered a normal variant given its high prevalence. Note numerous shadowing stones ➡ within the gallbladder neck.* (Right) *Axial T2WI FSE MR in a 32-year-old woman with chronic abdominal pain shows an incidental phrygian cap ➡.*

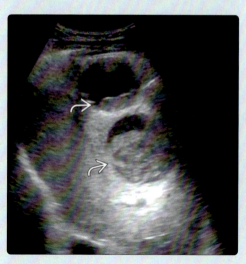
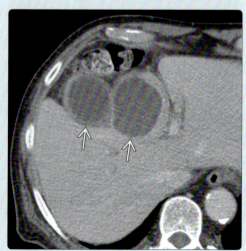

(Left) *Ultrasound of a 79-year-old debilitated man with right upper quadrant pain shows dependent sludge ➡ within both lobes of a bilobed gallbladder.* (Right) *CECT of the same patient shows 2 separate thick-walled gallbladders ➡. Both lobes of a bilobed gallbladder share a common cystic duct. Persistent abdominal pain and leukocytosis prompted cholecystostomy drainage of the more superficial gallbladder. Both lumina were successfully decompressed.*

IMAGING

General Features
- **Congenital anomalies of gallbladder (GB)**
  - Agenesis of GB: Congenital absence (rare)
  - Hypogenesis of GB: Rudimentary, very small GB
  - Bilobed GB: 2 completely divided GB cavities with shared cystic duct
  - Phrygian cap: Folding of GB fundus; considered normal variant given its high prevalence
  - Congenital diverticulum: Outpouching from GB lumen
  - Left-sided GB: Isolated or associated with situs inversus
  - Intrahepatic GB: Subcapsular GB partially or completely embedded within liver
  - Horizontal GB: Ectopic GB within porta hepatis; usually deeply embedded within liver
  - Retrodisplaced GB: Retrohepatic or retroperitoneal
  - Cholecystomegaly (enlarged GB)
    - Acquired anomaly or abnormality
    - Seen in patients with diabetes, sickle cell disease, or pregnancy as well as after truncal vagotomy
  - Microgallbladder
    - Acquired, most often in cystic fibrosis patients
- **Normal biliary anatomy**
  - Right hepatic duct (HD) is relatively short, has 2 branches
    - Anterior (ventrocranial) branch drains segments VI and VIII and has horizontal course extending lateral and towards right from right HD
    - Posterior (dorsocaudal) branch drains segments VI and VII, has vertical course upward from right HD
    - Right posterior duct fuses to right anterior duct from medial approach
  - Left HD formed by segmental branches from segments II-IV
  - Duct from caudate lobe can join origin of left or right HD
  - Right and left HD converge at porta hepatis to form common hepatic duct (CHD)
  - Cystic duct usually joins CHD just below confluence of right and left HD
  - Only central intrahepatic ducts seen on MRCP in normal patients (≥ 3 mm): Visualization of too many intrahepatic ducts raises concern for ductal strictures or dilation
- **Most common variants**
  - Most common variants involve aberrant right HD
    - Usually aberrant posterior branch, which can drain into left HD ("crossover anomaly"), CHD, common bile duct (CBD), cystic duct, or GB
      □ Most frequent is right posterior duct draining into left HD (13-19% of population)
      □ 2nd most common variant is right posterior duct fusing with lateral (right) aspect of right anterior duct (~ 12% of population)
    - **May complicate or preclude living donor right liver transplantation**
    - **May result in bile leak or stricture following cholecystectomy**
  - Abnormal junction of HDs
    - Trifurcation pattern ("triple confluence"), with single junction of left HD with anterior and posterior branches of right HD (11% of population)
      □ Right HD nonexistent in this pattern

- Accessory HDs seen in 2% of patients
- Anomalous insertion of cystic duct
  - Low insertion into CBD (10% of population)
  - May insert into right HD
  - May insert into medial aspect of common duct
  - May follow parallel course to CHD over several cm
  - **Must be recognized at cholecystectomy to avoid iatrogenic biliary injuries**
- Duplication of cystic duct or CBD: Rare
- **Pancreaticobiliary junction variants**
  - Separate entrance of CBD and main pancreatic duct into duodenum
  - Long (> 8 mm) common channel of distal CBD and pancreatic duct
  - CBD may enter side of pancreatic duct
    - > 1.5 cm proximal to ampulla of Vater
    - Commonly seen in type I choledochal cyst
    - Associated with higher prevalence of cholangiocarcinoma, GB carcinoma, choledocholithiasis, and chronic pancreatitis
- **Persistent postoperative dilation of bile ducts**
  - Affects common duct more commonly than intrahepatic ducts
  - Common duct > 8 mm in diameter
  - Most common in elderly patients following cholecystectomy
  - Especially common in patients who had choledocholithiasis and dilated common duct prior to surgery
    - Also seems to occur without precholecystectomy dilation (controversial)
  - No need for additional evaluation in absence of clinical or laboratory signs of biliary obstruction

Imaging Recommendations
- Best imaging tool
  - ERCP or MRCP
    - MRCP is noninvasive but more susceptible to artifacts, which can result in misinterpretation
    - Artifacts may simulate biliary strictures or stones
    - Any potential ductal stricture or filling defect should be confirmed on other MR sequences

DIAGNOSTIC CHECKLIST

Image Interpretation Pearls
- Careful depiction of biliary anatomy is crucial for planning partial liver resection transplantation
- Pseudocalculi and other MR artifacts are common in biliary tree, making familiarity with artifacts critical to avoid unnecessary intervention

SELECTED REFERENCES
1. Ragab A et al: Correlation between 3D-MRCP and intra-operative findings in right liver donors. Hepatobiliary Surg Nutr. 2(1):7-13, 2013
2. Griffin N et al: Magnetic resonance cholangiopancreatography: the ABC of MRCP. Insights Imaging. 3(1):11-21, 2012

(Left) *Transverse ultrasound of a neonate shows a completely intrahepatic gallbladder* ➡. *(Right) Sagittal ultrasound of the same patient shows liver surrounding the walls of an intrahepatic gallbladder* ➡. *As an isolated finding, this is not clinically significant, although the location of the gallbladder may make cholecystectomy exceedingly difficult.*

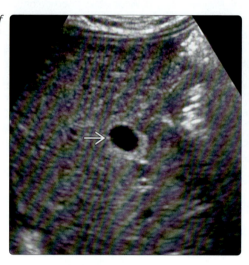 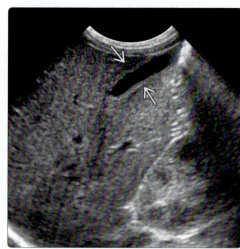

(Left) *Upper left-hand graphic (A) shows the conventional arrangement of the bile ducts. Variations are common, especially with aberrant insertion of the right posterior duct, as seen in figures D-F. This may lead to inadvertent ligation or transection at surgery.* (Right) *Graphic shows common variations in the course and insertion of the cystic duct, leading to difficulty in isolation and ligation at cholecystectomy. The cystic duct may be mistaken for the common hepatic or common bile duct.*

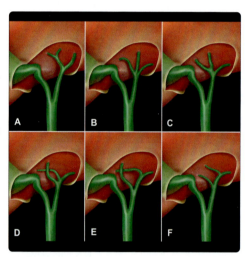 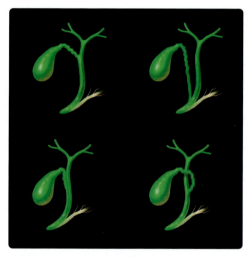

(Left) *Intraoperative cholangiogram shows a peculiar bilobed cystic dilation of the distal common duct* ➡, *presumably a type 3 choledochal cyst or choledochocele. Also noted is aberrant drainage of the posterior lobe bile duct* ➡ *into the common hepatic duct.* (Right) *Coronal MRCP with MIP reconstruction demonstrates separate origins of the right anterior and posterior ducts from the common duct. MRCP has a very high concordance with ERCP for identifying biliary tree variants.*

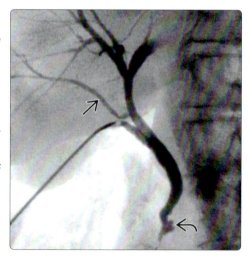 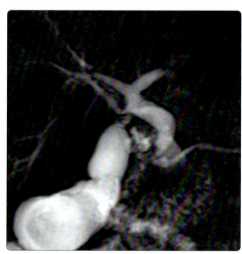

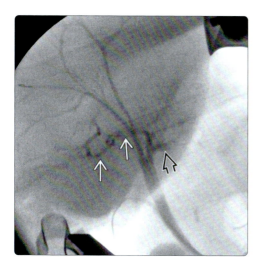
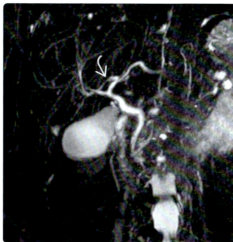

(Left) *Intraoperative cholangiogram obtained prior to right lobe liver donation shows insertion of the right posterior duct* ➡ *into the proximal left bile duct* ⊟. (Right) *Coronal MRCP with MIP reconstruction demonstrates the right posterior duct* ➡ *arising from the left hepatic duct. This is the most common biliary anatomic variant and is found in 13-19% of the population.*

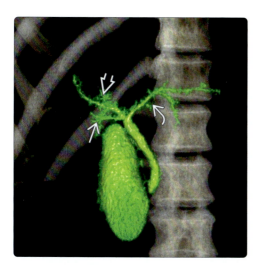
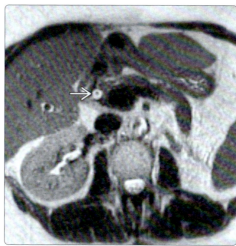

(Left) *Coronal 3D reconstruction CT cholangiogram of a potential liver donor shows trifurcation of the common duct into left* ➡, *right anterior* ➡, *and right posterior* ➡ *ducts. This anatomy may require more complex biliary reconstruction during transplantation or may preclude donation.* (Right) *Axial T2WI shows a small signal void in the middle of the distal common duct* ➡. *There was no proximal ductal dilation. Flow artifacts like these are more common when using single-shot technique.*

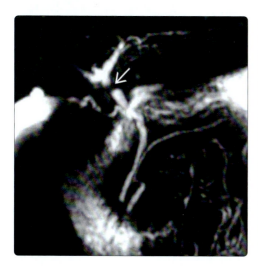
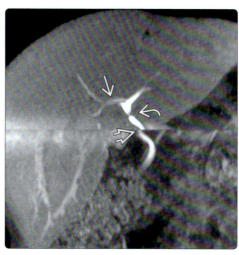

(Left) *Coronal MRCP shows a signal void* ➡ *in the common hepatic duct that simulates a stone. Note the absence of dilation of the ducts upstream from this point.* (Right) *MR cholangiogram performed after administration of Eovist in a potential right lobe liver donor shows drainage of the right posterior duct* ➡ *into the proximal left hepatic duct. Note the pulsation artifact proximal to the bifurcation* ➡ *and a motion-reconstruction artifact along the mid common duct* ➡.

TERMINOLOGY

- Spectrum of congenital malformations and deformities of gallbladder (GB)
  - **Agenesis of GB**: Congenital absence of GB
  - **Hypogenesis of GB**: Rudimentary GB
  - **Bilobed GB**: 2 completely divided GB cavities with common cystic duct
  - **Duplicated GB**: Duplicated GB and cystic duct
  - **Phrygian cap**: Folding of GB fundus; considered normal variant given its high prevalence
  - **Congenital diverticulum**
  - **Left-sided GB**: Isolated or associated with situs inversus
  - **Intrahepatic GB**: Subcapsular GB partially or completely embedded in liver
  - **Horizontal GB**: Ectopic GB within porta hepatis; usually deeply embedded in liver
  - **Retrodisplaced GB**: Retrohepatic or retroperitoneal ectopic GB

TOP DIFFERENTIAL DIAGNOSES

- Postcholecystectomy
- Cholecystitis, chronic
- Hartmann pouch of GB
- Hyperplastic cholecystoses
- Abdominal collection

CLINICAL ISSUES

- Most are of no clinical significance
- Rarely predispose to biliary stasis, inflammation, and stone formation

DIAGNOSTIC CHECKLIST

- Consider ectopic location or agenesis whenever GB is not visualized

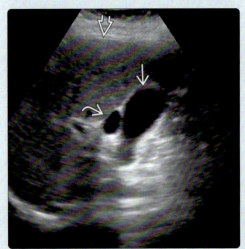
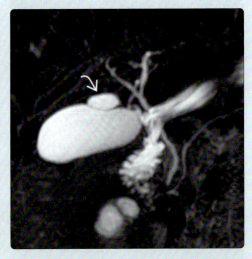

(Left) Ultrasound of a 24-year-old female patient with nonspecific abdominal pain shows an elongated, anechoic, cystic structure ➘ between the gallbladder ➘ and liver ➘. (Right) Coronal MRCP of the same patient shows a cystic structure ➘ adjacent to the gallbladder. The configuration of the "cyst" is characteristic of gallbladder duplication. Both the gallbladder and the "cyst" partially opacified via separate cystic ducts on a follow-up gadoxetate ("Eovist") enhanced MRCP.

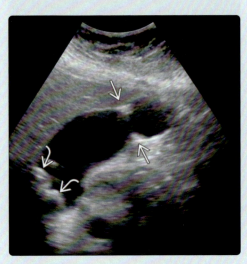
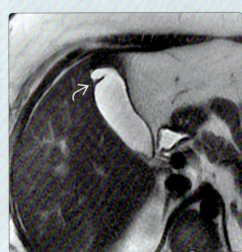

(Left) Ultrasound of a 51-year-old female patient shows a prominent fold ➘ (a phrygian cap) within the gallbladder fundus. Although a congenital abnormality, it is considered a normal variant given its high prevalence. Note numerous shadowing stones ➘ within the gallbladder neck. (Right) Axial T2WI FSE MR in a 32-year-old female patient with chronic abdominal pain shows an incidental phrygian cap ➘.

Congenital Abnormalities of the Gallbladder

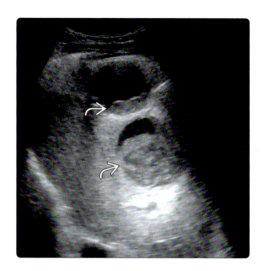

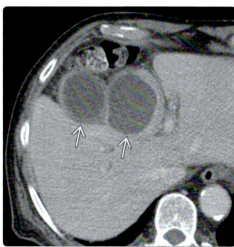

(Left) Ultrasound of a 79-year-old debilitated man with right upper quadrant pain shows dependent sludge ⟳ within both lobes of a bilobed gallbladder. (Right) CECT of the same patient shows 2 separate thick-walled gallbladders ➔. Both lobes of a bilobed gallbladder share a common cystic duct. Persistent abdominal pain and leukocytosis prompted cholecystostomy drainage of the more superficial gallbladder. Both lumina were successfully decompressed.

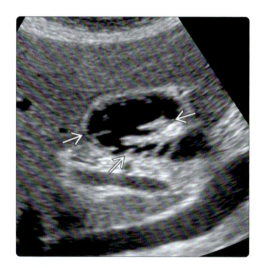

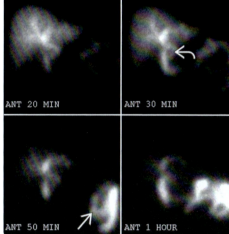

(Left) Ultrasound of a 68-year-old male patient with elevated liver function tests shows multiple thin septa ➔ within the gallbladder lumen. The honeycomb appearance is thought to be due to incomplete vacuolization of the gallbladder bud. (Right) Coronal Tc-99m HIDA scan of a 54-year-old woman with abdominal pain shows progressive filling of the bile duct ➔ and proximal small bowel ➔ but no gallbladder activity. The patient had no operative history and multiple imaging studies confirmed gallbladder agenesis.

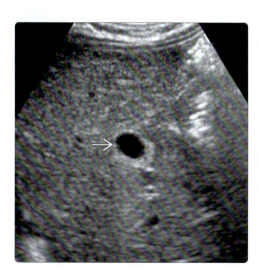

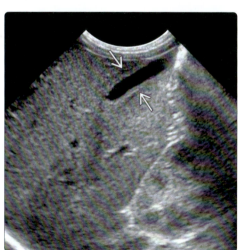

(Left) Transverse ultrasound of a neonate shows a completely intrahepatic gallbladder ➔. (Right) Sagittal ultrasound of the same patient shows liver surrounding the walls of an intrahepatic gallbladder ➔. As an isolated finding, this is not clinically significant, although the location of the gallbladder may make cholecystectomy exceedingly difficult.

KEY FACTS

TERMINOLOGY

- **Caroli disease**: Congenital, multifocal, segmental, saccular dilation of large intrahepatic bile ducts (IHBDs)
  ○ Type V choledochal cyst (Todani classification)
- **Caroli syndrome** (more common variant): Cystic bile duct dilation plus hepatic fibrosis (± portal hypertension)

IMAGING

- **MRCP ± IV gadoxetate (Eovist)**
  ○ **Usually definitive, obviating more invasive studies**
- CECT or MR: Enhancing dots (portal vein branches) surrounded by cystic spaces (dilated ducts) = "central dot" sign (characteristic)
  ○ **Cystic structures fill with contrast in gadoxetate (Eovist) MR, hepatobiliary phase**
- Calculi are focal signal voids within ducts
- ERCP findings: Saccular dilatation of IHBDs, stones, strictures

- Caroli syndrome is frequently associated with autosomal recessive polycystic kidney disease
- Other manifestations of congenital fibropolycystic disease (can occur in any combination)
  ○ **Congenital hepatic fibrosis**
    – Hepatic fibrosis in Caroli syndrome is ~ always diffuse
  ○ **Autosomal dominant or recessive polycystic liver and kidney disease**
    – Larger cysts that do not communicate with bile ducts
  ○ **Biliary hamartomas**
    – Small (< 15 mm) irregular cystic lesions: No biliary connection
  ○ **Choledochal cyst**

CLINICAL ISSUES

- Symptoms/signs related to cholangitis or biliary stasis
  ○ Pain, fever, jaundice
- Symptoms/signs related to hepatic fibrosis
  ○ Hepatomegaly and portal hypertension

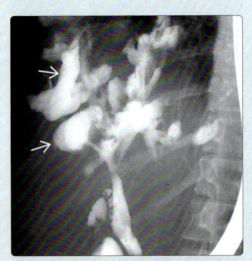
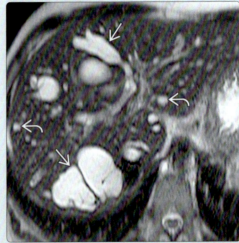

(Left) ERCP shows saccular dilatation of the intrahepatic bile ducts ➡. (Right) Axial T2WI MR shows cystic and fusiform dilation ➡ of the intrahepatic bile ducts. Also noted are innumerable small, spherical, "cystic" foci ➚, representing biliary hamartomas, which often occur as part of the same congenital disorder. The hamartomas do not communicate with bile ducts.

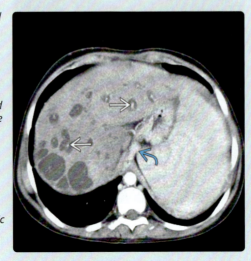
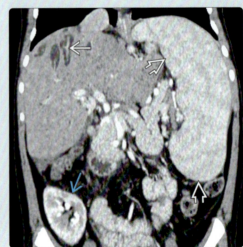

(Left) This young man has had a renal transplantation and has progressive liver failure. Axial CT shows typical features of Caroli syndrome with the portal vein branches ➡ surrounded by dilated bile ducts. Note splenomegaly and varices ➘. (Right) In the same patient, note the enhancing portal vein branch ➡ within one of the cystic spaces. Also note the enlarged spleen ➘ and renal allograft ➘. This patient has Caroli syndrome with hepatic fibrosis and autosomal recessive polycystic kidney disease.

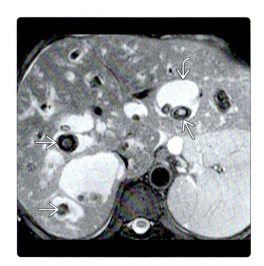

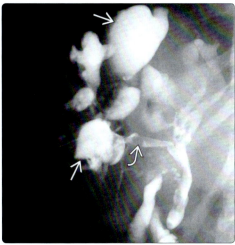

(Left) *Axial T2WI MR shows saccular dilation of the intrahepatic bile ducts* ➡, *many of which contain large, hypointense calculi* ➡. **(Right)** *ERCP shows opacification of the cystic spaces* ➡, *confirming their biliary origin. Also note the filling defects* ➡, *representing biliary calculi.*

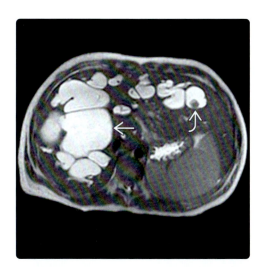

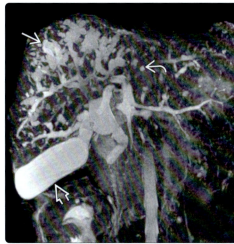

(Left) *Axial T2WI FSE MR of a 14-year-old boy shows massive saccular dilation of the intrahepatic biliary ducts* ➡ *and a stone within a peripheral left bile duct* ➡. **(Right)** *Coronal MRCP of a 22-year-old male liver transplant candidate with Caroli syndrome shows marked bilobar intrahepatic biliary ductal dilatation* ➡ *and a normal-appearing gallbladder* ➡. *This patient also has known hepatic fibrosis and biliary hamartomas* ➡, *the small spherical "cysts" that do not communicate with the biliary tree.*

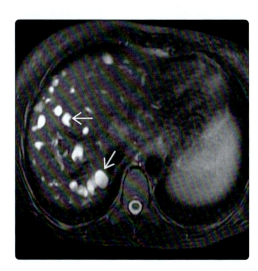

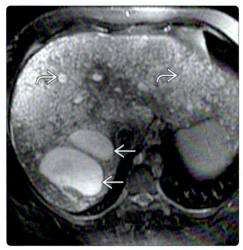

(Left) *Axial T2WI FSE MR of young man with Caroli syndrome (saccular biliary ductal dilatation and hepatic fibrosis) shows marked right lobe-predominant intrahepatic biliary ductal dilation* ➡. **(Right)** *Axial T2WI FSE MR of a 35-year-old woman with Caroli syndrome shows saccular dilation of posterior segmental ducts* ➡ *and innumerable, coalescent hyperintense biliary hamartomas* ➡, *the tiny spherical hyperintense foci. Hepatic fibrosis was also confirmed on liver biopsy.*

TERMINOLOGY

- Congenital segmental dilation of intrahepatic or extrahepatic bile ducts, most commonly affecting main portion of common duct (CD)
  - Most common congenital lesion of large bile ducts

IMAGING

- Type I: Solitary fusiform or cystic dilation of CD
  - Constitutes 50-85% of choledochal cysts
- Type II: Extrahepatic supraduodenal diverticulum
- Type III: Choledochocele
  - Dilation of distal common bile duct in wall of duodenum
- Type IVa: Fusiform CD and intrahepatic cysts
  - Comprises 40% of cases diagnosed in adults
- Type IVb: Dilation of CD with choledochocele
- Type V: Fusiform dilation of intrahepatic bile ducts, Caroli disease
- **MRCP or ERCP: Best imaging tools**
  - Best depiction of all types of choledochal cysts
- Often show aberrant early junction of common bile duct with pancreatic duct
- Ultrasonography: Not as useful as MR
  - Shows anechoic fluid-containing lesion with acoustic enhancement
  - Can be confused with dilated gallbladder or hepatic cyst, unless entire route of bile ducts is traced

CLINICAL ISSUES

- Rare and usually diagnosed in childhood (80%)
  - Can present even in older adults
- Infants: Intermittent jaundice and abdominal mass
- Adults: Recurrent right upper quadrant pain, jaundice, palpable mass
- Complications: Calculi, cholangitis, carcinoma

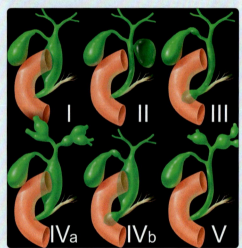

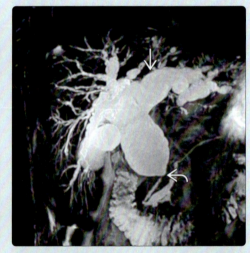

(Left) Todani classification of choledochal cysts is shown. Type I is fusiform dilation of the common duct (CD). Type III is an isolated, distal choledochocele. Type IV is fusiform dilation of the CD and intrahepatic ducts. Type V is synonymous with Caroli disease. (Right) Coronal MRCP shows massive dilation of the intrahepatic and proximal extrahepatic bile ducts ➡ with a sudden transition to a normal distal bile duct ➡. This is a type IV choledochal cyst.

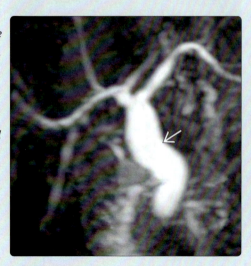

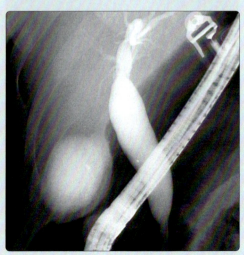

(Left) Coronal MRCP shows diffuse fusiform dilation of the extrahepatic CD ➡, a type I choledochal cyst in the Todani classification. This is the most common type of choledochal cyst. (Right) Film from an ERCP in the same patient shows the same fusiform dilation of the CD with normal intrahepatic ducts. ERCP offers more detailed visualization of the ductal anatomy but is usually redundant to MRCP, unless endoscopic intervention is being considered.

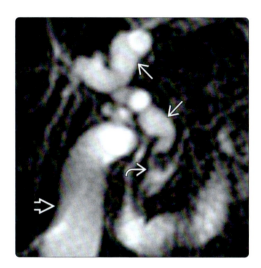

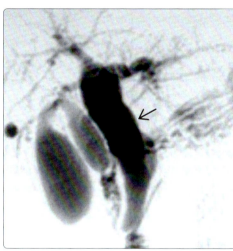

(Left) *MRCP shows dilation of the intra- and extrahepatic bile ducts ➡, constituting a type IV choledochal cyst. Note the abnormal entry of the distal common bile duct into the side of the pancreatic duct ➡, a finding often seen in choledochal cysts. The gallbladder ➡ is marked for orientation.* (Right) *Coronal MRCP shows diffuse dilation of the extrahepatic CD ➡, plus moderate irregular dilation of the right and left main ducts, a type IVa choledochal cyst.*

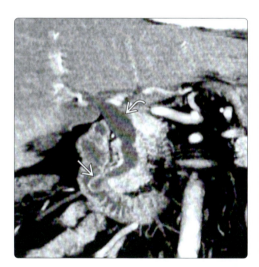

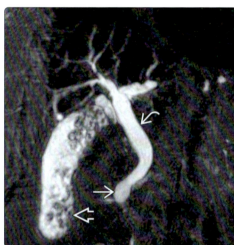

(Left) *Curved multiplanar CECT reformation along the length of the CD shows a small, distal choledochocele ➡ protruding into the duodenal lumen and mild dilation of the common bile duct ➡. This is either a type III or IVb choledochal cyst, depending on whether the CD is considered to be involved.* (Right) *Coronal MRCP in the same patient shows the choledochocele ➡ protruding into the duodenal lumen and the mildly dilated CD ➡ along with numerous stones in the gallbladder ➡.*

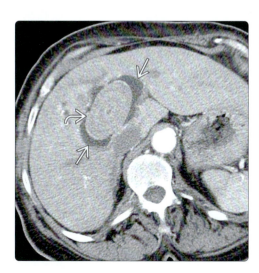

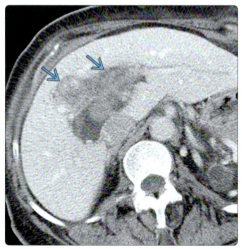

(Left) *Axial CECT shows a huge laminated stone ➡ within a type IV choledochal cyst with marked dilation of the intrahepatic ➡ and CDs (better seen on lower section).* (Right) *Axial portal venous-phase CECT in the same patient shows an enhancing soft tissue mass ➡ arising from the wall of the choledochal cyst. Both stones and cholangiocarcinoma are recognized complications of longstanding choledochal cysts.*

KEY FACTS

IMAGING

- **Multiphasic MR with MRCP is best noninvasive imaging test**
  - **Direct cholangiography is useful for diagnosis and biliary stent placement**
  - Abnormal bile duct wall thickening and enhancement
    - Abnormal arborization or branching pattern: Cannot follow branching ducts on sequential images
    - Multifocal strictures, segmental ectasia (dilation), and irregular beading of intra- and extrahepatic bile ducts
  - "Dominant stricture": Marked dilation of duct upstream from tight, long stricture [raises concern of cholangiocarcinoma (CCa)]
  - Intrahepatic biliary calculi: Calcific density adjacent to portal veins (present in ~ 8%)
  - MR or CT: Best to assess extent of liver injury and associated disease (CCa, cirrhosis, bowel disease, pancreatitis)

- Cirrhosis due to primary sclerosing cholangitis (PSC) has characteristic appearance, unlike other causes of cirrhosis
  - Dysmorphic liver; hypertrophy of caudate and deep right lobe; atrophy of peripheral liver
  - With dilation of intrahepatic ± extrahepatic ducts
- Ultrasonography
  - Ductal wall thickening (2-5 mm), segmental dilation, &/or stenosis of lumen
  - Brightly echogenic portal triads: Periportal edema and fibrosis

DIAGNOSTIC CHECKLIST

- Check for history or imaging evidence of inflammatory bowel disease (especially ulcerative colitis) or autoimmune pancreatitis (IgG4 diseases)
  - IgG4-related cholangiopathy is indistinguishable from PSC by imaging

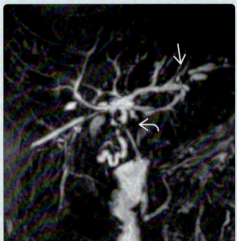
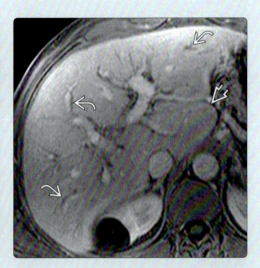

(Left) MRCP of a 31-year-old man with documented primary sclerosing cholangitis (PSC) shows beaded and irregular intrahepatic ducts ➡ and a stricture of the proximal common duct ➡. Involvement of intra- and extrahepatic ducts is characteristic of PSC. (Right) Axial T1WI C+ FS MR of a 45-year-old man with PSC shows mild intrahepatic biliary ductal dilatation ➡. Note the enlargement of the caudate ➡, an early manifestation of cirrhosis. Rapid progression of biliary cirrhosis prompted a liver transplant evaluation 3 years later.

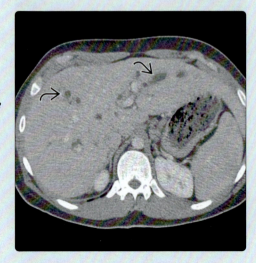
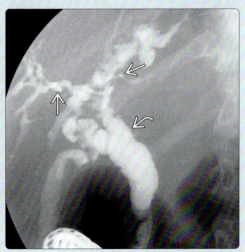

(Left) Axial CECT shows dilation and abnormal arborization of the intrahepatic ducts ➡. The peripheral ducts are dilated but cannot be followed into larger, more central ducts, as expected. (Right) ERCP of the same patient shows a "shaggy" extrahepatic duct ➡, strictures and dilation of the right and left ducts, beading of the intrahepatic ducts, and scattered diverticula ➡.

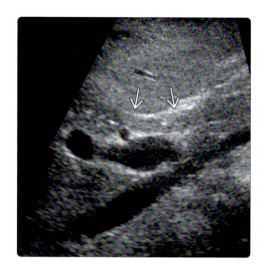
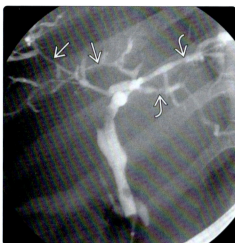

(Left) *Baseline ultrasound of a 19-year-old man with ulcerative colitis, abnormal liver function tests, and PSC shows diffuse thickening of the common duct ➡. CECT (not shown) was normal.* (Right) *ERCP of the same patient performed 4 years later shows long ➡ and short ➡ intrahepatic biliary ductal strictures. The biliary strictures are not specific, but a history of inflammatory bowel disease strongly suggests PSC. A dominant or progressing stricture on surveillance MRCP may indicate cholangiocarcinoma.*

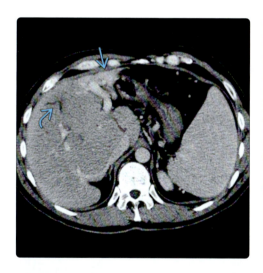
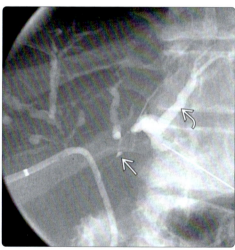

(Left) *Axial CECT shows marked atrophy of the lateral segment ➡ and mild, irregular dilation of the intrahepatic bile ducts ➡, typical findings when longstanding PSC has caused chronic liver damage.* (Right) *Percutaneous transhepatic cholangiography shows multifocal strictures and dilatations of the right intrahepatic bile duct. There is a long, dominant stricture ➡ of the main left duct and marked dilatation of the left intrahepatic bile duct ➡, raising concern for cholangiocarcinoma.*

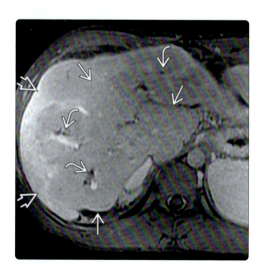
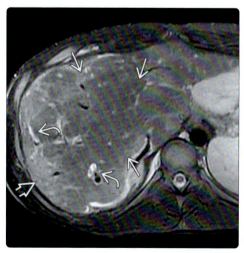

(Left) *T1WI C+ FS MR of the same patient shows similar central liver/caudate enlargement ➡, relative enhancement of atrophic, fibrotic peripheral liver ➡, and scattered dilated intrahepatic ducts ➡.* (Right) *T2WI FSE MR of the same patient shows characteristic morphologic changes of advanced PSC. Note relative enlargement of the central liver ➡ and scattered, irregular biliary ductal dilatation ➡. Subtle peripheral T2 hyperintensity ➡ is due to peripheral atrophy and fibrosis.*

Biliary System

TERMINOLOGY

- Inflammation of intra- &/or extrahepatic bile ducts (IHBDs), common bile duct (CBD) due to ductal obstruction and infection

IMAGING

- **Diagnosis often suggested by US or CT**
  - **Best depicted by MRCP or ERCP**
- Ultrasound: Stones within gallbladder are common and well seen
  - Stones and gas in CBD are not as well seen
  - US can show duct wall thickening
- CT: Shows dilation of IHBs and CBD (if present)
  - Often with irregular contours and branching pattern
  - Duct wall thickened with increased enhancement
  - Often detects abnormal periductal hepatic enhancement
  - ± liver abscess (1/4 of cases) or portal vein thrombosis

TOP DIFFERENTIAL DIAGNOSES

- Primary sclerosing cholangitis: More often associated with multifocal strictures of IHBDs and CBD
- Recurrent pyogenic cholangitis: Gross dilation of IHBDs and CBD with pigment stones and pus

CLINICAL ISSUES

- Pathogenesis: Stone/stricture → obstruction → bile stasis → ↑ biliary pressure → infection
  - Obstructing stone (~ 80%); tumor (~ 10%)
  - Incompetent sphincter of Oddi or prior duct-enteric anastomosis are additional causes
- Charcot triad (seen in 50-75%): Pain, fever, jaundice
- Initially described as life-threatening condition; however, its severity can range from mild to severe
- Treatment: Antibiotics; biliary decompression; percutaneous drainage of hepatic abscess

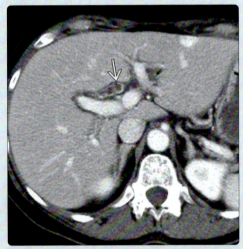
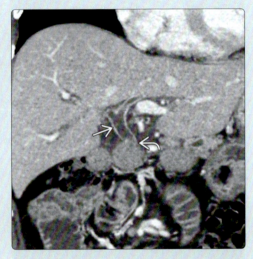

(Left) Axial CECT of a 57-year-old man with right upper quadrant pain, leukocytosis, and fever post Whipple procedure shows mild ductal dilatation. Note thickening and enhancement of the common duct wall ➡. (Right) Coronal reformatted CT of the same patient shows the choledochojejunostomy ➡ and subtle thickening and hyperenhancement of the biliary mucosa ➡. These imaging and clinical findings are characteristic of ascending cholangitis.

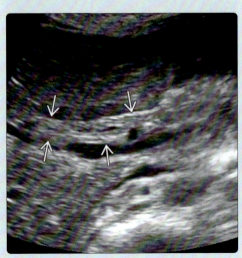
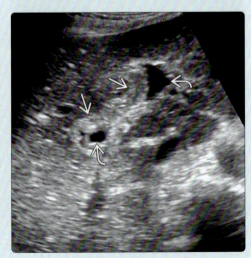

(Left) Longitudinal oblique ultrasound in a 33-year-old woman with right upper quadrant pain, leukocytosis, and jaundice shows a markedly thick-walled common duct ➡. (Right) Axial oblique ultrasound in the same patient shows marked circumferential wall thickening of the proximal right and left hepatic ducts ➡ adjacent to the right and left portal veins ➡, characteristic of cholangitis.

TERMINOLOGY

- Repeated bouts of cholangitis, intra- and extrahepatic biliary ductal dilatation, and biliary calculi, typically in inhabitants of or immigrants from Southeast Asia

IMAGING

- **Multiplanar, multiphasic MR is optimal imaging tool (CT as alternative)**
  - For detection of ductal dilatation, strictures, calculus burden, complications
  - Disproportionate dilatation of extrahepatic and central intrahepatic bile ducts
  - Ductal walls are thickened and contrast enhancing (due to inflammation)
  - Common duct and intrahepatic duct stones without stones in gallbladder
    - Rapid tapering of dilated intrahepatic ducts with arrowhead configuration
    - ↓ arborization of peripheral ducts
  - Hyperintense bile within obstructed ducts and low-signal calculi on T2WI + MRCP
    - Has ability to show ducts proximal to obstruction (advantage over ERCP)
  - May be associated with pyogenic liver abscesses, bilomas, steatosis, segmental atrophy with chronic biliary obstruction, cholangiocarcinoma
  - Atrophic liver segment may be iso- or hyperintense to normal liver on T2WI
- **Ultrasound**: Often initial imaging modality and useful for follow-up
  - Excellent sensitivity for detection of ductal dilatation, stricture, and calculi
  - Hepatolithiasis is seen in ~ 90% of cases (± acoustic shadowing)
    - Marked variability in echogenicity and acoustic shadowing of calculi
- **ERCP**: Provides diagnostic confirmation and therapy (stone extraction, sphincterotomy, duct decompression)

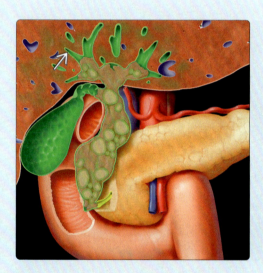

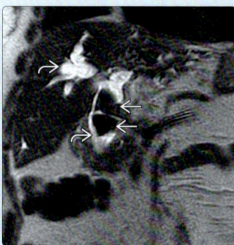

(Left) Graphic demonstrates marked dilation of the intrahepatic bile ducts with multiple common bile duct and intrahepatic stones. Note the rapid tapering of intrahepatic ducts with an arrowhead configuration ➡. (Right) In this elderly Chinese immigrant woman, coronal MRCP shows massive dilation of intrahepatic and extrahepatic bile ducts ➡ and large ductal calculi ➡ seen as signal voids within the ducts.

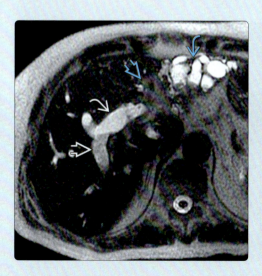

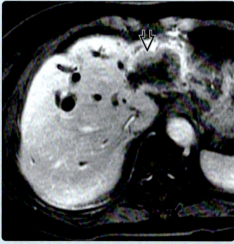

(Left) In the same patient, axial T2WI MR shows the dilated ducts in the central right lobe ➡ and massive dilation of ducts within an atrophic lateral segment ➡. Pus ➡ is present in the dependent ducts. A subtle mass ➡ is suggested encasing the left hepatic ducts. (Right) In the same patient, axial T1WI C+ MR shows a partially cystic and solid mass ➡; at surgery, a left hepatic lobectomy, the diagnoses of recurrent pyogenic cholangitis and cholangiocarcinoma, were confirmed.

Biliary System

TERMINOLOGY

- Gallstones: Concretions within biliary system [gallbladder (GB) and biliary ducts]
  - Cholesterol stones (75-80%)
  - Pigment stones (20-25%)
    - "Black" stones in sterile GB; small; common in cirrhosis and hemolytic states
    - "Brown" stones in infected bile (e.g., recurrent pyogenic cholangitis)
- Sludge: Suspension of particulate material, crystals, and bile within GB
- Choledocholithiasis: Presence of stones in common bile duct (CBD); usually originate in GB

IMAGING

- **Plain films**: Detect only 10-20% of cholesterol stones but most pigment stones
- **US** detects ~ all GB stones; often misses CBD stones

- Gallstone: Mobile mass with reflective echo and acoustic shadow within dependent GB
- Sludge: Mobile, low-level echoes that layer in dependent portion of GB with no acoustic shadow
- **CT** detects ~ 80% of gallstones in GB, fewer in CBD
  - Density varies
    - Gas density within central fissures of large cholesterol stones ("Mercedes Benz" sign)
    - Cholesterol stones are isodense to bile (not detected without rim or nidus of calcification)
    - Higher density in pigment (calcium bilirubinate) stones
  - Sludge: Nonenhancing layered material with attenuation ≥ bile
    - Often not evident on CT (US is more sensitive)
- **MR** detects ~ all stones in GB and CBD
  - Usually as signal void; may have bright T2WI signal if stone contains bile
  - **MRCP is best for diagnosis of CBD calculi**

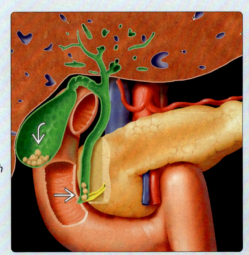
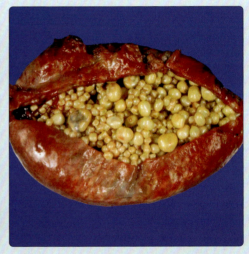

(Left) Coronal illustration shows cholelithiasis ➋ and choledocholithiasis ➡. While most gallstones are asymptomatic, migration of stones to the cystic duct and common duct may cause numerous complications, including biliary colic, cholecystitis, biliary obstruction, and pancreatitis. (Right) Gross photograph shows a gallbladder filled with numerous smooth, yellow cholesterol stones. The gallbladder wall is mildly thickened and hyperemic. (Courtesy G.F. Gray, MD.)

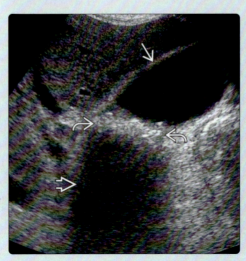
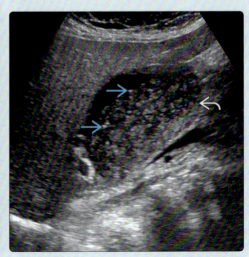

(Left) Ultrasound shows multiple asymptomatic gallstones ➋ with posterior acoustic shadowing ➋. The gallbladder wall is normal ➡. (Right) Ultrasound of a 66-year-old woman receiving total parenteral nutrition (TPN) shows nonshadowing sludge ➋ and tiny echogenic crystals ➡ within a distended gallbladder. Decreased gallbladder motility associated with TPN results in supersaturation of bile, mucus, and crystals.

TERMINOLOGY

Definitions

- Gallstones: Concretions within biliary system [gallbladder (GB) and biliary ducts]
  - Cholesterol stone (75-80%): Cholesterol is main constituent
  - Pigment stone (20-25%): Calcium-bilirubinate is main constituent
    - "Black" stone
      - Usually pigment stone in sterile GB; small and tar-like stones frequently associated with cirrhosis and hemolytic states
    - "Brown" stone
      - Usually pigment stone in infected bile duct, associated with cholestasis and biliary infections (e.g., recurrent pyogenic cholangitis)
- Choledocholithiasis: Presence of stones in common bile duct (CBD)
- Sludge: Suspension of particulate material and bile in GB

IMAGING

General Features

- Best diagnostic clue
  - Gallstone: Mobile mass with reflective echo and marked acoustic shadow within GB
  - Sludge: Mobile, low-level echoes that layer in dependent portion of GB with no acoustic shadow
- Location
  - Cholesterol and "black" stones form within GB
  - "Brown" stones form within bile ducts
    - Type typically seen in recurrent pyogenic cholangitis
  - Small stones (either cholesterol or pigment) may pass into CBD
  - Stones usually found in dependent portion of GB
- Size
  - Cholesterol stones are often multiple and range up to several centimeters in diameter
  - "Black" stones are usually numerous and < 1.5 cm
  - Can entirely fill GB with innumerable stones or 1 large stone
- Morphology
  - Surfaces of stones may be round or faceted
  - Rim calcification: Adsorbed rings of calcium in and on stone

Imaging Recommendations

- Best imaging tool
  - US (> 95% sensitivity and accuracy) is method of choice for GB stones
  - ERCP and MRCP have better accuracy for bile duct stones
- Protocol advice
  - US harmonic imaging decreases side lobe, near-field reverberation artifact

Radiographic Findings

- **Only 10-20%** of cholesterol stones have enough calcium to be visible on plain films
  - 50-75% of "black" stones are radiopaque
  - Majority of "brown" stones are radiolucent

- Mercedes Benz sign: Gas density within central fissures of large stones
  - Does not imply infection or complication

CT Findings

- 20% of stones are not identified on CT
  - Pure cholesterol stones are isodense to bile
  - Common duct stones, especially within nondilated duct
- Primarily used for complications of gallstones
  - e.g., gangrenous cholecystitis, gallstone ileus
- Single or multiple filling defects in GB or ducts
- Density varies: Calcium density, soft tissue density, or lucent (pure cholesterol or gas containing)
- Pattern of calcification: Uniformly calcified, laminated, rim calcification, or central nidus of calcification
- Sludge: Nonenhancing layered material with attenuation ≥ bile
  - Often not evident on CT (US is more sensitive)

MR Findings

- T2WI
  - Multiple signal void filling defects in GB or CBD
  - May have high T2 signal (bile within stone)
  - MRCP is best noninvasive test for ductal calculi

Ultrasonographic Findings

- Gallstones: Highly reflective echo from anterior surface of stone
  - Marked posterior acoustic shadowing
    - Small stones may not shadow
  - Mobility of stone on repositioning patient
  - Wall-echo-shadow sign: Seen when GB is filled with stones
    - Only anterior wall and superficial layer of stones are visible; rest of stones and posterior wall are not visible (due to marked acoustic shadow)
- Sludge: Low-level echoes layering in dependent portion of GB
  - No acoustic shadow; shifts slowly with repositioning patient
  - Can simulate mass (tumefactive sludge): No vascularity demonstrated on Doppler US

SELECTED REFERENCES

1. Bergman S et al: Gallstone disease in the elderly: are older patients managed differently? Surg Endosc. 25(1):55-61, 2011
2. Bär F et al: Gallstone ileus. Clin Gastroenterol Hepatol. 9(10):A22, 2011
3. Gurusamy K et al: Systematic review and meta-analysis of intraoperative versus preoperative endoscopic sphincterotomy in patients with gallbladder and suspected common bile duct stones. Br J Surg. 98(7):908-16, 2011
4. Yeh BM et al: MR imaging and CT of the biliary tract. Radiographics. 29(6):1669-88, 2009
5. Catalano OA et al: MR imaging of the gallbladder: a pictorial essay. Radiographics. 28(1):135-55; quiz 324, 2008
6. Chan WC et al: Gallstone detection at CT in vitro: effect of peak voltage setting. Radiology. 241(2):546-53, 2006
7. Bortoff GA et al: Gallbladder stones: imaging and intervention. Radiographics. 20(3):751-66, 2000
8. Ko CW et al: Biliary sludge. Ann Intern Med. 130(4 Pt 1):301-11, 1999
9. Barakos JA et al: Cholelithiasis: evaluation with CT. Radiology. 162(2):415-8, 1987

(Left) *Supine abdominal radiograph shows a gallbladder filled with innumerable opaque calculi ➡. Calcium bilirubinate stones are typically multiple, small, and radiopaque. A feeding tube ➡ marks the 2nd portion of the duodenum.* (Right) *Axial CECT shows gas ➡ with a "Mercedes Benz" sign shape within a large gallstone. The gas itself is of no diagnostic significance and is not a sign of infection. This patient has cholecystitis, evidenced by gallbladder wall thickening ➡.*

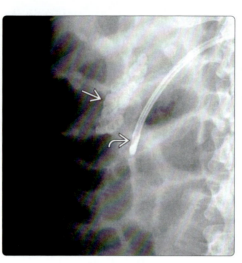
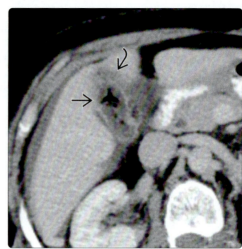

(Left) *MRCP shows 2 gallstones ➡ within the gallbladder but normal bile ducts. This patient had a CT scan on which these stones were not visible, since cholesterol stones are often isodense to bile.* (Right) *Ultrasound of a 39-year-old man with vague abdominal pain shows innumerable shadowing stones occupying the entire GB lumen. Note the wall-echo-shadow complex. A thin rim of hypoechoic bile demarcates a thin echogenic gallbladder wall ➡ and echogenic stones ➡ with an acoustic shadow ➡.*

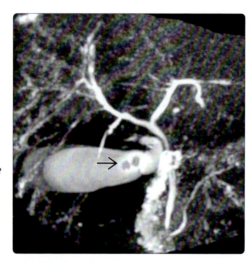
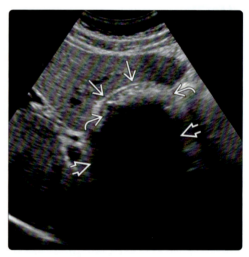

(Left) *Ultrasound of an 85-year-old man post ERCP and biliary stent placement shows extensive shadowing ➡ due to multiple layering stones ➡. Note "dirty" shadowing ➡ posterior to gas within the gallbladder lumen ➡ from the ERCP.* (Right) *Ultrasound of a 47-year-old man with primary sclerosing cholangitis shows tumefactive sludge ➡ within the gallbladder fundus. No flow was shown within the "mass" at color Doppler, and sludge eventually moved with changes in patient positioning.*

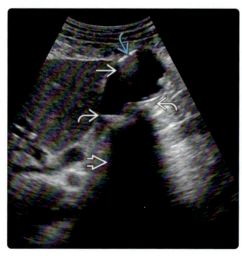
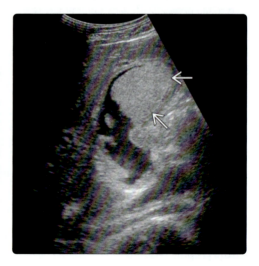

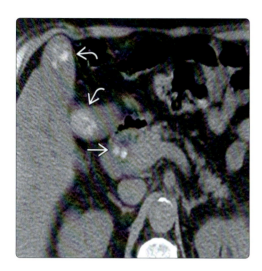

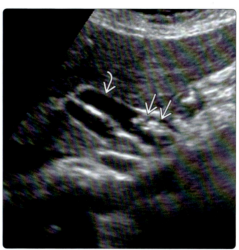

(Left) *NECT of an elderly man shows calcified, secondary, distal CBD stones ➡ and similar matrix gallstones ➡. Small distal duct calculi are often better shown on NECT than on CECT; ductal calculi may be obscured by oral contrast within the lumen of the duodenum or surrounding enhanced pancreas on CECT.* (Right) *Ultrasound of a 52-year-old woman post remote cholecystectomy shows multiple nonshadowing distal stones ➡ with the dilated CBD ➡. Primary pigment stones may not shadow despite their large size.*

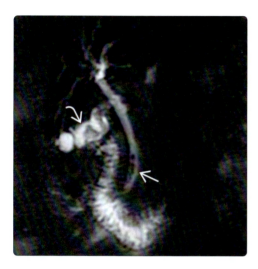

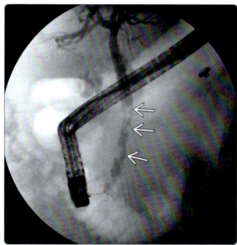

(Left) *Thick slab MRCP of an 83-year-old woman with acute pancreatitis shows multiple signal voids (stones) within a normal caliber CBD ➡. Note several stones within a collapsed gallbladder ➡.* (Right) *ERCP of the same patient confirms multiple corresponding radiolucent filling defects ➡. Pancreatitis resolved after papillotomy and balloon stone retrieval. ERCP can usually be reserved for therapeutic intervention once MRCP has demonstrated the relevant biliary disorder.*

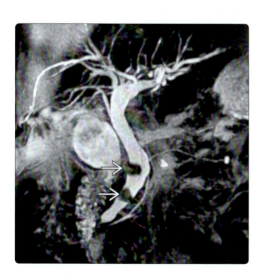

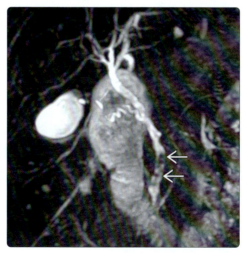

(Left) *Respiratory-triggered MRCP of a 71-year-old woman who presented with biliary colic demonstrates 2 stones as signal voids ➡ within a dilated CBD.* (Right) *Respiratory-triggered MRCP of a 91-year-old man with mild right upper quadrant pain and an elevated alkaline phosphatase shows multiple small calculi ➡ within a normal-caliber distal CBD. The high sensitivity/specificity of MRCP makes this study the noninvasive modality of choice for patients with suspected choledocholithiasis.*

Gallbladder Hydrops and Empyema

TERMINOLOGY

- Definition
  - Hydrops: Distended gallbladder (GB) secondary to chronic obstruction (commonly impacted stone) filled with watery mucoid material; content is usually sterile
  - Empyema: Pus filling inflamed and distended GB secondary to intraluminal infection

IMAGING

- **Ultrasound is 1st-line imaging test**
  - **Distended GB filled with anechoic mucoid content (hydrops) or echogenic pus (empyema)**
  - Markedly distended GB (up to 1,000 mL)
  - Gallstones usually; but may also be acalculous
  - Echogenic pus in lumen (empyema), similar in echogenicity to sludge
  - Intraluminal membranes from sloughed mucosa if gangrenous GB
  - Loss of GB wall reflectivity if gangrenous

- CT and MR show similar features
  - Thin or normal wall (hydrops)
  - Empyema: GB wall thickening, adjacent inflammatory infiltration, ± signs of wall perforation, abscess
  - High-signal edema in GB wall on T2WI sequences (empyema)

TOP DIFFERENTIAL DIAGNOSES

- Gangrenous cholecystitis
- Emphysematous cholecystitis
- Courvoisier GB (palpable, nontender GB)
  - Malignant obstruction of common bile duct

CLINICAL ISSUES

- Treatment
  - Hydrops: Cholecystectomy (if symptomatic)
  - Empyema: Antibiotic therapy; urgent cholecystectomy or cholecystostomy

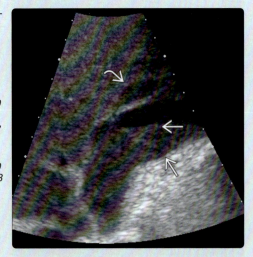
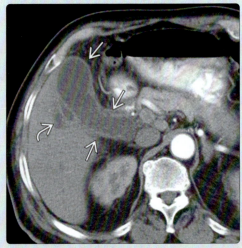

(Left) Ultrasound of a 79-year-old male patient with generalized abdominal pain, sepsis, and gallbladder (GB) empyema shows layering echoes within the GB lumen ➡ and a poorly defined pericholecystic fluid collection along adjacent liver ➡. (Right) Axial CECT in the same patient shows GB wall thickening ➡ and a pericholecystic fluid collection ➡. A perforated, pus-filled GB and an adjacent abscess were identified at laparotomy and cholecystectomy.

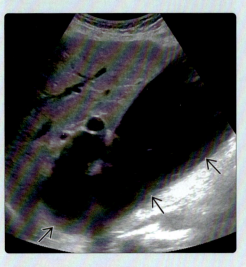
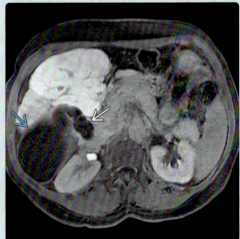

(Left) Surveillance ultrasound of a 63-year-old woman with primary sclerosing cholangitis shows a hydropic GB. Low-level echoes within the inferior aspect of the GB are due to side lobe artifact ➡. (Right) Delayed T1WI C+ FS MR with gadoxetate ("Eovist") in the same patient shows an unopacified, hydropic GB ➡ and a dilated cystic duct ➡. Lack of contrast within the GB on the delayed phase indicates that this chronic asymptomatic hydrops is due to a cystic duct obstruction.

Emphysematous Cholecystitis

TERMINOLOGY

- Rare form of acute cholecystitis caused by secondary infection with gas-forming organisms

IMAGING

- **Imaging protocols: CT is most sensitive and specific**
  - Plain films and US are specific but less sensitive
- CT: Gas in GB wall is curvilinear
  - Gas within GB lumen with air-fluid level
  - Gallstones identified by CT in < 50% of cases
  - With perforation of GB, may see pneumoperitoneum
  - Rarely, portal venous gas or gas within abscess
- US: Gas in gallbladder (GB) wall results in highly echogenic reflections, casting "dirty" shadows
  - Also referred to as ring-down or comet tail artifact
  - Gallstones seen in ~ 50% of cases
  - Highly echogenic gas in GB lumen may be misinterpreted as overlying gas-filled bowel or as stone-filled GB

- On real-time US, intraluminal gas bubbles may rise up to nondependent wall like bubbles of champagne

TOP DIFFERENTIAL DIAGNOSES

- Gangrenous cholecystitis
- Biliary gas from enteric anastomosis or sphincterotomy
- Gas from erosion of gallstone into bowel (gallstone ileus)

PATHOLOGY

- Infection of GB with gas-forming organisms, such as *Clostridium welchii* and *Escherichia coli*
- Extensive hemorrhagic necrosis

CLINICAL ISSUES

- Epidemiology: 1% of all cases of acute cholecystitis
- Diabetic, elderly patients are at higher risk
  - Clinical presentation may be mild and insidious
- High risk of gangrene, perforation, and sepsis if untreated

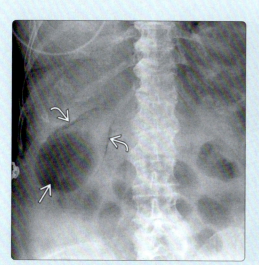
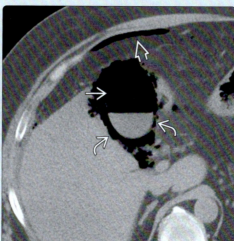

(Left) AP supine radiograph of a 72-year-old woman admitted with sepsis, right upper quadrant pain, and surgically confirmed emphysematous cholecystitis shows gas within the wall ➡ and lumen ➡ of the gallbladder (GB). (Right) NECT of a 57-year-old man with coronary artery disease, diabetes, and abdominal pain shows intraluminal ➡ and intramural ➡ GB gas. Note free intraperitoneal gas ➡, a manifestation of GB perforation. Transmural GB necrosis and gram-negative rods were shown at pathology.

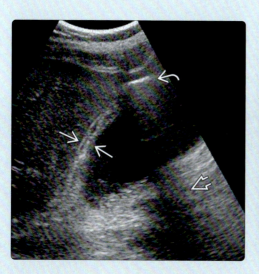
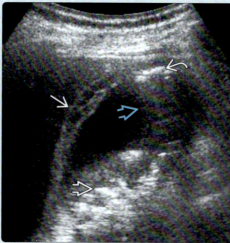

(Left) Ultrasound of a 79-year-old man with right upper quadrant pain shows wall thickening ➡ and intramural gas, the nondependent linear echogenicity ➡. Note "dirty" posterior shadowing ➡, an ultrasound artifact characteristic of gas. (Right) Longitudinal grayscale ultrasound of the GB in a 76-year-old man with diabetes and gram-negative septicemia reveals a thickened wall ➡ with echogenic intramural gas ➡ and posterior "dirty" shadows ➡, plus echogenic gallstones ➡.

Acute Calculous Cholecystitis

TERMINOLOGY

- Acute inflammation of gallbladder (GB) precipitated by impacted stone within GB neck or cystic duct

IMAGING

- **Best imaging tool: US (biliary scintigraphy, if necessary, for confirmation)**
- US
  - Sensitivity and specificity are both > 85%
  - Uncomplicated: Positive sonographic Murphy sign; stone impacted in GB neck or cystic duct; thickened GB wall (> 3 mm), pericholecystic fluid
  - Complicated: Gallstones, pericholecystic fluid/abscess, intraluminal membranes, gas in GB wall/lumen, asymmetric wall thickening
    - **Murphy sign may be absent in gangrenous cholecystitis**
- Biliary scintigraphy (HIDA scan)
  - Sensitivity & specificity similar to US

- Nonvisualization of GB (at 4 hours or after morphine administration) highly specific
  - False-positives due to fasting, hepatic failure, prior sphincterotomy
- CT
  - Not 1st-line tool for diagnosis
  - Can be helpful in atypical or complicated cases (e.g., gangrenous cholecystitis)
  - Misses at least 20% of gallstones that are isodense to bile
- MRCP
  - Not 1st-line for diagnosis of cholecystitis
  - Excellent depiction of choledocholithiasis
    - Focal signal void(s) within high intensity ("white") bile on T2WI & MRCP

DIAGNOSTIC CHECKLIST

- Consider perforated ulcer, pancreatitis, or hepatitis with secondary GB wall thickening

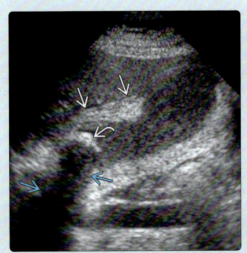
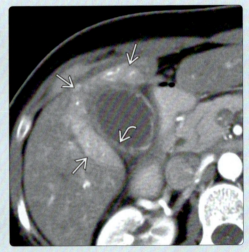

(Left) In this patient with right upper quadrant (RUQ) pain, nausea, vomiting, & an elevated white blood count, US shows marked GB wall thickening ➡ and sludge. A large stone ➡ within the neck of the GB was immobile at real-time examination. The stone is highly echogenic with a posterior acoustic shadow ➡. (Right) Axial CECT of a 37-year-old woman shows GB wall thickening ➡ & hyperemia of the surrounding hepatic parenchymal ➡, which is analogous to the rim sign of hepatobiliary scintigraphy.

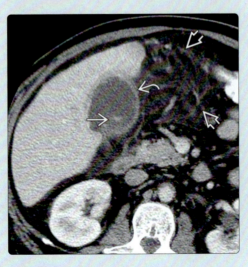
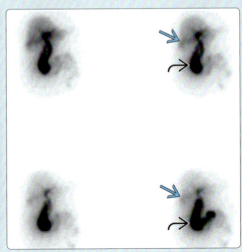

(Left) This CECT is of a 59-year-old man with clinical and CT features pathognomonic for acute cholecystitis. Note GB wall thickening, mucosal enhancement ➡, omental infiltration ➡, and subtle layering of calcified stones ➡. (Right) Hepatobiliary scan of a 48-year-old woman with RUQ pain and surgically confirmed acute cholecystitis shows the presence of tracer in the bowel ➡ but absence of GB activity and a subtle GB fossa rim sign ➡. Persistent pericholecystic activity may be due to hepatic inflammation and biliary stasis.

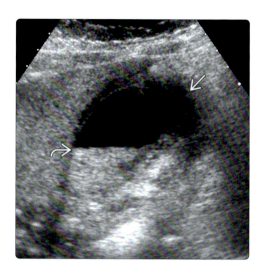
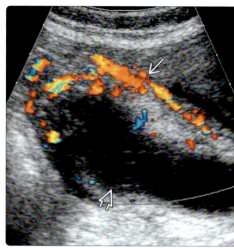

(Left) Ultrasound of a 67-year-old woman with RUQ pain and fever shows layering echogenic sludge ⮕ and focally absent reflectivity of the wall of the GB fundus ⮕, a characteristic finding of gangrenous cholecystitis. Color Doppler might also show absent flow in this setting. (Right) Color Doppler ultrasound of a 71-year-old woman who presented with a high fever, leukocytosis, and abdominal pain shows marked hyperemia ⮕ of the thickened wall of the GB ⮕.

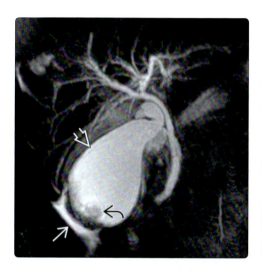
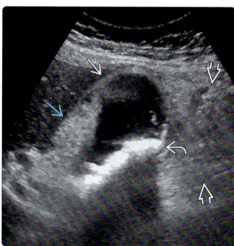

(Left) MRCP of a 27-year-old man with RUQ pain and fever (and ultimately surgically confirmed acute cholecystitis) shows a hydropic GB ⮕, gallstones ⮕, and pericholecystic fluid ⮕. (Right) Ultrasound of the same patient shows small, shadowing, layering calculi ⮕; mild GB wall thickening ⮕; and sludge ⮕. The omentum is infiltrated ⮕, and an unequivocal sonographic Murphy sign was easily elicited.

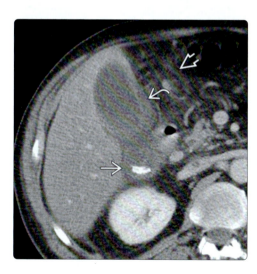
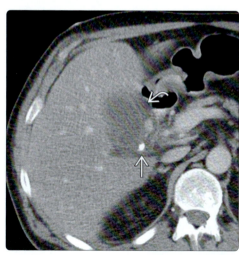

(Left) CECT of a man with fever, elevated white count, and RUQ pain shows layering calcified gallstones ⮕, mild GB wall thickening ⮕, and infiltration of the adjacent omentum & mesenteric fat ⮕. (Right) CECT of the same patient shows GB wall edema ⮕ and an obstructing, calcified cystic duct stone ⮕. Only 15-20% of gallstones will contain enough calcium to be perceived on radiographs, & not all are evident on CT. Nearly 100% are seen on sonography & MR.

Acalculous Cholecystitis

TERMINOLOGY

- Acute nongallstone-related necroinflammatory disease of gallbladder
- "Acute ischemic cholecystitis"

IMAGING

- **Best initial imaging: Ultrasonography**
- Findings similar to acute calculous cholecystitis except for absence of gallstones
  - Gallbladder wall thickening (> 3-4 mm)
  - Striated appearance of gallbladder wall (edema)
  - Mucosal sloughing
  - Gallbladder distention (> 5 cm in transverse plane)
  - Pericholecystic fluid/infiltration
  - Positive sonographic Murphy sign
- Nonvisualization of gallbladder at cholescintigraphy (hepatobiliary iminodiacetic acid scan)
  - Frequent false-positives in critically ill patients due to gallbladder dysfunction, bile stasis, and sludge

PATHOLOGY

- Bile stasis, gallbladder inflammation, and ischemia

CLINICAL ISSUES

- Accounts for 10% cases of acute cholecystitis
- Initially described in critically ill patients but also seen in outpatients with risk factors (e.g., diabetes, sepsis, renal insufficiency)
- Difficult clinical and imaging diagnosis in patients with multisystem organ failure
- High morbidity and mortality
  - ~ 50% risk of gangrene
  - ~ 10% risk of perforation
- Urgent percutaneous cholecystostomy or cholecystectomy may be required

DIAGNOSTIC CHECKLIST

- High degree of suspicion in patients with risk factors and abdominal sepsis

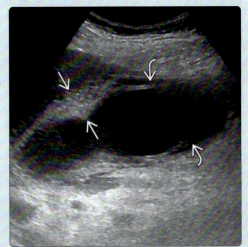
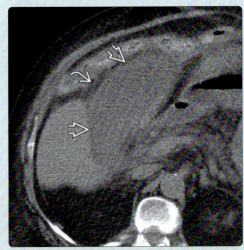

(Left) Ultrasound of an 87-year-old woman with abdominal sepsis and hypotension despite pressor support, post laparotomy for an incarcerated hernia shows irregular gallbladder (GB) wall thickening ➡ and a linear echogenic band adjacent to the wall ➡, features compatible with mucosal sloughing and acalculous, gangrenous cholecystitis.
(Right) Axial NECT in the same patient shows a distended GB ➡, irregular wall thickening, and pericholecystic fat infiltration ➡. The patient expired 1 day later.

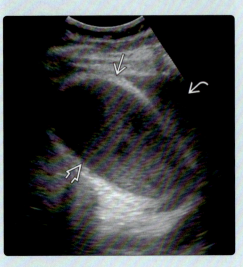
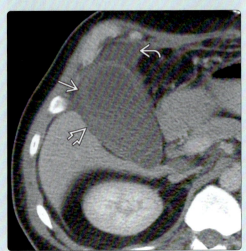

(Left) Ultrasound of a septic 57-year-old man 3 days post pancreatic debridement for hemorrhagic pancreatitis shows a distended, sludge-filled GB ➡, diffuse wall thickening ➡, and pericholecystic fluid ➡.
(Right) Axial CECT in the same patient shows a hydropic GB ➡, wall thickening ➡, and adjacent fluid ➡. Ongoing sepsis and persistent GB wall thickening on follow-up ultrasound exams prompted a percutaneous cholecystotomy. The aspirate was positive for Escherichia coli and Enterococcus faecalis.

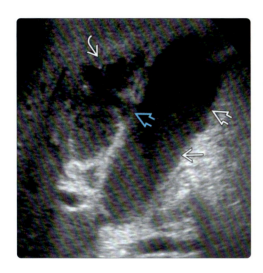

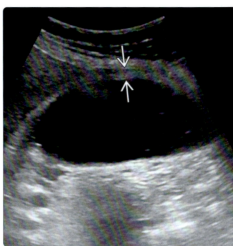

(Left) *ICU ultrasound of a 41-year-old man 3 weeks post trauma shows a distended GB ➡, sludge ➡, irregular wall thickening, a focal perforation ➡, and a complex pericholecystic fluid collection ➡. Acalculous, gangrenous cholecystitis was subsequently confirmed at surgery.* (Right) *Ultrasound of a 36-year-old man with chronic graft vs. host disease and acute onset of fever and pain shows GB hydrops and wall thickening ➡. Acalculous cholecystitis was confirmed at emergent cholecystectomy.*

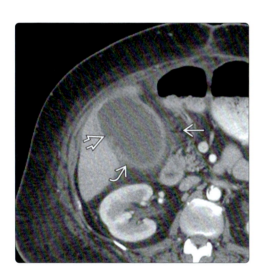

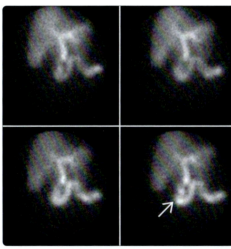

(Left) *CECT of a 55-year-old woman with diabetes and sepsis 4 days post laparotomy for a perforated duodenal ulcer shows a distended GB ➡, wall thickening ➡, and pericholecystic fat infiltration ➡. No gallstones were identified at ultrasound.* (Right) *Hepatobiliary (HIDA) scan of the same patient shows progressive small bowel filling ➡ but no GB activity 30 minutes post tracer administration. No GB activity was shown after morphine administration (an observation that increases exam specificity).*

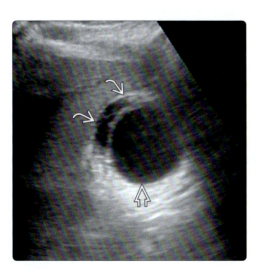

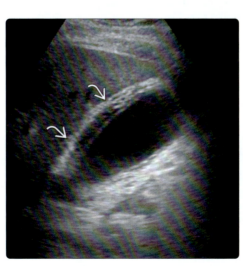

(Left) *Ultrasound of a 64-year-old man with ulcerative colitis, primary sclerosing cholangitis, hairy cell leukemia, fever, right upper quadrant pain, and leukocytosis shows asymmetric wall edema ➡ of the GB ➡.* (Right) *Sagittal ultrasound of the same patient shows asymmetric GB wall edema ➡ and no gallstones. A sonographic Murphy sign was elicited. Cholecystectomy revealed gangrenous, acute acalculous cholecystitis.*

Xanthogranulomatous Cholecystitis

TERMINOLOGY

- Rare form of gallbladder (GB) inflammation characterized by accumulation of lipid-laden macrophages and fibrous tissue

IMAGING

- **Multiplanar CT or MR**
  - GB wall thickening with intramural low-attenuation areas of foamy cell infiltrate
  - Adjacent focal hyperperfusion of liver: Transient hepatic attenuation difference
  - Gallstone(s): Always present though not always seen on CT
- MR: Areas of xanthogranulomatosis are iso- or slightly T2 hyperintense
  - Areas of necrosis and abscess are highly T2 hyperintense
  - Areas of xanthogranulomatous cholecystitis (XGC) demonstrate delayed enhancement on T1WI contrast-enhanced scans

- US: Hypoechoic nodules and bands within GB wall
  - Echogenic pericholecystic fat
  - Gallstones, sludge, echogenic intraluminal debris
- **Imaging findings favoring XGC over GB cancer**
  - Diffuse GB wall thickening with continuous mucosal line
  - Intramural low-attenuation nodules
  - Absence of invasion of adjacent organs or bile ducts
  - Presence of 3 findings leads to 83% sensitivity, 100% specificity, and 91% accuracy for differentiation of XGC from GB carcinoma

TOP DIFFERENTIAL DIAGNOSES

- GB carcinoma
- GB adenomyomatosis
- Acute cholecystitis (with perforation or abscess)

CLINICAL ISSUES

- RUQ pain, fever (similar to acute calculous cholecystitis)
  - May persist for years, leading to significant morbidity

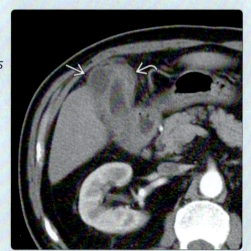
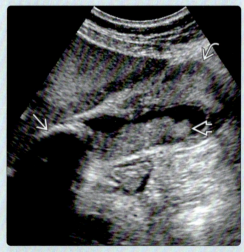

(Left) Axial CECT of an asymptomatic 75-year-old man shows irregular GB wall thickening ⬈ and intramural low attenuation ➡. (Right) US of the same patient shows asymmetric wall thickening ⬈, sludge ⬈, and an echogenic, shadowing stone ➡ within the GB neck. Preoperative differentiation between GB carcinoma and xanthogranulomatous cholecystitis is often difficult, but the absence of intrahepatic ductal dilatation may suggest a chronic inflammatory process rather than neoplasia.

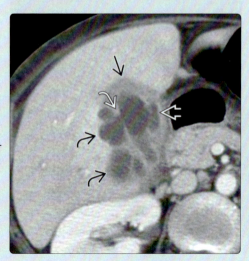
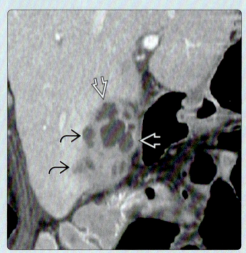

(Left) Axial CECT of a 79-year-old man with fever and right upper quadrant pain shows marked irregular GB wall thickening ➡, intramural low attenuation ⬈, a contained perforation ⬈, and several pericholecystic collections ➡. (Right) Coronal reformatted CECT of the same patient shows several intramural, low-attenuation nodules ⬈ and pericholecystic collections ➡. Low-attenuation intramural nodules are due to either abscesses or xanthogranulomas.

Mirizzi Syndrome

TERMINOLOGY

- Partial or complete obstruction of common hepatic duct (CHD) due to gallstone impaction in cystic duct, infundibulum, or Hartmann pouch of gallbladder (GB)

IMAGING

- **ERCP**: Extrinsic narrowing of CHD, dilated intrahepatic ducts, and lack of GB opacification
  - Impression on CHD is often concave to right
- **MR**: Dilated CHD and intrahepatic ducts with stricture at level of stone (signal void on all pulse sequences)
  - Site of CHD narrowing may appear thickened and hyperenhancing due to inflammation on T1WI C+
- **US**: Large, immobile gallstone impacted in cystic duct or infundibulum with dilated intrahepatic ducts

TOP DIFFERENTIAL DIAGNOSES

- Choledocholithiasis

- Cholangiocarcinoma, GB carcinoma, or regional lymphadenopathy
- Benign biliary stricture

PATHOLOGY

- Impaction of stone in cystic duct, infundibulum, or Hartmann pouch compressing bile duct at same level
  - Obstruction may be due to direct mass effect or development of stricture in CHD due to inflammation
- Predisposing factors: Long cystic duct running parallel to CHD or low insertion of cystic duct into common bile duct
- Cholecystocholedochal fistula may develop due to chronic inflammation/pressure necrosis with gallstones eroding from cystic duct into bile duct

CLINICAL ISSUES

- Common symptoms: Fever, jaundice, RUQ pain (symptoms of obstructive jaundice, acute cholecystitis, cholangitis)
- Definitive treatment is surgical with approach determined by type of Mirizzi syndrome

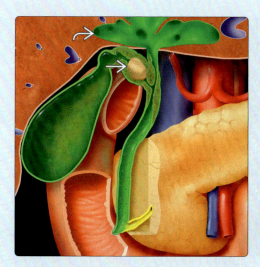
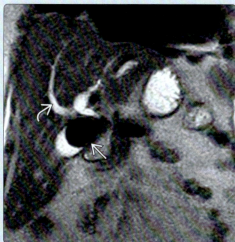

(Left) *Graphic of Mirizzi syndrome depicts a large cystic duct stone* ➡ *causing extrinsic compression of the common hepatic duct (CHD) and dilation of the intrahepatic bile ducts* ➡. (Right) *Coronal T2WI MR shows subtle intrahepatic bile duct dilation* ➡ *and a large gallstone* ➡ *impacted within the neck of the gallbladder (GB), causing extrinsic narrowing of the common duct.*

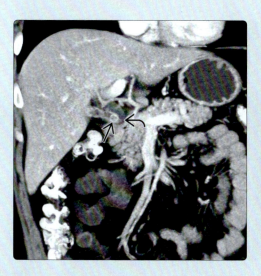
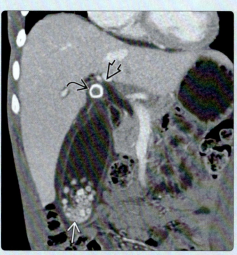

(Left) *Coronal CECT shows a cystic duct stone* ➡ *that causes extrinsic compression of the CHD* ➡. *The intrahepatic ducts were dilated, which was better seen on axial sections (not shown).* (Right) *Coronal CECT demonstrates a large gallstone* ➡ *in the GB neck compressing the adjacent CHD* ➡, *resulting in mild intrahepatic biliary dilatation (not shown). Note the dilated GB with multiple stones* ➡ *and mild wall thickening.*

Hyperplastic Cholecystoses

TERMINOLOGY

- Adenomyomatosis
  - Mural gallbladder (GB) wall thickening secondary to exaggeration of normal luminal epithelial folds (Rokitansky-Aschoff sinuses) in conjunction with smooth muscle proliferation
- Cholesterolosis
  - Deposition of foamy, cholesterol-laden histiocytes in subepithelium of GB; may coalesce into polyps

IMAGING

- **Best imaging tool: US for cholesterolosis; US or MRCP for adenomyomatosis**
- US; adenomyomatosis: Focal or diffuse GB wall thickening
  - Intramural diverticula containing high-amplitude echoes and comet-tail reverberation artifacts
  - String of echogenic pearls on US or MR
- US; cholesterolosis: Multiple small (< 10-mm), hyperechoic GB polyps on epithelial surface
- Also may show comet-tail or twinkle artifact (on Doppler), due to focal cholesterol deposits
  - **US: Accuracy of ~ 66% for Dx of adenomyomatosis**
- MRCP; adenomyomatosis: Bright, cystic spaces (Rokitansky-Aschoff sinuses) within thickened GB wall
  - Contrast-enhanced T1WI MR: Homogeneous intermediate signal for thickened wall
    - Nonenhancing cystic spaces within GB wall
- MR; cholesterolosis: Low-signal intraluminal filling defects attached to GB wall
- **MR is highly accurate in differentiation of adenomyomatosis from GB carcinoma**

CLINICAL ISSUES

- Often asymptomatic but may present with RUQ
- Cholecystectomy may be driven by symptoms or imaging overlap with GB carcinoma
- Management strategies (surveillance and size threshold for resection) are controversial

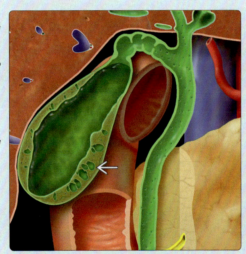
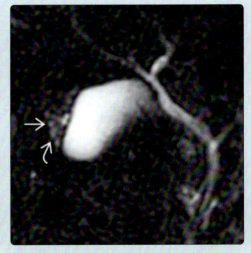

(Left) Schematic drawing of adenomyomatosis illustrates a thickened gallbladder (GB) wall with multiple intramural cystic spaces ➡. (Right) MRCP of a 51-year-old man with chronic right upper quadrant pain shows a fundal mass ➡ containing high-signal foci ➡ within dilated Rokitansky-Aschoff sinuses. This MR string of pearls sign is characteristic of fundal adenomyomatosis.

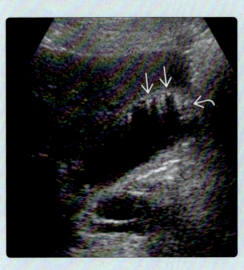
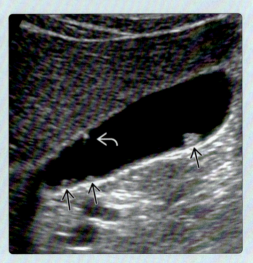

(Left) Ultrasound of a 66-year-old woman with right upper quadrant pain shows tiny echogenic foci ➡ within the anterior wall of the GB and posterior comet-tail artifacts ➡. This appearance is likely due to reverberation of the ultrasound pulse caused by cholesterol crystals within the GB subepithelium. (Right) Ultrasound of a 62-year-old woman shows comet-tail artifact ➡ and several minute, echogenic GB polyps ➡. Pathology showed cholesterolosis and hyperplastic (cholesterol) polyps.

Porcelain Gallbladder

TERMINOLOGY

- Calcification of gallbladder (GB) wall

IMAGING

- **Multiphasic, multiplanar CT is best for diagnosis, including possible GB carcinoma**
  - Curvilinear or granular calcification in GB wall
    - May involve entire wall or just segment
  - Distinguish from calcified surface of large cholesterol gallstone (very similar appearance)
  - Mural calcification is less evident on MR
    - But gallstones are more evident on MR than on CT
- **Ultrasonography**
  - Echogenic curvilinear structure in GB fossa with acoustic shadowing
  - May be difficult to distinguish from large echogenic gallstone that fills GB lumen
    - Wall-echo-shadow complex = large gallstone

TOP DIFFERENTIAL DIAGNOSES

- Large gallstone
  - Mimics porcelain GB on all modalities
- Cholecystitis, emphysematous
  - Echogenic crescent in GB with acoustic shadowing on ultrasound mimics GB wall calcification
  - CT can best distinguish gas from calcium
- Iatrogenic
  - Iodized oil in GB wall following hepatic chemoembolization

CLINICAL ISSUES

- Although association with adenocarcinoma is weaker than what was proposed in classic surgical series, ~ 15% prevalence is suggested in recent reviews
- Prophylactic cholecystectomy is recommended

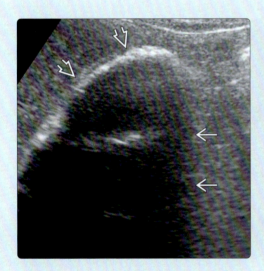
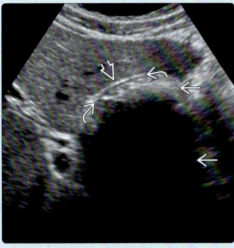

(Left) Ultrasound of a 63-year-old woman with right upper quadrant pain shows curvilinear shadowing echogenicity ➡ within the gallbladder (GB) wall (porcelain GB). Marked shadowing ➡ makes it impossible to assess the GB lumen. (Right) Ultrasound of a 43-year-old man shows a GB lumen filled with stones, a mimic of a porcelain GB. Note the wall-echo-shadow complex. A rim of hypoechoic bile ➡ between the GB wall ➡ and shadowing stones ➡ leads to a correct diagnosis of gallstones, not porcelain GB.

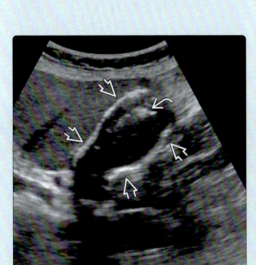
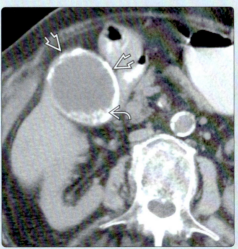

(Left) Ultrasound of a 73-year-old woman with abdominal pain shows increased echogenicity throughout the GB wall ➡ and a partially obscured mass ➡ within the fundus. Chronic cholecystitis, intramural calcification, and GB adenocarcinoma were identified at pathology. (Right) Axial NECT shows a rind of calcification in the GB wall ➡ and dependent calcified stones ➡. The association between porcelain GB and carcinoma is weaker than suggested in early surgical series, but cholecystectomy is still advocated.

Chemotherapy-Induced Cholangitis

TERMINOLOGY

- Chemotherapy-induced sclerosing cholangitis (or biliary sclerosis)
- Iatrogenic cholangitis following intraarterial chemotherapy for hepatic malignancies

IMAGING

- **MR with MRCP is best imaging test**
  - Segmental strictures of variable length (similar to those seen in primary sclerosing cholangitis)
- Strictures of common hepatic and larger intrahepatic ducts
  - Frequently involves common hepatic duct and biliary confluence but not distal common bile duct
- Ductal abnormalities may include
  - Duct wall thickening and luminal narrowing
  - Dilation of intrahepatic bile ducts upstream from strictures
  - Periductal edema
  - Hepatic perfusion abnormalities

- CT or MR may be necessary to differentiate cholangitis from extrinsic duct compression by lymph nodes or tumor

TOP DIFFERENTIAL DIAGNOSES

- Primary sclerosing cholangitis
- Autoimmune (IgG4-related) pancreatitis-cholangitis syndrome
- Extrinsic compression (liver masses)
- Chemical hepatitis

CLINICAL ISSUES

- Cholangiographic abnormalities reported in 7-30% of patients undergoing intraarterial chemotherapy
- Severe complications
  - Acute or subacute hepatic failure or death
- Treatment
  - Immediate cessation of intraarterial floxuridine; surgical or percutaneous drainage of biliary tree; endoscopic balloon dilation of strictures ± stenting

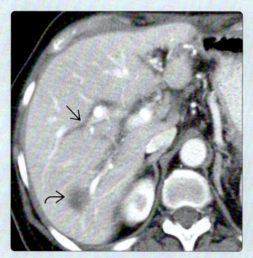
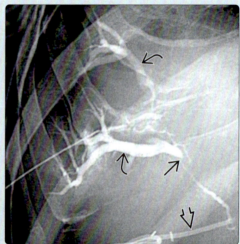

(Left) *Axial CT shows a liver metastasis ➡ that is low in attenuation, likely as a result of necrosis. Note the dilated ducts ➡ that resulted from a stricture of the biliary bifurcation and common hepatic duct, also due to chemotherapy.* (Right) *Transhepatic cholangiogram in the same patient shows gross dilation of the intrahepatic ducts ➡ with abrupt, high-grade stenosis at the confluence of the right and left ducts ➡. This patient had received floxuridine through an hepatic arterial catheter ➡.*

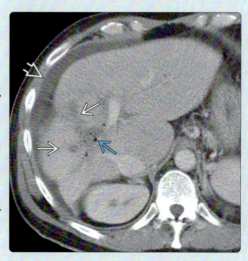
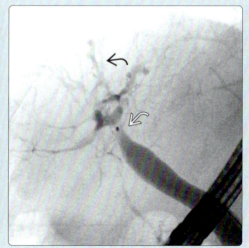

(Left) *CT of a patient with carcinoid (neuroendocrine) liver metastases after 8 courses of transcatheter arterial chemoembolization shows irregular right periductal low attenuation ➡, pneumobilia ➡, posterior segment atrophy, and ascites ➡. The appearance is compatible with chemotherapy-induced sclerosing cholangitis.* (Right) *ERCP of the same patient shows a proximal common duct stricture ➡ and irregular, strictured intrahepatic ducts ➡.*

TERMINOLOGY

Synonyms

- Chemotherapy-induced sclerosing cholangitis (CISC): Biliary sclerosis

Definitions

- Iatrogenic cholangitis following intraarterial chemotherapy for hepatic malignancies or metastases
  - Complication of hepatic artery infusion pump (HAIP) or transarterial chemoembolization (TACE)

IMAGING

General Features

- Location
  - Distribution of strictures in biliary tree reflects hepatic arterial supply to bile ducts
  - Commonly affects common hepatic duct and biliary confluence (~ 50%)
  - Rarely causes peripheral intrahepatic stricture
  - Distal common bile duct is not involved
  - Gallbladder and cystic duct may be involved
- Morphology
  - Stenosis or complete obstruction of involved ducts
    - ± dilation of upstream intrahepatic ducts
    - Associated fibrosis may impede ductal dilatation

Radiographic Findings

- ERCP
  - Abnormalities range from minimal duct wall irregularity to marked duct wall thickening with near obliteration of lumen

CT Findings

- CT (or MR) essential to differentiate cholangitis from extrinsic duct compression by lymph nodes or tumor
- Shows mildly dilated intrahepatic bile ducts
- May show periductal edema, mural thickening and enhancement of affected bile ducts, and fat stranding in hepatoduodenal ligament

MR Findings

- MRCP
  - Segmental strictures of variable length (similar to those seen in primary sclerosing cholangitis)

Imaging Recommendations

- Best imaging tool
  - CT, MRCP, and ERCP; may be used in concert to differentiate this entity from other causes of jaundice
    - e.g., compression by hepatic tumor, porta hepatis adenopathy, and chemotherapy hepatotoxicity

DIFFERENTIAL DIAGNOSIS

Primary Sclerosing Cholangitis (PSC)

- Skip dilations, stenosis, beading, pruning, irregular thickening of wall of intra- and extrahepatic bile ducts
  - Less common in chemotherapy cholangitis
- Gallbladder and cystic duct are usually more severely involved in chemotherapy cholangitis than in PSC

Autoimmune Pancreatitis-Cholangitis Syndrome

- Imaging findings are almost identical to those of PSC
- No history of prior chemotherapy

Extrinsic Compression (Liver Masses)

- May compress common hepatic duct
- Usually no short segment strictures

Chemical Hepatitis

- Clinically presents with jaundice mimicking cholangitis; however, there are no laboratory or imaging findings of biliary pathology

PATHOLOGY

General Features

- Etiology
  - Ischemic cholangiopathy &/or direct toxicity
    - Direct chemical toxic effects of drug on duct &/or occlusion of peribiliary vascular plexus with resultant biliary fibrosis
    - Toxic effects of fluoropyrimidines (floxuridine and 5-FU)
      □ Rarely from other drugs (e.g., mitomycin-C)

CLINICAL ISSUES

Presentation

- Most common signs/symptoms
  - Intermittent or progressive jaundice and cholestasis; cholangitis (pain, fever)
  - ↑ bilirubin, alkaline phosphatase

Demographics

- Epidemiology
  - Cholangiographic abnormalities reported in 7-30% of patients undergoing intraarterial chemotherapy

Natural History & Prognosis

- Complications: Acute hepatic failure, ischemic cholecystitis, biliary cirrhosis (rare)
- Mortality rate: 1%

Treatment

- Reduction or cessation of intraarterial chemotherapy
- Biliary decompression with endoscopic balloon dilation of strictures ± stenting
- Equivocal role of intraarterial steroids
- In rare cases, surgical resection of affected segment of bile duct or liver transplantation may be indicated

SELECTED REFERENCES

1. Ito K et al: Biliary sclerosis after hepatic arterial infusion pump chemotherapy for patients with colorectal cancer liver metastasis: incidence, clinical features, and risk factors. Ann Surg Oncol. 19(5):1609-17, 2012
2. Torrisi JM et al: CT findings of chemotherapy-induced toxicity: what radiologists need to know about the clinical and radiologic manifestations of chemotherapy toxicity. Radiology. 258(1):41-56, 2011
3. Kato Y et al: Chemotherapy-induced sclerosing cholangitis as a rare indication for resection: report of a case. Surg Today. 39(10):905-8, 2009
4. Menias CO et al: Mimics of cholangiocarcinoma: spectrum of disease. Radiographics. 28(4):1115-29, 2008
5. Alazmi WM et al: Chemotherapy-induced sclerosing cholangitis: long-term response to endoscopic therapy. J Clin Gastroenterol. 40(4):353-7, 2006
6. Phongkitkarun S et al: Bile duct complications of hepatic arterial infusion chemotherapy evaluated by helical CT. Clin Radiol. 60(6):700-9, 2005

KEY FACTS

IMAGING

- Biliary injuries are increasing in frequency
  - Imaging plays crucial role in identification & management
- **Direct Cholangiography**
  - ERCP is best for evaluation of injury to major hepatic duct branches & CBD
    - Also guides therapeutic intervention (sphincterotomy & stent placement)
- **CT**: Accurately depicts presence and extent of hepatic parenchymal injuries
  - Active bleeding is accurately depicted
  - Hepatic arterial (HA) occlusion may be depicted or suggested
  - Injuries to GB & bile ducts are suggested only indirectly
    - Presence of lower density (attenuation) fluid in GB fossa & peritoneal cavity
- **Eovist (Primovist) enhanced MR**

- Valuable in evaluation of patients with known or suspected biliary injuries
- Superior to hepatobiliary scintigraphy (greater anatomic detail & spatial resolution)
- **Hepatobiliary Scintigraphy**
  - Variations of Tc-99m "HIDA" scan (hepatobiliary iminodiacetic acid)
  - Look for extraluminal collections (bile leak) on sequential images over 60-120 minutes
  - SPECT (single photon emission computed tomography): Greater anatomic detail & spatial resolution
- **Recommended imaging protocol**
  - CT is optimal for initial evaluation of hepatobiliary injuries
  - Hepatobiliary scintigraphy is useful when clinical suspicion of biliary injury is relatively low
  - MR with MRCP and gadoxetate enhancement is optimal noninvasive test when clinical suspicion is high
  - ERCP or PTC is most accurate for diagnosis and guidance for therapy

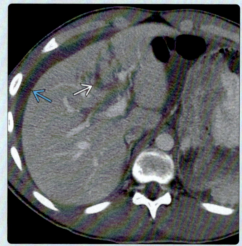
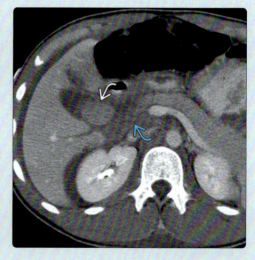

(Left) In this patient, injured in a motor vehicle crash, CT shows a deep hepatic laceration ➔ and free intraperitoneal fluid ➔ that was less dense than blood. (Right) In the same case, CT shows clotted blood ➔ and lower density fluid in the gallbladder fossa, as well as a heterogeneous lesion ➔ in the groove between the pancreatic head and 2nd portion of the duodenum, suggesting a traumatic injury.

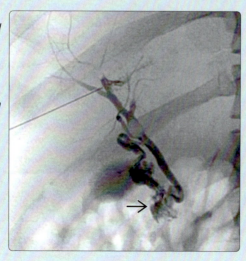
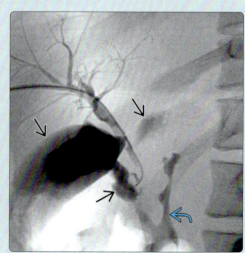

(Left) The same patient developed abdominal pain and a suggestion of peritonitis. Concern about a biliary injury prompted transhepatic cholangiography (PTC), which showed transection of the distal common bile duct within the pancreatic head, and extravasation of bile ➔. (Right) A 2nd image from the same PTC shows further accumulation of opacified bile ➔. This was treated with open choledochoenteric anastomosis. (Contrast-opacified urine is present in the kidney ➔ from the preceding CT scan.)

IMAGING

Traumatic and Iatrogenic Biliary Injuries

- Increasing in frequency due to increased prevalence of
  - Nonoperative management of hepatic trauma
  - Laparoscopic, rather than "open," surgical approach to gallbladder and biliary surgery
  - Resection of hepatic neoplasms
  - Hepatic transplantation
- Difficulty in diagnosis
  - Nonspecific clinical signs and symptoms
  - Delays in diagnosis and repair lead to increased morbidity and mortality
  - Imaging plays crucial role in identification and management of biliary injuries

Radiographic Findings

- **Direct Cholangiography**
  - ERC (endoscopic retrograde) or PTC (percutaneous transhepatic) cholangiography
  - Most accurate localization of leaks and strictures
    - Not 1st-line choice for diagnosis due to invasiveness & expense
      - □ Diagnosis of biliary injury usually suggested 1st by clinical presentation plus CT, MR or hepatobiliary scintigraphy
  - ERCP is best for evaluation of injury to major hepatic duct branches & CBD
  - PTC may detect injury to smaller ducts not reachable via ERCP
  - Also guides therapeutic intervention (sphincterotomy & stent placement)

CT Findings

- Accurately depicts presence and extent of hepatic parenchymal injuries
  - Deep lacerations invariably transect some branches of biliary tree & blood vessels
  - Active bleeding is accurately depicted as extravasation of fluid isodense to contrast-opacified blood
    - Confirmed & treated via catheter angiography with embolization
  - Hepatic arterial (HA) occlusion may be depicted or suggested
    - Occlusion of main hepatic artery is seen on contrast-enhanced CT or CT angiography
    - In liver transplantation setting
      - □ Strongly suggested by development of peribiliary fluid collections (due to biliary necrosis)
      - □ Confirmed, possibly treated, by catheter angiography
    - Following hepatobiliary surgery
      - □ Iatrogenic occlusion of HA branch
      - □ Suggested by ischemia or infarction of hepatic segment(s) supplied by occluded vessel
- Injuries to gallbladder and bile ducts are **suggested only indirectly by CT and ultrasonography**
  - Presence of lower density (attenuation) fluid
    - Hemoperitoneum typically measures ~ 35-45 HU
    - Blood-tinged bile (as ascites) measures ~ 15-25 HU

- Deep hepatic, duodenal, or pancreatic traumatic injury, placing bile ducts and gallbladder at risk
  - Coupled with suggestive clinical or imaging features
    - □ e.g., persistent or progressive signs of peritonitis
    - □ Persistent or ↑ intra- or extrahepatic fluid collections

MR Findings

- MR with conventional gadolinium-based contrast media
  - Shows same hepatic injuries and fluid collections as CT
  - Not 1st-line modality in acute trauma setting
    - Lengthy exam with unstable, agitated patient
- MR using hepatobiliary MR contrast agent (gadoxetate; Eovist, Primovist, Bayer HealthCare Pharmaceuticals)
  - Valuable in evaluation of patients with known or suspected biliary injuries
    - Superior to hepatobiliary scintigraphy
  - Biliary excretion of gadoxetate on delayed phase can accurately detect presence and site of biliary leaks and strictures
    - Imaging in multiple planes with greater anatomic detail & spatial resolution
    - Dynamic images over time may aid in recognition & estimation of rate of biliary leak

Nuclear Medicine Findings

- Hepatobiliary scintigraphy
  - Variations of Tc-99m "HIDA" scan (hepatobiliary iminodiacetic acid)
    - Uptake and excretion by liver & bile ducts into gallbladder (if present) & bowel
    - Look for extraluminal collections (bile leak) on sequential images over 60-120 minutes
      - □ Or delayed/absent bowel activity to indicate biliary stricture/obstruction
    - SPECT (single photon emission computed tomography)
      - □ Provides better spatial localization & accuracy than conventional planar imaging due to tomographic sections

Imaging Recommendations

- Best imaging tool
  - CT is optimal for initial evaluation of hepatobiliary injuries
    - Best depiction of extrahepatic injuries, ascites, etc.
  - Hepatobiliary scintigraphy is useful when clinical suspicion of biliary injury is relatively low
  - MR with MRCP and gadoxetate enhancement is optimal noninvasive test when clinical suspicion is high
  - ERCP or PTC is most accurate for diagnosis and guidance for therapy
- Protocol advice
  - Multimodality imaging is often necessary, guided by clinical signs and symptoms

SELECTED REFERENCES

1. Melamud K et al: Biliary imaging: multimodality approach to imaging of biliary injuries and their complications. Radiographics. 34(3):613-23, 2014
2. Thompson CM et al: Management of iatrogenic bile duct injuries: role of the interventional radiologist. Radiographics. 33(1):117-34, 2013

(Left) *In this patient who had recent laparoscopic cholecystectomy, CT shows clips ⇨ from the cholecystectomy and fluid in the gallbladder fossa ➡.* **(Right)** *A more caudal CT section in the same case shows a larger component of the fluid collection ➡ with a contrast-enhancing capsule, interpreted as a probable bile leak and confirmed by percutaneous catheter drainage. ERCP confirmed leak from the cystic duct remnant and a biliary stent was placed with resolution of the leak.*

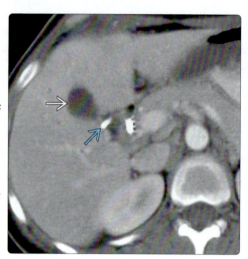
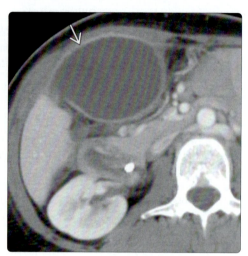

(Left) *In this young woman with pain & hyperbilirubinemia following cholecystectomy, planar images from a hepatobiliary scintigraphy (HIDA) study show progressive pooling of the radiotracer within the gallbladder fossa ⇨ & right paracolic gutter ➔, indicating bile leak.* **(Right)** *ERCP confirms the leak ➡ from the cystic duct remnant. ERCP guided placement of a stent that allowed resolution of the leak.*

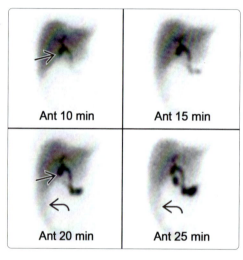

Ant 10 min   Ant 15 min

Ant 20 min   Ant 25 min

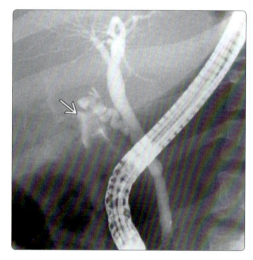

(Left) *In this elderly man with pain & hyperbilirubinemia following cholecystectomy, an Eovist (gadoxetate)-enhanced MR shows contrast opacification of the common bile duct ➡ and a separate collection of opacified bile ➔ that filled the gallbladder fossa on delayed images, confirming a bile leak.* **(Right)** *ERCP confirmed a leak from the cystic duct and guided placement of a stent ➡, resulting in resolution of the leak.*

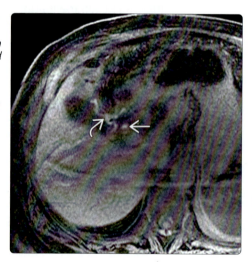
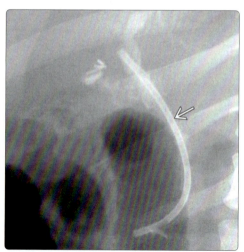

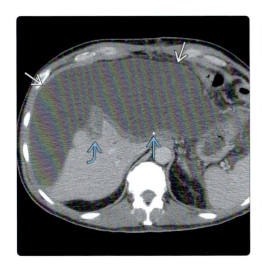

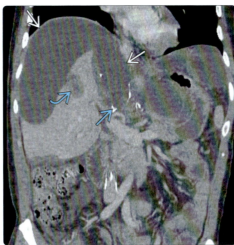

(Left) *This man had chemotherapy followed by surgical resection and ablation of hepatic metastases from colon cancer. Ten days later, he developed abdominal pain & fever. CT shows a large subcapsular and perihepatic fluid collection ➡ adjacent to surgical clips ➡ & ablation sites ➡.* (Right) *A coronal-reformatted CT in the same patient shows the large, low-density fluid collection ➡, clips ➡, and ablation sites ➡, suggesting a bile leak.*

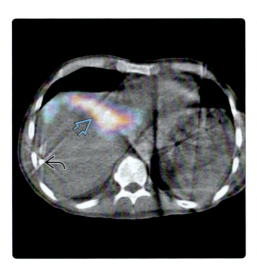

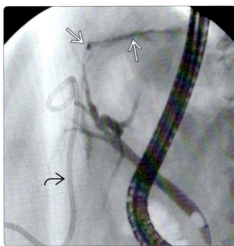

(Left) *Following percutaneous drainage of the fluid via US-guided catheter placement, an axial SPECT hepatobiliary scintigraphy study shows accumulation of the radiotracer ➡ along the left hepatectomy margin. Artifacts from the biliary drain are noted ➡.* (Right) *ERCP shows the drainage catheter ➡ & extravasation of contrast ➡ from one of the bile ducts. During the same procedure, a sphincterotomy was performed and a biliary stent was placed with complete resolution of the leak.*

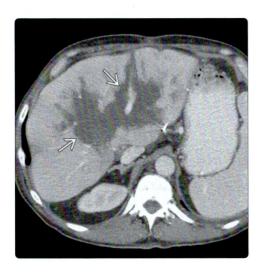

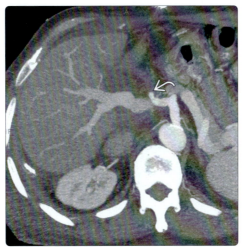

(Left) *In this hepatic transplant recipient, CT shows a large, intrahepatic, low-density branching fluid collection ➡ that parallels the biliary tree, characteristic of biliary necrosis.* (Right) *An MIP reconstruction from the same CT study shows occlusion of the main hepatic artery ➡, which accounted for the biliary necrosis seen as the peribiliary hepatic fluid collection. Urgent retransplantation was required.*

Gallbladder Polyps

TERMINOLOGY

- Polypoid or sessile lesion protruding from gallbladder mucosa

IMAGING

- **Ultrasonography is 1st line and usually sufficient for evaluation**
  - Nonmobile, hyperechoic mass protruding from gallbladder mucosa without acoustic shadowing
- Protocol advice
  - Grayscale and color Doppler ultrasound with 6-MHz transducer
- Ultrasonographic findings
  - Highly echogenic foci within polyp indicate likely cholesterol polyp
  - Large polyps may have internal vascularity on color Doppler ultrasound

TOP DIFFERENTIAL DIAGNOSES

- Tumefactive sludge
- Gallstone
- Polypoid gallbladder carcinoma
- Gallbladder metastases (e.g., melanoma)

PATHOLOGY

- Classification
  - Neoplastic (minority of lesions): Adenoma, adenoma-carcinoma, miscellaneous (fibroma, lipoma, etc.)
  - Nonneoplastic (majority): Cholesterol polyp, adenomyoma, inflammatory polyp, choristoma

CLINICAL ISSUES

- Size is most important predictor of malignancy
  - 88% of malignant polyps are > 10 mm
  - Almost 100% of polyps > 20 mm are malignant
  - 94% of benign polyps are < 10 mm
- Most are asymptomatic, incidental findings on ultrasound

(Left) Ultrasound of a 41-year-old man with chest pain shows two 4-mm gallbladder (GB) polyps ➡. Their small size, echogenicity, multiplicity, and stability at follow-up sonography indicate hyperplastic (cholesterol) polyps. (Right) Ultrasound of a 49-year-old woman shows multiple incidental polyps ➡ involving the anterior GB wall and the fundus; no acoustic shadowing from the polyps is demonstrated. Management strategies for small (< 1 cm) polyps are controversial, though most authors advocate ultrasound surveillance.

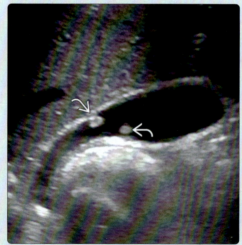
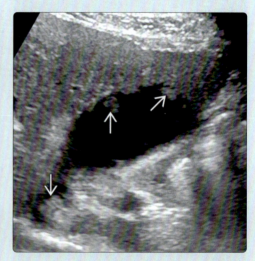

(Left) Ultrasound of a 47-year-old woman shows a 1-cm, pathologically confirmed adenomatous polyp ➡. The likelihood of neoplasia increases with polyp size, but most GB polyps are hyperplastic. (Right) Ultrasound of a 55-year-old woman shows a 1.8-cm polyp ➡ within the GB fundus. Loss of reflectivity of the adjacent GB wall ➡ might suggest a neoplastic polyp. This and the size of the polyp prompted elective cholecystectomy, which revealed a solitary but large cholesterol polyp.

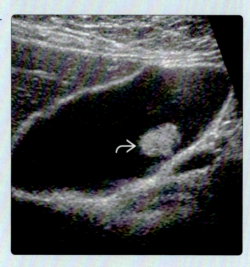
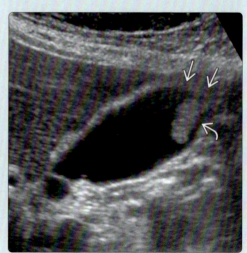

Biliary Papillomatosis

TERMINOLOGY

- Rare disorder characterized by multiple adenomatous papillary tumors of biliary tree
  - May be same entity as biliary intraductal papillary mucinous neoplasm (IPMN)

IMAGING

- **MRCP and ERCP are 1st-line tests**
- Multiple round or oval filling defects within biliary tree
  - Majority are within extrahepatic ducts
- Typically present with large intraductal mass (with ductal dilatation) at time of diagnosis

TOP DIFFERENTIAL DIAGNOSES

- Choledocholithiasis
- Cholangiocarcinoma
- Pneumobilia
- Duct invasive hepatocellular carcinoma

PATHOLOGY

- Postulated pathogenesis
  - Incited by chronic inflammation from choledocholithiasis, infection, or pancreatic juice reflux
  - Categorized into nonmucin and mucin-producing types
    - Pathology overlaps with IPMN of biliary ducts
  - Considered premalignant lesion
    - Frankly malignant polypoid lesion is typically identified at clinical presentation

CLINICAL ISSUES

- Repeated episodes of abdominal pain, jaundice, cholangitis
- Extremely rare lesion
  - Most cases have been reported from Far East Asia
- Treatment of multifocal, premalignant disease is difficult
  - Resection, liver transplantation, palliative stenting have been reported

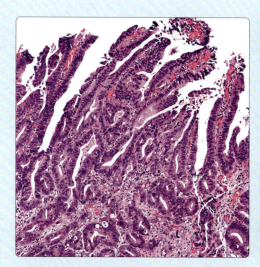

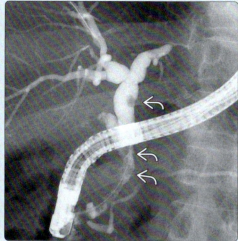

(Left) Biliary papillomatosis features numerous polypoid adenomatous lesions. This one, present in the common duct, resembles an intestinal-type tubulovillous adenoma. (Courtesy L. Lamps, MD.) (Right) ERCP of a patient with elevated liver function tests shows polypoid filling defects ➜ within the extrahepatic duct. Mild dysplasia was identified at resection. Biliary papillomatosis (like biliary IPMN) is considered a premalignant lesion and is often frankly invasive at diagnosis. (Courtesy M. Kanematsu, MD.)

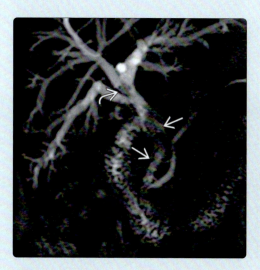

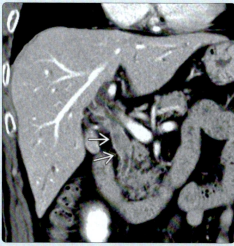

(Left) MRCP of a patient with jaundice shows multiple small common ➡ and anterior segmental ➡ ductal polypoid lesions (and mild intrahepatic ductal dilatation). Resection of this premalignant, multifocal disease is often impossible. (Courtesy S. Yeon Kim, MD.) (Right) Coronal CT reconstruction of the same patient again shows filling defects within the common duct ➡. Bile duct resection confirmed multiple papillary neoplasms associated with invasive carcinoma. (Courtesy S. Yeon Kim, MD.)

Gallbladder Carcinoma

TERMINOLOGY

- Malignant epithelial neoplasm arising from gallbladder (GB) mucosa; usually adenocarcinoma
- Most common biliary malignancy

IMAGING

- **Ultrasound: Most common method of diagnosis**
  - Gallstones; moderately echogenic polypoid intraluminal or mural mass
  - Mass with indistinct margins with adjacent liver
- **Contrast-enhanced CT or MR, ± PET/CT: Most comprehensive imaging**
  - Best test for depicting total extent of tumor (e.g., nodal, peritoneal, hematogenous metastases)
  - Hypovascular mass infiltrating GB fossa; invading adjacent liver; porta hepatis adenopathy
  - "Porcelain GB": Calcified wall; importance as precursor to GB carcinoma is debatable

TOP DIFFERENTIAL DIAGNOSES

- Chronic cholecystitis
- Complicated acute cholecystitis
- GB polyps
- Adenomyomatosis
- Xanthogranulomatous cholecystitis
- Metastatic disease to GB fossa: Especially melanoma

CLINICAL ISSUES

- Major risk factors: Cholelithiasis (seen in 70-90%), chronic inflammation/infection
- Nodal spread to porta hepatis, peripancreatic and retroperitoneal nodes
  - Direct and hematogenous spread to liver
  - Transmural spread to peritoneal cavity and omentum
- Very poor prognosis (5-year survival: 1-5%)

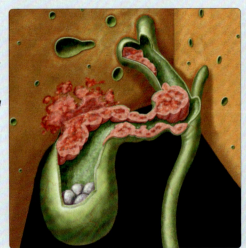
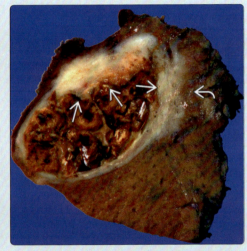

(Left) Schematic drawing of gallbladder (GB) carcinoma shows gallstones and a focal mural mass arising from the GB wall, invading the adjacent liver, and obstructing the common hepatic duct. (Right) Gross pathological section of a central liver specimen from a 55-year-old woman with confirmed invasive GB adenocarcinoma shows focal GB wall thickening ➡ and direct invasion of the adjacent liver by tumor ➡, a typical pattern of local spread of GB carcinoma. The GB lumen is filled with stones.

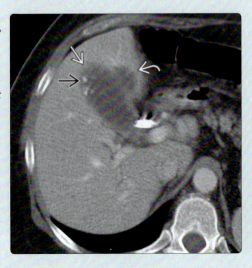
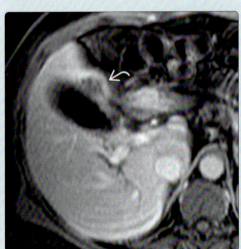

(Left) Preoperative CECT of the same patient shows subtle thickening of the wall of the GB fundus ➡, several adjacent partially calcified stones ➡, and focal invasion of the medial hepatic segment ➡. (Right) T1WI C+ FS MR of the same patient shows local invasion of the medial segment ➡. Recent work has suggested that delayed enhanced MR may play a role in staging early-stage (T1, T2) disease, although most patients with GB carcinoma present with at least transserosal (T3) tumor, as in this case.

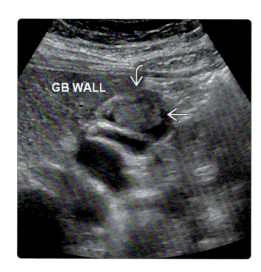

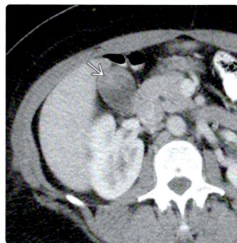

(Left) *Ultrasound of a 58-year-old woman with vague right upper quadrant pain shows a 2.2-cm polypoid mass* ➡ *within the GB fundus. Subtle loss of fundal wall reflectivity* ➡ *suggests transmural spread of tumor despite the small size of the lesion.* (Right) *CECT of the same patient shows a polypoid mass* ➡ *within the GB fundus. Direct liver invasion and peritoneal metastases were identified at laparoscopy. Early-stage GB carcinomas are typically only discovered serendipitously at cholecystectomy.*

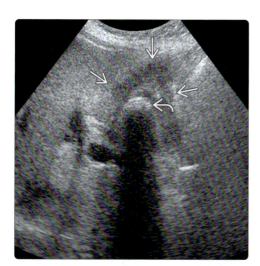

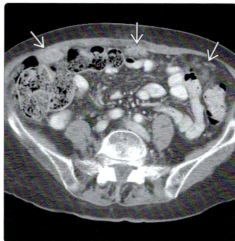

(Left) *Ultrasound of an 84-year-old woman with right upper quadrant pain and jaundice shows a GB fossa mass* ➡ *and a shadowing stone* ➡*. The mass is inseparable from adjacent liver. CT (not shown) demonstrated biliary duct dilatation and local invasion of the central liver by GB carcinoma.* (Right) *CECT of the same patient shows omental metastases* ➡*. The patient expired 10 months later. The 5-year survival rate for GB carcinoma is dismal, and most patients have metastases at the time of diagnosis.*

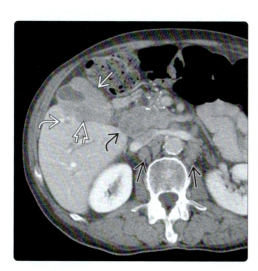

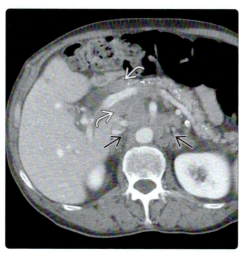

(Left) *CECT of a 69-year-old woman with right upper quadrant pain and weight loss shows marked irregular GB wall thickening* ➡*, direct liver invasion* ➡*, a subtle satellite liver metastasis* ➡*, and peripancreatic or portocaval* ➡ *and retroperitoneal* ➡ *adenopathy.* (Right) *CECT of the same patient shows peripancreatic* ➡ *and retroperitoneal* ➡ *adenopathy. Lymphatic spread along the hepaticoduodenal ligament is characteristic of GB carcinoma.*

IMAGING

- **Classification**: Based on anatomy and radiography
  - Intrahepatic ("peripheral") (10%)
    - Appears as intrahepatic mass, usually with obstruction of intrahepatic bile ducts (IHBDs)
  - Perihilar (50%)
    - **Klatskin tumor**: Small hilar tumor involving confluence of hepatic ducts
  - Distal (40%)
    - Extrahepatic; distal CBD
    - May appear as short stricture or small polypoid mass
- **MR with MRCP is best noninvasive imaging study**
  - Superior to CT for detection of small hilar tumors, intrahepatic & periductal tumor infiltration
  - Shows location of obstruction and dilation of upstream ducts
- **Contrast-enhanced CT**

- Venous phase: Minimal enhancement of tumor (small mass or thickened duct wall)
- Delayed phase: Persistent enhancing tumor (due to fibrous stroma)
- **Direct cholangiography** [percutaneous transhepatic (PTC) or ERCP]
  - Important to determine extent of intra- and extrahepatic duct involvement
  - Extension up right or left duct often precludes surgical resection
- **Ultrasonography**
  - May demonstrate tumor as ductal mass or abrupt stricture
- **Endoscopic ultrasound (EUS)**
  - Reported higher sensitivity than CT, US, and MRCP
  - May guide biopsy or brushing for tissue confirmation

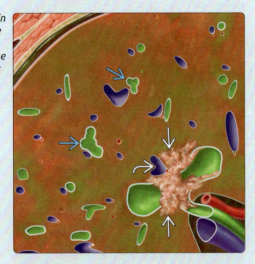
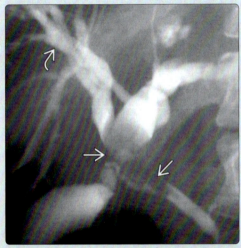

(Left) Graphic shows a Klatskin tumor ➡, a small mass at the confluence of the main right and left bile ducts invading the adjacent liver and the hepatic vein ➡. The intrahepatic ducts are dilated ➡, and the liver is bile stained. (Right) Cholangiogram shows a polypoid mass ➡ at the confluence of the main right and left ducts with marked dilation of the intrahepatic bile ducts ➡. The common hepatic duct is involved, but the cystic and common bile ducts are not.

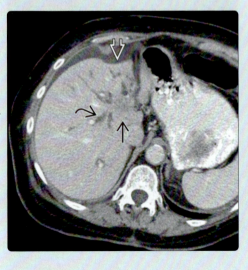
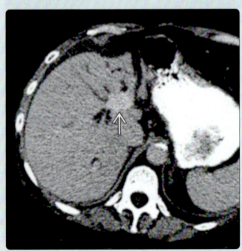

(Left) Axial, venous-phase CECT shows intrahepatic bile duct dilation ➡ ending abruptly at a small mass ➡ near the hepatic hilum. The lateral segment atrophy ➡ is a secondary sign of longstanding biliary obstruction. (Right) Axial CECT in the same patient on a 10-minute delayed scan shows delayed retention of contrast in the tumor ➡, reflecting the fibrous stroma component that is typical of cholangiocarcinomas. This is a classic example of a Klatskin tumor with direct hepatic invasion.

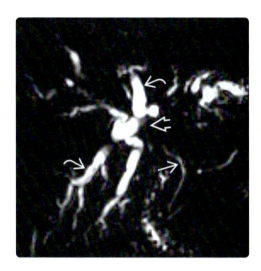

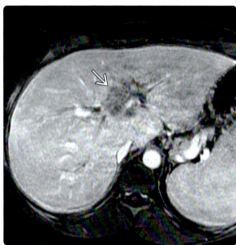

(Left) Coronal MRCP shows gross dilation of the intrahepatic bile ducts ⮰ but a normal-sized common duct ⮀. The biliary tree is abruptly obstructed ⮲ just beyond the confluence of right and left main ducts. (Right) Axial T1WI MR in the same patient during the hepatic parenchymal (portal venous) phase of enhancement shows the small infiltrative mass ⮀. This is a typical example of a Klatskin (hilar) cholangiocarcinoma.

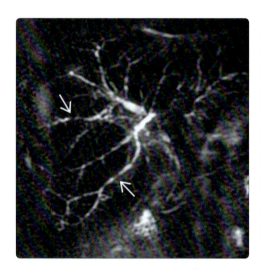

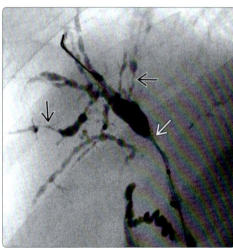

(Left) Coronal MRCP in the same patient with primary sclerosing cholangitis (PSC) shows irregular strictures of the intrahepatic ducts ⮀ with the right lobe ducts dilated more than the left. (Right) ERCP in the same patient with PSC shows irregular biliary strictures ⮲ and abrupt narrowing of the right hepatic duct ⮀ due to cholangiocarcinoma. Detailed anatomic depiction of involvement of common hepatic, right, and left ducts is critical to determine operability.

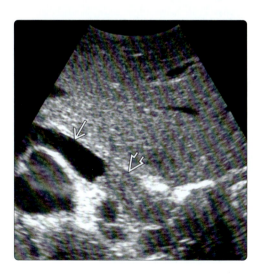

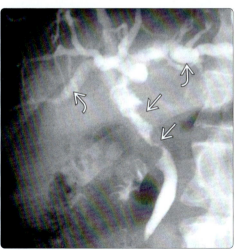

(Left) Longitudinal oblique ultrasound shows a markedly dilated common bile duct ⮀, which is obstructed by a mass ⮲ with homogeneous echogenicity and no acoustic shadowing. (Right) In the same case, ERCP shows an "apple core" stricture ⮀ of the common duct due to cholangiocarcinoma. The ducts upstream from the tumor are all dilated ⮰.

Ampullary Carcinoma

TERMINOLOGY

- Malignant epithelial neoplasm (adenocarcinoma) arising from ampulla of Vater

IMAGING

- **Multiplanar, multiphasic CECT or MR with MRCP for diagnosis**
  - Small ampullary mass with dilated common bile duct and pancreatic duct; nodal or liver metastases in advanced cases
  - Double duct sign with obstruction of common bile duct and pancreatic duct
- ERCP for confirmation and biopsy proof

TOP DIFFERENTIAL DIAGNOSES

- Pancreatic head carcinoma invading ampulla
- Adenoma of ampulla
- Distal cholangiocarcinoma
- Mesenchymal tumor of ampulla

- Duodenal carcinoma (adenocarcinoma)

PATHOLOGY

- Lobulated soft tissue mass arising from ampulla of Vater
- Markedly increased incidence in hereditary polyposis syndromes (e.g., familial adenomatosis coli, hereditary nonpolyposis colon cancer, etc.)

CLINICAL ISSUES

- Jaundice (80%), weight loss (61%), abdominal pain, and back pain (46%) are most common symptoms
- Better prognosis than periampullary carcinoma of biliary or pancreatic origin

DIAGNOSTIC CHECKLIST

- Duodenal distension with water on CECT or MR is key to identifying lesion
- Perform dedicated CT/MR pancreatic protocol when ampullary lesion suspected

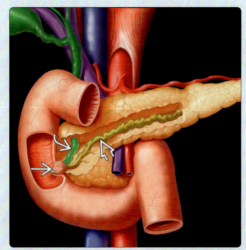
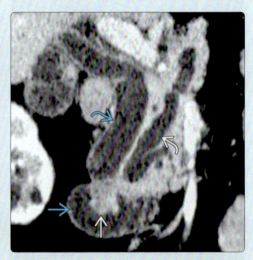

(Left) Graphic of an ampullary carcinoma ➡ causing obstruction of both the common bile duct ➡ and the pancreatic duct ➡ is shown. (Right) In this patient with painless jaundice, coronal minimum-intensity CT reconstruction shows a polypoid mass (carcinoma) ➡ in the ampullary region within the duodenum ➡. The double duct sign is evident with dilation of the common bile duct ➡ and pancreatic duct ➡.

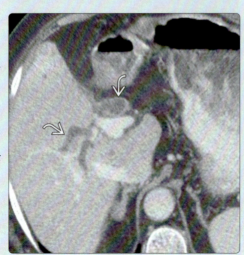
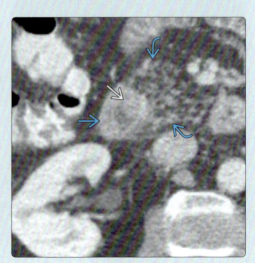

(Left) In a patient presenting with painless jaundice and concern for a pancreatic cancer, axial CECT shows dilated intra- and extrahepatic bile ducts ➡. (Right) In the same patient, axial CECT shows a small ampullary mass ➡ bulging into the lumen of the duodenum ➡. The pancreatic head ➡ is somewhat fatty infiltrated but otherwise normal. Surgery revealed a small ampullary carcinoma.

Biliary Metastases and Lymphoma

TERMINOLOGY

- Metastatic deposits involving gallbladder (GB) or bile duct (BD) wall

IMAGING

- Best diagnostic clue: Polypoid GB mass > 1.5 cm in patient with known melanoma (or lymphoma)
- **Ultrasound for initial diagnosis**
  - **CECT or MR for global view of abdomen**
- Morphology
  - Metastases: Polypoid mass in GB wall; BD wall mass ± luminal obstruction
  - Lymphoma: Bulky GB and porta hepatis mass with generalized lymphadenopathy

TOP DIFFERENTIAL DIAGNOSES

- Benign intramural GB polyp
- GB carcinoma
- Adenomyomatosis

PATHOLOGY

- Metastases
  - Melanoma is most common primary tumor
  - Renal cell and other cancers have been reported
- Lymphoma
  - Most cases are non-Hodgkin lymphoma

CLINICAL ISSUES

- Most patients are asymptomatic
  - Lesions are usually discovered as part of CT staging
  - Right upper quadrant pain or jaundice may result from BD metastases; rarely from lymphoma
- Metastases carry poor prognosis; usually part of widespread and advanced disease
- Treatment
  - Surgery for isolated GB metastasis
  - Radiation and chemotherapy for lymphoma

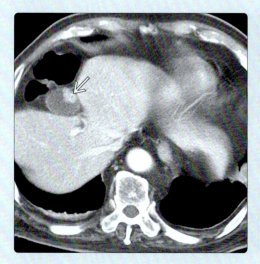

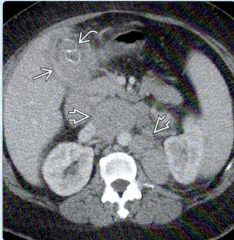

(Left) Axial CECT in a 55-year-old man with a history of scalp melanoma 2 years prior, now presenting with weight loss and fatigue, demonstrates 1 of several enhancing masses ➡ in the wall of the gallbladder, proven to be metastases from melanoma. (Right) Axial CECT in a 48-year-old woman with weight loss and jaundice shows a soft tissue mass ➡ within the gallbladder wall and lumen along with gallstones ➡. Also noted is massive lymphadenopathy ➡, all due to non-Hodgkin lymphoma.

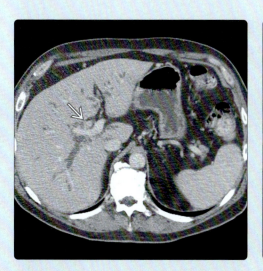

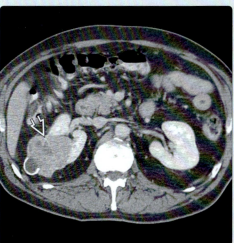

(Left) Axial CECT in a 54-year-old man with jaundice shows an enhancing mass ➡ causing obstruction of the bile ducts at the hepatic hilum. This lesion is indistinguishable by imaging from a Klatskin cholangiocarcinoma but proved to be metastasis from renal carcinoma. (Right) Axial CECT in the same patient shows primary renal cell carcinoma ➡ that caused the hilar biliary obstruction due to metastasis.

Biliary IPMN

TERMINOLOGY

- Mucin-producing papillary neoplasm of biliary mucosa
  - Analogous to pancreatic intraductal papillary mucinous neoplasm in imaging and pathology
- Overlap with biliary papillomatosis (same entity?)

IMAGING

- **Best imaging tools: Multiplanar CECT, MRCP**
  - Segmental or diffuse dilation of bile ducts ± polypoid or nodular intraductal mass
- **ERCP: Mucin-filled bile ducts** may result in nonvisualization of affected segment(s)
  - Extrusion of clear mucin from bulging ampulla
  - Clearing ducts of mucin helps define lesions [papillary mass(es)]
  - MRCP is not impaired by presence of mucin

TOP DIFFERENTIAL DIAGNOSES

- Cholangiocarcinoma (usual form)
  - Infiltrative or nodular mass with biliary stricture; does not produce excess mucin
- Recurrent pyogenic cholangitis
- Choledochal cyst (type IV)

PATHOLOGY

- Spectrum: Adenomatous dysplasia to frank invasive adenocarcinoma; often coexist
- Premalignant lesion with high potential for malignancy

CLINICAL ISSUES

- Most common signs/symptoms: Intermittent abdominal pain, fever, chills, jaundice
- Clinical profile: Asian patient with recurrent episodes of abdominal pain and fever
- Surgical resection of involved lobe or segment is curative for adenoma or dysplasia; may be curative for cancer limited to resected ducts and liver

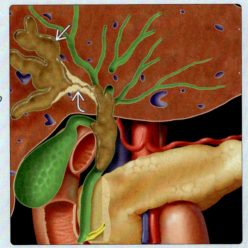
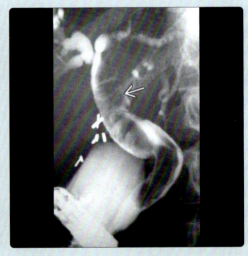

(Left) Graphic of biliary IPMN demonstrates segmental distension of the right lobe intrahepatic ducts ➡, which are filled with mucin, and a mucosal mass ⇗ arising from the ductal epithelium. The common bile duct (CBD) is also distended with mucin "downstream" from the mass, a unique feature of this disorder. (Right) ERCP obtained in a patient who presented with RUQ discomfort and elevated serum bilirubin demonstrates a grossly dilated CBD filled with amorphous mucin ➡.

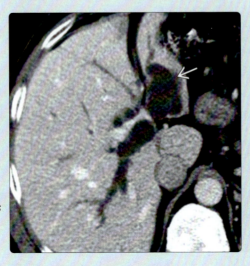
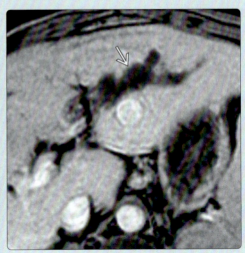

(Left) Axial CECT in a 49-year-old woman presenting with RUQ pain and elevated alkaline phosphatase demonstrates atrophy of the left lobe and marked dilation of the left bile duct ➡, more than the right. ERCP and subsequent surgery revealed a left duct IPMN. (Right) Axial T1WI with gadolinium enhancement in a 61-year-old woman with midepigastric pain and elevated alkaline phosphatase shows fusiform dilatation of the left bile ducts ➡, which proved to be biliary IPMN at surgery.

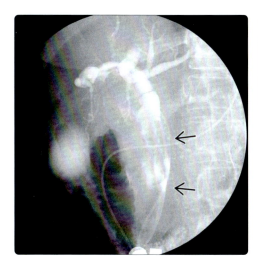

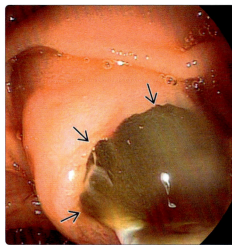

(Left) *ERCP of a patient with jaundice shows amorphous linear filling defects* ➡ *within a dilated common duct. CECT (not shown) revealed marked asymmetric right and CBD dilatation. (Courtesy S. Yeon Kim, MD.)* **(Right)** *The endoscopic image of duodenum in the same patient shows green mucin* ➡ *draining from a patulous, bulging papilla. The final diagnosis after right hepatectomy and bile duct resection was biliary IPMN associated with invasive carcinoma. (Courtesy S. Yeon Kim, MD.)*

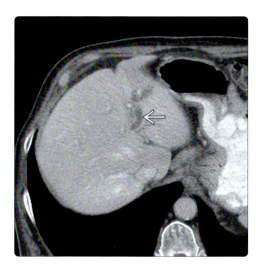

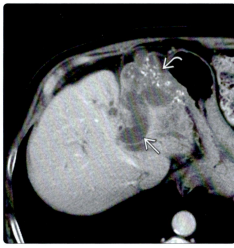

(Left) *CECT of a 75-year-old man shows mild left intrahepatic biliary ductal dilatation* ➡. *An ERCP performed previously reported a mucus plug.* **(Right)** *CECT of the same patient performed 6 years later shows marked left biliary ductal dilatation* ➡, *lobar atrophy, and calcifications* ➡. *Biliary IPMN and mucinous adenocarcinoma were identified at left hepatectomy. Biliary IPMN is a premalignant lesion and is considered a precursor for papillary cholangiocarcinoma.*

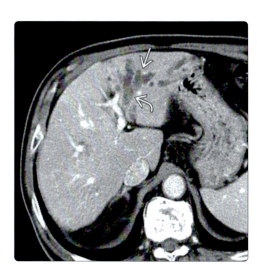

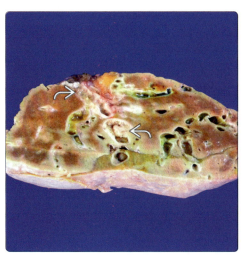

(Left) *CECT shows asymmetric left biliary ductal dilatation* ➡ *and subtle enhancing nodularity within the proximal left duct* ➡. *(Courtesy S. Yeon Kim, MD.)* **(Right)** *In this gross specimen from the same patient, multiple lateral segment intraductal papillary lesions* ➡ *are shown. Intraductal cholangiocarcinoma and background biliary IPMNs were identified at histology. Multifocal papillary proliferation and mucin hypersecretion are features shared with pancreatic IPMN. (Courtesy S. Yeon Kim, MD.)*

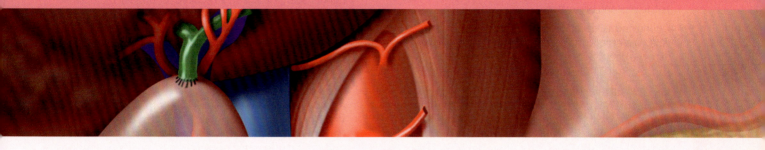

Embryology and Normal Variants

The body-tail segment of the pancreas develops from the embryologic dorsal pancreatic bud, while the head-uncinate segments develop from the ventral bud, which also gives rise to the liver and biliary tree.

During normal development, the ventral bud migrates clockwise around the fetal duodenum and eventually merges with the dorsal bud to form the pancreas with the branching pancreatic and biliary ducts in communication.

Variations in this process are relatively common, including many variations of the pancreatic duct branching pattern. Among the most common is **pancreas divisum**, in which there is no communication between the accessory duct of Santorini and the main duct of Wirsung that drains the pancreatic head.

Errors of rotation and fusion may also result in a completely circumferential or **annular pancreas**, which may be associated with pancreatitis as well as obstruction of the duodenal lumen.

As a result of their separate embryologic origins, the ventral and dorsal pancreatic segments may exhibit varying morphology, ranging from variations in the degree of fatty lobulation to complete absence of the dorsal pancreas. Both may simulate serious pathology unless one is familiar with these normal variants.

Pancreatic size and the degree of fatty lobulation vary substantially within the population based on patient age, body habitus, and other factors. In patients over the age of 70, the parenchyma atrophies, often develops small foci of calcification, and the pancreatic duct dilates slightly. These **senescent changes** should not be interpreted as evidence of chronic pancreatitis without corroborating clinical evidence.

Imaging Protocols

US may be the 1st study performed in the evaluation of abdominal pain. The pancreas, however, is often incompletely evaluated secondary to overlying bowel gas. If a cystic mass is identified, color Doppler should always be performed to rule out a vascular lesion. For most lesions, the pancreas is far better evaluated with **CT and MR using multiphasic and multiplanar imaging**.

Most ductal carcinomas are best detected as hypoenhancing masses relative to the normal pancreas, while endocrine (islet cell) tumors are hypervascular. Both types of tumors may be evident only on the arterial or pancreatic parenchymal phase of imaging (~ 35- to 45-second delay). Hepatic metastases from endocrine tumors may also be evident only on arterial-phase images. Portal venous (hepatic parenchymal)-phase images remain necessary in order to evaluate hypovascular metastases, venous involvement, and other anatomic features.

CT protocol: We often obtain a series of noncontrast scans through the liver and pancreas to help in recognition of small foci of calcification and degree of tumor enhancement and to help in localization for subsequent series. Since some hypervascular tumors (e.g., gastrinoma) may arise in the wall of the duodenum, and because multiplanar CT angiography is so often a useful adjunct, it is best to give **only water or a neutral oral contrast agent** rather than barium or iodinated contrast that may obscure intramural lesions or make CT angiography difficult.

Multiphasic scanning: Arterial (pancreatic parenchymal)-phase images should be obtained through the liver and pancreas as contiguous 0.65- to 1.25-mm images, reconstructed for viewing as 2.5- to 5.0-mm thick sections. The thinner source images are required for optimal multiplanar reformations. Portal venous (hepatic parenchymal)-phase images should be obtained through the liver and pancreas as well, using the same parameters.

Multiplanar reformations are very useful in recognizing and characterizing pancreatic disease. Curved planar reformations along the pancreatic duct offer the most compelling evidence of abrupt narrowing by a tumor mass or chronic pancreatitis. Variations of coronal and sagittal planes frequently make peripancreatic nodal involvement and local invasion more evident and may even be essential in recognizing a lesion as being intra- or peripancreatic in origin (e.g., an accessory spleen vs. a neuroendocrine tumor in the tail of the pancreas).

MR protocols: There are many vendor-specific pancreatic protocols, but the basic examination should include gradient-echo T1-weighted imaging in and out of phase, T2-weighted images, and dynamic gadolinium-enhanced gradient-echo images with fat suppression. An MRCP should be performed in cases of suspected pancreatic pathology to evaluate both the pancreatic and biliary ducts.

Approach to Abnormal Pancreas

Unlike other abdominal organs, the pancreas has only a thin capsule that is easily breached by inflammatory and neoplastic processes. Processes that originate within the pancreas can easily spread to adjacent structures, including other viscera within the anterior pararenal space, such as the duodenum and vertical colon segments. Pancreatitis, for instance, often affects the duodenal lumen and may cause inflammation of the descending colon as well. Pancreatic malignancies commonly invade the adjacent viscera, and even more commonly adjacent vessels and nerves, largely accounting for their poor prognosis. Invasion into the lumen of the splenic vein, which runs within the pancreas, leads to liver metastases; while occlusion of the splenic vein leads to characteristic perigastric varices in the absence of esophageal varices or cirrhosis. This may constitute the most obvious sign on imaging of a small primary tumor.

Obstruction or dilation of the pancreatic &/or common bile duct is another indirect but useful sign of pancreatic disease. Pancreatic ductal dilation is most frequently due to ductal carcinoma or chronic pancreatitis but may also result from intraductal papillary mucinous neoplasm (IPMN), neuroendocrine tumor, or even metastases to the pancreas.

Obstruction of the intrapancreatic bile duct may result from the same inflammatory and neoplastic processes of the pancreas. Obstruction of only the distal common bile duct with a normal pancreatic duct is more likely the result of primary inflammatory, infectious, neoplastic, or calculous disease originating in the biliary system.

Pancreatic ductal carcinomas are hypovascular tumors and often present on imaging as hypodense (hypointense) masses with abrupt obstruction of the ducts. Metastases to the pancreas from primary tumors, such as lung, breast, or melanoma, may simulate a primary ductal cancer.

Neuroendocrine tumors are more often hypervascular and may be simulated by metastases from hypervascular primary tumors, such as renal cell carcinoma.

Cystic pancreatic masses are discovered frequently on CT, MR, or US, making a pragmatic approach to their evaluation mandatory. Clinical history is necessary, as is consideration of the age, gender, and presence of laboratory evidence of pancreatitis. For example, mucinous cystic neoplasms occur almost exclusively in young or middle-aged women, while solid and papillary epithelial neoplasms occur in girls and young women. Pseudocysts are often indistinguishable from cystic tumors by imaging alone but usually occur in patients with known pancreatitis and evolve in size much more rapidly than tumors. Certain cystic tumors may have a characteristic appearance, allowing confident diagnosis and management; others will require further evaluation with endoscopic US emerging as the single most accurate means of guiding diagnosis and management in more complex cases.

Aneurysmal dilation of a peripancreatic artery (or varix) should be considered in the differential diagnosis of any cystic pancreatic mass. The presence of flowing blood must be determined by rapid IV administration of contrast medium for CT or MR or by color Doppler sonography.

Pancreatitis and complications of pancreatitis are commonly encountered in abdominal imaging. Because the pancreas is separated from the lesser sac by only the posterior parietal peritoneum, acute pancreatitis often results in exudation of fluid into the lesser sac, which should not be mistaken for a pseudocyst. These fluid collections usually resolve quickly, while pseudocysts take longer to resolve and have, by definition, a fibroinflammatory wall.

The tail of the pancreas is the distal few centimeters of the gland that lies within the splenorenal ligament and is actually intraperitoneal. Acute inflammation of the pancreatic tail may result in an intrasplenic pseudocyst and pancreatic ascites. Tumors arising from the pancreatic tail can easily invade the spleen without crossing an anatomic boundary. An important potential pitfall in this area is the accessory spleen, which may be located within the tail and mimic a hypervascular pancreatic mass.

Differential Diagnosis

Hypovascular Solid Pancreatic Mass
Common
- Pancreatic ductal carcinoma
- Acute or chronic pancreatitis
- Normal variants, pancreas (mimic)
- Peripancreatic lymphadenopathy

Less Common
- Serous cystadenoma, pancreas
- Ampullary carcinoma
- Pancreatic metastases and lymphoma
- Cholangiocarcinoma
- Pancreatic neuroendocrine tumor
- Solid and papillary epithelial neoplasm
- Autoimmune (IgG4-related) pancreatitis
- Groove pancreatitis
- Gastric tumors (mimic)
- Adrenal mass (mimic)
- Adjacent masses (mimic)
- Atypical and rare pancreatic tumors

Hypervascular Pancreatic Mass
Common
- Pancreatic neuroendocrine tumor
- Accessory spleen (mimic)

Less Common
- Pancreatic metastases
- Serous cystadenoma, pancreas
- Vascular lesions, peripancreatic
- Pheochromocytoma (mimic)
- Renal cell carcinoma (mimic)
- Gastric stromal tumor (mimic)
- Carcinoid tumor (mimic)
- Splenic tumors (mimic)

Cystic Pancreatic Mass
Common
- Pancreatic pseudocyst
- Lesser sac ascites (mimic)
- Mucinous cystic pancreatic tumor
- IPMN, pancreas
- Duodenal diverticulum (mimic)

Less Common
- Polycystic disease
- Cystic fibrosis, pancreas
- von Hippel-Lindau disease
- Serous cystadenoma, pancreas
- Solid and papillary epithelial neoplasm
- Pancreatic neuroendocrine tumor
- Epithelial (true) cyst, pancreas
- Pseudoaneurysm (mimic)
- Portal vein aneurysm (mimic)
- Metastases and lymphoma, pancreas
- Gastric stromal tumor (mimic)
- Choledochal cyst (mimic)
- Lymphangioma (peripancreatic, mimic)
- Pancreatic abscess

Rare but Important
- Hydatid cyst
- Teratoma, retroperitoneum
- Anaplastic carcinoma, pancreas
- Duplication cyst, duodenum (mimic)

Dilated Pancreatic Duct
Common
- Pancreatic ductal carcinoma
- Chronic pancreatitis
- Senescent change, pancreas
- IPMN, pancreas

Less Common
- Ampullary carcinoma
- Duodenal carcinoma
- Choledocholithiasis

Pancreatic Calcifications
Common
- Chronic or hereditary pancreatitis
- Pancreatic pseudocyst
- Senescent change, pancreas
- Vascular lesions, peripancreatic
- Choledocholithiasis (mimic)

Less Common
- Mucinous cystic pancreatic tumor
- Cystic fibrosis, pancreas
- Pancreatic neuroendocrine tumor
- Serous cystadenoma, pancreas
- Solid and papillary epithelial) neoplasm
- IPMN, pancreas

(Left) Graphic shows the ventral pancreas developing as an outpouching of the hepatic-biliary diverticulum. As the stomach and duodenum elongate, the ventral pancreas and bile ducts rotate clockwise and posteriorly to fuse with the dorsal pancreas. (Right) Coronal MRCP shows the normal CBD ➡ entering the duodenum and crossing the main pancreatic duct ➡, which continues as the duct of Santorini to the minor papilla, diagnostic of pancreas divisum. Fluid within the gastric fundus ➡ and small bowel is bright on this T2WI.

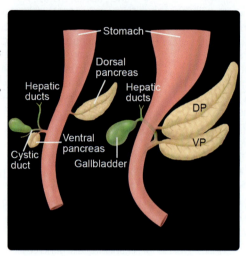
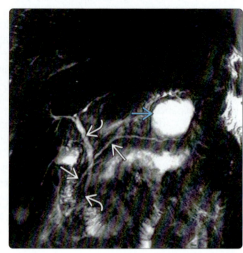

(Left) In this elderly man with painless jaundice, axial CT shows a hypodense mass ➡ in the head of the pancreas and a distended gallbladder ➡. The biliary tree was also dilated (not shown). (Right) Coronal CT reformation shows the dilated pancreatic duct ➡ interrupted as it enters the hypodense mass ➡, a typical presentation of pancreatic ductal carcinoma.

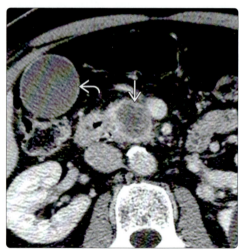
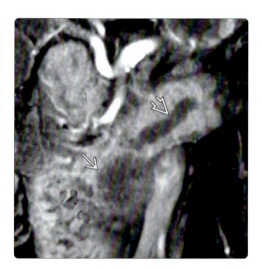

(Left) This 35-year-old man also presented with jaundice and weight loss with CT showing a hypodense mass ➡ in the head of the pancreas causing biliary obstruction and dilation of the gallbladder ➡. (Right) Curved planar reformation of the CT in the same patient shows the pancreatic "mass" ➡ causing partial obstruction of the bile duct ➡, while the pancreatic duct ➡ is only mildly dilated. Further evaluation, including biopsy, confirmed a diagnosis of autoimmune (IgG4-related) pancreatitis.

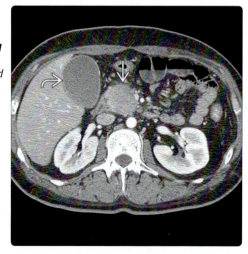
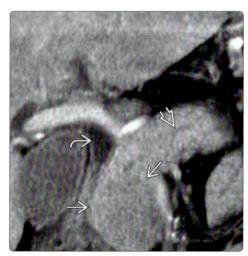

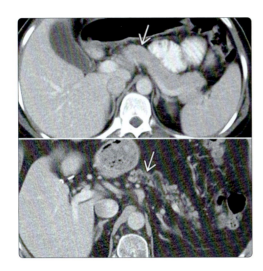

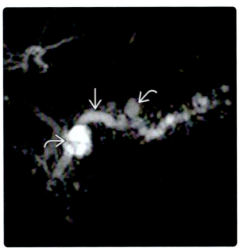

(Left) *The top CECT is from a 30-year-old woman, and the bottom image is from a 78-year-old man. With aging, the pancreas ➡ decreases in size with increased fatty lobulation. Small calcifications and mild ductal dilatation may also be seen.* (Right) *MRCP shows dilation of the main duct ➡ as well as the side branches ➡. This appearance could be due to chronic pancreatitis, but main and side branch intraductal papillary mucinous neoplasm (IPMN) was confirmed on endoscopic sonography.*

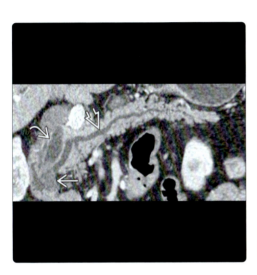

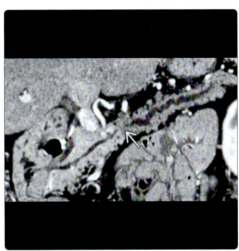

(Left) *In this 81-year-old man with painless jaundice, a curved planar reformatted CT shows mild dilation of the CBD ➡ and pancreatic duct ➡ due to a small hypodense ampullary carcinoma ➡.* (Right) *Curved planar CT reformation shows a sharp transition from a normal to dilated pancreatic duct ➡ caused by a small, subtle pancreatic cancer. Multiplanar imaging greatly enhances the ability to evaluate pancreatic masses.*

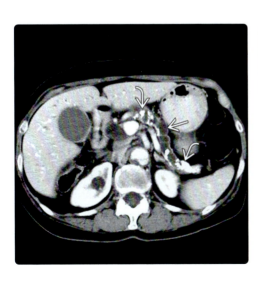

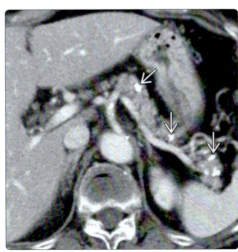

(Left) *Axial CT shows marked atrophy of the pancreatic parenchyma and dilation of the pancreatic duct ➡ with extensive calcifications ➡ within the ducts and parenchyma, typical features of chronic pancreatitis.* (Right) *In this 88-year-old woman with no clinical signs of chronic pancreatitis, CT shows multiple focal calcifications ➡ within the pancreas that are separate from vascular calcifications. There is no pancreatic ductal dilation, and these are considered normal senescent changes.*

Pancreas

(Left) *CT in the arterial phase shows a hypervascular pancreatic mass ➡ and innumerable hypervascular liver lesions ➡. All findings are typical of a malignant neuroendocrine tumor of the pancreas, a glucagonoma, in this case.* **(Right)** *In this elderly man, CT shows a bulky, hypervascular mass ➡ originating from the pancreas with direct invasion of the splenic vein ➡, typical features of a malignant neuroendocrine tumor.*

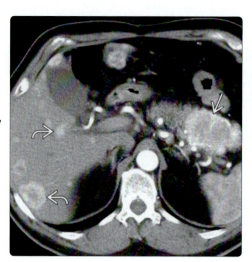
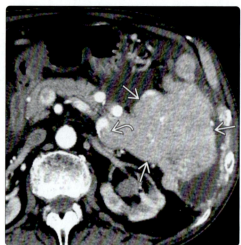

(Left) *In this 62-year-old woman who had a renal cell carcinoma (RCC) resected 10 years previously, CT shows surgical absence of the left kidney but no evidence of recurrence in the surgical bed. Hypervascular mass ➡ proved to be metastatic RCC. Pancreatic parenchyma is atrophic, and the duct ➡ is dilated upstream from the metastasis.* **(Right)** *Axial CT shows a mass ➡ in pancreatic tail that is isodense to spleen ➡, a typical appearance of an accessory spleen, which may be mistaken for a pancreatic tumor.*

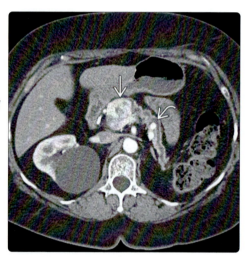
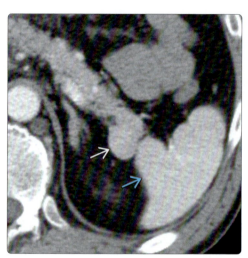

(Left) *In this 50-year-old man who had a multivisceral organ transplantation, a pseudoaneurysm ➡ of the arterial graft anastomosis simulates a hypervascular pancreatic mass.* **(Right)** *In this 52-year-old man with cirrhosis and portal vein thrombosis, CT shows a mass of varices ➡ in and around the pancreatic head that might be mistaken for a hypervascular tumor of the pancreas.*

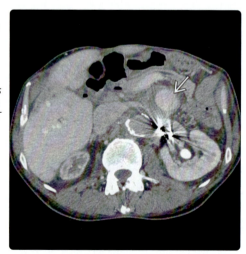
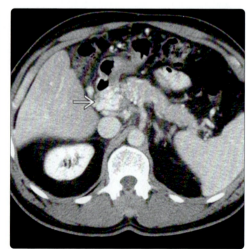

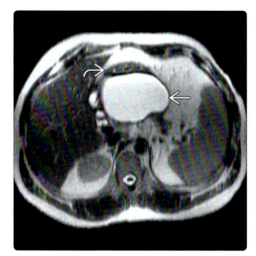

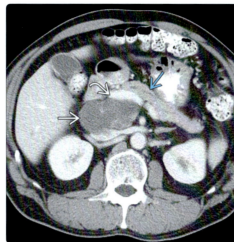

(Left) In this 45-year-old man, axial T2WI MR shows a retrogastric pseudocyst ➡ ➡ that displaces the stomach ➡. (Right) In this 62-year-old man, CT shows a multiseptate mass ➡ that abuts the pancreas ➡, duodenum, and portal vein ➡. The mass is not in the pancreas but is peripancreatic and is a benign lymphangioma.

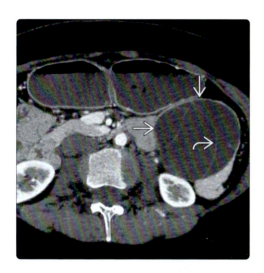

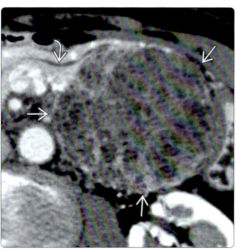

(Left) In this 33-year-old woman, CT shows an encapsulated cystic mass ➡ within the body-tail of the pancreas. Note the septa ➡ dividing it into several large, noncommunicating cystic spaces, a classic presentation for mucinous cystic neoplasm. (Right) In this 57-year-old woman, CT shows a large, encapsulated cystic pancreatic mass ➡ that displaces, but does not involve, the pancreatic duct ➡. The mass has a honeycomb or sponge appearance, characteristic of serous microcystic adenoma.

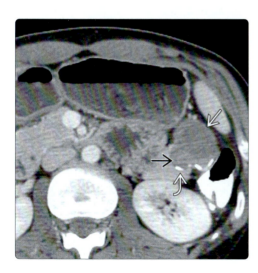

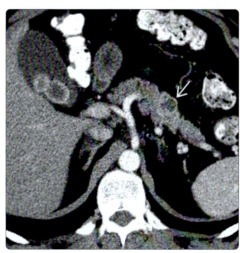

(Left) In this 21-year-old woman, CT shows a complex cystic mass ➡ in the tail of the pancreas with peripheral rim calcification ➡ and solid mural nodularity ➡, typical features of a solid and papillary neoplasm of the pancreas. (Right) Axial CECT shows a small mass ➡ in the pancreatic body with a brightly enhancing rim and central necrosis, representing a cystic pancreatic neuroendocrine tumor.

Agenesis of Dorsal Pancreas

TERMINOLOGY

- Complete or partial pancreatic agenesis, aplasia, or hypoplasia of dorsal pancreas

IMAGING

- Absence of pancreatic tissue in expected location of neck, body, and tail segments
- ERCP: Filling of ventral duct without identifiable dorsal ducts or minor papilla in agenesis of entire dorsal pancreas
- CT: Short pancreas, normal pancreatic head, with complete or partial absence of body and tail segments
- MRCP: In complete agenesis of dorsal pancreas, accessory and dorsal duct system are not observed
  - Small accessory duct of Santorini may be seen in partial agenesis

TOP DIFFERENTIAL DIAGNOSES

- Pancreatic ductal carcinoma
  - Abrupt, irregular obstruction of pancreatic duct seen on ERCP
  - Pancreatic duct dilated upstream from mass
- Pancreas divisum
  - Contrast injection into minor papilla fills dorsal duct
- Chronic pancreatitis
  - Parenchyma in body/tail often atrophic
  - Ductal and parenchymal calcifications are common

PATHOLOGY

- Associated conditions
  - Complete pancreatic agenesis (very rare); correlated with stillbirth or early neonatal death
  - Polysplenia syndrome (7 cases reported)
  - Bowel malrotation

CLINICAL ISSUES

- Usually asymptomatic, incidental finding
- May have increased incidence of pancreatitis

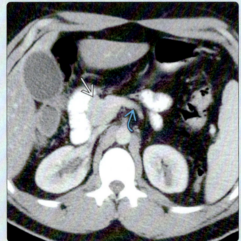
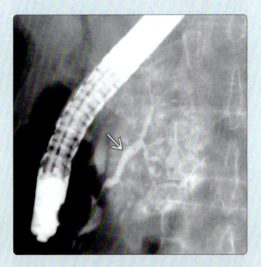

(Left) Axial CECT shows a normal-appearing pancreatic head ➡, but neither body nor tail (which normally lie ventral to the splenic vein ➡) are present. This patient has congenital absence of the dorsal pancreas and has had at least 1 episode of acute pancreatitis. (Right) ERCP shows filling of the pancreatic duct ➡ within the head and uncinate but not in the absent pancreatic body. The pancreatic acini are filled with contrast due to forceful injection, which can induce pancreatitis.

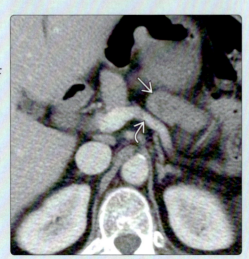
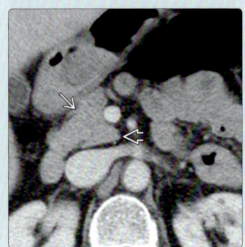

(Left) Axial CECT demonstrates absence of the body and tail of the pancreas, which normally lie anteriorly along the course of the splenic vein ➡. In the expected anatomic location normally occupied by the pancreatic body, there is only fat and a segment of small bowel ➡. (Courtesy H. Harvin, MD.) (Right) Axial CECT in the same patient demonstrates a normal head of pancreas ➡ and uncinate process ➡. (Courtesy H. Harvin, MD.)

Annular Pancreas

TERMINOLOGY

- Pancreatic tissue that almost or completely encircles descending portion of duodenum

IMAGING

- **CT or MR evidence of pancreatic tissue and annular duct encircling descending duodenum**
  - Large pancreatic head partially or completely encircling 2nd duodenum (marked by gas, enhanced mucosa, or oral contrast)
- MR with MRCP is most complete imaging test
  - Duct draining pancreatic head encircles duodenum
- Fluoroscopic barium study (UGI)
  - Concentric narrowing of 2nd part of duodenum ± dilated proximal duodenum

TOP DIFFERENTIAL DIAGNOSES

- Postbulbar peptic ulcer
  - Similar findings on UGI but not on CT or MR

- Pancreatic ductal carcinoma
  - Can mimic annular pancreas on UGI or CT
- Duodenal carcinoma
  - Attenuation of duodenal carcinoma is usually different than that of pancreas

PATHOLOGY

- Associated congenital anomalies in up to 75% of pediatric cases
  - e.g., atresia of esophagus, duodenum, or anus

CLINICAL ISSUES

- 50% of cases become clinically evident in infancy
  - Neonates: Persistent vomiting since birth
- 50% of cases are diagnosed in adults
  - Minimal symptoms of nausea, early satiety, pain
- Complications
  - Gastric and duodenal ulcers (26-48%)
  - Pancreatitis (15-30%)

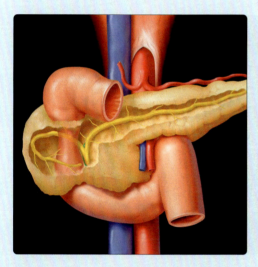

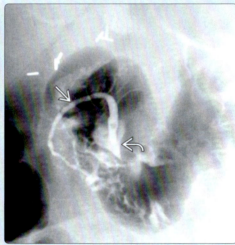

(Left) *Graphic shows concentric duodenal luminal narrowing by the encircling pancreatic tissue. The pancreatic head duct also encircles the descending duodenum. Note the dilatation of the proximal duodenum.* (Right) *ERCP shows a pancreatic head duct ➡ originating on the right anterior surface of the duodenum, encircling it and emptying into the main pancreatic duct near the ampulla ➡.*

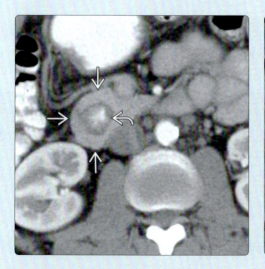

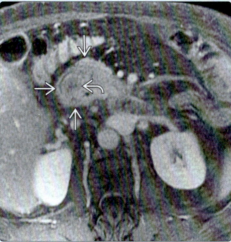

(Left) *Axial CECT shows the 2nd portion of the duodenum ➡ completely encircled by pancreatic tissue ➡. The duodenal lumen is marked by oral contrast medium.* (Right) *Gadolinium-enhanced MR demonstrates a thin rim of pancreatic tissue ➡ encircling the 2nd duodenum ➡. There is no significant narrowing of the lumen of the duodenum and this adult patient was asymptomatic. Note that the thin rim of pancreatic tissue lateral to the duodenum enhances exactly as the rest of the pancreatic head tissue.*

Pancreas Divisum

TERMINOLOGY

- Failure of ventral and dorsal pancreatic buds to fuse
  - Most common congenital anatomic variant of pancreas
- Head and uncinate process of pancreas: Drained by ventral pancreatic duct of Wirsung via major papilla
- Body and tail of pancreas: Drained by dorsal pancreatic duct of Santorini via minor papilla

IMAGING

- **Best imaging tool: MRCP before and after secretin stimulation**
  - Multiplanar CT shows same anatomy, though less clearly
  - ERCP may be useful for confirmation and treatment, though technically difficult to cannulate minor papilla
- Shows course and drainage pattern of dorsal and ventral pancreatic ducts
  - Dorsal duct: Long and narrow entering minor papilla; crosses distal common bile duct
  - Ventral duct: Short, entering major papilla

- No communication between dorsal and ventral ducts in 85% of cases
- Secretin-induced ductal dilatation occurs in 72% of symptomatic patients due to stenotic minor or accessory papilla
- 2 distinct pancreatic moieties separated by fat cleft (not commonly seen)
  - Unfused ductal system on thin collimation scans
  - Pancreatic head may be large with abnormal contour

CLINICAL ISSUES

- Young patient with history of recurrent idiopathic pancreatitis episodes

DIAGNOSTIC CHECKLIST

- Rule out other causes of pancreatic duct obstruction on ERCP, such as pancreatic ductal carcinoma

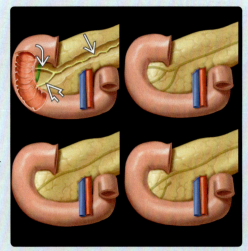
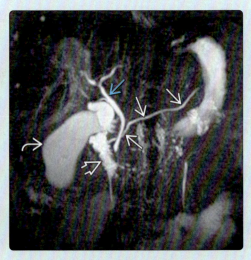

(Left) Graphic shows several common variations in the arrangement of the main pancreatic duct ➡, accessory duct of Santorini ➡, and duct of Wirsung ➡. The upper left image is normal, while the lower right image shows complete pancreas divisum. (Right) Coronal MRCP shows pancreas divisum with the dorsal pancreatic duct ➡ crossing the common bile duct ➡ to drain into the expected location of the minor papilla. The diminutive ventral duct is not seen. Note the distended gallbladder ➡ and fluid within the duodenum ➡.

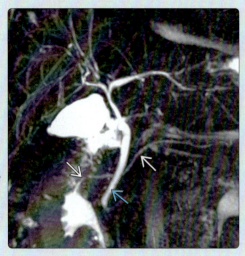
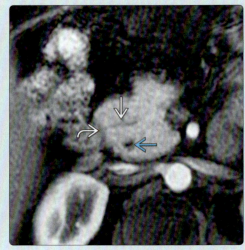

(Left) MRCP shows the main pancreatic duct ➡ entering the minor papilla, and the common bile duct ➡ entering the duodenum at the major papilla. The relationship between the pancreatic and common duct is referred to as the crossing duct sign. (Right) Axial gadolinium-enhanced T1WI MR scan in the same patient demonstrates the main pancreatic duct ➡ entering the duodenum via the minor papilla ➡. The common bile duct ➡ is seen posteriorly as its enters the duodenum via the major papilla.

Ectopic Pancreatic Tissue

TERMINOLOGY

- Ectopic pancreatic tissue (EPT)
- Pancreatic tissue located outside normal confines of pancreas and lacking any anatomic or vascular connection with it
  - Locations: Stomach > duodenum > Meckel diverticulum > ileum

IMAGING

- Upper GI series may show narrowed pyloric channel ± polypoid or sessile mass
- Diagnostic: Small intramural gastric mass with central umbilication (45%)
  - Central umbilication: Orifice of rudimentary duct within ectopic pancreas through which EPT opens and drains into gastric lumen
  - Stomach: Typically 1-2 cm in diameter, along greater curvature or posterior aspect of antrum, within 6 cm of pylorus

- CT: EPT is usually too small to be detected
  - Rarely, intramural solid or cystic lesion in stomach or duodenum

TOP DIFFERENTIAL DIAGNOSES

- Gastric ulcer (on upper GI series)
  - Round ulcer, smooth mound of edema, radiating folds to ulcer edge, Hampton line, ulcer collar
- Gastric carcinoma
  - Polypoid or circumferential mass ± ulceration, focal wall thickening with mucosal irregularity, focal infiltration of wall
- Gastric metastases and lymphoma
  - Bull's-eye sign: Ulceration in center of lesion
  - Multiple lesions are likely malignant, not ectopic pancreas
- Gastric GI stromal tumor
  - Large, lobulated, submucosal mass with ulceration; requires biopsy and histologic diagnosis

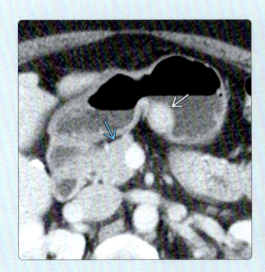
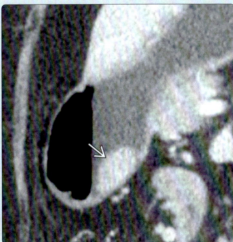

(Left) Axial CECT demonstrates a mural mass ➡ in the body of the stomach. Note that the mass is of soft tissue attenuation and enhances similarly to the normal pancreas ➡. (Right) Sagittal CECT reformation in the same patient shows the mural mass ➡ to have a broad base of attachment to the gastric wall and obtuse angles with the gastric lumen, suggesting a submucosal location for the mass. Endoscopic biopsy revealed ectopic pancreatic tissue.

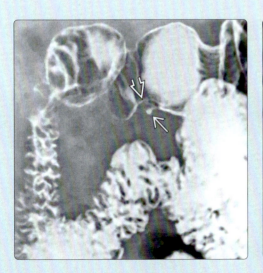
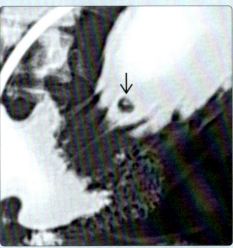

(Left) Upper GI series spot film shows a small antral mass ➡ with intact mucosa. A central "dot" of barium ➡ can be seen filling a rudimentary duct. (Right) Upper GI series spot film shows a small mass ➡ with central umbilication. This is an unusual location for an ectopic pancreas. A bull's-eye lesion of this type and location would raise concern for a metastatic lesion, Kaposi sarcoma, or lymphoma.

IMAGING

- **Interstitial edematous pancreatitis (IEP)** (70-80% of cases): Normal enhancement of pancreas without necrosis
  - Pancreas typically enlarged and edematous
  - Peripancreatic fat stranding, edema, and free fluid
  - Mild edematous pancreatitis can appear normal on CT
- **Necrotizing pancreatitis (NP)** (20-30% of cases): Areas of nonenhancing parenchymal necrosis
  - May necrose pancreatic duct as well
  - Necrosis usually develops within 3-4 days after symptom onset
- Complications
  - **Infected pancreatic necrosis**: Ectopic gas, in absence of intervention, is highly suggestive of infected necrosis
  - **Central necrosis**: Necrosis of central portion of gland/duct with intact pancreas/duct in head and tail
  - **Pseudoaneurysm**: Most common locations are splenic (50%) and gastroduodenal (20%) arteries

- **Venous thrombosis**: Splenic vein most common, but portal vein or superior mesenteric vein can be involved
- **Fluid collections**: Nomenclature depends on age of collection and edematous vs. NP
  - **Acute peripancreatic fluid collection**: Fluid collection within first 4 weeks after acute IEP
  - **Pseudocyst**: Fluid collection persisting > 4 weeks
  - **Acute necrotic collection**: Nonloculated but containing internal necrotic debris and blood
  - **Walled-off necrosis**: Loculated, complex fluid collection persisting > 4 weeks after NP

DIAGNOSTIC CHECKLIST

- Multiphasic/multiplanar CT is best for initial evaluation
- MR with MRCP is better for evaluation of pancreatic duct and complex fluid collections

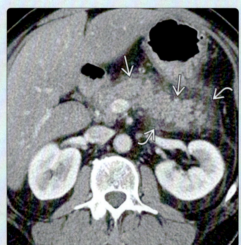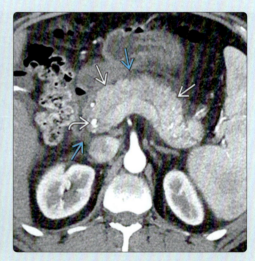

(Left) Axial CECT in a patient with abdominal pain shows enlargement and edema of the pancreas ➡ with surrounding fluid and stranding ⤴, compatible with acute edematous pancreatitis. The gland enhances normally without evidence of necrosis. (Right) Axial CT in a patient following ERCP placement of a biliary stent ➡ shows enlargement of the pancreas ➡, edema, and peripancreatic fat stranding ➡ and fluid, compatible with acute interstitial edematous pancreatitis (IEP).

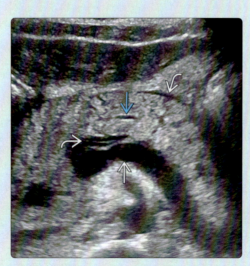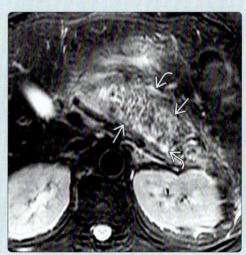

(Left) Transverse US demonstrates mild diffuse enlargement of the pancreas. The pancreatic duct ➡ is normal in size. The main sign of acute pancreatitis is fluid ➡ anterior to the pancreas and anterior to the splenic vein ➡. (Right) Axial T2 MR shows marked heterogeneity of the pancreas ➡ with parenchymal edema and peripancreatic fluid ➡ consistent with IEP. Fat-suppressed T2WI is the best pulse sequence for highlighting changes of acute pancreatitis on MR.

IMAGING

CT Findings

- 2 primary subtypes of acute pancreatitis
  - **Interstitial edematous pancreatitis (IEP)** (70-80%)
    - Pancreas typically enlarged and edematous
    - Peripancreatic fat stranding, edema, and free fluid
    - Usually involves entire gland but can be focal
    - Normal enhancement of pancreas without necrosis
    - Normal CT does not exclude pancreatitis
  - **Necrotizing pancreatitis (NP)** (20-30% of cases): Areas of parenchymal necrosis that are either nonenhancing or severely hypoenhancing (usually < 30 HU)
    - Usually more peripancreatic inflammation than IEP
    - Necrosis may not be present initially but can develop within 3-4 days after symptom onset
      □ Early CT can underestimate or miss necrosis
- Necrosis both parenchymal and peripancreatic in 75%, peripancreatic alone in 20%, parenchymal alone in 5%
- Complications
  - **Infected pancreatic necrosis**
    - Implies superinfection of necrotic parenchyma
    - Ectopic gas in pancreatic bed, in absence of intervention or fistula, is virtually diagnostic
  - **Central necrosis (disconnected duct syndrome)**
    - Necrosis of parenchyma and duct in body with intact pancreas/duct in head and tail
    - Results in encapsulated fluid/debris collection with continual leakage of pancreatic fluid into collection
  - **Extrapancreatic fat necrosis**
    - Pancreatic enzymes cause fat necrosis
    - Usually low density with heterogeneous fluid and solid components but can appear nodular and mass-like, mimicking carcinomatosis
  - **Pseudoaneurysm**
    - Small contrast-filled outpouching arising next to artery ± adjacent hematoma (due to leak or rupture)
    - Mostly splenic (50%) and gastroduodenal (20%) arteries
  - **Venous thrombosis**
    - May occur due to direct intimal injury or mass effect from adjacent collections
    - Splenic vein > portal vein or superior mesenteric vein (SMV)
  - **Fluid collections**
    - **Acute peripancreatic fluid collection**: Fluid collection first 4 weeks after acute IEP
      □ Simple, nonloculated with no internal debris
    - **Pseudocyst**: Fluid collection persisting > 4 weeks
      □ Loculated with well-defined, enhancing wall usually in lesser sac or pararenal spaces
      □ Simple fluid attenuation with no internal debris
    - **Acute necrotic collection**: Fluid collection within first 4 weeks after acute NP
      □ Nonloculated but contains internal necrotic debris and blood
    - **Walled-off necrosis (WON)**: Loculated fluid collection persisting > 4 weeks after NP
      □ Heterogeneous collection with well-defined wall and internal necrotic debris/blood products

MR Findings

- Pancreas appears enlarged with increased signal on T2WI and abnormally low signal on T1WI due to edema
- T1WI C+ images similar to CECT in detection of necrosis and nonenhancement
- T2WI offers advantage (over CT) of allowing differentiation of simple fluid collections from those with internal solid debris (i.e., WON)
- MRCP can evaluate integrity of pancreatic duct, unlike CT
  - May delineate communication between collection and pancreatic duct
  - Very sensitive for gallstones and other biliary pathology

Ultrasonographic Findings

- Enlarged, hypoechoic pancreas with adjacent free fluid
- Ultrasound often performed to look for gallstones

Imaging Recommendations

- Best imaging tool
  - **Multiphasic/multiplanar CT is best initial study**
  - **MR with MRCP helpful problem-solving tool to assess pancreatic duct or composition of fluid collections**

DIFFERENTIAL DIAGNOSIS

Infiltrating Pancreatic Carcinoma

- Heterogeneous, hypoenhancing mass with abrupt obstruction of upstream pancreatic duct and upstream pancreatic atrophy
- Pancreatic cancer may present with pancreatitis in ~ 5% of cases
- Focal pancreatitis can appear mass-like and mimic malignancy

Shock Pancreas

- Shock, hypotensive complex can include peripancreatic edema (similar to pancreatitis)
- Usually history of hypotension and other imaging stigmata of shock, such as shock bowel

Lymphoma

- Lymphoma can rarely diffusely infiltrate and enlarge pancreas, superficially mimicking pancreatitis
- Usually associated with regional lymphadenopathy, and pancreatic involvement appears mass-like
- No evidence of ductal or vascular obstruction

DIAGNOSTIC CHECKLIST

Consider

- Pancreatic duct obstruction should suggest presence of underlying mass

SELECTED REFERENCES

1. Baker ME et al: ACR appropriateness criteria acute pancreatitis. Ultrasound Q. 30(4):267-73, 2014

(Left) *Initial axial CT of a patient with abdominal pain demonstrates early necrotizing pancreatitis with pancreatic edema and significant peripancreatic free fluid* ➡ *but also with relative hypoenhancement of the pancreatic neck/body* ➡. (Right) *Axial CECT acquired 3 days later due to clinical deterioration demonstrates worsening necrosis* ➡ *with only a small portion of the pancreatic body* ➡ *still enhancing. Early CT (< 72 hours) can miss or underestimate pancreatic necrosis.*

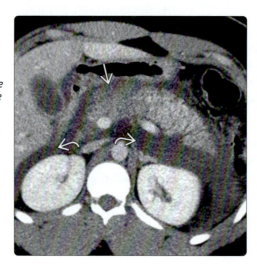
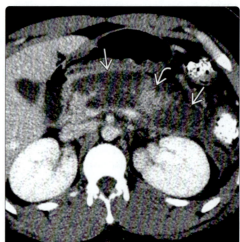

(Left) *Axial T2 FS MR in the same patient demonstrates diffuse abnormal T2 signal due to necrotizing pancreatitis. The neck and tail* ➡ *are more heterogeneous-appearing on MR than on CT, better demonstrating the complexity of the acute necrotic collections. The viable body* ➡ *is slightly less heterogeneous.* (Right) *Axial T1 C+ MR in the same patient better demonstrates severe necrotizing pancreatitis* ➡ *with only a small portion of the body* ➡ *still enhancing and viable.*

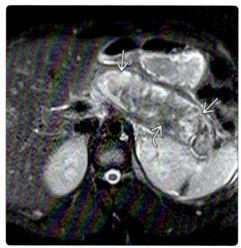
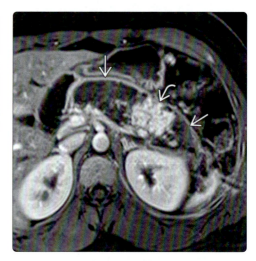

(Left) *Coronal MRCP in a patient with extensive necrosis shows that the pancreatic duct* ➡ *is still intact. Evaluation of the pancreatic duct is a significant advantage of MR over CT. Gallstones* ➡ *are seen within the gallbladder, and passage of ductal stones caused the pancreatitis.* (Right) *Axial CECT demonstrates the characteristic findings of infected pancreatic necrosis with nonenhancement of the entire pancreas* ➡ *and multiple foci of ectopic gas* ➡ *in the pancreatic bed.*

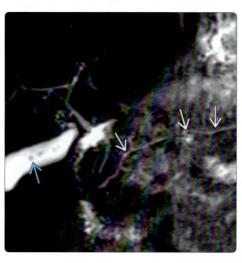
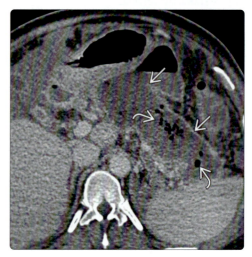

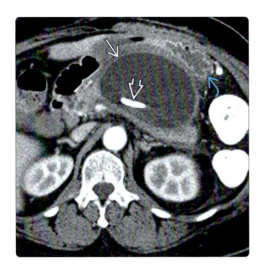

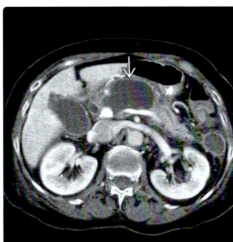

(Left) Axial CT shows a loculated fluid collection ➡ in the lesser sac with a well-defined wall and simple internal contents after a bout of pancreatitis, in keeping with a pseudocyst. An endoscopic cyst-gastrostomy ➡ has been performed to relieve the mass effect on the stomach ➡. (Right) Axial CECT shows WON ➡ in the body of the pancreas with absence of normally enhancing pancreatic parenchyma in this location. The central necrosis in this patient raises concern for disconnected duct syndrome.

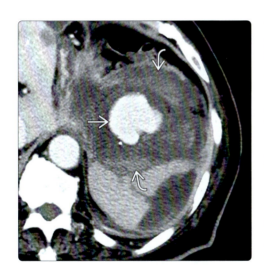

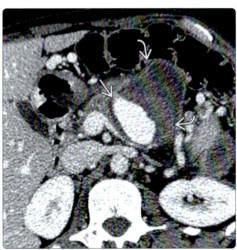

(Left) Axial CECT shows a high-attenuation (same as the aorta), rounded structure ➡ in the expected location of the splenic artery with surrounding acute hemorrhage ➡. This patient suffered a life-threatening hemorrhage from the ruptured splenic artery pseudoaneurysm resulting from pancreatitis. (Right) Axial CECT demonstrates a large pseudoaneurysm ➡ with hemorrhage ➡ into an acute necrotic collection in a patient with pancreatitis. Pancreatic enzymes can digest arterial walls, leading to rupture.

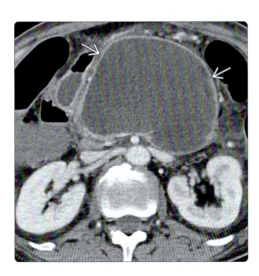

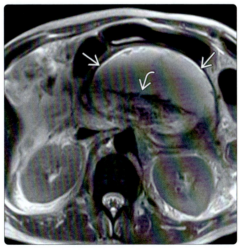

(Left) Axial CECT several months after a bout of pancreatitis demonstrates a large, relatively simple-appearing loculated fluid collection ➡ with a well-defined wall filling the pancreatic bed. (Right) Axial T2 MR in the same patient shows that the collection ➡ is not simple but contains internal solid debris ➡, suggesting this is WON rather than a pseudocyst. WON often requires a large bore catheter for drainage or necrosectomy. MR is much better than CT to characterize internal contents.

TERMINOLOGY

- Irreversible fibroinflammatory damage to pancreas, usually evident on imaging or functional testing

IMAGING

- **Imaging protocols: Multiplanar multiphasic CT or MR (fat-suppressed images), MRCP**
  - MR with secretin stimulation is most comprehensive (anatomic & functional) imaging study
  - ERCP mostly for intervention (stone extraction, stent, etc.)
- Atrophy of gland, dilated main pancreatic duct (MPD), intraductal & parenchymal calculi
  - Fibroinflammatory mass: Common in pancreatic head
- May have double duct sign (stricture of distal CBD and pancreatic duct, resulting in dilation of ducts upstream)
  - Not pathognomonic of pancreatic carcinoma
  - Long, smooth taper of CBD (not abrupt, as with carcinoma)

- **Secretin-stimulated MRCP is most complete imaging test (anatomical & functional)**
  - MPD is irregularly dilated; fails to respond normally to secretin stimulation
  - Less than expected secretion of fluid into duodenum
    - Due to decreased exocrine function
- Splenic vein thrombosis, splenomegaly, gastric varices
  - May progress to thrombosis of portal vein
- Pseudoaneurysm of gastroduodenal or other arteries
  - Detected by US, CTA, or MRA
  - Coil embolization of pseudoaneurysms is therapy of choice

TOP DIFFERENTIAL DIAGNOSES

- Pancreatic ductal carcinoma
- Pancreatic IPMN (main duct)
- Senescent change (in elderly patients)
  - Parenchyma atrophies to some degree and duct dilates
  - May also have small foci of calcification

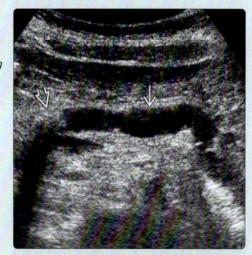 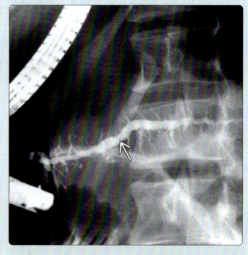

(Left) Transverse grayscale ultrasound of the pancreas demonstrates a dilated main pancreatic duct (MPD) ⇨ upstream from an obstructing intraductal stone ⇨. (Right) ERCP shows irregular dilatation of the main pancreatic duct ⇨ and side branches characteristic of chronic pancreatitis.

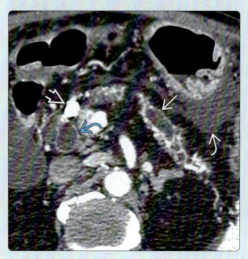 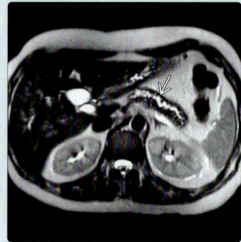

(Left) Axial CECT shows marked parenchymal atrophy and dilation of the main pancreatic duct ⇨. Note the large intraductal stone ⇨ in the neck of the pancreas as well as a dilated common bile duct ⇨. There is fluid in the lesser sac ⇨ from acute pancreatitis. This is an example of acute and chronic pancreatitis. (Right) Axial T2WI MR shows an irregularly dilated main pancreatic duct ⇨ and glandular atrophy in the body-tail segments of the pancreas.

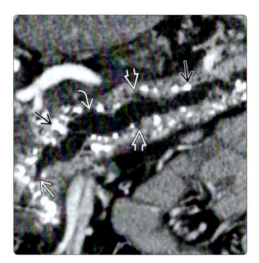

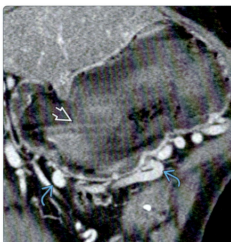

(Left) Coronal curved planar reformation from a CECT shows dilatation of the pancreatic duct ⇨ upstream from a stricture ⇨. Note the dilated side branches of the pancreatic duct ⇨ and extensive parenchymal calcifications ⇨, diagnostic of chronic pancreatitis. (Right) In this patient with chronic pancreatitis, coronal CT shows varices ⇨ along the greater curvature and high-density blood ⇨ within the stomach. The patient had hematemesis from the gastric varices that resulted from splenic vein occlusion.

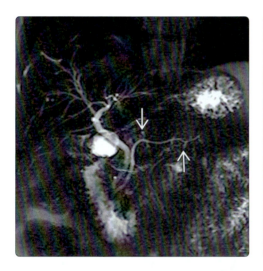

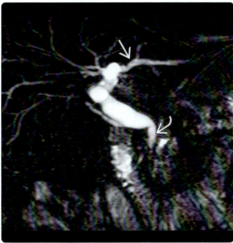

(Left) Coronal MRCP reconstruction in a patient with chronic abdominal pain demonstrates subtle dilatation of a few scattered pancreatic duct side branches ⇨, an early sign of chronic pancreatitis, subsequently confirmed using endoscopic ultrasound. (Right) Coronal MRCP in a patient with chronic pancreatitis demonstrates smooth tapering of the distal common bile duct ⇨ as it traverses the pancreatic head. There is minimal dilatation of the intrahepatic bile ducts ⇨.

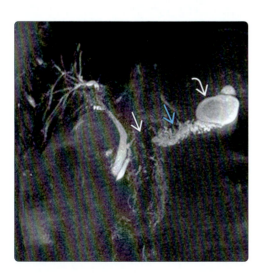

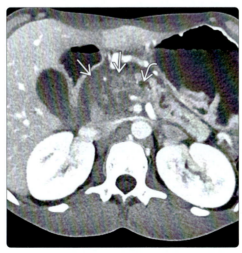

(Left) Coronal MRCP shows changes of "big duct" chronic pancreatitis, including a dilated main duct ⇨ and side branches, a stricture ⇨ in the downstream duct, and a pseudocyst ⇨. (Right) Axial CECT demonstrates an infiltrative hypodense pancreatic mass ⇨ with a dilated upstream pancreatic duct ⇨. A few calcifications were present in the parenchyma (not shown). The patient underwent Whipple procedure due to concern for malignancy, where this mass was found to be due to chronic pancreatitis.

Groove Pancreatitis

TERMINOLOGY

- Synonym: Cystic dystrophy of duodenal wall
- Chronic segmental pancreatitis in groove between duodenum and pancreatic head
  - Distal common bile duct (CBD) traverses posterior aspect of groove

IMAGING

- **MR is best; multiplanar CT is good alternative**
  - Thickened duodenal wall with narrowed lumen ± cysts in wall (better shown on MR)
  - Sheet-like mass between pancreatic head and C loop of duodenum
  - Groove is hypointense (T1WI MR) or hypodense (CT) relative to pancreas
  - Delayed enhancement of affected tissue (typical feature of fibrotic tissue)
  - Long, smooth narrowing of intrapancreatic CBD and distal pancreatic duct

PATHOLOGY

- Fibroinflammatory mass in groove with stenosis of terminal CBD and pancreatic duct
- Inflamed duodenal wall (± cysts) with stenosis of lumen
- **Etiology unknown; theories**
  - Alcohol consumption leads to ↑ viscosity of pancreatic juice → Brunner gland hyperplasia → occlusion of minor papilla
  - Chronic inflammation of duodenal wall (e.g., from peptic ulcer) → fibroinflammatory scarring
  - Ectopic pancreatic tissue in duodenal wall

CLINICAL ISSUES

- More common in middle-aged men with history of alcohol consumption
- Postprandial abdominal pain, vomiting
- Weight loss; jaundice (usually mild and intermittent)
- **Clinical and imaging features may be identical to pancreatic carcinoma** (may require resection)

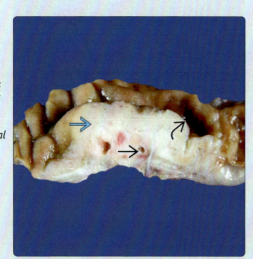
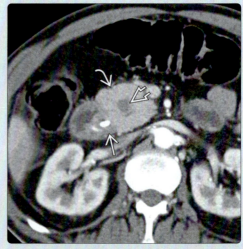

(Left) Gross photograph of a pancreaticoduodenectomy specimen shows a mass-like lesion beneath the duodenal mucosa ➡. Note the paraduodenal zone of fibrosis ➡ with numerous small cysts ➡. (Right) Axial CECT shows subtle soft tissue thickening ➡ in the pancreaticoduodenal groove, as well as mass-like pancreatic head ➡ enlargement with an internal cyst ➡. This was found to be segmental (given pancreatic head involvement) groove pancreatitis at surgery.

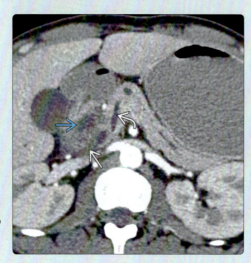
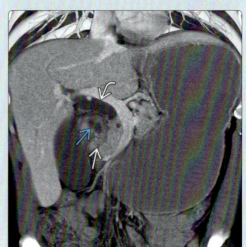

(Left) Axial CECT demonstrates a hypodense soft tissue mass ➡ in the pancreaticoduodenal groove with associated cystic spaces ➡, resulting in upstream pancreatic ductal dilation ➡. (Right) In the same case, coronal CECT demonstrates the hypodense soft tissue mass ➡ in the pancreaticoduodenal groove with associated cystic spaces ➡. Note the dilated common bile duct ➡. Initially suspected to represent malignancy, this was found to be groove pancreatitis at surgery.

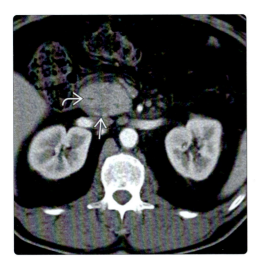

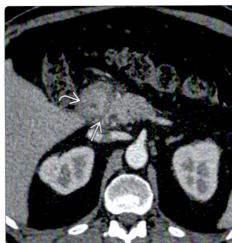

(Left) *Axial CECT demonstrates subtle stranding and induration* ➡ *in the pancreaticoduodenal groove, which persisted on follow-up examinations. The lumen of the duodenum* ➡ *was constricted.* (Right) *Axial CECT from the same patient again demonstrates induration* ➡ *in the pancreaticoduodenal groove, and duodenal wall thickening* ➡. *Initially suspected to represent a duodenal malignancy, this was found to be groove pancreatitis at surgery.*

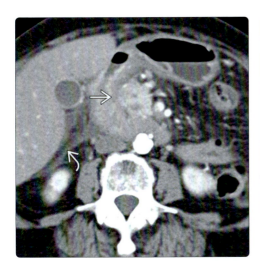

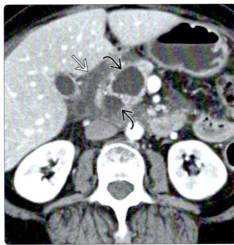

(Left) *Axial CECT shows focal soft tissue thickening* ➡ *in the pancreaticoduodenal groove, which persisted over multiple follow-up studies. There is also some fluid* ➡ *tracking from the groove into the right anterior pararenal space.* (Right) *Axial CECT in the same patient shows thickening* ➡ *in the groove, with several cysts* ➡ *present in the pancreatic head. This was found to be groove pancreatitis at surgery, but the presence of fluid tracking in the retroperitoneum is atypical and more common with acute edematous pancreatitis.*

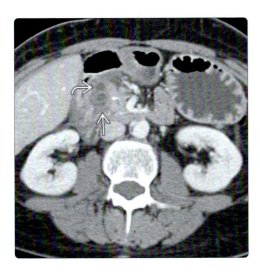

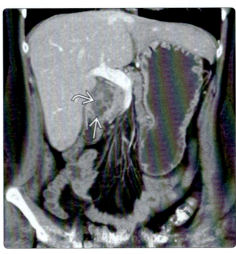

(Left) *Axial CECT demonstrates focal soft tissue thickening* ➡ *in the pancreaticoduodenal groove with multiple internal cystic spaces* ➡. (Right) *Coronal volume-rendered CECT from the same patient again demonstrates focal soft tissue thickening* ➡ *in the pancreaticoduodenal groove with multiple internal cystic spaces* ➡. *While this was suspected to represent groove pancreatitis, a Whipple procedure was performed to exclude underlying malignancy, a common outcome in these cases.*

TERMINOLOGY

- Immune-mediated fibroinflammatory disease primarily involving pancreas responding to steroid therapy

IMAGING

- **Contrast-enhanced, multiphasic MR with MRCP (or CT)**
- Diffuse form
  - Sausage-like enlargement of pancreas (with smooth contour) and loss of normal pancreatic lobulations
  - Hypoattenuating halo or capsule around pancreas
  - Absence of retroperitoneal fluid, fluid collections/pseudocysts, or inflammation
  - Less enhancement than expected in arterial phase; parenchyma/capsule may show delayed enhancement
  - MRCP: Multiple discontiguous MPD/bile duct strictures that resolve after secretin (duct penetrating sign)
- Focal form
  - Focal mass or localized enlargement of pancreas (usually head/uncinate) with delayed enhancement

- Lack of biliary or pancreatic ductal dilatation

TOP DIFFERENTIAL DIAGNOSES

- Pancreatic ductal adenocarcinoma
- Chronic pancreatitis
- Acute edematous pancreatitis

PATHOLOGY

- 2 distinct histologic subtypes
  - Type I: Lymphoplasmacytic sclerosing pancreatitis
    - Positive IgG4 tissue staining; serum IgG4 elevated
    - Extrapancreatic organ involvement common (~ 60%); inflammatory bowel disease in only 2-6%
    - Older patients (usually > age 60) with M > F
  - Type II: Idiopathic duct-centric pancreatitis
    - No IgG4 tissue staining; serum IgG4 not elevated
    - No extrapancreatic organ involvement; inflammatory bowel disease in 30%
    - Younger patients (mean age: 43) with M = F

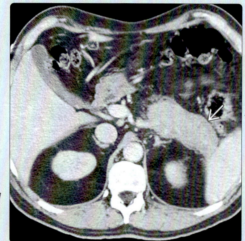
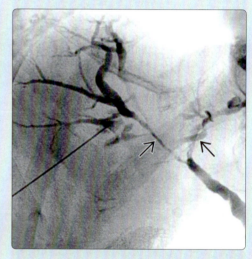

(Left) Axial CECT shows diffuse infiltration and enlargement of the pancreas with loss of normal fatty lobulation. There is a hypodense halo or capsule ➡️ around the pancreas, with relatively little spread into adjacent tissues, compatible with autoimmune pancreatitis (AIP). All symptoms and signs resolved with steroid therapy. (Right) Transhepatic cholangiogram in a patient with autoimmune pancreatitis shows multifocal strictures ➡️ indistinguishable from those of primary sclerosing cholangitis.

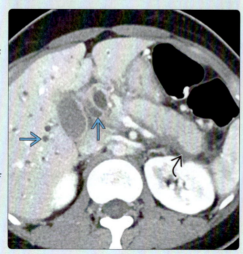
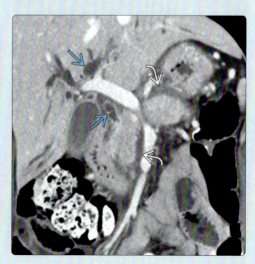

(Left) Axial CECT demonstrates a diffusely enlarged pancreas with a low-attenuation halo ➡️ around its margin. Intra- and extrahepatic bile ducts ➡️ are dilated. (Right) Coronal CECT from the same patient shows similar findings with a low-attenuation capsule ➡️ around the enlarged pancreatic margin. Note the presence of biliary dilation ➡️ in this patient with a history of biliary strictures, often associated with autoimmune pancreatitis.

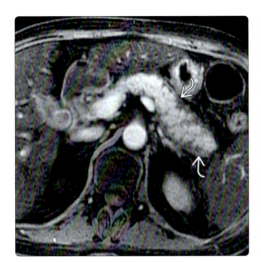
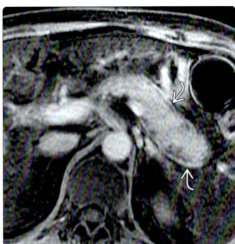

(Left) *Axial T1 C+ MR in the arterial phase demonstrates diffuse pancreatic enlargement with a subtle low-signal rim or capsule ➡ around the margin of the pancreas.* (Right) *Axial T1 C+ MR in a more delayed phase demonstrates that the capsule ➡ now shows avid delayed enhancement, a characteristic feature of autoimmune pancreatitis. The fatty lobulation of the pancreas is also lost on these images.*

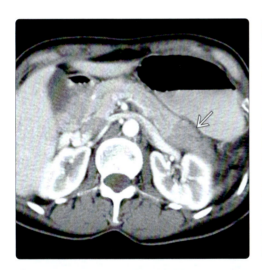
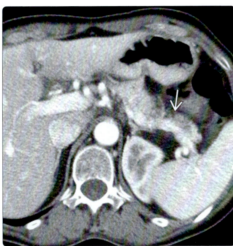

(Left) *Initial axial CECT shows a focal hypodense mass ➡ in the tail of the pancreas. Serologic testing (IgG4) suggested the diagnosis of autoimmune pancreatitis, and steroid therapy was started.* (Right) *Repeat axial CECT in the same patient 10 months later shows substantial decrease in the size of the inflammatory mass ➡ and slight atrophy of the affected pancreatic tail segment.*

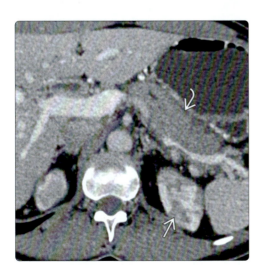
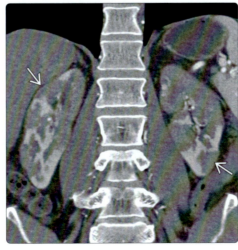

(Left) *Axial CECT demonstrates mild enlargement of the pancreas with a subtle low-density capsule ➡ in a patient with an elevated IgG4, compatible with autoimmune pancreatitis. Note the low-density wedge-shaped lesions ➡ in the left kidney.* (Right) *Coronal CECT in the same patient better demonstrates the full extent of the wedge-shaped low density lesions ➡ in both kidneys. Renal lesions, likely a manifestation of autoimmune disease, are a frequent associated finding in patients with AIP.*

IMAGING

- Surgical approach determined by location of pathology
  - Whipple resection for lesions in head, neck, and uncinate process
  - Distal pancreatectomy for lesions in body or tail
  - Central resection for lesions of pancreatic neck
  - Laparoscopic enucleated for small lesions, such as neuroendocrine tumors lying superficial to main pancreatic duct
- **Multiplanar CECT or MR for preoperative planning**
  - **CT for postoperative complications** (e.g., leak, hemorrhage, infection, pseudoaneurysm)
  - Small, unencapsulated fluid collections in pancreatic bed in perioperative period are expected finding
- Interval enlargement of soft tissue in pancreatic bed is best indication of local tumor recurrence
- Abscesses are rim-enhancing fluid collections with mass effect; may or may not have gas bubbles

- Fat necrosis in omentum or mesentery may have enhancing rim and mass effect, mimicking abscess
- Fat attenuation noted centrally

CLINICAL ISSUES

- Immediate postoperative complications
  - Abscess (rim-enhancing fluid collection); biliary leak
  - Hemorrhage (high-density fluid collection)
- 1-6 months following Whipple resection
  - Stricture of either biliary or pancreatic anastomosis (ductal dilation on imaging)
  - Pancreatic leak; pseudocyst; pancreatic fistula (e.g., to pleural space)
- Late complications
  - Tumor recurrence in pancreatic bed; liver, peritoneal, or distant metastases
  - Anastomotic strictures (pancreatic ductal dilation; pancreatic insufficiency)

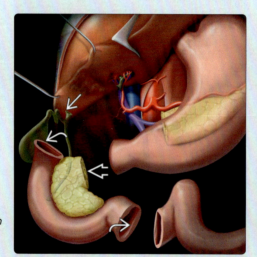 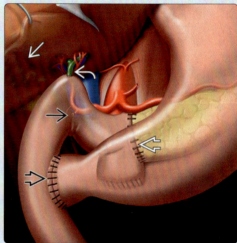

(Left) Illustration shows the pylorus-sparing Whipple (pancreaticoduodenectomy) procedure. Note the common bile duct margin ⇒, pancreatic margin ⇒, and intestinal margins ⇒. (Right) Graphic depicts pylorus-sparing Whipple anatomy: Pancreaticojejunostomy ⇒, choledochojejunostomy ⇒, gastrojejunostomy or duodenojejunostomy ⇒, and cholecystectomy ⇒. The pylorus may be removed or preserved, depending on extent of disease and surgeon preference. Note the ligated gastroduodenal artery ⇒.

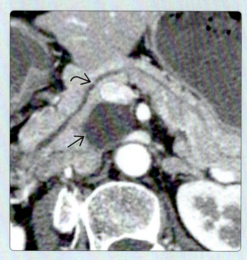 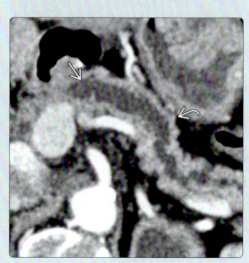

(Left) Curved planar reformation of the normal pancreatic duct ⇒ shows a cystic mass ⇒ in an uncinate process that at surgery was a benign side branch IPMN. (Right) Six months after a Whipple resection, the same patient returned with rising glucose levels. Curved planar reformation of the pancreatic duct shows marked ductal dilation ⇒ from a stricture at the pancreatic ductal anastomosis. Note the pancreatic parenchymal atrophy ⇒ accounting for the patient's abnormal glucose levels.

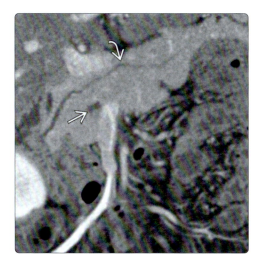

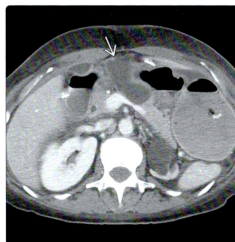

(Left) *Curved planar reformation from a CECT shows a small cystic lesion in the neck of the pancreas ➡ and a normal caliber pancreatic duct ➡.* (Right) *The same patient underwent a central pancreatectomy to remove the cystic lesion, which proved to be a benign side branch IPMN. Axial image from a postoperative CECT shows a loculated pancreatic duct leak with an enhancing rim ➡ at the site of the central pancreatic resection.*

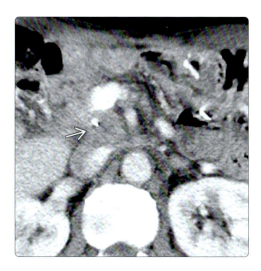

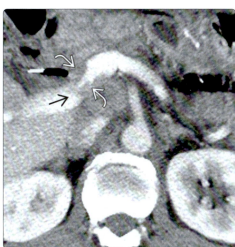

(Left) *Axial CECT shows recurrent malignant lymphadenopathy ➡ in the portocaval space 8 months after Whipple resection for carcinoma of the pancreatic head.* (Right) *At a more cranial level in the same patient, note the periportal malignant nodes ➡ both anterior and posterior to the splenoportal confluence, causing marked narrowing ➡ of the portal vein.*

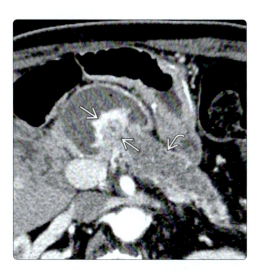

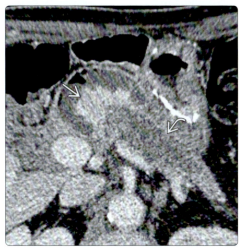

(Left) *Axial arterial phase of a CECT 11 months after Whipple resection for a neuroendocrine tumor (NET) shows a hypervascular mass ➡ obstructing the anastomotic site of the pancreatic duct, consistent with a recurrent NET. The pancreas is atrophic, and the duct ➡ is dilated.* (Right) *Axial venous-phase CECT in the same patient shows enhancing tissue ➡ within the markedly dilated pancreatic duct ➡. EUS-guided biopsy confirmed the anastomotic recurrence as well as intraductal growth of the NET.*

Pancreatic Transplantation

IMAGING

- Normal imaging appearance
  - **CT**: Homogeneous soft tissue mass in right abdomen with adjacent suture line at duodenal stump
  - **MR**: Normal pancreatic parenchyma is isointense to renal cortex on T1WI and isointense to muscle on T2WI
  - **US**: Normal pancreas allograft is homogeneous and hypoechoic to adjacent mesenteric fat
- Imaging of major complications
  - **Allograft pancreatitis**: Edema, enlargement, and heterogeneous pancreas with peripancreatic fluid
  - **Acute rejection**: Enlargement and edema of graft with increased T2WI signal on MR
  - **Chronic rejection**: Small and atrophic graft with decreased T1WI and T2WI signal on MR
  - **Vascular complications**: Venous thrombosis is more common than arterial
    - Arterial thrombosis on US: No Doppler flow within artery or graft parenchyma

- Venous thrombosis on US: Echogenic intraluminal thrombus, absent vascular flow, and high-resistance arterial waveforms with reversed diastolic flow
  - Graft infarction on US: Enlarged avascular transplant
  - **Intraabdominal fluid collections**: May represent abscess, seroma, lymphocele, urinoma, or pseudocyst

PATHOLOGY

- Goal of pancreas transplantation is treatment of diabetes by restoring endogenous insulin secretion

CLINICAL ISSUES

- Graft survival is better with combined pancreas-kidney transplant than with pancreas alone
- Graft pancreatitis is common after transplantation
  - 35% experience mild, self-limited pancreatitis; usually related to reperfusion injury after surgery
- Chronic rejection is leading cause of late allograft loss
- Vascular thrombosis is 2nd leading cause of graft dysfunction (usually in acute postoperative setting)

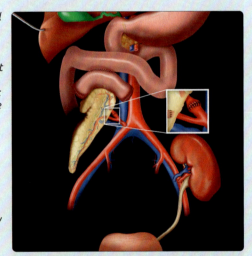
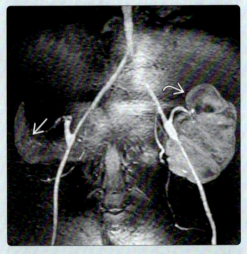

(Left) Graphic shows the usual surgical anatomy of a combined pancreas-kidney transplant with pancreatic-enteric drainage. The recipient iliac artery is anastomosed to the donor superior mesenteric and splenic arteries to perfuse the pancreatic allograft (inset). The venous drainage can be to the iliac vein (as drawn) or the superior mesenteric vein. (Right) Coronal MRA of a kidney-pancreas transplantation reveals that the renal ➘ and pancreatic allografts ➡ show normal perfusion and parenchymal enhancement.

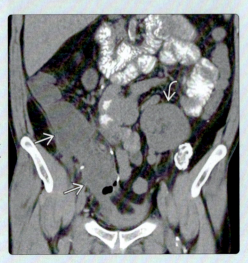
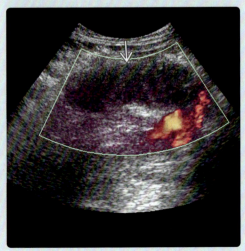

(Left) Coronal nonenhanced CT shows that the right lower quadrant pancreatic allograft ➡ is enlarged and hypodense with adjacent fat stranding and induration. Based on the CT findings, this could represent either graft ischemia or pancreatitis. The renal allograft is marked ➘. (Right) Sagittal power Doppler ultrasound in the same patient shows that the pancreatic allograft ➡ is enlarged and diffusely hypoechoic, without appreciable internal vascularity, compatible with infarction.

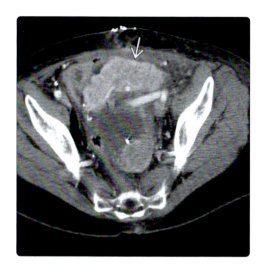

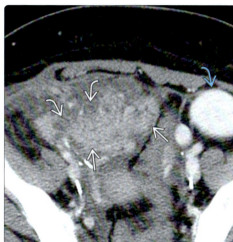

(Left) *Axial CECT shows the pancreatic allograft* ➡️ *with mild swelling of the gland and peripancreatic stranding, indicating mild pancreatitis, a finding seen frequently in the immediate posttransplant period.* (Right) *Axial CECT shows diffuse pancreatic allograft* ➡️ *enlargement and heterogeneity with scattered areas of decreased enhancement* ➡️ *and perigraft infiltration, consistent with posttransplant pancreatitis. Note the normally enhancing renal allograft* ➡️ *in the left lower quadrant.*

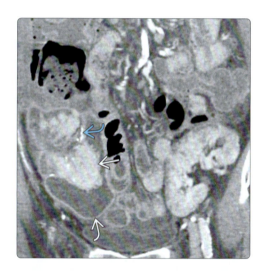

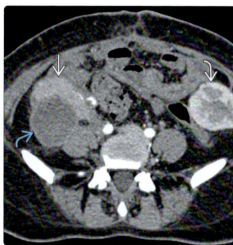

(Left) *Coronal CECT shows a rim-enhancing fluid collection* ➡️ *surrounding the pancreatic allograft* ➡️*. The location of the fluid collection near the anastomotic staple line* ➡️ *correctly suggested an anastomotic leak, confirmed at urgent surgery.* (Right) *Axial CECT demonstrates a loculated fluid collection* ➡️ *adjacent to the pancreatic allograft* ➡️ *in a patient with a history of pancreatitis, compatible with a pseudocyst. A renal allograft* ➡️ *is noted in the left lower quadrant .*

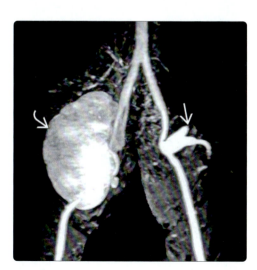

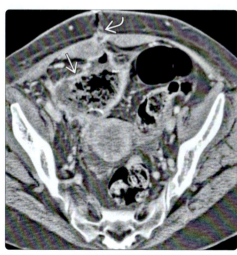

(Left) *Coronal MRA shows the normal appearance and enhancement of the right lower quadrant renal allograft* ➡️ *while the branching arterial supply to the pancreatic allograft* ➡️ *is totally occluded. The infarcted pancreatic allograft was then resected.* (Right) *Axial CECT in a patient with infected necrosis shows gas and fluid* ➡️ *replacing the pancreatic allograft in the right iliac fossa with a fistulous tract to the skin* ➡️*. Infected necrosis of the pancreatic allograft was noted at resection.*

KEY FACTS

TERMINOLOGY

- Group of nonneoplastic, noninflammatory, benign pancreatic cysts of different etiologies
- Includes congenital, true (epithelial) pancreatic cysts; lymphoepithelial cysts and several "syndromic" cysts

IMAGING

- **Best imaging tool: Multiplanar CT or MR, with endoscopic US-guided aspiration, if needed**
- Imaging features can show some variability, since this category encompasses several distinct types of nonneoplastic cysts
  - Usually unilocular, well-defined cyst with sharp margin and thin, imperceptible wall
    - Typically no internal complexity, septations, nodularity, or calcifications
    - No communication with pancreatic duct
    - Usually single cyst, except in patients with underlying syndrome

- Less commonly, imaging features can overlap with neoplastic pancreatic cysts, and lesions can demonstrate more complexity (multiloculation, calcifications, etc.)
  - Lymphoepithelial cysts are more commonly complex, multiseptate; may contain fat

CLINICAL ISSUES

- Syndromes account for most nonneoplastic cysts diagnosed in clinical practice
  - von Hippel-Lindau disease (VHL), autosomal dominant polycystic kidney (ADPKD), and cystic fibrosis (CF)
  - Simple-appearing cysts in setting of known syndrome (VHL, ADPKD, CF) are almost certainly benign
- Simple-appearing cysts < 2 cm are generally safe to follow, especially in older patients
  - Larger lesions or lesions with worrisome morphologic features require endoscopic US and cyst aspiration with possible surgical resection

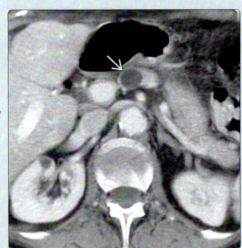
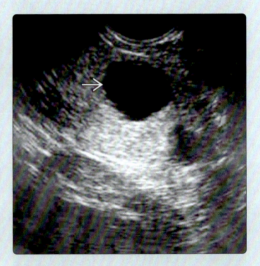

(Left) Axial CECT in an asymptomatic patient demonstrates a small, simple-appearing, thin-walled cyst ➡ in the pancreatic neck with no communication with the pancreatic duct. (Right) Endoscopic US in the same patient shows a simple cyst ➡ in the neck of the pancreas with no mural nodularity or other sign of complexity. Aspiration demonstrated clear serous fluid with no elevated tumor markers. This cyst has remained stable for several years and is presumably a nonneoplastic simple cyst.

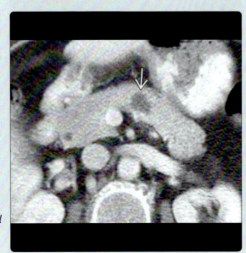
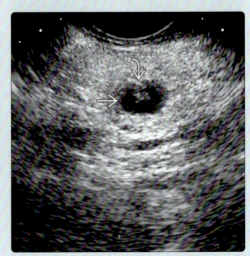

(Left) Axial CECT shows a water-density cystic lesion ➡ in the pancreatic body that has a slightly irregular margin. (Right) Endoscopic US in the same patient shows an anechoic cyst ➡ with a small mural nodule ➡. Needle aspiration yielded clear fluid with borderline elevated CEA and cellular atypia. This was interpreted as equivocal for malignancy, and a laparoscopic distal pancreatectomy was performed. The excised specimen showed an epithelial lining and was classified as a true cyst of the pancreas.

Nonneoplastic Pancreatic Cysts

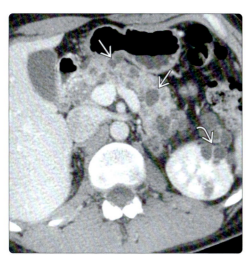
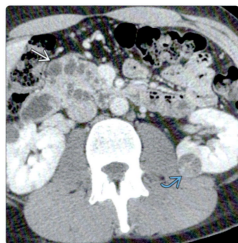

(Left) *Axial CECT in a patient with von Hippel-Lindau syndrome shows multiple small pancreatic cysts* ➡ *as well as multiple renal cysts* ➡. (Right) *Axial CECT in the same patient at a more caudal level again shows multiple simple pancreatic cysts* ➡ *in the pancreatic head. In addition, there is small renal cell carcinoma in the left kidney* ➡.

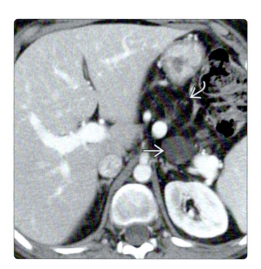
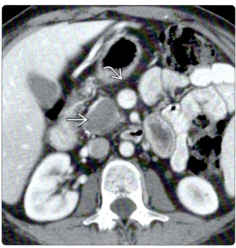

(Left) *Axial CECT in a patient with cystic fibrosis shows fatty replacement and pseudohypertrophy of the pancreas* ➡, *characteristic of pancreatic involvement with this disease. Notice also the thin-walled retention cyst in the tail of the pancreas* ➡. (Right) *Axial CECT of the same patient at the level of the head of the pancreas shows the fatty replacement and pseudohypertrophy of the pancreas* ➡ *as well as a simple-appearing cyst* ➡. *Patients with cystic fibrosis may have solitary, multiple, or innumerable pancreatic cysts.*

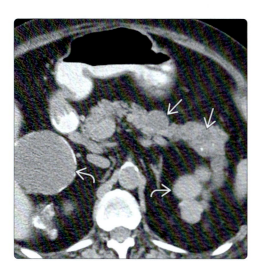
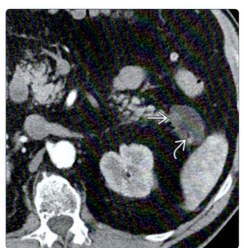

(Left) *Axial NECT in a patient with autosomal dominant polycystic kidney disease shows multiple renal cysts* ➡, *some with calcified walls. Also present are several pancreatic cysts* ➡, *usually of no clinical importance.* (Right) *Axial CECT demonstrates a cyst in the pancreatic tail. Notice the internal complexity within the cyst, including possible mural nodularity* ➡ *and a small focus of internal fat density* ➡. *This was found to be a lymphoepithelial cyst at resection, as these lesions can sometimes demonstrate internal fat.*

TERMINOLOGY

- Benign pancreatic tumor lined by glycogen-rich cells that arise from acinar cells

IMAGING

- **MR is best imaging tool; EUS with aspiration for definitive diagnosis**
  - MR better characterizes internal morphology than CT with ↑ sensitivity for microcysts
- 3 primary morphologies
  - **Microcystic adenoma** (classic serous cystadenoma)
    - Honeycomb or sponge pattern with innumerable internal tiny cysts, enhancing septa, central scar
    - Peripheral rim (capsule) enhancement
    - Calcifications common; peripheral, central, or septal
    - T2WI: Hyperintense cystic components and hypointense fibrous components/central scar
  - **Macrocystic (oligocystic) serous cystadenoma**
    - Single or few cystic components or locules

- "Solid" serous adenoma (~ 5% of serous tumors)
  - Enhancing septa predominate over cystic spaces, producing solid hyperenhancing lesion on imaging
    □ Mimics pancreatic neuroendocrine tumors
  - **Transabdominal US** is more prone to misinterpretation as solid neoplasm
- Rare, vascular, biliary or pancreatic ductal obstruction
- **Endoscopic US**: May better delineate internal cysts, sponge morphology, central scar, and internal calcification
  - Can guide aspiration and biopsy, if necessary

TOP DIFFERENTIAL DIAGNOSES

- Mucinous cystic pancreatic tumor (fewer, larger cystic spaces)
- Pancreatic neuroendocrine tumors
  - Solid serous adenomas appear solid/hypervascular and indistinguishable from neuroendocrine tumors

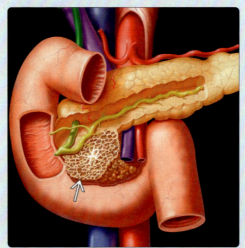
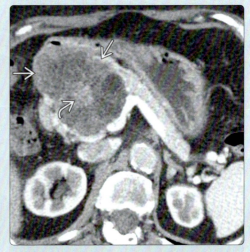

(Left) Graphic shows a mass ➡ in the pancreatic head. The mass has a sponge or honeycomb appearance and is characterized by innumerable small cysts, a central scar, and no obstruction of the pancreatic or bile duct. (Right) Axial CECT in an elderly woman with vague abdominal pain shows a large, lobulated mass ➡ in the pancreatic head. Note the sponge-like appearance with multiple tiny cystic spaces surrounding an enhancing fibrous scar ➡, typical of a microcystic serous cystadenoma.

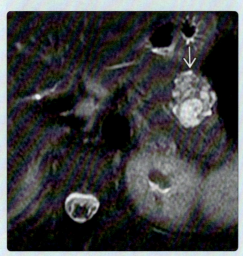
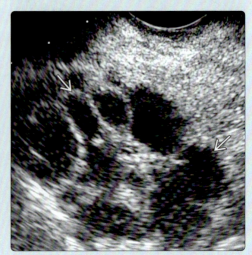

(Left) Axial T2 FS MR of a pancreatic lesion thought to be indeterminate on CT (not shown) demonstrates a cystic mass ➡ composed of many tiny internal cysts, classic for a microcystic serous cystadenoma. (Right) Endoscopic US of a serous cystadenoma demonstrates the characteristic multiple tiny cysts ➡. Aspiration of the cyst contents revealed thin, glycogen-rich fluid with no cellular atypia or elevated tumor markers.

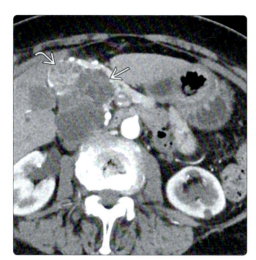

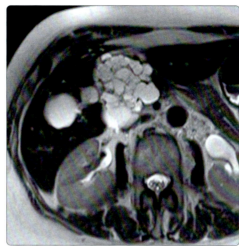

(Left) *Axial CECT demonstrates a mixed cystic and solid mass ➡️ arising from the pancreatic head. Note that there are areas of more solid-appearing hyperenhancement ➡️, reflecting many enhancing septa predominating over cystic spaces.* (Right) *Axial T2 MR in the same patient better demonstrates the microcystic morphology of the lesion, characteristic of a serous cystadenoma. MR can be very helpful for better delineating the internal morphology of these lesions when indeterminate on CT.*

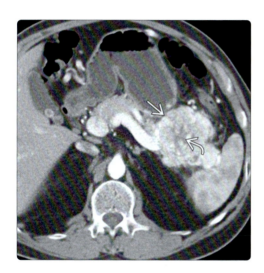

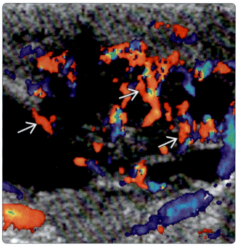

(Left) *Axial CECT in the arterial phase demonstrates an avidly hypervascular mass ➡️ in the pancreatic body with a central scar ➡️. Innumerable tiny cysts are suggested by CT.* (Right) *Transverse intraoperative color Doppler US in the same patient demonstrates the highly vascular nature of the mass with multiple intrinsic blood vessels ➡️. The cystic spaces and vascularity are quite typical of a benign serous cystadenoma.*

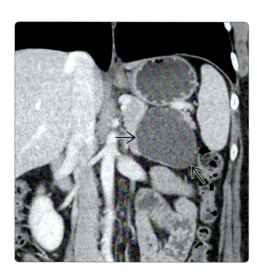

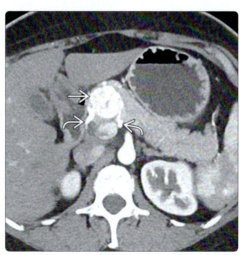

(Left) *Coronal CECT shows a simple-appearing cystic lesion ➡️ arising from the pancreatic tail. While the differential diagnosis includes a mucinous cystic neoplasm, this was found to be a unilocular (oligocystic) serous cystadenoma at surgery.* (Right) *Axial CECT in the arterial phase demonstrates a markedly hypervascular mass ➡️ in the pancreatic head with hypertrophied feeding vessels ➡️. This solid serous adenoma would be difficult to distinguish from a pancreatic neuroendocrine tumor by imaging alone.*

Pancreatic Ductal Carcinoma

IMAGING

- **Multiplanar, multiphasic CT or MR**
- **CT**: Poorly marginated, hypodense mass with tendency to infiltrate posteriorly into retroperitoneum
  - Strong tendency to obstruct pancreatic and common bile ducts, with abrupt ductal cutoff at site of obstruction
  - Pancreatic parenchymal atrophy upstream from mass
  - Soft tissue infiltration to involve adjacent vessels and organs (e.g., duodenum, bowel, stomach, and adrenals)
  - Most common sites of distant metastatic disease are liver, peritoneum, and lungs
  - Arterial involvement quantified as < 180° or ≥ 180° tumoral involvement of vessel circumference
  - Venous involvement may involve abutment, encasement, narrowing, or occlusion
- **MR**: Tumor conspicuous on T1WI, appearing low signal and juxtaposed against high-signal pancreatic parenchyma
  - T2WI less useful, as tumors are isointense to pancreas

- Conspicuity on contrast-enhanced T1WI similar to CT with tumors showing progressive delayed enhancement

CLINICAL ISSUES

- Most common malignant tumor of exocrine pancreas and accounts for > 95% of pancreatic malignancies
- Most common symptoms are jaundice, weight loss, abdominal pain, and back pain
  - Often asymptomatic until late in course, particularly body/tail tumors that do not cause jaundice
- Only potentially curative treatment is complete surgical resection with negative surgical margins
- Only 15-20% of patients are candidates for surgery at presentation, with 5-year survival of ~ 20% after surgery
- 5-year survival rate is < 5% without surgery with median survival of 3.5 months

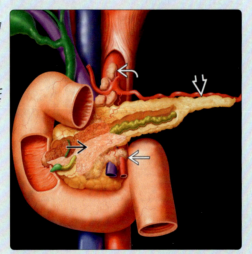

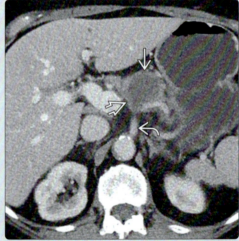

(Left) *Graphic shows pancreatic head carcinoma ⇒ encasing and obstructing the pancreatic and distal bile ducts. There is encasement of the superior mesenteric vessels ⇒ and spread to celiac nodes ⇒. Note the atrophy of the distal body/tail segments ⇒.* (Right) *Axial CECT in the venous phase demonstrates a poorly marginated hypodense mass ⇒ in the pancreatic body, typical for pancreatic adenocarcinoma. The mass abuts the distal celiac trunk ⇒ and the hepatic artery ⇒, with < 180° involvement of each.*

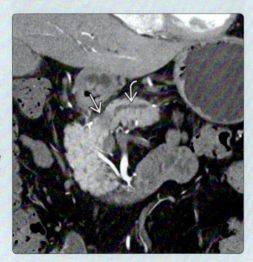

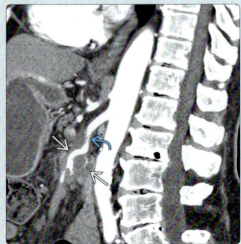

(Left) *Coronal CECT demonstrates a subtle hypodense mass ⇒ in the pancreatic neck resulting in obstruction and upstream dilatation of the pancreatic duct ⇒. The presence of pancreatic ductal dilatation and abrupt cut-off should always prompt careful search for a pancreatic mass.* (Right) *Sagittal CECT demonstrates a poorly marginated pancreatic cancer ⇒ encasing the SMA ⇒, with 360° involvement. This degree of encasement almost certainly makes this tumor unresectable.*

Pancreatic Ductal Carcinoma

TERMINOLOGY

Synonyms

- Pancreatic adenocarcinoma, pancreatic cancer

Definitions

- Malignancy arising from ductal epithelium of exocrine pancreas

IMAGING

General Features

- Best diagnostic clue
  - Poorly marginated, hypoenhancing mass with abrupt obstruction of pancreatic duct ± common bile duct
- Location
  - Head (60%), body (20%), diffuse (15%), tail (5%)

CT Findings

- CT sensitivity for pancreatic cancer is excellent (~ 97%)
  - Excellent modality for determining unresectability (positive predictive value for unresectability of 89-100%)
  - Less effective in determining resectability, as only 60-91% of tumors judged to be resectable on CT are actually resectable at surgery
- Poorly marginated, hypodense mass with tendency to infiltrate posteriorly into retroperitoneum
  - Tumor most conspicuous in portal venous (~ 70 seconds) and pancreatic (~ 40 seconds) contrast phases
  - ~ 5% of tumors are isodense to pancreas on all phases, requiring attention to secondary signs of tumor
  - Tumor virtually never calcifies in absence of treatment
- Secondary signs of tumor
  - Strong tendency to obstruct pancreatic and common bile ducts with abrupt ductal cutoff at site of obstruction
  - Pancreatic parenchymal atrophy upstream from mass
  - Abnormal contour of pancreas with loss of normal fatty lobulation and texture
  - Soft tissue infiltration to involve adjacent vessels and organs (e.g., duodenum, bowel, stomach, and adrenals)
- Distant metastatic disease
  - Most common sites are liver, peritoneum, and lungs
  - Regional lymph nodes frequently involved, but CT is not accurate for involvement (sensitivity < 20%)
- CT is best modality for determining vascular invasion
  - Arterial involvement quantified as < 180° or ≥ 180° tumoral involvement of vessel circumference
  - Venous involvement determined based on degree of contact between tumor and vessel, and described as abutment, encasement, narrowing, or occlusion
    - Distinction between < 180° or ≥ 180° involvement of veins no longer as important with advent of venous reconstruction
    - Superior mesenteric vein or splenic vein narrowing often results in mesenteric or gastroepiploic collateral veins
  - Tumor thrombus in mesenteric veins very uncommon (much more common with neuroendocrine tumors)
- Pancreatic adenocarcinoma classically causes hypercoagulability: Look for evidence of incidental pulmonary emboli or deep venous thrombosis

MR Findings

- Normal pancreas
  - Diffuse high signal intensity on T1WI (≥ liver)
  - Parenchyma variable in signal on T2WI
  - Pancreas enhances avidly and homogeneously on T1WI C+ (hyperintense to liver on arterial phase and isointense on delayed phase)
- MR is particularly helpful in identifying small group of tumors that are isodense to normal pancreas on CT
- Tumor conspicuous on T1WI, appearing low signal and juxtaposed against high-signal pancreatic parenchyma
  - Atrophic pancreas upstream from tumor often abnormally low signal on T1WI
- T2WI generally not useful for tumor detection, as tumors often isointense to pancreas
- Conspicuity on T1WI C+ similar to CT with hypovascular tumors often demonstrating progressive delayed enhancement
- Tumors often demonstrate restricted diffusion with lower ADC values than adjacent normal pancreas
  - DWI not helpful in differentiating tumors from other entities (such as autoimmune pancreatitis)
- MRCP and T2WI can demonstrate abrupt cutoff and obstruction of pancreatic and common bile ducts
- MR generally 2nd choice (behind CT) for evaluating vascular involvement

Ultrasonographic Findings

- Hypoechoic mass with only minimal internal color Doppler flow vascularity
- Biliary dilation and pancreatic ductal dilatation upstream from tumor
- Endoscopic ultrasound: Similar to conventional ultrasound findings with inferior accuracy compared to CECT for locoregional staging or determining vascular involvement
  - Helpful in **excluding** malignancy in patients with indeterminate CT findings (↑ negative predictive value)
  - Can help guide biopsy of pancreatic masses

Nuclear Medicine Findings

- PET/CT
  - PET alone (without diagnostic CT) is not effective for diagnosis of primary tumor (sensitivity as low as 72%)
    - Possible role in differentiating malignant from benign lesions, as FDG-avid lesions have ↑ risk of malignancy
      - May help differentiate pancreatic adenocarcinoma, which shows avid focal uptake in mass, from focal autoimmune pancreatitis, which shows diffuse uptake throughout pancreas and within salivary glands
    - Effective in judging response to treatment (chemoradiation), whereas CT may not differentiate posttreatment fibrosis from residual tumor
  - PET not helpful for vascular involvement or locoregional staging (e.g., lymph nodes) due to poor spatial resolution
  - Helpful for distant staging, and may change resectability status of ~ 20% of patients compared to CECT

Radiographic Findings

- ERCP
  - Shows ductal obstruction; guide biopsy & stent placement

(Left) *In a patient with painless jaundice, coronal MRCP demonstrates the typical double duct sign associated with pancreatic cancer, with abrupt occlusion of the pancreatic duct* ➡ *and common bile duct* ➡ *at the level of the patient's pancreatic head mass.* (Right) *ERCP in the same patient demonstrates an irregular stricture* ➡ *of the common bile duct. The abrupt, irregular narrowing of the duct at the stricture is a characteristic feature for malignancy. A biliary stent was placed during this procedure.*

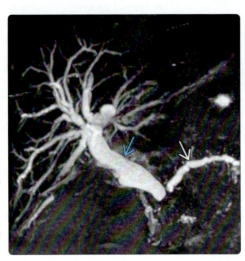
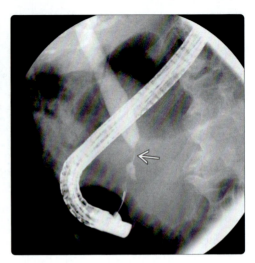

(Left) *Coronal CECT demonstrates a poorly marginated hypodense mass* ➡ *in the pancreatic head/neck, typical of pancreatic adenocarcinoma. Note that the tumor encases the portal vein* ➡*, portal/SMV confluence, and the SMV* ➡*.* (Right) *Coronal volume-rendered CECT in the same patient demonstrates that the mass* ➡ *has occluded the SMV over several centimeters extending from the confluence* ➡*, with development of multiple collaterals with a patent SMV seen more inferiorly* ➡*.*

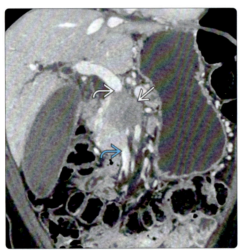
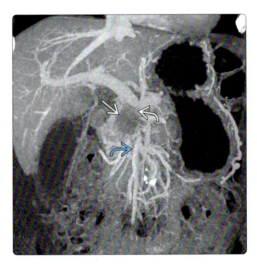

(Left) *Axial T1-enhanced MR in the arterial phase demonstrates a hypodense mass* ➡ *in the pancreatic tail, compatible with pancreatic adenocarcinoma. Several metastases* ➡ *are present in the liver.* (Right) *Axial enhanced MR in the delayed phase from the same patient shows that the mass* ➡ *now demonstrates considerable delayed enhancement. Delayed enhancement, which is much easier to appreciate on MR compared to CT, is a fairly common feature of pancreatic adenocarcinoma.*

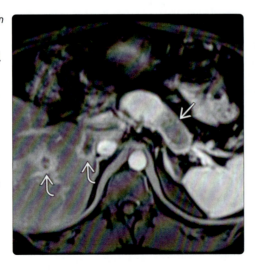
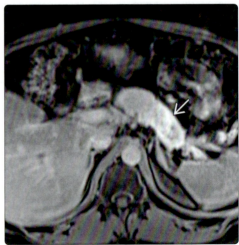

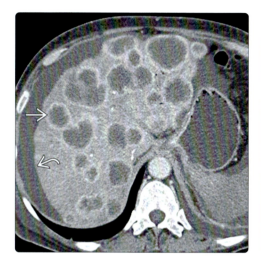
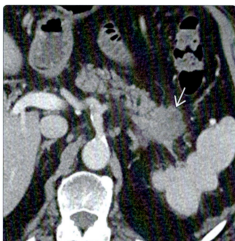

(Left) *Axial CECT in a patient with pancreatic cancer demonstrates peripherally enhancing metastases ⇒ throughout the liver, and ascites ⇗. The liver is almost always the 1st site of distant metastasis for pancreatic adenocarcinoma.* (Right) *Axial CT in the same case shows an infiltrative, hypodense mass ⇒ in the pancreatic tail, suggestive of pancreatic ductal carcinoma. Pancreatic tail cancers typically do not involve vital vasculature and often come to attention later than pancreatic head cancers due to lack of jaundice.*

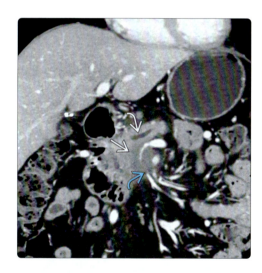
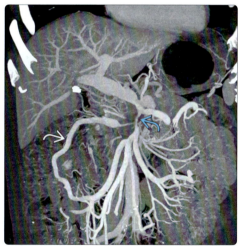

(Left) *Coronal CECT demonstrates an infiltrative hypodense mass ⇒ in the pancreatic head with upstream pancreatic ductal dilatation ⇒ & parenchymal atrophy. The mass encases and severely narrows the SMV ⇗.* (Right) *Coronal volume-rendered CECT in the same patient demonstrates severe narrowing of the SMV ⇗ with the development of large venous collaterals ⇒. The presence of venous collaterals in a pancreatic cancer patient should always suggest the presence of venous narrowing or occlusion.*

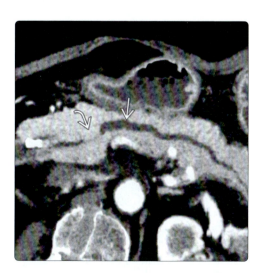
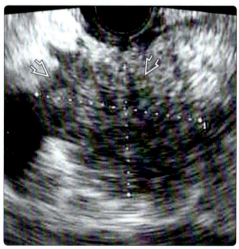

(Left) *Axial curved MinIP shows upstream dilatation of the pancreatic duct ⇒ proximal to a focal stricture ⇒ in the pancreatic duct. No mass is evident.* (Right) *Endoscopic ultrasound of the strictured area reveals a solid mass ⇒ that was biopsied and shown to be adenocarcinoma. Any focal stricture of the main pancreatic duct should be considered as an isodense carcinoma until proven otherwise, and should lead to endoscopic ultrasound interrogation and biopsy.*

Mucinous Cystic Neoplasm (Pancreas)

TERMINOLOGY

- Thick-walled, uni-/multilocular neoplasm composed of large, mucin-containing cysts
  - Considered premalignant or frankly malignant

IMAGING

- **Multiplanar MR or CT is best for detecting lesion**
  - **Endoscopic US for cyst aspiration, and biopsy is definitive**
- Large mass (2-12 cm) encapsulated by thick fibrous capsule
  - Typically located in body/tail segment of pancreas
- Fewer (< 6) and larger (> 2 cm) cystic spaces than serous ("microcystic") adenoma
- Enhancement of internal septa and cyst wall ± calcification
  - Solid papillary projections protrude into interior of tumor (suggests frank malignancy)
- Cyst contents: Hyperintense on T2 MR; septa and calcifications hypointense

- **MRCP**: Depicts displacement, possible narrowing and prestenotic dilation of pancreatic duct
- **US**: Multiloculated cystic mass with echogenic internal septa
- **Endoscopic US**: Best for depicting complexity of cystic mass
  - Cyst aspiration and analysis for tumor markers are highly sensitive and specific for diagnosis

CLINICAL ISSUES

- Probably most common type of cystic pancreatic neoplasm
- **Striking female predominance (9:1)**
  - Commonly affects women in child-bearing years (30s and 40s)

DIAGNOSTIC CHECKLIST

- Multiloculated cystic mass with enhancing septa in pancreatic body or tail
  - Usually requires resection; may not warrant additional imaging after initial imaging detection

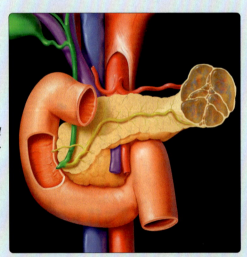
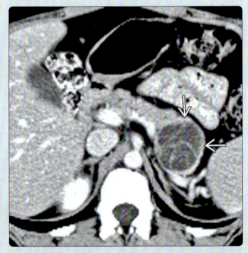

(Left) Graphic of a mucinous cystic neoplasm (MCN) shows a multiseptate, mucin-filled, cystic mass in the pancreatic tail that displaces the pancreatic duct. (Right) Axial CECT in a 40-year-old woman with vague abdominal discomfort shows a cystic tumor ➡ in the pancreatic tail with multiple enhancing septa. The clinical and imaging features are so characteristic of MCN that additional imaging and biopsy may not be warranted; complete surgical resection is needed.

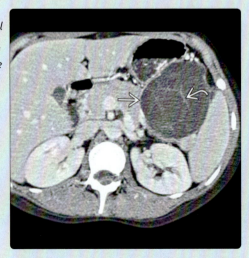
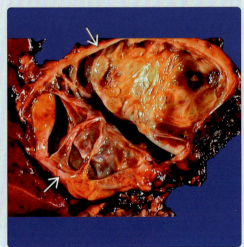

(Left) Axial CECT in a 50-year-old man with vague abdominal pain shows a large complex cystic mass ➡ in the body/tail segment of the pancreas. Note the septa ➡ and the large, relatively few cystic spaces within the mass. Most MCNs occur in women (9:1 predominance). (Right) Gross pathology from the same patient shows that the resected mass ➡ was full of mucinous fluid and had thickened septa. Histologic exam showed cellular atypia, and the lesion was considered a low-grade malignancy.

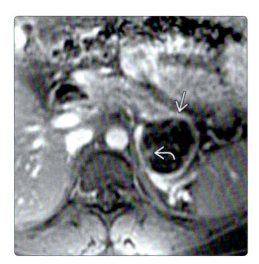

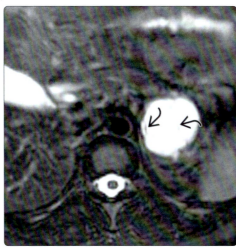

(Left) Axial gadolinium-enhanced MR in a 61-year-old woman shows a well-defined cystic mass ⮕ in the pancreatic tail. Note the enhancing wall and septa ⮕. (Right) Axial T2 MR in the same patient reveals thin septa ⮕ within the cystic mass with high-signal fluid content. Surgical resection was performed and a benign MCN was found.

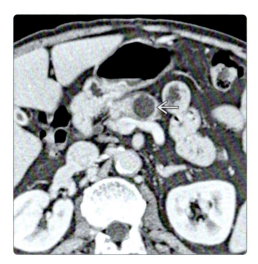

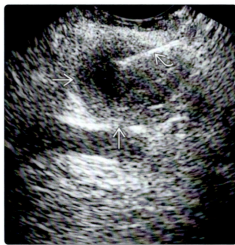

(Left) Axial CECT shows a small, spherical, cystic mass ⮕ that appears relatively simple, although it has a visible wall. (Right) Endoscopic ultrasound in the same patient demonstrates more apparent wall thickening ⮕. Needle aspiration ⮕ yielded mucinous fluid. Resection showed a MCN with malignant foci in the wall.

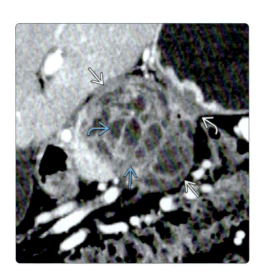

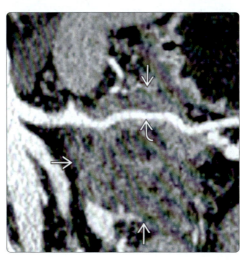

(Left) Coronal CECT in a 75-year-old woman shows a complex cystic mass ⮕ in the body of the pancreas containing both solid ⮕ and cystic ⮕ elements. Note that the mass invades into the adjacent serosa of the stomach ⮕, causing focal mural thickening. (Right) Curved planar reformation of the splenic artery in the same patient shows vascular encasement ⮕ confirming that this mass ⮕ is a mucinous cystadenocarcinoma.

Pancreatic Intraductal Papillary Mucinous Neoplasm (IPMN)

TERMINOLOGY

- Mucin-producing papillary tumor arising from epithelium of main pancreatic duct (MPD) or duct side branches

IMAGING

- **Side branch IPMN**
  - Well-defined cystic lesion with variable morphology: Unilocular, multicystic, or tubular
  - Communication with adjacent MPD is key to diagnosis (may be more visible on MR than CT)
  - Dilation of adjacent MPD should raise concern for main duct involvement
  - Multiplicity is strong clue to diagnosis: Often multiple small cysts scattered throughout pancreas
- **Main duct IPMN**
  - Markedly dilated, tortuous MPD often with bulging ampulla filled with fluid (mucin)
  - Dilation may be segmental or diffuse
  - Polypoid nodularity in MPD worrisome for malignancy
  - Amorphous calcifications may be seen within duct
  - Pancreas often atrophic overlying dilated duct
- **Combined IPMN**
  - Cystic lesion in contiguity with dilated MPD (shares imaging features of main duct and side branch IPMN)

CLINICAL ISSUES

- EUS cyst aspiration: Elevated cyst fluid CEA (> 192 ng/mL)
- Most patients asymptomatic (incidental imaging finding) but can result in repetitive bouts of pancreatitis
- Risk of transformation into invasive carcinoma with main duct involvement associated with ↑ risk of malignancy
- Management of IPMN based on 2012 IAP guidelines
  - Worrisome features: Cyst size ≥ 3 cm, MPD dilatation 5-9 mm, peripheral wall thickening, nonenhancing mural nodularity, abrupt change in main duct caliber with upstream pancreatic atrophy
  - High-risk features: MPD dilatation ≥ 1 cm, enhancing solid mural nodularity, or biliary obstruction

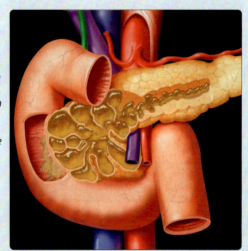

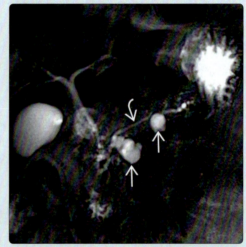

(Left) Graphic shows a combined main and side branch intraductal papillary mucinous neoplasm (IPMN) with gross dilation of all ducts by mucin, which pours out of a bulging papilla into the duodenum. The parenchyma in the pancreatic head is atrophic. (Right) Coronal MRCP demonstrates 2 discrete side branch IPMNs ➡ and their direct connection with the adjacent normal-sized pancreatic duct ➡.

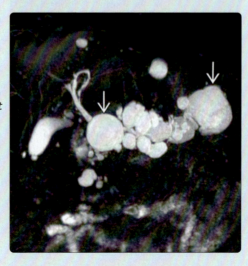

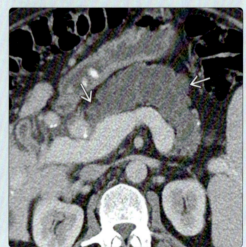

(Left) Coronal MRCP with MIP reconstruction demonstrates multiple cysts ➡ throughout the pancreas compatible with multiple side branch IPMN. Multifocality is characteristic of IPMN, and multiple discrete cystic lesions are often present in the same patient. (Right) Coronal CECT demonstrates innumerable pancreatic cysts ➡, compatible with multiple side branch IPMNs. No worrisome individual cyst or solid mass was seen, but EUS findings were considered worrisome, and the patient was found to have invasive carcinoma at surgery.

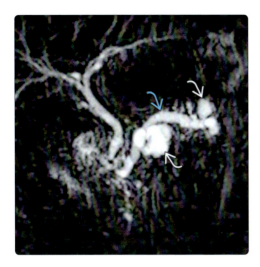
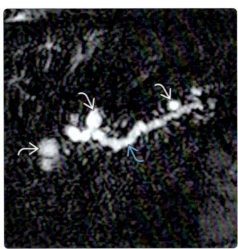

(Left) Coronal MRCP demonstrates numerous cyst-like focal dilations of the side branches ⇗ and diffuse dilation of the main pancreatic duct ⇘ (combined main and branch duct IPMN). MRCP is an excellent noninvasive method to evaluate suspected pancreatic IPMNs. (Right) Coronal MRCP shows dilation of the main pancreatic duct ⇗ as well as the side branches. Note the cyst-like focal dilations of side branches ⇗ in this case of main and branch duct IPMN.

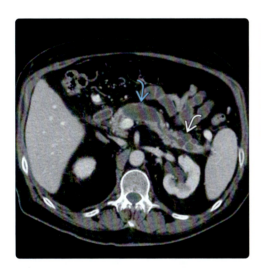
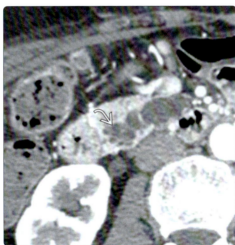

(Left) Axial CECT shows massive dilation of the main pancreatic duct ⇗ and some of the side branches ⇗ along with parenchymal atrophy in this case of main and branch duct IPMN. (Right) Axial CECT demonstrates a cluster of grapes appearance of multiple small cystic areas ⇗ in the uncinate process of the pancreas, representing branch duct IPMNs.

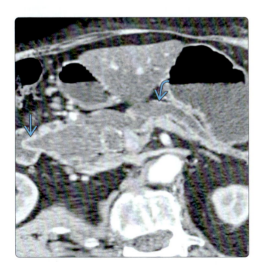
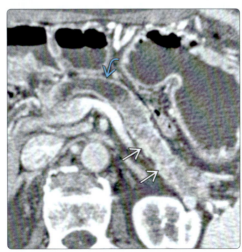

(Left) Axial CECT with curved planar reformation shows a diffusely dilated main pancreatic duct ⇗ with a bulging ampulla ⇘, a characteristic feature of main duct IPMN. Note the parenchymal atrophy. (Right) Axial CECT demonstrates a markedly dilated main pancreatic duct ⇗ that contains intraductal solid tissue ⇘ characteristic of a malignant main duct IPMN.

Pancreatic Solid and Pseudopapillary Epithelial Neoplasm

IMAGING

- **Multiplanar enhanced CT or MR is 1st-line imaging test**
- Well-defined, heterogeneous, large mass with thick, enhancing capsule
  o Most often solid but can have variable internal cystic components and intratumoral hemorrhage
- Capsule enhances on CECT and T1 C+ MR and appears as rim of low T2 signal intensity
- Frequent peripheral or central calcification (45-50%)
- Presence of internal hemorrhage highly characteristic feature and may result in fluid-fluid or hematocrit levels
  o Internal hemorrhage is easier to perceive on MR
- Usually no biliary or pancreatic ductal obstruction
- Metastatic disease is very uncommon but may metastasize to liver and locoregional lymph nodes

PATHOLOGY

- Rare: < 3% of all pancreatic tumors

- Previously thought to have separate benign and malignant subtypes, but recent WHO classification defines all solid and pseudopapillary neoplasm (SPEN) as low-grade malignancies
  o Low malignant potential (< 10% metastasize or recur)

CLINICAL ISSUES

- > 90% occur in women
- Almost always arises in patients < 35 years (rarely reported in older adults)
  o Accounts for 8-16% of pancreatic tumors in children
- Possible predilection for African Americans and Asians
- Most patients are symptomatic with abdominal pain most common presenting symptom
- Treatment: Complete surgical resection

DIAGNOSTIC CHECKLIST

- **Consider SPEN when confronted by encapsulated solid pancreatic mass in young woman**

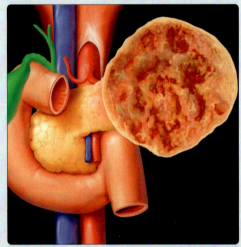
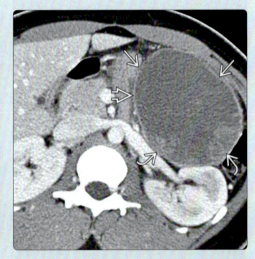

(Left) Graphic shows a large, encapsulated mass arising from the pancreatic tail with prominent solid and cystic or hemorrhagic components. (Right) Axial CECT in a 15-year-old girl presenting with a palpable LUQ mass demonstrates a large predominantly cystic mass ➡ with peripheral solid components ➡. The mass is well circumscribed with an enhancing peripheral capsule ➡. The lesion was found to be a solid and pseudopapillary neoplasm (SPEN).

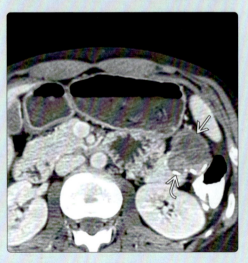
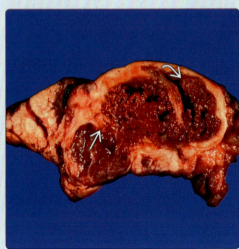

(Left) Axial CT in a 21-year-old woman shows a complex cystic-solid mass ➡ with peripheral rim calcification ➡ in the tail of the pancreas. Endoscopic ultrasound (not shown) confirmed a complex cystic mass. Needle aspiration of the mass at ultrasound yielded fluid that had few cells and no elevated tumor markers. The fluid was not mucoid. (Right) Resected mass shows areas of hemorrhage and necrosis ➡, surrounded by tissues with solid and pseudopapillary projections ➡, compatible with a SPEN.

Pancreatic Metastases and Lymphoma

IMAGING

- **Multiplanar CT of chest, abdomen, pelvis provides best assessment of etiology and extent of tumors**
  - **PET/CT for FDG-avid tumors** helps detect other sites of metastasis (which are usually present)
- Pancreatic metastases
  - Uncommon (2% of pancreatic malignancies)
  - Solitary (78%) or multiple (17%) discrete mass(es)
  - Enhancement pattern is variable; mimics primary tumor
  - Hypervascular: Usually from renal cell cancer (RCC)
  - Hypovascular: Lung, breast, colon, melanoma
  - Concomitant intraabdominal metastases
    - Liver, nodes, adrenal (each ~ 30%)
  - Obstruction of pancreatic or bile duct uncommon (33%)
- Pancreatic lymphoma
  - Homogeneous soft tissue mass or masses with little enhancement
  - Diffuse enlargement of pancreas with infiltrating tumor ± peripancreatic fat involvement; may simulate acute pancreatitis
  - Associated lymphadenopathy is common
  - May encase but rarely obstructs pancreatic or bile ducts or vessels

TOP DIFFERENTIAL DIAGNOSES

- Pancreatic ductal carcinoma: Usually focal, rarely diffuse
  - More likely than metastases or lymphoma to obstruct biliary and pancreatic ducts or blood vessels
- Pancreatic neuroendocrine tumor
  - Usually hypervascular; can have same appearance as metastases from RCC

CLINICAL ISSUES

- **Renal cell metastases may occur 5-15 years after initial diagnosis**
  - **May be isolated only to pancreas, amenable to resection**

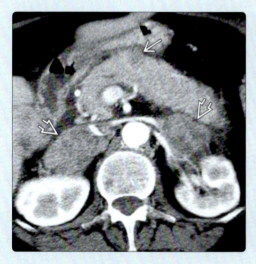

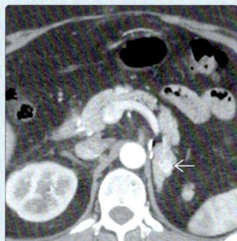

(Left) In this patient with metastatic melanoma, axial CECT shows predominantly solid, bilateral adrenal metastases ➡ as well as metastasis ➡ in the body of the pancreas. In most cases, pancreatic metastases are accompanied by metastases to other sites. (Right) In this patient who is 12 years post left nephrectomy for renal cell carcinoma, CT shows 1 of several hypervascular metastases ➡. The appearance of this lesion is indistinguishable from a pancreatic neuroendocrine tumor.

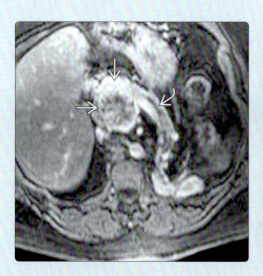

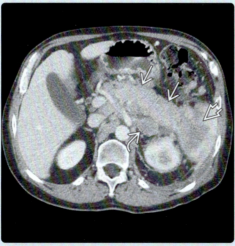

(Left) Axial T1 C+ MR shows an enhancing mass ➡ with central necrosis in the pancreatic head. The pancreatic duct ➡ is slightly dilated upstream. Note the posterior position of the pancreatic tail as a result of a prior left nephrectomy for renal cell carcinoma, the primary source of this metastasis. (Right) Axial CECT shows diffuse infiltration of the pancreas ➡ and invasion of the spleen ➡ by non-Hodgkin lymphoma. Also note the associated peripancreatic lymphadenopathy ➡.

Pancreas

IMAGING

- **Protocols: Multiphasic, multiplanar CECT or MR**
- **Anaplastic carcinoma**: Large, heterogeneous, **moderately enhancing**, exophytic lesion with areas of necrosis
  - Usually in body-tail segments
  - Locally invasive with lung and liver metastases
  - 2-7% of all pancreatic primary malignancies
  - Extremely aggressive with rapid local and distant spread
  - Mean survival from time of diagnosis: 2-3 months
- **Small cell carcinoma**: Large, homogeneous, **mildly enhancing** mass with confluent lymphadenopathy
  - Pancreatic head; homogeneous, hypovascular
  - Resembles lymphoma by imaging
  - Indistinguishable from metastatic small cell carcinoma
  - 1.0-1.4% of all pancreatic cancers
  - Prolonged or complete remissions have been reported with chemotherapy ± radiotherapy

- **Giant cell carcinoma**: Large, heterogeneous exophytic mass with hemorrhage, septation, and calcification
  - May be largely cystic ± hemorrhagic
  - Local invasion and distant metastases are uncommon
  - < 1% of all pancreatic cancers
- **Acinar cell carcinoma**
  - 1% of all pancreatic cancers
  - Rounded exophytic mass with central necrosis
- Others: e.g., peripancreatic sarcoma; nerve sheath tumors; myeloma (plasmacytoma)
  - **No characteristic imaging features**
  - **Diagnosis requires image-guided biopsy**

TOP DIFFERENTIAL DIAGNOSES

- Pancreatic neuroendocrine tumors
- Metastatic renal cell carcinoma
- Pancreatic ductal carcinoma
- Mucinous cystic neoplasm
- Non-Hodgkin lymphoma, pancreas

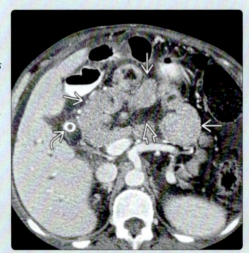
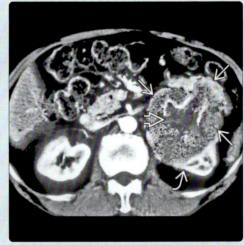

(Left) Axial CECT in a patient with anaplastic carcinoma shows a bulky mass ⟶ involving the body of the pancreas with central necrosis ⟶. Note the obstruction of the common duct, which contains a metallic stent ⟶. (Right) Axial CECT in a patient with anaplastic carcinoma shows a large mass ⟶ arising from the pancreatic tail with moderate vascularity and central necrosis ⟶. Note the invasion of the left kidney ⟶ by the mass.

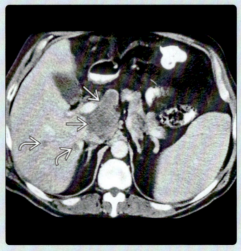
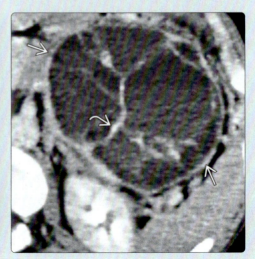

(Left) In a patient with small cell carcinoma, axial CECT shows a hypodense mass ⟶ in the pancreatic head. The mass is homogeneously & minimally enhancing and conforms to the contours of adjacent structures. There is no biliary obstruction; however, multiple liver metastases ⟶ are noted. (Right) Axial CECT in a patient with giant cell carcinoma shows a multiseptate, complex cystic mass ⟶ arising from the tail of the pancreas. Note the focal calcification in one of the septa ⟶. Mucinous cystic neoplasm could have the same appearance.

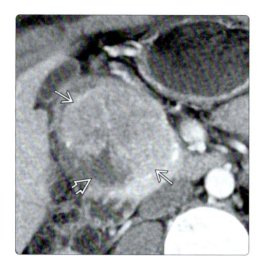 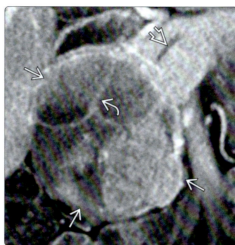

(Left) *Axial CECT shows a rounded, heterogeneously enhancing mass in the head of the pancreas ➡ with areas of central necrosis ⊞.* **(Right)** *Coronal volume-rendered CECT in the same patient demonstrates that the mass ➡ contains septations ↗ and does not obstruct the upstream pancreatic duct ⊞. Percutaneous biopsy of the heterogeneous mass revealed acinar cell carcinoma. The fact that the pancreatic duct is not obstructed should suggest possibilities other than ductal adenocarcinoma.*

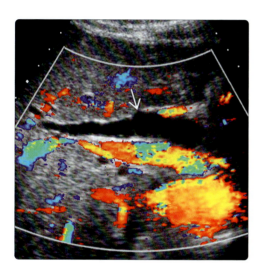 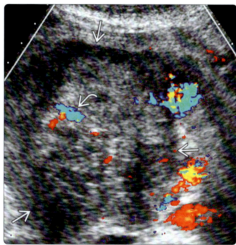

(Left) *In this patient with abnormal liver function, sagittal color Doppler ultrasound shows a dilated common bile duct ➡.* **(Right)** *In the same patient, color Doppler of the head of the pancreas shows a large hypoechoic mass ➡ that contains intrinsic vascularity ↗. The differential diagnosis of such a large, solid pancreatic mass includes neuroendocrine tumors and lymphoma. The history of multiple myeloma was key in suggesting that this mass was a plasmacytoma, which was confirmed on biopsy.*

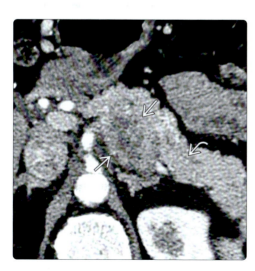 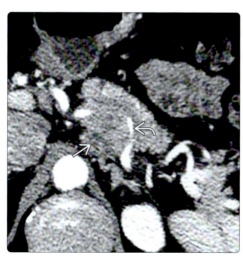

(Left) *Axial CECT shows a heterogeneously enhancing mass ➡ involving the posterior aspect of the body of the pancreas. Note that there is no upstream dilation of the pancreatic duct ↗.* **(Right)** *Axial CECT in the same patient at a more cranial level demonstrates that the mass ➡ encases the splenic artery ↗. Percutaneous biopsy of the mass revealed leiomyosarcoma invading the pancreas. The appearance of this hypodense mass with vascular encasement mimics primary ductal adenocarcinoma.*

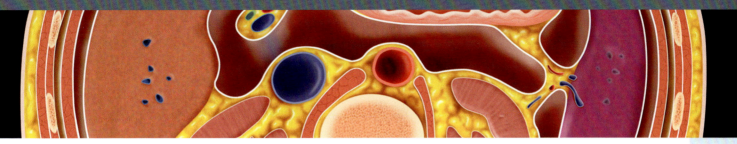

INDEX

INDEX

INDEX

INDEX

INDEX

INDEX

H

J

K

INDEX

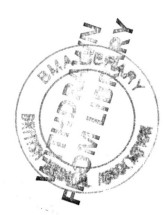